Oxford textbook of clinical pharmacology and drug therapy

Oxford textbook of clinical pharmacology and drug therapy

D. G. Grahame-Smith, MBBS, PhD, FRCP

Rhodes Professor of Clinical Pharmacology, University of Oxford; Honorary Director, Medical Research Council Unit of Clinical Pharmacology; Honorary Consultant Physician to the Oxfordshire Health Authority

and

J. K. Aronson, MBChB, DPhil, FRCP

Clinical Reader in Clinical Pharmacology (Wellcome Lecturer), University of Oxford; Honorary Consultant Physician to the Oxfordshire Health Authority

Second edition

OXFORD   NEW YORK   TOKYO
OXFORD UNIVERSITY PRESS
1992

Oxford University Press, Walton Street, Oxford OX2 6DP

Oxford New York Toronto
Delhi Bombay Calcutta Madras Karachi
Kuala Lumpur Singapore Hong Kong Tokyo
Nairobi Dar es Salaam Cape Town
Melbourne Auckland Madrid

and associated companies in
Berlin Ibadan

Oxford is a trade mark of Oxford University Press

Published in the United States
by Oxford University Press Inc., New York

First published 1984. Reprinted 1985
Reprinted 1987 (with corrections), 1990, 1991
Second edition published 1992

A catalogue record for this book is available from the British Library

Library of Congress Cataloging in Publication Data
Grahame-Smith, David Grahame.
Oxford textbook of clinical pharmacology and drug therapy / D.G.
Grahame-Smith and J.K. Aronson. — 2nd ed.
Includes bibliographical reference and index.
1. Pharmacology. 2. Chemotherapy. I. Aronson, J.K. II. Title.
III. Title: Oxford textbook of clinical pharmacology and drug therapy.
[DNLM: 1. Drug Therapy. 2. Pharmacology, Clinical.   WB 330 G742o]
RM300.G715   1992   615.5'8—dc20   92–13006
ISBN 0-19-261676 5 (hbk)
ISBN 0-19-261675 7 (pbk)

Typeset by
The Charlesworth Group, Huddersfield, UK
Printed in Great Britain by
Butler & Tanner Ltd, Frome

Preface to the second edition

That there has been a demand for a second edition of this textbook is evidence that our approach to the subject of clinical pharmacology and drug therapy has found some favour. We have not therefore altered the general format from that of the first edition. However, we have made many alterations which we feel improve upon the original text.

Firstly, where advances have occurred we have brought up to date the relevant information. The most important aspect of this has been the revision of the chapters in Section III on the drug therapy of diseases. Conscious of increasing specialization in the diagnosis and treatment of disease we have thought it wise to recruit the assistance of specialists in their fields, one for each area of therapeutic practice described in Chapters 22–37. These specialists have reviewed our revised text and have made suggestions on further revisions. The final text has been based on those suggestions. We are exceptionally grateful to our colleagues for the speed and efficiency with which they have performed this task. Their help has been inestimable, and we have acknowledged our debt to them by naming them as co-authors of the relevant chapters. However, in all cases the responsibility for the final text has been ours, and if there are any errors of fact or judgement we are the ones to blame. We are also grateful to Dr Cheryl Smith, Principal Pharmacist of the Oxford Regional Drug Information Centre, for help in updating the bibliography in Chapter 20.

Secondly, we have made the coverage of some areas more comprehensive. For example, the information originally contained in Chapter 11 on the use of drugs in pregnancy has been transferred to a completely new chapter on drugs and reproduction. This new chapter (Chapter 12) also contains new material on methods of contraception, the treatment of infertility, and the drug management of labour, in addition to some material on the adverse effects of drugs in reproduction (teratogenesis and breast-feeding) which has been incorporated from the original Chapter 9. We have also expanded Chapter 6, which deals with the practical applications to drug therapy of the basic principles of clinical pharmacology, to include a description of the practical application of pharmacokinetic principles to the development of drug dosage regimens.

Finally, we have reorganized some material in what we feel is a more logical way. This applies particularly to the reorganization of Chapter 4 (The pharmacodynamic process), with the incorporation of some of its material into Chapter 5 (The therapeutic process), and the introduction of new material into both. This includes a description of stereoisomerism and drug action.

In the preface to the first edition we invited readers to make constructive criticisms and suggestions. We should like here to express our gratitude to those who did. Several of the changes to this edition have been made in response to such critical suggestions. We hope that readers of this edition will respond in a similar fashion to a repetition of our original invitation.

Oxford
July 1992

D.G.G.-S.
J.K.A.

Preface to the first edition

We have written this book with the needs of medical students in their clinical years paramount in our minds. Nevertheless, medical education is not restricted to the pre-qualification years, and we hope that the text may also prove of interest to those with more experience. The book is composed of four sections. In Section I we have dealt with the general aspects of clinical pharmacology, our aim being to provide a scientific basis upon which a knowledge and understanding of drug therapy can be built.

Section II is brief and deals mainly with practical aspects of prescribing.

Section III is the drug therapy section, in which we have described the role of drugs in the treatment of disease. We have restricted ourselves to discussing drugs, and have not generally dealt with other matters concerned with the management of illness.

Section IV is a Pharmacopoeia. In this we have tried to bring together essential information about the majority of drugs mentioned elsewhere in the text. We felt that it was important to have this information in a separate section, but complementing the information about the use of drugs in disease. Too often the sciences of basic and clinical pharmacology are divorced from the practice of medicine, and one of our particular aims in writing this book has been to marry the scientific disciplines with the practical approach to drug therapy. The Pharmacopoeia will enable the student to recall those aspects of the basic and clinical pharmacology of individual drugs strictly relevant to the use of the drug in treatment, while the complementary drug therapy section will provide the means for understanding the role that each drug plays in the overall drug therapy of disease, interpreted in the light of the basic principles outlined in Section I.

We hope that this method of organization of the book, in addition to the information it contains, will enable the student to gain both the knowledge which is essential to the practice of safe and effective drug therapy and the understanding of how to effect that practice.

Some may be surprised that we have not included references. We did not feel this to be necessary. Instead we have included in Section II a chapter on sources of information, which for the interested student will lead to further reading.

We are conscious that in our approach to the subject we may not have hit on the ideal format first time round, and that there will be room for improvements. We shall welcome constructive criticism and suggestions.

There is a great deal of detailed information about drugs in this book, and we have tried very hard to make it accurate. However, it is always possible that errors have been missed, particularly in regard to the important matter of dosages. Furthermore, dosage schedules are constantly being revised and new adverse effects and drug interactions being described. For these reasons we urge all who use this book to consult pharmaceutical manufacturers' Data Sheets or other sources of information before prescribing or administering the drugs described in this book, or indeed any drugs. One cannot be too careful.

Oxford
June 1984

D.G.G.-S.
J.K.A.

Drug dosages and availability

We have made every effort to check that the drug dosages listed in this book are correct. Nevertheless, it is possible that mistakes may have occurred and been missed in the checking. Furthermore, new dosage regimens are constantly being devised and previously unrecognized adverse effects and interactions are being described.

We therefore urge all those who use this book to consult pharmaceutical manufacturers' data sheets or other sources of information (see Chapter 20) before prescribing or administering the drugs described in this book, or indeed any drugs.

All the drugs mentioned in this book in the context of drug therapy were available for prescription in the UK at the time of going to press. However, the availability of drugs varies considerably, both world-wide and from time to time, and the local availability of drugs may have to be checked and may influence prescribing.

Contents

Section II Practical prescribing

Section III   The drug therapy of disease

Section IV   Pharmacopoeia

Co-authors

J. Carmichael BSc, MD, MRCP (Chapter 36)
Consultant in Clinical Oncology,
ICRF Clinical Oncology Unit,
Churchill Hospital,
Oxford

C. P. Conlon MBBS, MRCP (Chapter 22)
Senior Registrar in Infectious Diseases,
Department of Infectious Diseases,
John Radcliffe Hospital,
Oxford

T. R. Cripps DM, MRCP (Chapter 23)
Senior Registrar in Cardiology,
Department of Cardiovascular Medicine,
John Radcliffe Hospital,
Oxford

H. R. Dalton BSc, MBBS, MRCP (Chapter 25)
Research Fellow in Gastroenterology,
Gastrointestinal Unit,
Radcliffe Infirmary,
Oxford

J. Efthimiou BSc, MD, MRCP (Chapter 24)
Senior Registrar in Chest Medicine,
Osler Chest Unit,
Churchill Hospital,
Oxford

J. D. Firth DM, MRCP (Chapter 26)
Lecturer in Medicine,
Nuffield Department of Clinical Medicine,
John Radcliffe Hospital,
Oxford

M.E. Haines BSc, PhD, MBBS, MRCP,
MRCPath (Chapter 28)
Senior Registrar in Haematology,
Department of Haematology,
John Radcliffe Hospital,
Oxford

R. M. Hillson MD MRCP (Chapter 27)
Consultant Physician,
Hillingdon Hospital,
Uxbridge,
Middlesex

H. J. McQuay DM, FFA RCS (Chapter 32)
Clinical Reader in Pain Relief,
Oxford Regional Pain Relief Unit,
ICRF Building,
Churchill Hospital,
Oxford

A. G. Mowat MBChB FRCP FRCP(E)
(Chapter 29)
Consultant Rheumatologist,
Department of Rheumatology,
The Nuffield Orthopaedic Centre,
Oxford

P. K. Panegyres BMedSci, MBBS, FRACP
(Chapter 30)
Registrar in Neurology,
University Department of Clinical Neurology,
Radcliffe Infirmary,
Oxford

D. J. M. Reynolds BMBCh, MRCP (Chapter 35)
Clinical Lecturer in Clinical Pharmacology,
University Department of Clinical
Pharmacology,
Radcliffe Infirmary,
Oxford

P. J. Robson MBBS, MRCP, MRCPsych
(Chapter 34)
Consultant Psychiatrist,
Department of Addictive Behaviour,
Chilton Clinic,
Warneford Hospital,
Oxford

J. W. Sear BSc, PhD, MBBS, FFA RCS,
DObst RCOG (Chapter 33)
Clinical Reader in Anaesthetics,
Nuffield Department of Anaesthetics,
Radcliffe Infirmary,
Oxford

G. P. Spickett DPhil, MRCP, MRCPath
(Chapter 37)
Consultant and Senior Lecturer in Clinical
Immunology,
Regional Department of Immunology,
Newcastle General Hospital,
Newcastle upon Tyne

N. J. White BSc, MD, FRCP (Chapter 22)
Faculty of Tropical Medicine,
Mahidol University,
Bangkok,
Thailand

A. J. Wood DM, MRCP, MRCPsych
(Chapter 31)
Clinical Lecturer in Psychiatry,
University Department of Psychiatry,
Warneford Hospital,
Oxford

Section I

Clinical pharmacology: the scientific basis of drug therapy

1 The four processes of drug therapy

The processes of drug therapy are very complex, although not more complex than those processes which underlie the illness for which therapy is being given. Historically, modern drug therapy has developed from the herbal and folklore medicine of the past, with its mixture of magic, empirical pharmacology, and faith of the patient in the doctor. Some cynics might hold that not much has changed. However, there have been changes, even though the apparent magic of drug therapy is still a potent force in its success. The changes which have occurred are in the understanding of the mechanisms of action of the drugs we use and in the optimal application of those drugs to the treatment of disease. Underlying all this is an immense amount of research in the sciences of basic and clinical pharmacology.

The rationalization of drug therapy has lagged behind the understanding of disease processes, for obvious reasons. The rational person wants to be able to understand a pathological process, and to make a precise diagnosis, before instituting treatment. Until relatively recently, few specific and effective therapies were available, and it is not therefore surprising that medical education has in the past concentrated on the art and science of diagnosis and the minute understanding of disease processes, neglecting, to a great extent, their treatment with drugs. The art and science of surgical treatment was not so neglected, because manifestly it is profoundly effective in appropriate cases and demonstrates in a most dramatic way the doctor's concern and masterly activity on behalf of his or her patients.

In recent years, however, drug therapy has been undergoing a process of increasing rationalization. Advances in the understanding of the detailed events underlying the pathology of diseases have allowed their manipulation with drugs.

Conversely, the empirical development of drugs useful in the treatment of specific diseases has led to improvements in our understanding of those diseases. For example, the discovery of the precise biochemical abnormality in Parkinson's disease has led to the introduction of specific therapy with levodopa, while the study of the mechanisms of action of psychotropic drugs has been one of the major factors in promoting the biochemical and pharmacological investigation of brain function in relation to mental illness.

One of the main aims of the approach to therapeutics we shall outline here is to provide a method of analysis of drug therapy within a discipline as strict as that by which a diagnosis is reached. It does not matter that in the course of this analysis there may arise questions to which there are at present no answers, for only by asking such questions can we begin to understand the extent of our own knowledge and ignorance.

The approach which we shall describe is one in which drug therapy is analysed step by step from the time of the formulation of a drug by a pharmaceutical manufacturer to the time of the eventual therapeutic outcome in the patient. The scheme we shall outline can be applied to any type of drug therapy, to answer any questions about drug therapy in an individual patient, and to optimize that patient's drug therapy.

There are four main processes involved in drug therapy (Fig. 1.1). They are:

(1) the pharmaceutical process;

(2) the pharmacokinetic process;

(3) the pharmacodynamic process;

(4) the therapeutic process.

These four processes can be represented by simple questions, one for each process:

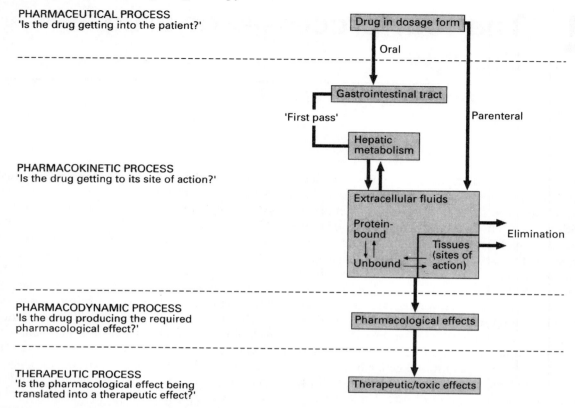

PHARMACEUTICAL PROCESS
'Is the drug getting into the patient?'

Oral

Gastrointestinal tract

'First pass'

Parenteral

Hepatic metabolism

PHARMACOKINETIC PROCESS
'Is the drug getting to its site of action?'

Drug in dosage form

Extracellular fluids

Protein-bound

Unbound

Tissues (sites of action)

Elimination

PHARMACODYNAMIC PROCESS
'Is the drug producing the required pharmacological effect?'

Pharmacological effects

THERAPEUTIC PROCESS
'Is the pharmacological effect being translated into a therapeutic effect?'

Therapeutic/toxic effects

■ **Fig. 1.1** The four main processes involved in drug therapy. Compare this figure with Fig. 6.2, in which more detail is given.

1. Is the drug getting into the patient?
2. Is the drug getting to its site of action?
3. Is the drug producing the required pharmacological effect?
4. Is the pharmacological effect being translated into an appropriate therapeutic effect?

1.1 The pharmaceutical process: is the drug getting into the patient?

The pharmaceutical process is concerned with all those factors inherent in the pharmaceutical formulation and presentation of a drug formulation, which determine whether or not it is absorbed from the gut (in the case of oral or rectal adminis-

tration), from the skin (in the case of topical administration), or from the subcutaneous tissues or muscle (in the case of subcutaneous and intramuscular injections). Strictly speaking, we are not concerned here with the process of absorption itself, but with the properties of the drug formulation, for example the amount of drug in a tablet, drug crystal size, tablet compression, excipients (i.e. supposedly inactive ingredients used to bulk out a formulation and to confer on it certain properties), and the predictability of certain properties of the formulation, for example rates of disintegration and dissolution of tablets.

Although it is not strictly relevant to the pharmaceutical process it is convenient here to remember to consider the question of patient compliance, since that is an important determinant of whether or not the drug gets into the patient.

1.2 The pharmacokinetic process: is the drug getting to its site of action?

The pharmacokinetic process is concerned with the absorption, distribution, and elimination (by metabolism and excretion) of drugs. It can be studied by measuring the concentrations of drug and metabolite in blood and/or urine over periods of time after dosing. It is evident that, however many structural and metabolic barriers drug molecules have to pass, the concentration of a drug at its site of action must have the blood concentration as one of its determinants. Thus, a proper mathematical description of the pharmacokinetic characteristics of a drug can provide a great deal of information of relevance to its pharmacological effects and to its therapeutic or toxic effects.

By studying the pharmacokinetic process, individual and interindividual variability in absorption, distribution, metabolism, and excretion of drugs can be defined. Such studies have contributed much to our understanding of the variability of responses to drugs.

cokinetic and pharmacodynamic processes is not always simple, as a few examples will show.

1. Some drugs combine with their receptors quickly and dissociate from them quickly. For such drugs the pharmacological effects wax and wane in time with the concentration of drug in the plasma. An example is the use of intravenous sodium nitroprusside in the control of blood pressure, for example during neurosurgery.

2. Other drugs combine with their receptors but do not readily dissociate from them, so that the pharmacological effect persists despite a falling plasma concentration, and the two are not directly related to each other. The irreversible monoamine oxidase (MAO) inhibitors provide an example.

3. Yet other drugs combine with their receptors and, irrespective of their rates of association or dissociation, set in train a sequence of events which runs on despite a falling plasma concentration. An example is that of the anti-inflammatory effects of corticosteroids.

It can be very difficult to sort out the relationships between the plasma concentrations of drugs and their pharmacological effects with drugs of types 2 and 3 above.

1.3 The pharmacodynamic process: is the drug producing the required pharmacological effect?

When the drug reaches its site of action it has a pharmacological effect, and it is with this effect that the pharmacodynamic process is concerned. The pharmacodynamic process encompasses not only those pharmacological effects which may be responsible for an eventual therapeutic effect, but also those responsible for the adverse effects, as well as some effects which may be of no practical clinical relevance. The link between the pharma-

1.4 The therapeutic process: is the pharmacological effect being translated into an appropriate therapeutic effect?

If the patient is to benefit from drug therapy the pharmacological effect of the drug must be translated into clinical benefit. Of course this presumes that the detailed nature of the pharmacological effect responsible for the therapeutic action of the drug is known, and that is not always so, as in the case of tricyclic antidepressants in depression. One of the problems here is that the question: Is the pharmacological effect being translated into an appropriate therapeutic effect? can be countered by two further questions.

1. What do you consider to be the pharmacodynamic effect of a drug?
2. What do you mean by the therapeutic effect?

In case the reader thinks that this is unnecessary obscurantism, an example will illustrate the point. Consider the treatment of asymptomatic hypertension with, say, propranolol, a non-selective β-adrenoceptor antagonist. There is no doubt that propranolol lowers the blood pressure, but how does it do it (i.e. what is its pharmacodynamic effect)? Presumably β-blockade in the heart is involved, but is the hypotensive effect exerted through the fall in cardiac output or through subsequent adaptive changes, such as alterations in ventricular muscle performance, baroreceptor reflex arcs, or the renin-angiotensin system (via renal β-adrenoceptor blockade)? The practical person will be interested only in the observation that propranolol lowers the blood pressure, and that will be considered to be the pharmacodynamic action of the drug. Indeed, in the management of the hypertensive patient this is plainly the correct attitude. However, the clinical scientist will be forgiven for pondering on the exact mechanism by which propranolol produces its effects, because hidden in the response to the drug are the mechanisms causing the hypertension, the clues to why some patients respond better than others, and the details from which the relationships among the pharmacokinetic, pharmacodynamic, and therapeutic processes can be elucidated.

The answer to the question: What is the therapeutic effect? may in this case appear to be obvious, but in fact there are several possible answers. One might, for example, consider a lowering of the blood pressure to be the therapeutic effect, but lowering the blood pressure does not make patients feel any better, since they are asymptomatic; indeed, it may make them feel worse. In any case, the lowering of the blood pressure is only the first step towards the ultimate goal, which is to reduce the risk of myocardial infarction, stroke, heart failure, and renal failure. So the lowering of the blood pressure produced by the treatment is probably closer to the pharmacodynamic action than to the therapeutic action, which in an individual patient will be virtually impossible to calculate. Assessment of the long-term therapeutic outcome in this case depends upon the results of large-scale clinical trials of the efficacy of antihypertensive drugs in the prevention of the complications of hypertension, evaluated by statistical methods. It will probably never be possible for any one practitioner to know from his or her own experience whether or not the treatment of asymptomatic hypertension produces any real benefit in an individual patient or even in the total population of patients whom he or she treats during a working lifetime.

Consideration of this example of a very common therapy reveals many problems. It is the analysis of drug therapy in this way which brings these sorts of problems to light. In the following four chapters we shall consider the approach of analysing drug therapy through the pharmaceutical, pharmacokinetic, pharmacodynamic, and therapeutic processes, and we shall see how this approach can impose upon drug therapy the same kind of academic discipline as exists for the process of diagnosis, with its component processes of history-taking, physical examination, and investigation. That in its application in the clinical setting unanswerable questions may be raised is all to the good. The only word of caution is that one should not allow one's ignorance of the answers to such questions to interfere with the treatment of a patient with a drug which has been shown, however empirically, to be definitely effective.

2 The pharmaceutical process

Is the drug getting into the patient?

The two important factors which determine whether a drug gets into the patient are:

(1) patient compliance;
(2) systemic availability (bioavailability).

2.1 Patient compliance

A prescription is a complicated, often rather imprecise set of instructions. Consider the following list of drugs prescribed for a 60-year-old woman with atrial fibrillation, heart failure, hypertension, diabetes mellitus, osteoarthritis, depression, insomnia, and a urinary tract infection.

propranolol 80 mg t.d.s.
bendrofluazide 10 mg daily
digoxin 0.25 mg daily
ibuprofen 400 mg t.d.s.
chlorpropamide 250 mg daily
co-trimoxazole tablets 2 twice daily
amitriptyline 25 mg t.d.s.
nitrazepam 5 mg o.n.
(For the meanings of the abbreviations used here see p. 214).

There may have been every medical justification for the prescription of each of these drugs at the time they were first prescribed. However, it was a formidable task for the patient to organize herself to remember to take 18 tablets a day, three drugs to be taken three times a day, one drug twice a day, three drugs once a day in the morning, and one at bedtime. Indeed, it is likely that on most days she would have failed to do all this correctly.

It is not surprising that patient compliance with complicated prescriptions is poor, as numerous studies have shown. However, poor compli-ance also extends to simple prescriptions. It is not easy to put a precise figure on the frequency of non-compliance in general, because the problem is difficult to study. This is reflected in the results of studies which have shown that the prevalence of non-compliance varies between about 10 per cent and 90 per cent of patients. Non-compliance is so common that it should be the first matter to check when drug therapy appears ineffective. Similarly, mistakes in medicine-taking should be sought in the event of unexpected drug toxicity. Simple therapeutic regimens, patient education, manipulation of drug formulations, and the avoidance of adverse effects are all measures which might be expected to improve patient compliance. These matters are discussed in more detail in Chapter 13.

2.2 Systemic availability (bioavailability)

Systemic availability (commonly known as bioavailability) is a term used to describe the proportion of administered drug which reaches the systemic circulation and is thus available for distribution to the site of action. The term is usually applied in reference to formulations given by the oral route, although it can also refer to other routes of administration, such as intramuscular or transdermal. The precise meaning of the term is best explained by considering Fig. 2.1, in which the several steps involved are defined.

1. When an intravenous dose of a drug is given it all enters the systemic circulation. It thus has a systemic availability of 100 per cent. From the plot of plasma concentration of the drug against time, with or without urinary or other tissue drug concentration analyses, the way the body handles

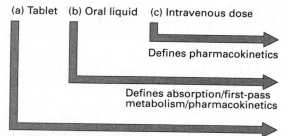

■ **Fig. 2.1** A diagrammatic definition of systemic availability (or bioavailability). The systemic availability of a drug formulation can be defined as the amount of the administered drug which reaches the systemic circulation, and hence the site of action, as a proportion of the dose. This definition should also incorporate some notion of the rate at which this happens.

the drug (its pharmacokinetics) can be defined. This is illustrated in Fig. 2.1(c), and discussed in detail in Chapter 3.

2. When a liquid solution of the drug is given orally all the drug is theoretically available to the gastrointestinal mucosa for absorption. The plot of plasma concentration versus time, and analysis of the concentrations of drug and its metabolites in the urine compared with the corresponding intravenous data, will give an index of the degree of absorption and the metabolic effect of the liver as it passes through for the first time (the so-called 'first-pass effect'). This is illustrated in Fig. 2.1(b).

3. When a tablet or capsule is given orally, by following the plot of plasma concentration versus time, and the cumulative urinary excretion of the drug and its metabolites, and by comparing these data with those collected after dosage with a liquid form, one can define those factors intrinsic to the formulation which affect its ultimate systemic availability. These factors include the rate of disintegration of the tablet and the rate of dissolution of the drug particles in the intestinal fluid. This may be termed 'pharmaceutical availability'. This is illustrated in Fig. 2.1(a).

Prescribing doctors generally depend upon the skills of the pharmacist and pharmaceutical chemist to provide formulations of drugs of high stability and predictable pharmaceutical availab-

ility, which should reach the standards laid down in national pharmacopoeias, such as *The British Pharmacopoeia* (see p. 218). The physical factors which have to be taken into account and controlled are:

1. Tablet compression and excipients. These factors affect the rate of tablet disintegration.

2. Other tablet excipients. These affect the interaction of the drug with aqueous gastrointestinal juices, and therefore the rate of dissolution.

3. The form of the drug. The rate of dissolution will also partly depend on the form the drug is in, such as crystalline or salt forms, or complexed with a tablet constituent.

4. Particle size. Smaller drug particles generally dissolve more quickly.

If two formulations are of equal systemic availability they are said to be bioequivalent. If formulations differ in their systemic availability they are said to be bioinequivalent. There have been cases in which problems of bioinequivalence caused by manufacturing factors have had serious clinical consequences. For example, in Australia in 1968 an outbreak of phenytoin toxicity occurred because of a switch from calcium sulphate to lactose as an apparently inert tablet excipient. This change rendered the phenytoin more soluble and increased its systemic availability, with a consequent increase in plasma concentrations and an increased incidence of toxicity. Variability in the systemic availability of digoxin led in 1975 to the imposition of new pharmacopoeial standards for digoxin tablets in both the UK and the USA. This problem came to light because of the use of plasma digoxin concentration measurements after their introduction in 1968, when variable systemic availability of digoxin from different formulations was discovered.

Alterations in pharmaceutical availability are of particular importance for drugs with a low therapeutic index (i.e. drugs for which the dose which will have a toxic effect is very little more than the dose which will have a therapeutic effect). Phenytoin and digoxin are examples of such drugs. If a patient is taking a formulation of low pharmaceutical availability which is producing a good therapeutic effect, switching to a formulation of high availability can tip the patient into toxicity.

The definition of systemic availability given at the beginning of this section incorporates the process of absorption, which is dealt with further in Chapter 3. The pharmaceutical and chemical skills used in drug development are aimed not only at providing formulations which will deliver the drug in a soluble form to the site of absorption, but also, before that stage, at producing a molecule which, in the case of oral administration, is stable in the gastrointestinal juices and capable of absorption.

The process of drug absorption from oral formulations involves passage of the drug across the gastrointestinal mucosa, into the mesenteric circulation. For the sake of discussion here (and it is merely a matter of arbitrary definition and not some absolute truth) absorption will be taken to mean only the process of passage across the gastrointestinal mucosa into the capillary blood of the mesenteric circulation, and not to include the appearance of the drug in the systemic circulation (see Fig. 6.1). This distinction is made because between the gut and the systemic circulation lies the liver, the great 'poison trap', protecting the systemic circulation from numerous potential toxins which enter the gastrointestinal tract. Evolutionary experience of environmental toxins has provided the liver with an extraordinary range of detoxifying mechanisms for natural toxins, mechanisms which are also active in detoxifying many drugs. However, the very presence of the trap means that for many drugs not all that is absorbed reaches the systemic circulation intact. This is known as the 'first-pass effect' (the second and subsequent passes being when the drug comes round again in the hepatic artery as part of the systemic circulation, and therefore in much lower concentrations).

As far as drug therapy is concerned the most practical definition of systemic availability is that which incorporates some guide to the rate and extent of appearance of the drug in the systemic circulation, but it is most important to understand the various component parts of the process, so that they may be analysed separately. The scheme outlined above will help in the understanding of those component parts.

2.3 Special drug formulations

Before leaving the subject of systemic availability it is worthwhile considering some factors involved in the systemic availability of certain formulations. These include subcutaneous, intramuscular, and local injections, sublingual, buccal, and rectal formulations, inhalations, transdermal formulations, slow-release formulations, and combination formulations.

2.3.1 Subcutaneous, intramuscular, and local injections

Control of the absorption of insulin from the site of subcutaneous injection is achieved by differences in the physical state of the insulin (for example, crystalline or non-crystalline), in the zinc or protein content, and in the nature and pH of the buffer in which the insulin is suspended. At one end of the scale is insulin BP, which is soluble and amorphous (i.e. non-crystalline). Soluble insulin has a rapid onset and short duration of action (about 6 h); at the other end of the scale is ultralente insulin, which has large crystals of insulin and a high zinc content, suspended in a solution of sodium acetate/sodium chloride (pH 7.1–7.5), with an onset of action at about 7 h, and a duration of action of about 36 h.

The absorption of drugs from intramuscular injection sites may be retarded by the use of thick oils, which slow down diffusion of the drug from the site of injection; for example, vasopressin tannate in oil in the treatment of diabetes insipidus and fluphenazine decanoate in oil in the treatment of schizophrenia.

Superficially one might think that intramuscular administration would always provide better systemic availability than oral administration. However, this is not always so, the prime example being phenytoin. The plasma phenytoin concentrations achieved after intramuscular injection are about half of those achieved after the oral administration of the same dose, because of precipitation at the site of injection. This should be borne in mind when changing the patient from oral to intramuscular phenytoin or vice versa, or when using intramuscular phenytoin to prevent epilepsy after intracranial operations. Another example is chloramphenicol, which is also poorly absorbed after intramuscular injection.

Some formulations of local anaesthetics contain adrenaline which, by causing vasoconstriction, prevents the local anaesthetic, say lignocaine, from being carried away by the circulation from the site of injection. It thus prolongs the effect of the local anaesthetic, but incidentally provides a potential interaction with tricyclic antidepressants and MAO inhibitors.

2.3.2 Inhalations

Inhaled formulations come in several forms, with different intentions. Sodium cromoglycate is formulated as a powder for inhalation, designed to have a local effect on the bronchioles in the treatment and prevention of bronchial asthma. Salbutamol aerosol, on the other hand, is designed to produce bronchodilatation by a metered dose (100 micrograms) of droplets, whose size (2–5 μm) allows them to penetrate down the bronchial tree to bronchiolar level. Just how much drug reaches the site of action directly is uncertain. Plainly it will depend in part on the type of inhaler and how the patient uses it, including the depth of inspiration and how much of the drug is swallowed, among other factors (see p. 308). However, it is thought that only about 10 per cent of any drug in an aerosol or other form for inhalation reaches the bronchial tree, the rest being lost in the air, absorbed from the oropharynx, or swallowed. In acute severe asthma the use of a nebulizer, to provide continuous aerosolized salbutamol or other drugs, is now routine.

An ergotamine aerosol is available for the treatment of migraine. The metered dose is 360 micrograms, which is close to the usual dose for intramuscular or oral administration. However, in migraine the nausea and vomiting associated with the illness may impair the absorption of a drug given orally, and ergotamine tends to be most effective when given very early following the onset of an attack. The aerosol is designed to produce rapid absorption from the tracheobronchial mucosa, thus avoiding the absorption problems posed by the oral route of administration.

2.3.3 Sublingual, buccal, and rectal formulations

Drugs which are absorbed through the oral or rectal mucosa enter the venous circulation and pass into the systemic circulation intact, avoiding first-pass metabolism in the liver. For example, glyceryl trinitrate is taken sublingually, and is then effective in doses about ten times less than those required by the oral route. In addition, sublingual administration results in a very rapid therapeutic effect.

Corticosteroids may be given by the rectal route for a direct effect on the large bowel, and in the past aminophylline was sometimes given by suppository, the object being to avoid gastric irritation and to produce controlled release of drug overnight. However, aminophylline suppositories frequently caused proctitis and have been superceded by modern slow-release oral formulations.

2.3.4 Transdermal formulations

Some drugs are absorbed well via the skin, and their transdermal administration via so-called patches allows controlled release of small amounts of drug over a period of hours. Drugs which have been used in this way include glyceryl trinitrate in the long-term treatment of angina pectoris, transdermal hyoscine in the treatment of travel sickness, and oestradiol in hormone replacement therapy.

These and many other examples illustrate the several ways in which pharmaceutical chemists can manipulate drug formulations in order to meet a particular therapeutic objective.

2.3.5 Controlled-release formulations

Different types of controlled-release formulations (for example delayed-release and slow-release formulations) are being used increasingly, through the development of advanced pharmaceutical technology. Some of these formulations are useful for specific reasons, good examples being enteric-coated aspirin, whose release is delayed until the tablet reaches the small intestine, thus reducing the risk of gastric erosions, and slow-release formulations of quinidine, which allow less frequent administration than would be possible with conventional formulations. Other examples of drugs which may usefully be prescribed as slow-release formulations include theophylline and nifedipine, because of their relatively short durations of action.

Many such formulations are of undoubted value in drug therapy. However, it is sometimes difficult to know whether or not the use of some controlled-release formulations is a real contribution to therapeutic practice. Take, for instance, the slow-release formulations of the β-adrenoceptor antagonists propranolol and oxprenolol. There is much evidence that once-daily therapy with ordinary formulations of these drugs is as effective in the treatment of hypertension as with slow-release formulations, and that the latter may therefore be unnecessary. For procainamide there is evidence, albeit currently inconclusive, that it may cause neutropenia more often in slow-release than in ordinary formulations.

2.3.6 Combination products in oral therapy

Combination products for oral use are widely available, but only under certain circumstances may they be acceptable or even preferable. These circumstances arise when the following minimum criteria are met.

1. When the frequency of administration of the two drugs is the same.

2. When the fixed doses in the combination product are therapeutically and optimally effective in the majority of cases (i.e. when it is not necessary to alter the dose of one drug independently of the other).

Good examples of well-tried combination products are:

1. Aspirin or paracetamol plus codeine. Here two agents achieve their analgesic effects through different mechanisms and summate therapeutically but not with regard to their adverse effects.

2. Levodopa (L-dopa) plus a peripherally-acting dopa decarboxylase inhibitor (benserazide or carbidopa). Here the peripheral action of the decarboxylase inhibitor blocks the peripheral metabolism of L-dopa, which is free to enter the brain, where it is converted to the pharmacologically active product dopamine, producing the therapeutic effect in Parkinson's disease.

3. Combined oral contraceptives, which contain an oestrogen and a progestogen (see p. 147).

4. DTP vaccine, a combination of vaccines against diphtheria, tetanus, and pertussis.

5. Ferrous sulphate plus folic acid, used in the prevention of anaemia in pregnancy.

There are many other examples of valuable combinations (see Table 2.1), but there are also examples of what might be considered bad combinations currently on the market. These include

■ **Table 2.1**   Potential advantages of combination formulations

Potential advantages	Examples
Improved compliance	Antituberculous drugs (rifampicin + isoniazid)
	Ferrous sulphate + folic acid (pregnancy)
Ease of administration	Triple vaccine (diphtheria, tetanus, pertussis)
Synergistic or additive effects	Trimethoprim + sulphonamides (e.g. co-trimoxazole)
	Amoxycillin + clavulanic acid (co-amoxiclav)
	Aspirin + codeine (simple analgesia) (co-codaprin)
	Paracetamol + metoclopramide (migraine)
	Combined oral contraceptive (oestrogen + progestogen)
Decreased adverse effects	L-dopa + decarboxylase inhibitors (Parkinson's disease)
	Diuretics (potassium-wasting + potassium-sparing)

the combination of α-methyldopa 250 mg with hydrochlorothiazide 15 mg, for the treatment of hypertension, and the combination of amitriptyline 12.5 mg with chlordiazepoxide 5 mg, for the treatment of mixed anxiety and depression. In neither case is there flexibility of dosages, and the timing of administration of the two components differs. It is difficult to see how these combinations can be used optimally in the treatment of their supposed indications.

3 The pharmacokinetic process

Is the drug getting to its site of action?

In this chapter we shall deal with the principles underlying the ways in which drugs are handled by the body. In Chapter 6 we shall illustrate how these principles can be used in the development of dosage regimens.

The pharmacokinetic process comprises:

1. drug absorption and systemic availability;
2. drug distribution;
3. drug metabolism;
4. drug excretion.

3.1. Drug absorption and systemic availability

After oral administration a drug will reach the systemic arterial circulation only if it is absorbed from the gastrointestinal tract and if it escapes metabolism in the gastrointestinal tract, the liver, and the lungs. In practice, however, it can be difficult to characterize the separate contributions of absorption and pre-systemic metabolism to the changes in plasma drug concentrations with time after an oral dose. The concept of systemic availability, or bioavailability, has therefore been developed (see Fig. 2.1).

The systemic availability of a drug is defined in terms of (1) the amount of administered drug which reaches the systemic circulation intact, and (2) the rate at which that happens. The rate of availability depends on pharmaceutical factors (see Chapter 2) and gastrointestinal absorption, pre-systemic metabolism being relatively unimportant. On the other hand, the extent of availability depends on both the extent of absorption and the extent of pre-systemic metabolism.

These two components of systemic availability may be assessed by considering Fig. 3.1. The three curves shown represent the theoretical plasma concentrations resulting over a period of time after the oral administration of three different formulations of the same dose of the same drug. Each curve contains three features of interest:

(1) the peak concentration (C_{max});
(2) the time taken to reach the peak (t_{max});
(3) the total area under the curve (AUC).

The C_{max} and t_{max} are measures of the rate of availability, and the total AUC is a measure of its extent (i.e. the proportion of administered drug which reaches the systemic circulation intact). In the three hypothetical cases illustrated in Fig. 3.1 the rates of availability are clearly different. In the case of formulation I the systemic availability is fast, perhaps too fast, leading to potentially toxic plasma concentrations. Formu-

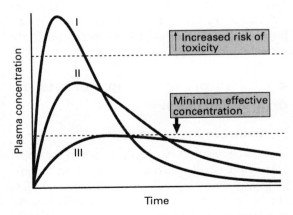

Fig. 3.1 The theoretical plasma concentrations resulting over a period of time after the oral administration of three different formulations of the same dose of the same drug. The profile in each case depends on both the rate and the extent of systemic availability.

lation II is not so quickly available and plasma concentrations are never in the potentially toxic range. Formulation III is slowly available and plasma concentrations after a single dose are always subtherapeutic. However, in contrast to the rate of availability, the extent of availability of these three formulations, as assessed by the AUC, is the same in each case.

For drugs whose action may depend on the threshold plasma concentration achieved after a single dose (for example analgesics) such differences may be important. Thus, for the rapid relief of pain a soluble aspirin formulation, giving a curve like that of formulation II, would be preferable to an enteric-coated formulation, giving a curve like that of formulation III. The latter would be more useful in the long-term treatment of rheumatoid arthritis, since accumulation could occur to therapeutic concentrations during repeated administration (see Fig. 3.9).

Sometimes a curve of type I can be therapeutically useful, for example if a very fast rate of absorption is needed in order to produce a quick therapeutic effect, as for sublingual glyceryl trinitrate in the relief of an acute attack of angina pectoris. With glyceryl trinitrate the fast rate of absorption of a large amount of drug leads to the rapid relief of symptoms, but also to the adverse effect of headache caused by dilatation of extracranial blood vessels.

For drugs whose action is related to a steady-state concentration during multiple dosing the differences in rate of availability become less important and the chief consideration is the extent.

3.1.1 Factors affecting the rate of drug absorption

(a) Gastrointestinal motility

Since drug absorption occurs mainly in the upper part of the small intestine, alterations in the rate of gastric emptying will result in corresponding alterations in the rate of absorption. For example, in migraine the rate of absorption of analgesics, such as paracetamol, may be reduced because of reduced gastric motility, and the response to oral analgesics may therefore be delayed. This delay can be reduced by giving at the same time meto-

clopramide, a drug which increases the rate of gastric emptying.

These changes in rate of absorption depend on rapid dissolution of the drug before it reaches the site of absorption. When the rate of dissolution is much longer than the rate of gastric emptying, enhanced gastrointestinal motility may reduce both the rate and extent of absorption, as in the case of enteric-coated formulations, which may on occasion pass through the gut intact.

(b) Malabsorptive states

Although one would expect drug absorption to be impaired in patients with malabsorptive states, that is not always the case. For example, the absorption of propranolol, co-trimoxazole, and cephalexin are increased in patients with coeliac disease, as is the absorption of propranolol in Crohn's disease. Digoxin, however, is less well absorbed from tablets in patients with coeliac disease, radiation-induced enteritis, and other forms of gastrointestinal disease, and thyroxine absorption is impaired in coeliac disease.

(c) Food

Food may either enhance or impair the rate of absorption of drugs and may also affect the extent of their absorption. For example, eggs impair iron absorption, and milk (and any calcium, aluminium, magnesium, or ferrous salt) impairs tetracycline absorption, by the formation of an insoluble chelate. The rate, but not the extent, of absorption of most penicillin antibiotics is impaired by food, while that of hydralazine, propranolol, metoprolol, and nitrofurantoin is increased. Fat specifically improves the absorption of griseofulvin. The mechanisms of these effects are mostly unknown. They are generally of little clinical importance.

3.1.2 First-pass metabolism

An important factor (separate from absorption across the gut wall) which is often a determinant of systemic availability is the extent of metabolism occurring before the drug enters the systemic circulation, the so-called 'first-pass' effect (see p. 8). The organs which may be involved in this pre-systemic or 'first-pass' metabolism are the gut lumen, the gut wall, the liver, and the lungs (the last being relatively unimportant).

(a) The gut lumen

Benzylpenicillin and insulin, for example, are both almost completely inactivated by gastric acid and proteolytic enzymes respectively.

(b) The gut wall

Chlorpromazine and isoprenaline, for example, are both sulphated in the gut wall. The metabolism of monoamines, such as tyramine, by gut wall monoamine oxidase (MAO) forms the basis of the interaction of amine-containing foods with MAO inhibitors (see Chapter 10).

(c) The liver

The liver is a more important site of first-pass metabolism than either the gut or the lungs, and there are many examples of drugs which are subject to pre-systemic metabolism in the liver. For instance, lignocaine is metabolized to two active compounds which have less anti-arrhythmic activity than lignocaine itself, but which are more toxic. Propranolol is metabolized to 4-hydroxypropranolol, which is pharmacologically inactive. Other examples can be found in Table 3.5 (p. 33), which contains a list of drugs with a high hepatic extraction ratio.

When first-pass metabolism results in the formation of compounds with less pharmacological activity than the parent compound then there is a decrease in efficacy of the drug after its oral administration by comparison with the effect that would be achieved following, say, intravenous (i.v.) administration. In some cases this may be surmountable by using an oral dose greater than that which is effective by the intravenous route. For example, by the i.v. route, propranolol produces a β-blocking effect in a single dose of about 5 mg, but a single dose of about 100 mg would be needed to produce a similar effect after oral administration.

In some cases metabolism is so extensive that it renders oral therapy impossible with conventional oral formulations (for example lignocaine and insulin). In such cases the drug must be given by another route, usually intravenously, intramuscularly, or subcutaneously. However, in some cases it may be possible to administer the drug via the gastrointestinal tract, for example, sublingually or rectally (see also p. 9). The sublingual route, for example, may be used for the administration of glyceryl trinitrate, since the drug will be absorbed via the oral mucosa directly into the systemic circulation. The rectal route, with drainage via the inferior rectal veins directly into the systemic circulation, offers a comparable alternative, but is more commonly used to achieve a topical effect on the rectum and colon (for example prednisolone enemas in the treatment of ulcerative colitis), or to minimize adverse effects occurring in the upper gut (for example indomethacin, which is more likely to cause gastric ulceration if given orally).

Hepatic drug metabolism is discussed in more detail below.

3.2 Drug distribution

3.2.1 Protein binding

Many drugs are bound to circulating proteins, usually albumin, but also globulins, lipoproteins, and acid glycoproteins. Only that fraction of the drug which is non-protein-bound can bind to cellular receptors, pass across tissue membranes, and gain access to cellular enzymes, thus being distributed to other body tissues, metabolized, and excreted (for example by the kidney). Thus, changes in protein binding may sometimes cause changes in drug distribution. However, for such changes to be important the following criteria must be met:

(a) The bound drug must constitute more than 90 per cent of the total drug in the plasma

This is because changes in protein binding are usually of the order of a few per cent. Thus, a decrease of 5 per cent binding for a drug which is only 20 per cent bound (for example digoxin) results in a change from 80 to 85 per cent of free drug, a negligible effect. In contrast, a similar change in binding of a drug which is 95 per cent bound (for example phenytoin) results in a change from 5 to 10 per cent of unbound drug, a relatively large and therefore important effect.

Protein binding is therefore important in practice for only a few drugs, principally phenytoin, warfarin, and tolbutamide. The extent of protein binding of some commonly used drugs is given in Table 3.1.

The factors which may cause an increase in the fraction of circulating unbound drug are:

1. Renal impairment, in which the characteristics of binding of drugs to albumin are altered by unknown mechanisms.

2. Hypoalbuminaemia. Drug binding is reduced when the plasma albumin concentration falls below 25 g/L.

3. The last trimester of pregnancy. There may be reduced protein binding during the last trimester of pregnancy, partly because of hypoalbuminaemia and partly because of other, as yet unidentified, factors.

4. Displacement by other drugs. Drugs may be displaced from their protein binding sites by other drugs (see Chapter 10).

5. Saturability of protein binding. For some drugs (for example clofibrate and disopyramide) protein binding is saturable and decreases at increasing plasma drug concentrations within the therapeutic range.

(b) The extent of distribution of the drug to the tissues must be small

If the drug is widely distributed to the body tissues, then even large increases in the amount of unbound drug in the plasma will be unimportant, since the increment of bound drug, small in comparison with total body content, will be readily redistributed in body tissues and the unbound concentration in the plasma will rise by a negligible amount.

3.2.2 Tissue distribution

The second aspect of drug distribution is that of distribution to the tissues of the body, the extent of which varies widely from drug to drug. Some drugs are distributed only to the body fluids, while others are bound extensively in body tissues. The apparent volume of distribution (see the later sections in this chapter on pharmacokinetic calculations) gives a mathematical measure of the extent of tissue distribution, but does not give any anatomical or physiological information about that distribution.

The following factors may influence the distribution of drugs to different tissues:

■ **Table 3.1** Values of percentage protein binding for some commonly used drugs

99% bound	95-99% bound	90-95% bound	50-90% bound	<50% bound
Phenylbutazone*†	Amitriptyline	Diazoxide	Aspirin*†	Alcohol
Thyroxine	Chlorpromazine	Disopyramide*	Carbamazepine	Aminoglycosides
Tri-iodothyronine	Clofibrate*	Glibenclamide	Chloramphenicol	Chlorpropamide
Warfarin‡	Diazepam	Phenytoin‡	Chloroquine	Digoxin
	Digitoxin	Propranolol	Disopyramide*	Disopyramide*
	Frusemide	Tolbutamide‡	Lignocaine	Insulin
	Gold salts	Valproate	Quinidine	Paracetamol
	Heparin		Sulphonamides†	Phenobarbitone
	Imipramine		Theophylline	Procainamide
				Trichloroethanol‡ (chloral metabolite)

*Protein-binding saturable. Disopyramide binding varies between 35 per cent at high therapeutic doses and 95 per cent at low doses.
†May be the precipitant drug in protein-binding displacement interactions (see Chapter 10).
‡May be the object drug in protein-binding displacement interactions (see Chapter 10).

(a) Plasma protein binding

This is discussed above.

(b) Specific receptor sites in tissues

For example, the binding of cardiac glycosides to Na^+K^+ ATPase in cell membranes throughout the body.

(c) Regional blood flow

Well-perfused organs, such as the heart, kidneys, and liver, tend to accumulate drugs to a greater extent than poorly perfused organs, such as fat and bone. For drugs which are highly extracted (have a high 'extraction ratio') from the blood by a particular tissue, small changes in tissue blood flow lead to large changes in the distribution of drug to that tissue (see p. 31).

(d) Lipid solubility

Since cell membranes are composed mostly of lipoproteins, non-polar drugs, which are relatively lipid-soluble, will distribute more readily to tissues than will polar compounds.

(e) Active transport

A few drugs are actively transported across cell membranes, for example the adrenergic neurone blocking drugs (see also (g) below).

(f) Diseases

Some diseases are associated with altered distribution characteristics of some drugs, the underlying mechanisms often being obscure. The effects of disease on plasma protein binding have been mentioned above. Renal failure, apart from its effect on protein binding, may also be associated with a decreased distribution of some drugs (for example insulin and digoxin), as is hyperthyroidism (cardiac glycosides). This change in distribution results, for example, in higher plasma digitalis concentrations than expected, but the interpretation of plasma digitalis concentrations in these circumstances is not clear (see Chapter 7). In cardiac failure the distribution of some antiarrhythmic drugs is decreased (for example disopyramide and lignocaine). Obesity influences the distribution of drugs which are highly fat soluble (for example anaesthetics).

(g) The effects of other drugs (see Chapter 10)

Tricyclic antidepressants inhibit the active transport of the adrenergic neurone blockers, reducing their access to the site of action in the brain, and thus reducing their efficacy. Quinidine decreases the distribution of digoxin by an unknown mechanism.

(h) Miscellaneous examples

These include the binding of tetracyclines to growing bones and teeth (because of the formation of a calcium chelate), resulting in mottling of the teeth and increased bone fragility in children, and the binding of chloroquine to retinal melanin with consequent retinopathy.

3.3 Drug metabolism

Most drug metabolism occurs in the liver, although some occurs elsewhere (for example suxamethonium in the plasma, insulin and vitamin D in the kidneys, cytosine arabinoside, cyclophosphamide, and other cytotoxic drugs in many cells, and acetylcholine and other neurotransmitters at synapses and within nerves).

Drug metabolism occurs in two phases:

1. Phase I metabolism involves chemical alteration of the basic structure of the drug, for example by oxidation, reduction, or hydrolysis. Oxidation reactions are further subdivided according to whether they are carried out by the cytochrome-linked mixed function oxidases or not. Examples of phase I reactions include: the *N*-demethylation of diazepam to desmethyldiazepam, an active metabolite with a long duration of action; the oxidation of theophylline to dimethyluric acid; the oxidation of ethanol to acetaldehyde; the hydrolysis of lignocaine to the toxic metabolites monoethylglycylxylidide and glycylxylidide.

2. Phase II metabolism involves conjugation, for example by sulphation, glucuronidation, methylation, or acetylation. Some drugs are conjugated without prior phase I transformation, while others undergo phase I metabolism before conjugation can take place. The end-products of conjugation are compounds which are more

water-soluble and therefore more rapidly eliminated from the body. They are usually, although
not always, pharmacologically inactive. Examples
of phase II reactions include: the glucuronidation
of paracetamol; the *N*-acetylation of hydralazine
and procainamide; the methylation of desipramine to its active metabolite imipramine. In some
cases a conjugated product may be further metabolized. For example, oestrogens may be deconjugated in the gut and reabsorbed after they have
been excreted via the bile.

The end result of drug metabolism is inactivation, although during the process compounds
with pharmacological activity may be formed.
There are three ways in which the activity of a
drug may be altered by its metabolism.

3.3.1 Metabolism of a pharmacologically inactive compound to one with pharmacological activity

Inactive drugs, administered for the known effects
of their active metabolites are called 'prodrugs'
and the reasons for their use are numerous.

(a) Altered absorption

Prodrugs may be better absorbed than the active
compounds to which they are metabolized. For
example, carfecillin and talampicillin are inactive
precursors of carbenicillin and ampicillin respectively, but are much better absorbed than the
active drugs.

Conversely, it may be desirable for a prodrug
to be poorly absorbed, if the desired site of action
is the large bowel. This is the case for sulphasalazine, which is poorly absorbed. When sulphasalazine reaches the large bowel it is hydrolysed by
colonic bacteria to mesalazine (5-aminosalicylic
acid), which is therapeutically active, and to
sulphapyridine, which contributes mostly to the
adverse effects of sulphasalazine. When this metabolic pathway was elucidated a safer prodrug,
sodium   diazosalicylate   (olsalazine),   was
developed; it is hydrolysed in the colon to two
molecules of mesalazine, thus avoiding the problems of adverse effects due to sulphapyridine.
Mesalazine itself is well absorbed, and cannot
therefore be given by mouth in conventional

formulations; to circumvent this problem special
enteric-coated and pH-sensitive formulations of
mesalazine have been developed as an alternative
to the use of the prodrug olsalazine.

(b) Prevention of an adverse effect in the gastrointestinal tract

For example, the incidence of diarrhoea is less
with talampicillin than with ampicillin, since the
former is better absorbed and does not alter large
bowel bacterial flora to the same extent as the
latter. The incidence of gastrointestinal bleeding
is less with benorylate than with aspirin, since
the direct action of a high concentration of
aspirin on the gastric mucosa is at least part of
the mechanism responsible for gastric erosion.

(c) Improved distribution

For example, dopamine is of no value in treating
Parkinson's disease, since it does not enter the
brain. Its precursor, L-dopa, does enter the brain,
where it is metabolized to dopamine.

(d) Chance

For example, the therapeutic effect of carbimazole depends on its conversion to methimazole.
There is no rational reason for preferring carbimazole in routine therapy, but in the UK it has
always been preferred, since it was discovered
first.

3.3.2 Metabolism of a pharmacologically active compound to other active compounds

In some cases the active metabolites of a drug
have equal or greater pharmacological activity
than the parent compound. Examples of parent
drugs with active metabolites include diamorphine (which is rapidly metabolized to morphine),
phenacetin (which, because of its adverse effects
on the kidney, has been supplanted by its active
metabolite paracetamol), and some benzodiazepines (such as diazepam and chlordiazepoxide,
which are metabolized to temazepam and
oxazepam, which have shorter durations of
action).

Some active compounds are metabolized to
toxic compounds. Examples include lignocaine

(the accumulation of whose toxic metabolites limits the duration of therapy possible with lignocaine), phenytoin (whose main metabolite may inhibit the further metabolism of phenytoin), and isoniazid (whose acetylated metabolite is hepatotoxic, resulting in an increased risk of liver damage in fast acetylators; but see p. 621).

3.3.3 Metabolism to pharmacologically inactive compounds

This is the most common type of metabolic transformation. Even active metabolites are usually eventually inactivated before excretion.

The following factors affect hepatic (and other) drug metabolism:

(a) Genetic

See Chapter 8.

(b) Other drugs

See Chapter 10.

(c) Hepatic blood flow

For drugs with a high extraction ratio (see pp. 31–2) small changes in hepatic blood flow result in large changes in hepatic clearance rates. Such effects are generally of little clinical importance.

(d) Liver disease

The capacity of the liver is so great that liver disease must be extensive before effects on drug metabolism become important. However, arteriovenous shunting, in the absence of much hepatocellular damage, may impair drug metabolism.

(e) Age

The metabolism of some drugs may be impaired in old people; similarly, babies under the age of about 6 months, particularly premature babies, are less able to metabolize some drugs than are adults (see Chapter 11). In both cases the impairment is due to reduced activity of the hepatic microsomal drug metabolizing enzymes. An example of the clinical importance of this is the effect of chloramphenicol in neonates. In the neonatal liver there is a low activity of UDP glucuronyl transferase, which conjugates chlor-

amphenicol. Neonates thus eliminate chloramphenicol more slowly, and may suffer peripheral circulatory collapse (the 'grey syndrome') when given chloramphenicol in weight-related doses which are non-toxic to adults.

3.4 Drug excretion

The kidney is the main route whereby drugs are excreted from the body. Other routes include: the lungs (important for paraldehyde); breast milk (see Chapter 12); sweat, tears, and genital secretions (alarming if the patient is not expecting the orange-red discoloration caused by rifampicin); bile (leading to the recirculation of some compounds, for example chloramphenicol (whose inactive metabolites are reactivated by hydrolysis in the gut), morphine, rifampicin, tetracyclines, and digitoxin); and saliva (sometimes used in monitoring drug concentrations in body fluids; see Chapter 7).

Renal excretion of drugs occurs chiefly by the following three processes (Fig. 3.2):

(1) glomerular filtration;

(2) passive tubular reabsorption;

(3) active tubular secretion.

Thus, total renal clearance = clearance by filtration + clearance by secretion − retention by reabsorption.

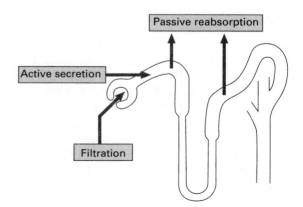

■ **Fig. 3.2** A diagrammatic representation of a nephron, showing the sites of the three major processes whereby drugs are excreted via the kidney.

If a drug is metabolized mainly to inactive compounds, then renal function will not greatly affect elimination of the active compound. However, if the drug or an active metabolite is excreted unchanged via the kidneys, then changes in renal function will influence its elimination.

3.4.1 Glomerular filtration

All drugs are filtered at the renal glomerulus. The extent of filtration is directly proportional to the glomerular filtration rate (GFR = 120 mL/min) and to the fraction of unbound drug in the plasma (f_u). Thus,

$$\text{Rate of clearance by filtration} = f_u \times \text{GFR}$$

If the total renal clearance of a drug is equal to $f_u \times \text{GFR}$, then it is principally cleared by filtration. It may, of course, also be affected by the other two mechanisms (secretion and reabsorption), but in that case those effects must balance each other. Examples of drugs whose clearance is similar to glomerular filtration rate (after correction for protein binding) are digoxin, gentamicin, procainamide, methotrexate, and ethambutol. Since creatinine is cleared principally by filtration, measurement of the rate of renal clearance of creatinine is useful in estimating the clearance rates of these drugs.

3.4.2 Passive tubular reabsorption

If the value of renal clearance of a drug is less than $f_u \times \text{GFR}$ then its clearance after filtration is being restricted by passive reabsorption by the renal tubules. The renal clearance of drugs with very low rates of renal clearance (i.e. approaching urine flow rate, or about 1–2 mL/min) will be significantly affected by changes in urine flow rate (since a doubling of urine flow rate will increase their rate of clearance by 1–2 mL/min, i.e. twofold). However, for weak acids and weak bases the principal factor affecting passive reabsorption is the pH of the renal tubular fluid, since the extent of their ionization (and therefore of their passive reabsorption) depends on the pH when seen in relation to the pK_a of the drug. For example, weak acids with a pK_a below 7.5, such as aspirin, are more highly ionized, and therefore less well reabsorbed, in an alkaline urine. The reverse is true for weak bases with a pK_a greater than 7.5, such as amphetamine, whose reabsorption is decreased, and whose clearance is therefore enhanced, by an acid urine. These principles are sometimes put to use in the treatment of drug overdose (see Chapter 35). Renal failure alters passive reabsorption indirectly, by alterations in urine flow rate and pH.

3.4.3. Active tubular secretion

If the value of renal clearance of a drug is greater than $f_u \times \text{GFR}$ then as well as being filtered it is also being cleared by active tubular secretion in the proximal tubule. Penicillin is an example of such a drug. Some drugs inhibit active tubular secretion, and this forms the basis of some drug interactions (see Chapter 10). For example, probenecid inhibits the active secretion of penicillin, prolonging its duration of action. Quinidine inhibits the active secretion of digoxin, leading to an increased risk of digoxin toxicity if the digoxin dosage is not reduced by about 50 per cent. Other examples of the effects of drugs on active tubular secretory processes are the effects of diuretics, aspirin, sulphinpyrazone, and probenecid on the secretion of uric acid. Some diuretics (for example frusemide, bumetanide, thiazides) and low doses of aspirin, sulphinpyrazone, and probenecid inhibit the secretion of uric acid, leading to its retention. Higher doses of sulphinpyrazone, probenecid, and aspirin also inhibit the active reabsorption of uric acid in the proximal tubule, and the net result is increased excretion of uric acid (see Fig. 29.4). In renal failure active tubular secretion of drugs is impaired.

In the two following parts of this chapter we shall deal with the ways in which pharmacokinetic calculations are made, first descriptively, and second mathematically. If you want to retain the thread of the four phases of drug therapy you should skip these two parts for the time being and go on to Chapter 4.

3.5 Simple pharmacokinetic calculations

Although a full description of the pharmacokinetic properties of a drug requires complex mathematical analysis of appropriately gathered data, it is possible to grasp the principles of pharmacokinetics using a simple approach, and to use those principles in tackling practical problems. The principles are outlined here, and in Chapter 6 we shall deal with the practical application of those principles in designing dosage regimens.

Pharmacokinetics is the science of interpreting data on changing concentrations or amounts of a drug and its metabolites in blood, plasma, urine, and other body tissues and fluids. In order to approach the methods used to analyse such data, we shall start by considering the meaning of 'order' in pharmacokinetics.

3.5.1 Kinetic 'order'

Kinetic processes are defined according to their 'order' (a term which simply means that the various processes are ranked in order of increasing complexity). The important kinetic processes which concern us here are those governing the entry of a drug into the blood, its distribution in body tissues, and its elimination from the body by metabolism and excretion. Such processes are generally of 'zero order' or 'first order'.

(a) Zero-order kinetics

A zero-order process is one which proceeds at a constant rate, the rate being independent of the amount of drug undergoing the process. For such a process the plot of drug plasma concentration against time is linear (see the example of ethanol in Fig. 3.3).

The following are examples of zero-order processes:

1. The entry of a drug into the circulation during intravenous infusion. The rate of administration of a drug in an infusion solution can be controlled at a constant value, that value being independent of the concentration of drug in the solution.

2. The absorption of many depot forms of administration. The incorporation of some drugs in formulations for depot administration ensures that for the majority of the time over which the drug is released from the formulation its release occurs at a uniform rate, independent of the amount of drug left in the formulation. Examples include fluphenazine decanoate in oil (used in

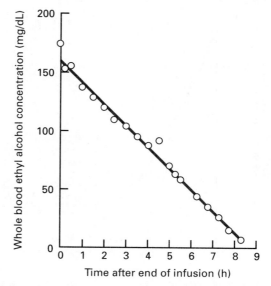

■ **Fig. 3.3** Whole blood concentrations of ethyl alcohol (ethanol) following the intravenous infusion of 15 per cent ethyl alcohol in 5 per cent dextrose. Note the linear scale of ethyl alcohol concentration on the vertical axis. For most of the time after administration the relationship between whole blood concentration and time is linear. (Adapted from Korsten *et al.* (1975). *New Engl. J. Med.* **192**, 386–9, with permission.)

the treatment of schizophrenia) and oestrogen pellet implants (used in hormone replacement therapy).

3. Saturable metabolism. When the concentration of a drug approaches a value at which its metabolizing enzymes are working at full capacity the enzymes are said to be saturated. When that happens the rate of metabolism of the drug by those enzymes becomes predominantly zero-order (Fig. 3.4). Examples of importance are those of ethanol (ethyl alcohol), whose metabolism is of zero order at virtually all plasma concentrations (Fig. 3.3), and both phenytoin and acetylsalicylic acid (aspirin), whose metabolism becomes predominantly of zero order within the therapeutic range of plasma concentrations.

The consequences of this peculiarity of metabolism on changes in plasma concentrations with changing dose in the therapeutic range of doses is illustrated in the case of phenytoin in Fig. 3.5. For a relatively small change in dose there may be a large change in plasma concentration if

(a)

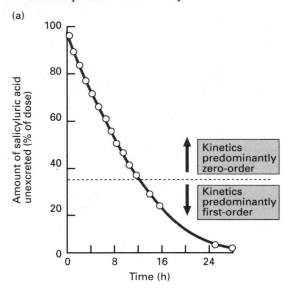

(b)

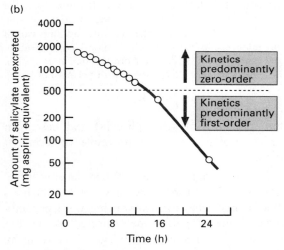

■ **Fig. 3.4** Mixed kinetics illustrated by the excretion of salicylate after an oral dose of aspirin (2 g). (a) The amount of salicyluric acid unexcreted (analogous to plasma concentrations) over the 28 h after the dose; the vertical axis is linear and the relationship is approximately linear for up to 12 h (i.e. zero-order kinetics), after which it becomes predominantly exponential (i.e. first-order kinetics). (b) Similar data, but the vertical axis is logarithmic: here the relationship is predominantly curvilinear to 12 h (i.e. zero-order kinetics), after which it becomes predominantly log-linear (i.e. first-order kinetics). (Adapted from Levy (1965). *J. Pharm. Sci.* **54**, 959–67, with permission.)

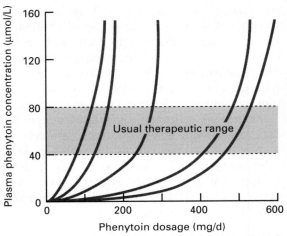

■ **Fig. 3.5** The relationship between daily phenytoin dosage and the associated steady-state plasma phenytoin concentrations in five patients. Each curve was constructed by making discrete measurements of steady-state concentrations at several different maintenance dosages. Note two important features: first, the large variability in steady-state phenytoin concentrations from patient to patient at any one dosage; and secondly, the non-linearity of the relationship: within the therapeutic dosage range small changes in dosage can cause large changes in plasma concentration. (Adapted from Richens and Dunlop (1975). *Lancet* **ii**, 247–8, with permission.)

metabolism is saturated (i.e. when the kinetics are predominantly of zero-order).

(b) First-order kinetics

Most kinetic processes affecting drug disposition in therapeutic practice are of first order. A first-order process is one whose rate is not uniform, but which is proportional to the amount of drug undergoing the process: the greater the amount of drug the faster the amount changes. For such a process the plot of, for example, drug plasma concentration against time is curvilinear (the higher it is the faster it falls). However, the logarithm of the plasma concentration plotted against time is linear. This is illustrated below for the case of ampicillin (Fig. 3.6). When semilogarithmic plots of this kind are linear the kinetics are first-order. That this is so is proved in the section in which the mathematics of these processes is outlined (see p. 34).

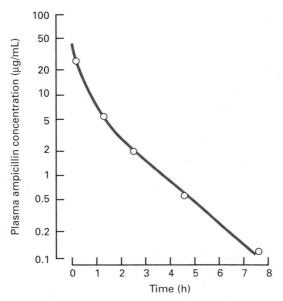

■ **Fig. 3.6** Plasma ampicillin concentrations during the 8 h after an intravenous dose of ampicillin (570 mg). Note that the vertical scale is logarithmic and that the relationship between plasma concentration and time is log-linear for most of the time (i.e. first-order kinetics). (Adapted from Jusko and Lewis (1973). *J. Pharm. Sci.* **62**, 69–76, with permission.)

3.5.2 Interpretation of plots of plasma drug concentrations against time

Consider what happens when a drug is given in a single intravenous bolus. We shall assume that the injection is given very rapidly, and that the drug distributes in the circulating plasma and throughout the tissues of the body within a few minutes. We shall also assume that first-order kinetics apply. If we take repeated small samples of blood at various times after injection and measure the concentration of the drug in the plasma, and if we then plot the plasma drug concentration against time, we shall find something like the result shown in Fig. 3.7(a).

At first the plasma concentration falls rapidly, and later on more slowly. The rate of fall at any time is proportional to the concentration at that time. If instead of using a linear scale for drug concentration we use a logarithmic scale, we find that the curve becomes a straight line

(Fig. 3.7(b)). This makes mathematical analysis of the data easier, since straight lines are easier to handle mathematically than curves. We can now define certain pharmacokinetic variables: the half-time, the apparent volume of distribution, and the clearance.

(a) Half-time (or half-life) ($t_{1/2}$)

Because the relationship between the logarithm of the drug concentration and time is linear, the rate of decline is logarithmically constant. Linear constancy would imply the subtraction of a constant amount in unit time; however, logarithmic subtraction is equivalent to linear division, so logarithmic constancy implies division by a constant amount in unit time. If we choose to define 'unit time' as the time it takes for the concentration to fall by an arbitrary factor of two, then that time can be called the 'half-time', i.e. the time it takes for the concentration to halve, no matter what the starting concentration. This is illustrated in Fig. 3.8. Each downstroke represents a halving of the plasma concentration, and each across-stroke is the time taken for that halving to occur, i.e. the half-time. In this case the half-time is 26 min. The half-times of some commonly used drugs, in patients with normal renal function, are given in Table 3.2.

The following are the uses of the half-time:

1. As a guide to the time it take for a drug to be eliminated from the body. The percentages of the total amount of drug in the body eliminated after one or more half-times without further administration of the drug are given in Table 3.3.

2. As a guide to the rate of accumulation of drug in the body during multiple dosing. The half-time is the only variable which determines the rate at which drug accumulates in the body during regular multiple dosing. Consider the regular oral administration of a drug which is rapidly absorbed (Fig. 3.9). After the first dose the concentration of drug in the plasma rises sharply as the drug is absorbed; it reaches a peak, and then starts to fall as the drug is distributed around the body and eliminated. After the second dose the rise in concentration to the next peak is the same as after the first dose, but because the new peak is higher than the first the rate of fall is faster (first-order kinetics). There is there-

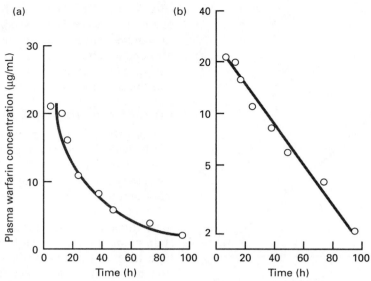

■ **Fig. 3.7** Plasma warfarin concentrations during the 100 h after an intravenous dose of warfarin (200 mg). In (a) the data are plotted in linear scale, and in (b) the same data are plotted in semilogarithmic scale (i.e. first-order kinetics). (Adapted from O'Reilly *et al.* (1971). *Thrombosis Diathesis Haemorr.* **25**, 178–86, with permission.) (Same data as in Fig. 3.8 and Fig. 3.14.)

fore a greater absolute fall in plasma concentration before the third dose is given than there was before the second. After each successive dose the increase in plasma concentration is the same, but because the peak is always higher the size of the fall after the peak becomes progressively larger with successive doses. Eventually the size of the fall in plasma concentration after the peak is as great as the size of the preceding rise, and a 'steady state' is reached. At steady state the amount of drug eliminated from the body in a single dosage interval is the same as the amount which enters it.

Strictly speaking this is not a true steady state, for two reasons. Firstly, because the plasma concentrations are fluctuating all the time. Secondly, because even the mean of those concentrations does not reach a true steady value until infinite time. However, for practical purposes a steady state can be said to have occurred after four to five half-times, when 94–97 per cent of the eventual steady-state value will have been reached.

If 'accumulated' is substituted for 'eliminated' in the heading above the right-hand columns in Table 3.3 the same percentage figures will apply.

This means that the time taken to reach steady state depends neither on the size of the dose nor on the frequency of its administration, but only on the half-time of the drug. The effect of varying the dose is shown in Fig. 3.10. Curves (a) and (b) show the plasma concentrations of a drug given once every half-time; the dose in case (a) is twice that in case (b). The time taken to reach steady state is the same in each case and the final plasma concentration is proportional to the dose.

The effect of varying the frequency of administration of the drug without altering the total daily dose is also shown in Fig. 3.10. Curve (a) shows the plasma concentrations of a drug given once every half-time, and curve c shows the concentrations of the drug when half the dose is given twice every half-time (i.e. the same total dose in both cases). In this instance both the time to steady state and the final mean plasma concentration are the same for the two cases. However, the degree of fluctuation is less when the drug is administered more frequently. The extreme case of the repeated administration of smaller amounts of drug at more frequent intervals is that of continuous intravenous infusion (Fig. 3.11). In this instance there is no fluctuation

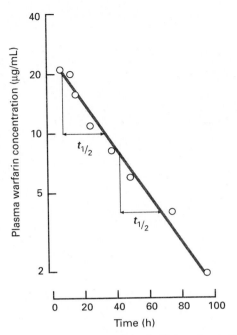

∎ **Fig. 3.8** The principle of the half-time ($t_{1/2}$). When plasma concentration versus time data are linear in a semilogarithmic plot the time it takes for the plasma concentration to fall from any value to half that value is a constant, the half-time. (Same data as in Figs. 3.7 and 3.14.)

3. As a guide to the relation between the loading dose and the maintenance dose. When a drug has a half-time greater than 24 h (for example digoxin 40 h, digitoxin 7 d, S(-)warfarin 32 h) it takes several days or weeks of regular administration of the same daily dose before the steady-state plasma concentration or amount of drug in the body is reached. Such a delay may be unacceptable if the eventual steady-state plasma concentration is that associated with a therapeutic effect. In such cases a loading dose may be given in order to boost the amount of drug in the body to the required level. This would then be followed by the administration of the regular maintenance dose to maintain the steady state (Fig. 3.13). Even when the half-time of a drug is short it may be necessary to give a loading dose if a very rapid effect is required. Take the example of lignocaine in the treatment of cardiac arrhythmias. The half-time of lignocaine is about 1 h. Because it would take about 4 h before a steady state was reached a loading dose is usually given, the treatment of arrhythmias being an urgent matter.

This is discussed further in Chapter 6 in relation to the development of dosage regimens.

(b) Apparent volume of distribution (*V*)

In Fig. 3.7 we saw how, with first-order kinetics, the plasma drug concentration falls linearly with time when plotted in semi-logarithmic scale. Let us assume that after intravenous administration there is instantaneous distribution of the drug throughout the body. If we now extrapolate the line back to the time of administration, the point at which it crosses the vertical axis represents the theoretical plasma concentration which would have occurred at a time when all the drug given was still in the body and uniformly distributed throughout it (Fig. 3.14).

In the illustrated case for warfarin the theoretical plasma concentration, $C(0)$, at zero time, the time of administration, is 25 µg/mL. The dose given was 200 mg. We can therefore calculate the theoretical volume of body fluid, equivalent to a theoretical volume of plasma, in which the drug is distributed: it is the ratio of the dose to the zero-time concentration:

$$V = \text{dose}/C(0) = 200 \text{ mg}/25 \text{ µg per mL}$$

$$= 8 \text{ L of plasma}.$$

in plasma drug concentration; it is as if infinitely small doses of the drug were being given at infinitely small dosage intervals. However, it still takes the same time to reach steady state.

Finally, consider what happens when the half-time of a drug is prolonged because its clearance from the body is reduced (Fig. 3.12). Because the half-time is prolonged it takes proportionately longer for a steady state to be reached. However, because less drug is being eliminated during a dosage interval the eventual steady-state plasma concentration is proportionately higher. This is what happens when, for example, renal digoxin elimination is reduced in renal failure: it takes longer to reach a steady state, and for a given dosage regimen the eventual steady-state plasma concentration is higher than it would be if renal function were normal. In such cases dosages must be reduced, and a delay in the onset of effect must be expected if no loading dose is given (see below).

■ **Table 3.2** Mean half-times of some drugs in patients with normal renal function

<1 h	1–4 h	4–12 h	12–24 h	1–2 d	>2 d	Dose dependent
Dobutamine	Aminoglycosides*	β-blockers (most)	Carbenoxolone	Allopurinol†	Amiodarone	Phenobarbitone (in overdose)
Dopamine	Bumetanide	Glibenclamide	Chlorpromazine	Carbamazepine	Chloroquine	Phenytoin
Insulin	Cephalosporins	Hydralazine	Clonidine	Chlorpropamide	Diazepam	Salicylates
Naloxone	Chloramphenicol	Quinidine	Doxycycline	Clonazepam	Digitoxin	
Nitroprusside	Colchicine	Sulphonamides (many)	Haloperidol	Diazoxide	Phenobarbitone	
Penicillins (most)	Diamorphine†	Tetracyclines (most)	Lithium	Digoxin	Thyroxine	
	Erythromycin	Theophylline	Minocycline	Tri-iodothyronine		
	Ethambutol	Tolbutamide	Ouabain	Warfarin		
	Frusemide	Trimethoprim	Spironolactone†			
	Heparin	Valproate				
	Isoprenaline					
	L-dopa					
	Lignocaine					
	Morphine					
	Paracetamol					
	Procainamide					

*But see the Pharmacopoeia.
†These drugs have shorter half-times than shown, but are listed under the half-times of their active metabolites.

■ **Table 3.3** The percentages of any amount of drug eliminated by first-order elimination after different numbers of half-times

Number of half-times	Percent eliminated	Total (%)
1	50	50.0
2	50 + 25	75.0
3	50 + 25 + 12.5	87.5
4	50 + 25 + 12.5 + 6.25	93.8
5	50 + 25 + 12.5 + 6.25 + 3.125	96.9

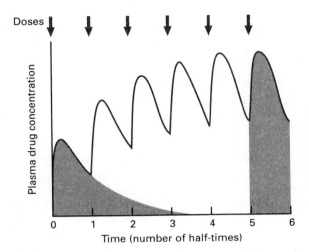

■ **Fig. 3.9** The theoretical plasma concentrations of a drug over a period of time during its repeated oral administration. After the administration of the drug (at the times indicated by the arrows, in this case once every half-time) the plasma concentration rises sharply as the drug is absorbed. Then, because of subsequent drug distribution and elimination, the concentration reaches a peak and starts to fall. Note that with repeated administration there is accumulation to an eventual steady state (97 per cent of which will be reached after five half-times), and that the area under the curve of plasma concentration versus time during a single dosage interval at steady state is equal to the area under the curve extrapolated to infinity after a single dose (hatched areas).

In this case the apparent volume of distribution of the drug is similar to that of the extracellular fluid. One might therefore postulate that the drug is evenly distributed throughout the extracellular fluid volume, in which its concentration would be the same as that in the plasma. Although it is sometimes the case that the apparent volume of distribution can be related to a known identifiable fluid volume in the body, more often the apparent volume of distribution is greater than even that of total body water (about 0.6 L/kg). For example, the apparent volume of distribution of propranolol is about 3 L of plasma per kg body weight. This theoretical volume simply gives an index of how extensively the drug is distributed to the tissues of the body compared with the plasma. Incidentally, we have attributed this volume to the plasma because the drug concentrations were measured in plasma; if the concentrations had been measured in, for example, serum or whole blood the volume would have been expressed in litres of serum or whole blood. The higher the apparent volume of distribution of a drug the more extensively it is distributed to the body tissues. The values of the apparent volumes of distribution of various commonly used drugs are listed in Table 3.4.

Intuitively we can see that the more highly protein-bound a drug is in the circulation the less readily will it distribute to the body tissues, and the lower will be its apparent volume of distribution. It should be remembered in this discussion that the protein-bound drug is not reckoned as being tissue-bound, since what is generally measured as plasma drug concentration includes both bound and unbound drug. Thus, the apparent volume of distribution of total drug (bound and unbound) must be roughly proportional to the extent to which the drug circulates in non-protein-bound form in the plasma (i.e. the unbound fraction).

In the tissues a drug may or may not be bound to tissue proteins, and the apparent volume of

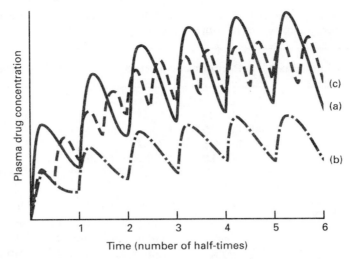

■ Fig. 3.10 The effects of varying the dose and frequency of administration on the time taken to reach steady state and the eventual steady-state plasma concentration.

1. The effect of varying the dose. Curve a represents the plasma concentrations which would occur during administration of a dose (which we shall term the 'standard dose') once every half-time (compare Fig. 3.9). Curve b represents the concentrations during administration of half the standard dose given at the same frequency. The time taken to reach steady state is the same in both cases, but the eventual steady-state concentration in case b is half that in case a, being proportional to the dose.

2. The effect of varying the frequency of administration. Curve a represents the plasma concentrations which would occur during administration of the standard dose once every half-time. Curve c represents the concentrations during administration of half the standard dose given twice as often (i.e. the total dose is unchanged). Neither the time taken to reach steady state nor the eventual mean steady-state concentration is affected. However, the fluctuations in plasma concentration during a dosage interval are reduced in case c (compare Fig. 3.11).

distribution will obviously also be inversely proportional to the non-tissue-protein-bound fraction. The relationship between the extent of a drug's apparent volume of distribution and its protein binding (a) in the plasma and (b) in the tissues is expressed by the following equation:

$$V = V_P + V_T \left(f_u / f_{uT} \right)$$

where V = the apparent volume of distribution; V_P = the volume of the plasma (i.e. about 3 L); V_T = the volume of the total body 'tissue fluid' (i.e. fluid other than the plasma, about 39 L); f_u = the fraction unbound in the plasma; and f_{uT} = the fraction unbound in the tissues. There is a slightly more complicated equation which can be used if one also wants to take into account the distribution of a drug in the total extracellular fluid and not just the plasma:

$$V = 7 + 8 f_u + V_T \left(f_u / f_{uT} \right)$$

where T, the 'tissue fluid,' now refers to the body fluids other than the plasma and the extracellular fluid (i.e. about 27 L).

The following are the uses of the apparent volume of distribution:

1. In planning dosage regimens. The use of the apparent volume of distribution in planning dosage regimens is discussed in Chapter 6.

2. In relating half-time to total clearance. The half-time of a drug is related to the apparent volume of distribution and the total body clearance in the following way:

Total clearance × half-time = volume × $\log_e 2$

(You will often see $\log_e$ written as ln, which stands for natural logarithm.)

It is important to note that clearance and volume are independent of each other. For

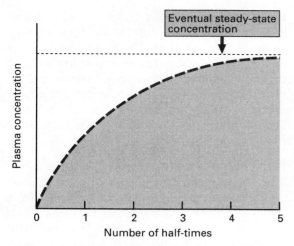

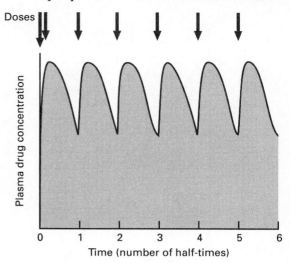

Fig. 3.11 The theoretical plasma concentrations which would occur during the continuous intravenous infusion of a drug. The plasma concentration rises steadily during infusion, but does not reach steady state any sooner than in the various cases of oral administration, such as those illustrated in Fig. 3.10.

Fig. 3.13 The effect of an initial loading dose. If the correct loading dose is given, a steady state can be achieved rapidly and then maintained by giving a smaller maintenance dose. In this example, because the drug is being given once every half-time the maintenance dose is half the loading dose. Compare this figure with Fig. 3.9.

example, the rate at which a drug is cleared from the plasma by glomerular filtration is obviously not dependent on the intracellular concentration in the heart. Since clearance and apparent volume of distribution are independent of each other, it follows that the half-time must depend on the independent values of clearance and volume.

Thus, a change in half-time implies a change in either clearance, or volume, or both. Furthermore, if one finds that the half-time of a drug is unchanged during a drug interaction or in the presence of some disease, that does not necessar-

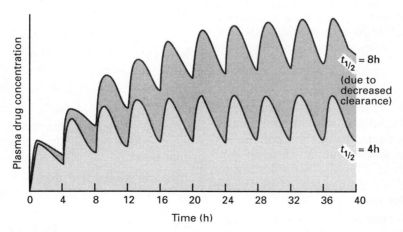

Fig. 3.12 The effect of reduced body clearance of a drug on the time taken to reach steady state and the eventual steady-state plasma concentration. Reducing the clearance has two effects: (1) Prolongation of the half-time; the time taken to reach steady state is prolonged proportionately. (2) Increased accumulation of the drug; the eventual steady-state plasma concentration is increased proportionately.

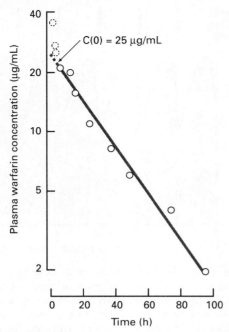

∎ **Fig. 3.14** Calculation of the apparent volume of distribution (same data as in Fig. 3.7 and Fig. 3.8). Extrapolation of the linear plasma concentration versus time curve to the vertical axis yields a value for the theoretical plasma concentration, $C(0)$, which would have occurred at the time of administration had there been uniform distribution of the drug throughout the body at that time. The apparent volume of distribution (V) is given by the expression $V = \text{dose}/C(0)$.

Note that the assumption of uniform distribution leads to an overestimate of the volume, since the warfarin concentrations (open circles) measured during the relatively short time before the linear phase (closed circles) were actually higher than $C(0)$. A better estimate would be given by the expression shown as equation 3.13 (p. 35).

ily imply that the pharmacokinetic properties of the drug are unaffected, since proportionately equal and independent changes in clearance and apparent volume of distribution will result in no change in half-time. This can happen when the protein binding of a drug is altered by another drug (see Chapter 10).

3. In the interpretation of drug interactions. When a new interaction between two drugs is described, the question of its mechanism always arises. One can confidently rule out protein-binding displacement interactions if one knows

that the object drug (see Chapter 10) has a high apparent volume of distribution (greater than about 30 L of plasma). This is because any rise in the free concentration of the object drug in the plasma will only be clinically obvious if the drug does not have to distribute through a large apparent volume of distribution, which would literally dilute out the effects of the increase in free drug concentration.

(c) Clearance (*CL*)

The clearance of a drug is defined as that fraction of the apparent volume of distribution from which the drug is removed in unit time. It is expressed in units of amount per time (for example mL/min), sometimes corrected for body weight (for example mL/min/kg).

Total body clearance is equal to the sum of the clearances by all routes of elimination, and it is usually subdivided into renal and non-renal clearances. The relationship between clearance and apparent volume of distribution has been given above.

(i) Renal clearance (*CL*$_R$)

Adapting the above definition of total clearance we can define renal clearance as that fraction of the apparent volume of distribution from which drug is removed by renal excretion in unit time. Thus:

CL_R = the fraction of the amount of drug in the body excreted in urine in unit time $\times V$
i.e.

$$CL_R = (A_e/A_{TOT}) \times V$$

where A_e = the amount excreted in unit time and A_{TOT} = the total amount in the body.

But $\qquad V = A_{TOT}/C$ (see above).
So $\qquad\qquad CL_R = A_e/C$

i.e. CL_R = (total drug excreted in the urine in unit time)/(mean plasma drug concentration during unit time).

You will have noted that this expression is precisely the same as that commonly used in renal physiology for the expression of renal clearance (for example of creatinine):

$$\text{renal clearance} = UV/P$$

where U = the urinary concentration of the compound; V = the volume of urine excreted per unit

■ **Table 3.4** Values of the apparent volumes of distribution of some commonly used drugs

<12 L	12-40 L	40-100 L	100-200 L	>200 L
Frusemide	Acetazolamide	Carbamazepine	Procainamide	Chlorpromazine
Phenylbutazone	Alcohol	Lignocaine	Propranolol	Cyclosporin
Sulphonyureas	Aminoglycosides	Lithium		Digoxin
(e.g. tolbutamide)	(e.g. gentamicin)	Paracetamol		Haloperidol
Warfarin	Digitoxin			Tricyclic antidepressants
	Insulin			(e.g. amitriptyline)
	Penicillin G			
	Phenytoin			
	Quinidine			
	Theophylline			
	Valproate			

time; and P = the mean plasma concentration of the compound.

Non-renal clearance is usually calculated as the difference between total clearance and renal clearance.

The mechanisms whereby drugs are cleared from the body have been discussed in the earlier part of this chapter.

(ii) Hepatic clearance (CL_H)

Adapting the definition of clearance we can define hepatic clearance as that fraction of the apparent volume of distribution from which drug is removed by metabolism and biliary excretion in unit time. As in the case of renal clearance we can derive an expression for hepatic clearance, as follows:

CL_H = (total amount of drug excreted in the bile + total amount of metabolite appearing in hepatic venous blood in unit time)/(mean drug concentration in the plasma entering the liver during unit time).

It is clear, however, that while we could easily measure separately the components of the corresponding equation for renal clearance, we cannot for practical purposes measure the variables in the equation for hepatic clearance. However, for those drugs whose non-renal clearance is entirely or almost entirely by the hepatic route (and that is the case for most drugs) the problem can be solved by measuring total clearance and renal clearance. Hepatic clearance will then be the difference between the two:

$$CL_H = CL_{TOT} - CL_R \text{ (assumption: } CL_H = CL_{NR})$$

Two factors influence the hepatic clearance of a drug: the rate of hepatic blood flow, and the extent of protein binding of the drug in the circulation. The extent to which either or both of these factors affects hepatic clearance depends on how well the liver is capable of removing drug from the incoming blood.

If we think of the liver as a reservoir (Fig. 3.15) into which drug in solution flows, and from which drug may either flow out unchanged or after metabolism, we can judge how these factors affect hepatic clearance.

Case 1. The ability of the liver to clear drug by metabolism or excretion into the bile is high

In this case, there is virtually no restriction to flow through either outlet from the reservoir (Fig. 3.15(a)). Thus, clearance will depend only on the rate of flow into the reservoir (i.e. total hepatic blood flow). The higher the rate of flow the higher the rate of clearance.

Case 2. The ability of the liver to clear drug by metabolism or by excretion into the bile is low

In this case, outflow via hepatic clearance is restricted and will not be affected by the rate of inflow (Fig. 3.15(b)). Instead the extent of protein binding becomes important, since it will determine how much drug is available for transport

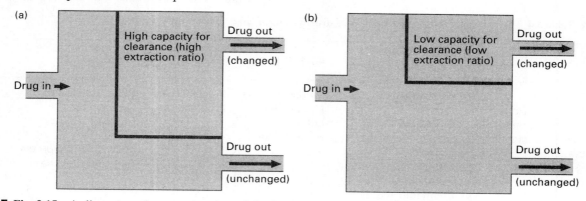

■ **Fig. 3.15** A diagrammatic representation of the factors affecting the rate of hepatic clearance of a drug. The liver is represented as a reservoir into which drug flows (i.e. 'drug in') either 'changed' (i.e. metabolized or excreted via the bile) or 'unchanged' (i.e. via the hepatic veins).

Case 1. If the ability of the liver to clear the drug is high (i.e. if the extraction ratio is high) then the rate-limiting factor is the speed with which it is presented to the sites of clearance, which in turn is equal to the rate of blood flow through the organ (i.e. for $E \Rightarrow 1$, $CL_H \approx Q_H$; see equation 3.26).

Case 2. If the ability of the liver to clear the drug is low (i.e. if the extraction ratio is low) the rate-limiting factor is the quantity of drug which is presented to the sites of clearance, and since only non-protein bound drug can be metabolized that in turn depends on the fraction of drug unbound in the plasma (i.e. for $E \Rightarrow 0$, $CL_H \approx CL_{int}$ and $CL_H \propto f_u$; see equations 3.27 and 3.29).

Case 3 (not illustrated). For drugs for which the liver has an intermediate capacity for clearance (i.e. $E \approx 0.5$) the rate of hepatic clearance will be affected by both hepatic blood flow and the unbound fraction of drug in the plasma.

to the sites of clearance. The higher the fraction of unbound drug in the blood, the higher the rate of clearance.

Case 3. The ability of the liver to clear drug by metabolism or by excretion into the bile is intermediate

In this case, both hepatic blood flow and protein binding will influence hepatic clearance.

Lists of drugs which are subject to high, low, or intermediate degrees of extraction by the liver are given in Table 3.5.

The following are the uses of the clearance:

(i) In assessing the mechanism of renal clearance

The magnitude of the renal clearance rate of a drug is related to its principal mechanism of renal excretion. This arises from the relationship:

Renal clearance $= (f_u \times GFR) - $ (rate of passive reabsorption) $+$ (rate of active secretion)

where $f_u =$ the fraction of drug unbound in the plasma and GFR = glomerular filtration rate (see p. 20).

If a drug has a renal clearance equal to $f_u \times GFR$ its principal mechanism of excretion is by filtration. That does not mean that the drug is not also subject to passive reabsorption and active secretion in the renal tubule: it may be subject to both, but in equal measure.

If the renal clearance of a drug is less than $f_u \times GFR$ it is both filtered and reabsorbed (and perhaps also secreted, but only to a small extent). This reabsorption is affected by the degree to which the drug is ionized, highly ionized compounds being poorly reabsorbed. Its excretion may therefore be influenced by alterations in the pH of the urine (although only if it is both lipophilic and either a weak acid or a weak base), since that will determine its degree of ionization.

If the renal clearance is greater than $f_u \times GFR$ then it is both filtered and secreted (and perhaps also reabsorbed, but only to a small extent). Its excretion may therefore be influenced by other drugs which alter tubular secretion.

▮ **Table 3.5** Drugs of low, intermediate, and high hepatic extraction ratio

Low	Intermediate	High
Chloramphenicol	Aspirin	Chlormethiazole
Diazepam	Codeine	Ergotamine*
Digitoxin	Quinidine	Glyceryl trinitrate
Isoniazid	Nortriptyline	Labetalol
Paracetamol		Lignocaine
Phenobarbitone		Morphine
Phenylbutazone		Pethidine
Phenytoin		Propranolol
Procainamide		
Theophylline		
Tolbutamide		
Warfarin		

*May reduce its own clearance.

(ii) In calculating dosage regimens

The use of the clearance in calculating dosage regimens is discussed in Chapter 6.

3.5.3 Non-linear kinetics

In section 3.5.2 we have been making the assumption that the pharmacokinetics of the drugs we were discussing were linear, i.e. obeyed first-order kinetics at all therapeutic, or even toxic, doses. If first-order (i.e. linear) kinetics hold, then kinetic variables, such as clearance, apparent volume of distribution, and half-time, are the same no matter what the dose. However, that is not always the case. In some cases a pharmacokinetic process (for example metabolism, protein binding) may be saturated at doses within the therapeutic range, and if that happens a mixture of first-order and zero-order kinetics occurs (see Fig. 3.4). The most important examples involve saturable metabolism and include phenytoin, alcohol, and acetylsalicylic acid. The example of phenytoin is illustrated in Fig. 3.5. For some drugs (for example clofibrate, disopyramide) there is saturable protein binding, and the kinetics of those drugs become non-linear at high doses or if there is hypoalbuminaemia.

There are several tests for non-linearity of pharmacokinetics, but the simplest is that of measuring steady-state plasma concentrations at different dosages. For most drugs steady-state concentrations vary in linear proportion to the dosage. If there are kinetic non-linearities this linear proportionality does not occur (see Fig. 3.5). Other methods of detecting kinetic non-linearities include measuring half-times or clearance rates at different doses. If the kinetics are linear these values should be the same at all doses. If there are kinetic non-linearities then half-time and clearance rate may change with changes in dose.

The details of this phenomenon of non-linear kinetics are discussed later in this chapter (p. 37), but it should be apparent that the change from predominantly first-order to predominantly zero-order kinetics with increasing dosage produces an unstable pharmacokinetic state. In such circumstances it may be important to measure plasma drug concentrations to monitor drug therapy when such drugs are used (see Chapter 7 for reference to phenytoin).

3.6 The mathematics of pharmacokinetics

In this section we shall describe the mathematical derivation of the principles outlined in the foregoing section.

3.6.1 Zero-order kinetics

A zero-order process is one whose rate is independent of the amount of drug undergoing the process. Thus:

$$\mathrm{d}A/\mathrm{d}t = -k_0 \qquad (3.1)$$

where A = the amount of drug, t = time, and k_0 = the zero-order rate constant. In this equation the rate of change of amount is expressed as a constant; the negative sign is used for this rate constant because drug amounts are taken to be falling with time.

Integration of equation (3.1) yields:

$$A(t) = -k_0 t + \text{constant} \qquad (3.2)$$

where $A(t)$ is the amount of drug yet to undergo the process at time t, and 'constant' is the constant of integration.

When $t = 0$, $A(t) = A(0)$ (the amount at time zero). Substitution in equation (3.2) yields:

$$A(t) = A(0) - k_0 t \qquad (3.3)$$

Equation (3.3) is the equation of a straight line relating $A(t)$ to t. The slope of the line is $-k_0$ (i.e. the rate of change, or the rate of elimination, for example 5 mL/min) and the intercept on the vertical axis is $A(0)$ (Fig. 3.16).

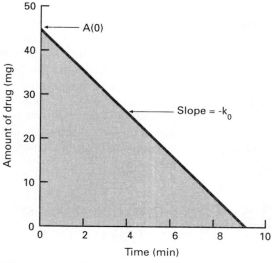

∎ **Fig. 3.16** Zero-order kinetics. The relationship between amount of drug and time. Note that the vertical scale is linear.

3.6.2. First-order kinetics

A first-order process is one whose rate is directly proportional to the amount of drug undergoing the process. Thus:

$$\mathrm{d}A/\mathrm{d}t = -kA \qquad (3.4)$$

(Note that this equation can also be written thus:

$$\mathrm{d}A/\mathrm{d}t = -kA^1$$

and that equation (3.1) can be written thus:

$$\mathrm{d}A/\mathrm{d}t = -kA^0, \text{ since } A^0 = 1.$$

In these forms these two equations indicate the origin of the terms 'first-order' and 'zero-order'.)

Integration of equation (3.4) yields:

$$\log_e A(t) = -kt + \text{constant} \qquad (3.5)$$

When $t = 0$, $A(t) = A(0)$. Substitution in equation (3.5) yields:

$$\log_e A(t) = \log_e A(0) - kt \qquad (3.6)$$

or

$$A(t) = A(0)\mathrm{e}^{-kt} \qquad (3.7)$$

In these equations $A(t)$ and $A(0)$ represent the amounts of drug yet to undergo the process at times t and zero respectively.

Equation (3.6) is the equation of the straight line relating $\log_e A(t)$ and t. The slope of the line is $-k$ and the intercept on the vertical axis is $\log_e A(0)$. Therefore, if one plots $\log_{10} A(t)$ against t (Fig. 3.17) the intercept on the vertical axis will be $A(0)$ and the slope $-k/2.3$ (since $2.3 = \log_e 10$).

In this case k is the first-order rate constant and it has units of reciprocal time (for example per hour or h^{-1}). This is to be contrasted with the zero-order rate constant k_0 (eqn 3.1), which has units of amount or volume per time (for example mL/min).

3.6.3. Half-time ($t_{1/2}$)

When $t = t_{1/2}$, $A(t) = A(0)/2$.

Substituting in equation (3.7) yields:

$$A(0)/2 = A(0)\,\mathrm{e}^{-kt_{1/2}} \qquad (3.8)$$

Thus:

$$\mathrm{e}^{-kt_{1/2}} = 1/2 \qquad (3.9)$$

$$kt_{1/2} = \log_e 2 \qquad (3.10)$$

$$t_{1/2} = \log_e 2/k \approx 0.7/k \qquad (3.11)$$

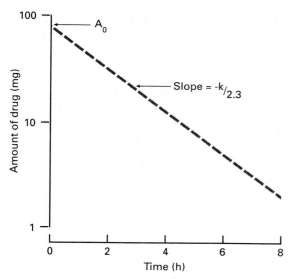

■ **Fig. 3.17** First-order kinetics. The relationship between amount of drug and time. Note that the vertical scale is logarithmic.

3.6.4 Apparent volume of distribution (V)

$$V = A(0)/C(0) = \text{dose}/C(0) \qquad (3.12)$$

where $C(0)$ = the theoretical concentration at zero time (compare Fig. 3.16). This is the so-called extrapolated volume (V_{extrap}).

In all the discussion so far we have assumed that the drug is evenly distributed throughout the body (i.e. that the body behaves as if it were a single 'compartment'). A glance at Fig. 3.14 will show that in the case of warfarin (and, it turns out, most other drugs) such an assumption is wrong: plasma concentration measurements, if taken early enough after a single intravenous dose, show concentrations higher than those predicted by instantaneous distribution. In the case of warfarin the error involved in this assumption is quite small. However, for other drugs the error is large, and in such cases other model-dependent methods of analysing drug distribution, multi-compartmental and physiological, have been developed. However, a discussion of their complexities is beyond the scope of this book. It is, in any case, usually simpler to derive the values of pharmacokinetic variables without recourse to formal theoretical models, using so-called com-partmental model-independent techniques. One such method for calculating the apparent volume of distribution is known as the area method, and the volume is called V_{area} since it is derived from the following relationship:

$$V_{area} = (f \times \text{dose})/(\text{area} \times k) \qquad (3.13)$$

where 'area' is the area under the curve of the plasma concentration plotted against time extrapolated to infinite time, and f is the fraction of the dose which reaches the systemic circulation intact. Applying this equation to the case of single-compartment distribution after intravenous administration discussed above yields:

$$\text{area} = \int_{\infty}^{0} C(0)e^{-kt}\,dt = C(0)/k \qquad (3.14)$$

Substituting in equation (3.13) yields:

$$V_{area} = \text{dose}/(C(0)/k) \times k \qquad (3.15)$$

Thus:

$$V_{area} = \text{dose}/C(0) \qquad (3.16)$$

So, for the single-compartment model $V_{extrap} = V_{area}$ (compare eqns 3.12 and 3.16). The same is not true if the data do not fit the single-compartment model well, when V_{extrap}, calculated on the assumption of a single compartment, is an overestimate of V_{area}, which is the more accurate measure of the apparent volume of distribution.

In calculating V_{area} it is sometimes helpful to make use of the observation (see Fig. 3.9) that the area under the curve of plasma concentration plotted against time extrapolated to infinity is the same as the area under the curve measured during a single dose at steady state.

Better still is the so-called steady-state apparent volume of distribution, V_{ss}. This can be calculated using either compartmental analysis or a model-independent method involving so-called moment theory. However, a discussion of these methods is beyond the scope of this book.

3.6.5 Clearance (CL)

$$CL = V_{area} \times k = V_{area} \times \log_e 2/t_{1/2} \qquad (3.17)$$

But $V_{area} = \text{dose}/\text{area} \times k$ [(eqn 3.13) with $f = 1$ for intravenous administration].

Thus:

$$CL = \text{dose/area} \qquad (3.18)$$

After oral administration one must allow for the possibility of incomplete absorption and first-pass metabolism and adjust the dose accordingly. The fraction of the orally administered dose which reaches the systemic circulation intact is usually designated f. Thus:

$$CL = f \times \text{dose/area} \qquad (3.19)$$

and:

$$V_{\text{area}} = f \times \text{dose/area} \times k \qquad (3.20)$$

(a) Renal clearance

$$CL_R = C_{\text{ur}} \times V_{\text{ur}}/(C_p \times t) \qquad (3.21)$$

where C_{ur} is the concentration of drug in the urine, V_{ur} is the volume of urine collected over a period of time (t), and C_p is the mean concentration of drug in the plasma over the collection period. For drugs with a long half-time relative to the collection period, and for which therefore the plasma concentration does not change much during the period of measurement, this equation gives a good approximation of the value of renal clearance when C_p is measured at the mid-point of the collection period, and that is what is done in routine clinical measurements of creatinine clearance. However, it is not so accurate for drugs whose half-times are short by comparison with the collection period, and in those cases alternative methods must be used. One such method is based on repeated plasma drug concentration measurements during the collection period:

$$CL_R = C_{\text{ur}} \times V_{\text{ur}}/\text{area} \qquad (3.22)$$

where 'area' is the area under the curve of the plasma concentration plotted against time during the urine collection period.

(b) Hepatic clearance

(i) Extraction ratio

The extraction ratio (E) of a drug is a measure of the extent to which the drug is removed by the liver (via metabolism and biliary excretion) from incoming blood (i.e. portal venous and hepatic arterial blood). It is thus the difference in drug concentration between incoming and outgoing blood ($C_{\text{IN}} - C_{\text{OUT}}$), expressed as a fraction of the incoming concentration:

$$E = (C_{\text{IN}} - C_{\text{OUT}})/C_{\text{IN}} \qquad (3.23)$$

If a drug is subject to a high degree of removal by the liver then the concentration in the outflowing blood (C_{OUT}) will be low, and E will approach the value of 1 ($E \Rightarrow 1$). If there is poor extraction, on the other hand, then C_{OUT} will be close in value to C_{IN}, and E will approach zero ($E \Rightarrow 0$).

(ii) The effect of hepatic blood flow

If the extent to which a drug is extracted by the liver is given by ($C_{\text{IN}} - C_{\text{OUT}}$) then the rate at which it is removed must be the product of this extent and the rate of hepatic blood flow:

$$\text{Rate of extraction} = Q_H(C_{\text{IN}} - C_{\text{OUT}}) \quad (3.24)$$

where Q_H is the rate of hepatic blood flow. Therefore, the hepatic clearance rate will be the rate of extraction expressed as a fraction of the incoming concentration:

$$CL_H = [Q_H(C_{\text{IN}} - C_{\text{OUT}})]/C_{\text{IN}} \qquad (3.25)$$

or:

$$CL_H = Q_H \times E \qquad (3.26)$$

However, this relationship is only strictly true at high degrees of extraction, i.e. for high values of E (see Fig. 3.15(a)). At low values of E the relationship between hepatic clearance and hepatic blood flow becomes more complex, and we must introduce another concept, that of intrinsic clearance.

(iii) Intrinsic clearance

The intrinsic clearance of a drug is a measure of the maximal ability of the liver to remove drug from the incoming blood, independent of the rate of hepatic blood flow. Intrinsic clearance is a complicated function, which depends partly on the activity of hepatic drug metabolizing enzymes, the rate of biliary excretion, the coefficient of partition of the drug between the liver and the outgoing blood, and the apparent volume of distribution of the drug in the liver (i.e. the extent of tissue protein binding). If one makes certain assumptions one can show, although the derivation is too complicated to give here, that hepatic blood flow, extraction ratio, and intrinsic clearance (CL_{int}) are related as follows:

$$E = CL_{int}/(Q_H + CL_{int}) \qquad (3.27)$$

Thus:

$$CL_H = Q_H \times E = Q_H \times CL_{int}/(Q_H + CL_{int}) \qquad (3.28)$$

Case 1 (see p. 31)
When

$$E \Rightarrow 1, \ CL_{int} \Rightarrow Q_H, \text{ and thus } CL_H = Q_H \qquad (3.29)$$

Case 2 (see p. 31)
When

$$E \Rightarrow 0, \ Q_H \Rightarrow CL_{int}, \text{ and thus } CL_H = CL_{int} \qquad (3.30)$$

Thus, for drugs with a high extraction ratio hepatic clearance is proportional to hepatic blood flow (eqn 3.29). For drugs with a low extraction ratio hepatic clearance is proportional to intrinsic clearance (eqn 3.30). For drugs with an intermediate extraction ratio both factors influence hepatic clearance. The extraction ratios of some commonly used drugs are listed in Table 3.5.

Intrinsic clearance can be measured by comparing the clearance of an intravenous dose of drug with the clearance of an oral dose of drug, but only for low extraction ratio drugs which are completely absorbed intact from the gut.

(iv) The relationship between CL_H and protein binding

$$CL_{TOT} \times C_{TOT} = CL_u \times C_u \qquad (3.31)$$

Thus:

$$CL_{TOT} = CL_u \times (C_u/C_{TOT}) = CL_u \times f_u \qquad (3.32)$$

where u indicates unbound drug.

Thus, at low values of E hepatic clearance is directly proportional to the fraction of drug which is bound to plasma proteins in the circulation. This is an important result when we come to consider the course of events during displacement of drugs from protein binding sites (see, for example, Chapter 10, p. 124).

3.6.6 The relationship between the loading dose and the maintenance dose during intermittent dosage

(a) At steady state

Let D_L = the maximum amount of drug in the body at steady state (i.e. the loading dose). Let D_M = the difference between the maximum amount of drug in the body at steady state and the amount left in the body at the end of a dosage interval (i.e. the amount required to replace losses during a dosage interval, the maintenance dose). Thus:

$$D_M = D_L - D_L \, e^{-kt} \qquad (3.33)$$

and thus:

$$D_M = D_L(1 - e^{-kt}) \qquad (3.34)$$

(b) During a continuous intravenous infusion

At steady state input = output. Thus, the rate of infusion (R_0) = the rate of elimination. Thus:

$$R_0 = CL \times V_{ss} \qquad (3.35)$$

But

$$CL = V_{area} \times k \text{ (eqn 3.17)}.$$

Thus:

$$R_0 = V_{area} \times k \times C_{ss} \qquad (3.36)$$

But

$$D_L = V_{area} \times C_{ss} \text{ (compare eqn 3.16)}.$$

Thus:

$$R_0 = D_L \times k \qquad (3.37)$$

and:

$$R_0 = D_L \times 0.7/t_{1/2} \qquad (3.38)$$

3.6.7 Non-linear kinetics

From the characteristics of the plot of steady-state plasma concentration versus dose, as shown in Fig. 3.18, one can define two features:

1. The D_{max}: the dose at which the curve becomes perpendicular (i.e. the asymptote at $y = $ infinity).

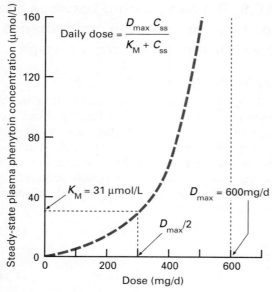

■ Fig. 3.18 Non-linear kinetics. The curve was constructed by measuring the steady-state plasma concentrations found at different daily maintenance doses of phenytoin in the same individual. Analysis of the curve (see Fig. 3.19) yielded values of D_{max} and K_M as shown. D_{max} is the asymptote of the curve and K_M is the steady-state plasma concentration found when the maintenance dose is half of the D_{max}.

2. The K_M: the steady-state plasma concentration which results from the administration of half the D_{max}.

These two features, which are constant in an individual, are related to the rate of dosing and the resultant steady-state plasma concentration (C_{ss}) as follows:

$$\text{Rate of dosing} = (D_{max} \times C_{ss})/(K_M + C_{ss}) \quad (3.39)$$

This equation is comparable with the Michaelis–Menten equation of enzyme kinetics, and with the equation of the dose response curve (eqn 4.11). The shape of the curve which it defines is shown in Fig. 3.18.

We can now consider what happens to equation (3.39) in two cases: at low dosages and at high dosages:

1. At very low doses, and therefore low values of C_{ss}, $K_M \gg C_{ss}$, and thus $K_M \approx C_{ss} + K_M$. Now

eqn (3.39) becomes:

$$\text{Rate of dosing} \approx (D_{max}/K_M) \times C_{ss}$$

$$= \text{constant} \times C_{ss} \quad (3.40)$$

Equation (3.40) is recognizable as a first-order equation (compare equation 3.4).

2. At very high doses, and therefore high values of C_{ss}, $C_{ss} \gg K_M$, and thus $K_M + C_{ss} \approx C_{ss}$. Now eqn (3.39) becomes:

$$\text{Rate of dosing} \approx D_{max} = \text{constant} \quad (3.41)$$

Equation (3.41) is recognizable as a zero-order equation (compare equation 3.1).

Thus, at low dosages (case 1) the pharmacokinetic properties are predominantly first-order, while at high dosages (case 2) they are predominantly zero-order. At intermediate dosages the kinetics are mixed.

Since equation (3.39) describes the curve in Fig. 3.18 it will be apparent that K_M and D_{max} cannot be calculated properly on the basis of a steady-state concentration measurement made during maintenance therapy with only one dosage of drug. To define the characteristics of the curve with a reasonable degree of accuracy one must make measurements at steady state during the administration of several different dosages. However, in practice one can calculate K_M and D_{max} approximately on the basis of only two such measurements. This can be done using any one of the classical linearizations of equation (3.39), such as the so-called Scatchard plot (i.e. by plotting dose/C_{ss} on the vertical axis and C_{ss} on the horizontal axis, in which case the slope of the line is equal to $-1/K_M$ and the intercept on the horizontal axis is equal to D_{max}). However, it is much simpler to use a plot known as the 'direct linear plot' (Fig. 3.19). In this plot, instead of plotting each value of C_{ss} and its corresponding daily dose as a single point, as on a conventional plot, each pair of values (C_{ss} and dose) is plotted as a straight line joining the two values: C_{ss} on the horizontal axis, conventionally to the left, and daily dose on the vertical axis. The point at which two such lines cross indicates the K_M (on the horizontal axis to the right) and the D_{max} (on the vertical axis).

In the example shown in Fig. 3.19(a) two doses

of phenytoin, 300 mg and 400 mg, were given daily until steady state was reached in each case. The corresponding steady-state plasma concentrations were 30 µmol/L and 60 µmol/L respectively. The two lines formed by these two pairs of values crossed at the point where $K_M = 31$ µmol/L and $D_{max} = 600$ mg/day.

Although accurate measurement of K_M and D_{max} depends on the measurement of C_{ss} at several different maintenance doses, one can use a single measurement of C_{ss}, in combination with the mean K_M calculated from studies on many individuals, to derive an approximate value of D_{max} in an individual, and hence to assess the appropriate daily dosage. That is because, while the values of D_{max} in individuals are very variable,

the values of K_M are much less so (see Fig. 3.5). The method for this calculation is shown in Fig. 3.19(b).

In the example illustrated, for phenytoin, a steady-state plasma concentration of 20 µmol/L was achieved at a daily maintenance dose of 200 mg. If we assume that the K_M for phenytoin in this patient is 22 µmol/L the D_{max} can be estimated at 382 mg/day. If one wanted to know the daily dose required to produce a steady-state plasma concentration of 60 µmol/L one would draw a line joining the point of (K_M, D_{max}) to 60 µmol/L on the horizontal axis. The point where the line crosses the vertical axis shows the daily maintenance dose required. Try it yourself. The answer is 300 mg.

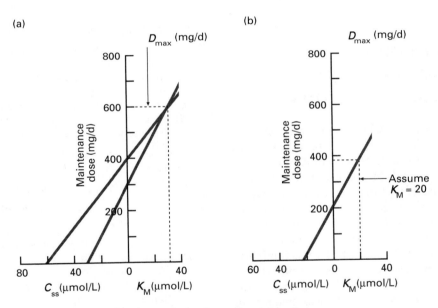

∎ **Fig. 3.19** The direct linear plot for the analysis of non-linear kinetics.

(a) Calculation of phenytoin D_{max} and K_M using two separate steady-state concentration measurements (same data as in Fig. 3.18). Each line is formed by joining the points indicating the steady-state plasma concentration (horizontal axis to the left) and the corresponding daily maintenance dose (vertical axis). The point where these extrapolated lines cross shows the K_M (horizontal axis to the right) and the D_{max} (vertical axis).

(b) Prediction (first approximation) of steady-state plasma concentrations at any daily maintenance dose from a single measurement. The line joining the daily dose of 200 mg to the measured steady-state phenytoin concentration has been constructed. Assume, for the first approximation, that the patient's K_M is 20 µmol/L. To calculate the D_{max}, construct the vertical line which passes through the value of 20 µmol/L on the horizontal axis to the right. From the point at which this line meets the first line, draw a horizontal line to meet the vertical axis (dotted line on the graph). This is the first approximation of the D_{max}. Using this construction, one can calculate the likely steady-state plasma concentration at a given maintenance dose or the maintenance dose which will be required to produce a pre-chosen steady-state plasma concentration.

4 The pharmacodynamic process

Is the drug producing the required pharmacological effect?

The pharmacodynamic process describes all those matters concerned with the pharmacological actions of a drug, whether they be determinants of therapeutic effects or of adverse effects.

4.1 The types of pharmacological actions of drugs

The different ways in which drugs may produce their pharmacological effects are classified in Table 4.1. As we unfold this classification it will be seen that several of the examples we shall quote cross the boundaries of the classification. For example, the cardiac glycosides may be considered as ligands which act by binding to their receptor (the Na^+K^+ ATPase), as inhibitors of an enzyme (the Na^+K^+ ATPase), or as inhibitors of a transport process (the Na^+K^+ pump). However, this should not be seen as a defect of the system of classification, but rather as evidence of the richness of drug action.

4.1.1 Drug action via a direct effect on a receptor

Receptors are specific proteins, situated either in cell membranes, or in some cases within the cellular cytoplasm. For each type of receptor there is a specific group of drugs or endogenous substances (known as ligands) which are capable of binding to the receptor and thereby producing

■ **Table 4.1** The types of pharmacological actions of drugs

---

1. Drug action via a receptor
   (a) Agonists
   (b) Antagonists
   (c) Partial agonists

2. Drug action via indirect alteration of the effect of an endogenous agonist
   (a) Physiological antagonism
   (b) Increase in endogenous release
   (c) Inhibition of endogenous re-uptake
   (d) Inhibition of endogenous metabolism
   (e) Prevention of endogenous release

3. Drug action via the inhibition of transport processes

4. Drug action via enzyme inhibition

5. Drug action via enzymatic action or activation of enzyme activity

6. Drug action via other miscellaneous effects
   (a) Chelating agents
   (b) Osmotic diuretics
   (c) Volatile general anaesthetics
   (d) Replacement drugs

---

a pharmacological effect. There are three types of ligand which can act by binding to a receptor – agonists, antagonists, and partial agonists.

(a) Agonists

Ligands which bind to a receptor and produce an appropriate response are called agonists. For example, the catecholamine adrenaline is an agonist at β-adrenoceptors. When it binds to β-adrenoceptors in the heart it increases the heart rate.

(b) Antagonists

Ligands which prevent an agonist from binding to a receptor, and thus prevent its effects, are called antagonists. However, antagonists do not themselves have any pharmacological actions mediated by receptors. For example, propranolol is a β-adrenoceptor antagonist. When it binds to β-adrenoceptors in the heart it prevents catechol-amine-induced tachycardia (for example in response to exercise).

(c) Partial agonists

A full agonist is one which is capable of produ-cing a maximal response, when it binds to a sufficient number of receptors. In contrast, a partial agonist cannot produce the maximal response of which the tissue is capable, even when it binds to the same number of receptors as a full agonist binds to when it produces a complete response. Since the effects of a ligand are generally produced by concentrations of the ligand which are well below those which would bind to all the receptors necessary to produce a complete response, this means that above a cer-tain level of binding a partial agonist may bind to receptors without producing any further increase in effect. However, in so doing it may prevent the action of other agonists, and may thus appear to be acting as an antagonist. It is this mixture of actions which is called partial agonism. For example, oxprenolol, which is a β-adrenoceptor antagonist is also a partial agon-ist. Thus, it may have less of an effect in slowing the heart rate than adrenoceptor antagonists which do not have partial agonist action.

In the case of β-adrenoceptor antagonists, the amount of β-blockade produced by a given dose of the β-blocker will vary according to how much endogenous sympathetic nervous system activity there is: the more activity the more β-blockade will result from the action of a partial agonist. This is clearly seen in the actions of the β-agonist/ antagonist xamoterol. Xamoterol acts as a β-ad-renoceptor agonist in patients with mild heart failure, and in them it improves cardiac contrac-tion. However, it acts as a β-blocker in patients with even moderate heart failure, and in them it worsens the heart failure. This problem greatly restricts the value of xamoterol in the treatment of heart failure.

In some cases a receptor may have subtypes, for which certain ligands may exhibit some degree of selectivity. For example, β-adrenoceptors exist in two subtypes, called β_1 and β_2, both of which can respond to adrenaline. However, the β-adren-oceptor antagonists may act at both subtypes or may have some selectivity for one or other of the subtypes. For example, propranolol is an antag-onist at both β_1 and β_2 receptors, while atenolol is relatively selective for β_1 receptors. Note that selectivity of this kind is only relative, and that while a drug such as atenolol acts primarily on β_1 receptors, at high enough concentrations it may have effects on β_2 receptors as well. This is discussed in more detail in the last section of this chapter (p. 54).

4.1.2 Short-term and long-term effects of drugs at receptors

The mechanisms whereby drugs and endogenous substances produce their pharmacological actions through binding to receptors are not fully under-stood. However, there are two types of action which are known to be involved in their short-term and long-term effects respectively.

(a) Short-term effects

Many drugs are used for their short-term effects. For example, dopamine is used as a renal arteri-olar vasodilator, diamorphine to relieve pain in the treatment of myocardial ischaemia, and nebu-lized salbutamol to reverse bronchoconstriction in the treatment of acute severe asthma.

Many agonist drugs acting on cellular recep-tors exert their effects through so-called second messenger systems, illustrated in Fig. 4.1. The regulation of these systems is currently assuming increasing importance in drug therapy.

(b) Long-term effects

Some drugs are given for long-term therapy. When that happens their short-term effects may be altered by adaptive responses which result from chronic therapy. Examples include L-dopa in Parkinson's disease, β-adrenoceptor agonists in chronic asthma, and benzodiazepines in chronic anxiety. These effects may be accompan-ied by either increases ('up-regulation') or decreases ('down-regulation') in receptor numbers during long-term therapy, and such changes may be responsible for both beneficial and adverse effects of drugs (see section 5.2).

The important receptor systems and the ligands which have their actions through binding to them are listed in Table 4.2. The mathematics of the interaction of a ligand with its receptor and the concept of the dose–response curve are discussed in section 4.5.

4.1.3 Drug action via indirect alteration of the effect of an endogenous agonist

Just as an antagonist can produce a therapeutic effect by directly opposing the action of an endo-genous agonist, so it is possible to alter the effect of an endogenous agonist in indirect ways.

(a) Physiological antagonism

A drug which produces the opposite physiological effect to that of an agonist will indirectly oppose the action of that agonist. For example, glucagon is a physiological antagonist of the actions of insulin.

(b) Increase in endogenous release

The action of an endogenous agonist may be enhanced if its release is increased. For example, amphetamines increase the release of mono-amines, such as dopamine, from nerve endings. Because amphetamines can cause a syndrome similar to schizophrenia, this action has led to

■ **Table 4.2** Some clinically relevant examples of important receptors and of their agonists and antagonists

Receptor type	Subtype	Site(s) in the body	Agonists	Antagonists
Cholinoceptors	Muscarinic	Tissues innervated by parasympathetic nerves	Acetylcholine and analogues (e.g. carbachol, bethanecol)	Atropine and analogues Benzhexol Orphenadrine Quinidine Disopyramide Tricyclic anti-depressants Pirenzepine (M_1 selective)
	Nicotinic	Neuromuscular junction Postganglionic cells in ganglia	Acetylcholine and some analogues (e.g. carbachol)	Neuromuscular blocking drugs Ganglion blocking drugs Quinidine Aminoglycoside antibiotics
Adrenoceptors	α/β		Adrenaline Noradrenaline	Labetalol
	α_1	Vascular smooth muscle Pupillary dilator muscle	Phenylephrine Dopamine (high doses)	Prazosin
	α_2	Presynaptic nerve terminals	Clonidine	Yohimbine

Receptor type	Subtype	Site(s) in the body	Agonists	Antagonists
Adrenoceptors	α_1/α_2		Phentolamine	
(*continued*)	β_1	Heart CNS	Dopamine (moderate doses) Dobutamine	Practolol Atenolol Metoprolol
	β_2	Smooth muscle (bronchiolar, vascular, uterine) Pancreatic islets	Salbutamol Terbutaline Rimiterol Fenoterol	Propanolol Oxprenolol
	β_1/β_2		Isoprenaline Dopamine	Propranolol Oxprenolol
Dopamine	Various	CNS Renal vasculature	Dopamine (low doses) Bromocriptine	Phenothiazines (e.g. chlorpromazine) Thioxanthenes (e.g. flupenthixol) Butyrophenones (e.g. haloperidol) Metoclopramide Domperidone Apomorphine
Histamine	H_1	Smooth muscle (bronchiolar, vascular, gastrointestinal)	Histamine	Antihistamines (e.g. mepyramine, promethazine)
	H_2	Stomach	Histamine	Cimetidine Ranitidine Famotidine Nizatidine
Opioid receptors	Various	CNS Vascular smooth muscle Gastrointestinal tract Biliary tract Genitourinary tract Pupillary muscle	Morphine and analogues (e.g. buprenorphine, diamorphine) β-endorphin Enkephalins Non-opioid narcotics (e.g. pentazocine)	Naloxone Naltrexone
5-hydroxy- tryptamine (5-HT) receptors	Various	CNS Vascular smooth muscle Gastrointestinal tract	5-HT Cyproheptadine	Methysergide Sumatriptan ($5\text{-}HT_1$-like) Ketanserin ($5\text{-}HT_2$) Ondansetron ($5\text{-}HT_3$)
GABA receptors	$GABA_A$/BDZ complex	CNS	GABA Benzodiazepines	Bicuculine
	$GABA_B$	CNS (presynaptic)	GABA	Baclofen

the idea that schizophrenia may be related to excess dopamine action in the brain.

(c) Inhibition of endogenous re-uptake

Conversely, if a drug inhibits the re-uptake of an endogenous agonist it will enhance its effects. For example, the tricyclic and other antidepressants inhibit the re-uptake by neurones of certain neurotransmitters, such as noradrenaline and 5-hydroxytryptamine (see Table 31.2).

(d) Inhibition of endogenous metabolism

If a drug inhibits the metabolism of an endogenous agonist it will enhance its effects. For example, the monoamine oxidase inhibitors inhibit the metabolism of monoamines such as adrenaline and noradrenaline, and thus enhance their actions.

(e) Prevention of endogenous release

Prevention of the release of an endogenous agonist will decrease its effects. For example, one of the proposed mechanisms whereby sodium cromoglycate produces its therapeutic effects is via inhibition of the release of inflammatory mediators from tissue mast cells. Angiotensin converting enzyme (ACE) inhibitors prevent the formation of angiotensin II; this prevents the endogenous release of aldosterone, whose effects are thereby reduced, resulting in potassium retention.

4.1.4 Drug action via the inhibition of transport processes

Because the transport and disposition of cations (such as sodium, potassium, and calcium) and of other substances (such as organic acids in the kidneys and neurotransmitters in the nervous system) play so many important roles in the maintenance of normal cellular function, the inhibition of their transport is an important type of mechanism whereby drug action may occur. Similar mathematical principles apply to the active transport of substances across cell membranes as to the binding of a ligand to its receptor (see section 4.5), and the concept of a dose–response curve can therefore be developed analogously. The following are examples of the ways in which

drugs may act through the inhibition of transport processes.

(a) Diuretics

Many diuretics act by the inhibition of sodium reabsorption in the renal tubules, although they do so by different mechanisms. For example, the loop diuretics, frusemide and bumetanide, act in the ascending limb of the loop of Henle by inhibiting the active transport system known as the $Na^+/K^+/Cl^-$ co-transport, which involves the transport of sodium, potassium, and chloride in the same direction across cell membranes. The potassium-sparing diuretic amiloride acts by inhibiting sodium channels in the distal segment of the distal convoluted tubule. The thiazide diuretics act by inhibiting a Na^+/Cl^- co-transport system in the proximal segment of the distal convoluted tubule. Although most of the diuretic effect of the cardiac glycosides occurs by virtue of increased cardiac output and therefore increased renal blood flow, part of its action occurs via inhibition of renal tubular Na^+K^+ ATPase.

However, some diuretics act by mechanisms other than direct actions on transport processes. For example, spironolactone is a competitive antagonist of the action of aldosterone at receptors in the distal convoluted tubule and acetazolamide is an enzyme inhibitor, inhibiting the action of carbonic anhydrase in the proximal convoluted tubule.

(b) Calcium antagonists

The calcium antagonists, such as verapamil, diltiazem, and the dihydropyridines (for example nifedipine), act by inhibiting the transmembrane transport of calcium through potential-operated channels in cell membranes. The different calcium antagonists have different specificities for calcium channels in different tissues, and because calcium plays so many important roles in these tissues, the calcium antagonists have several different actions, principal among which are an anti-arrhythmic action in the heart (for example verapamil), and a vasodilator action on peripheral arterioles (for example nifedipine).

(c) Insulin

One of the many actions of insulin is to increase the inward flux of glucose into cells by an action mediated via insulin receptors. In the treatment of hyperglycaemia in diabetes the rapid fall in blood glucose produced by insulin is undoubtedly due to this action. Insulin also causes an inward flux of potassium into cells, probably by stimulating the Na^+K^+ ATPase, and in the emergency treatment of hyperglycaemia with insulin this may result in hypokalaemia. For this reason the fluids infused intravenously during the emergency treatment of severe hyperglycaemia with insulin should usually contain potassium.

(d) Probenecid

Probenecid is an organic acid, a benzoic acid derivative, which was developed to reduce the tubular secretion of penicillin and thus to delay the excretion of penicillin from the body, prolonging its therapeutic action. It inhibits the transport of organic acids across epithelial barriers and not only blocks the active secretion of penicillin into the renal tubular lumen, but also blocks the active reabsorption of uric acid. It is now mainly used as a uricosuric agent in the treatment of gout, and occasionally to decrease the renal clearance of the penicillins or cephalosporins from the blood. This action can be of value, for example, in maintaining high blood penicillin concentrations in the treatment of infective endocarditis, although this is usually achieved without probenecid, simply by increasing the dose of penicillin.

(e) Drugs acting on potassium channels

Potassium channels in cell membranes control the rate of efflux of potassium from the cells, and this tends to stabilize the transmembrane potential. Drugs which open potassium channels will therefore tend to reduce the likelihood of activation of the cell, while drugs which close potassium channels will tend to increase the likelihood of activation of the cell.

Drugs which open potassium channels include vascular smooth muscle relaxants, such as minoxidil and hydralazine (used in the treatment of hypertension). Drugs which close potassium channels include the sulphonylureas, which thus increase the release of insulin from beta cells in the pancreas (used in the treatment of maturity-onset diabetes).

4.1.5 Drug action via enzyme inhibition

Many diverse types of drug action may be produced by inhibition of enzymes, and the precise action will depend on the role that the inhibited enzyme plays in normal function. The principles outlined in section 4.5 on the mathematics of the interaction of a ligand with its receptor apply equally to the interaction of an enzyme inhibitor with the relevant enzyme, and the concept of a dose–response curve can be developed analogously. The following are illustrative examples of the ways in which drugs may act by inhibiting enzymes.

(a) Neostigmine

Neostigmine is a reversible cholinesterase inhibitor. It is used in the treatment of myasthenia gravis because of its effect in increasing the concentration of acetylcholine at the muscle motor end-plate, thereby alleviating the block in neuromuscular transmission which occurs in this condition.

(b) Allopurinol

Xanthine and hypoxanthine are oxidized to uric acid by the enzyme xanthine oxidase, which is inhibited by allopurinol. Allopurinol therefore decreases the synthesis of uric acid. This effect is produced mainly by its active metabolite, alloxanthine (or oxypurinol), which is a non-competitive inhibitor of xanthine oxidase. The decrease in uric acid production reduces the risks of attacks of acute gouty arthritis, decreases the incidence of chronic gouty arthritis, and prevents the occurrence of uric acid stones (gouty nephropathy). Xanthine and hypoxanthine are considerably more water-soluble than uric acid and their urinary excretion is rapid.

(c) Monoamine oxidase (MAO) inhibitors

The monoamine oxidase inhibitors inhibit the metabolism of the monoamines 5-hydroxytryptamine, noradrenaline, and dopamine in the brain, and it is presumably by this action that they produce their antidepressant action. Isocarboxazid and phenelzine bind irreversibly to MAO and new enzyme molecules must be synthesized in order to restore to normal the metabolism of monoamines, a process which takes about two weeks. In contrast, the inhibition of MAO by tranylcypromine is reversible.

Just as drugs which act via receptors may be specific for one subtype of a receptor or another, so MAO inhibitors may be specific for one of the subtypes of MAO. For example, selegiline is a specific inhibitor of MAO type B; it therefore inhibits the metabolism of dopamine in the brain and thereby enhances the action of L-dopa in the treatment of Parkinsonism. However, because MAO in the gut is principally of type A, selegiline does not produce the 'cheese reaction' that other MAO inhibitors do (see Chapter 10, p. 129).

(d) Cardiac glycosides

The actions of the cardiac glycosides are probably brought about by their inhibition of the sodium/potassium-activated adenosine triphosphatase (Na^+K^+ ATPase), a membrane-bound enzyme which is responsible for the major part of the active transport of potassium into cells and of sodium out of them, thus maintaining the normal transmembrane gradients of these ions. The actions of the cardiac glycosides are thought to operate via this inhibition, perhaps through a secondary alteration in calcium disposition within cells.

(e) Lithium

Lithium alters the turnover of the second messenger system involving phosphoinositides (see Fig. 4.1) by inhibition of one of the enzymes of that system. However, it is not yet certain whether or not that is the mechanism whereby lithium produces its therapeutic effects in the treatment of manic-depressive illness.

(f) Other examples

Other drugs which act via enzyme inhibition include the following:

(1) warfarin, which inhibits vitamin K epoxide reductase;

(2) aspirin and other non-steroidal anti-inflammatory drugs, which inhibit the enzymes involved in prostaglandin synthesis;

(3) captopril and related drugs, which inhibit the angiotensin converting enzyme;

(4) disulfiram, which inhibits alcohol dehydrogenase;

(5) some anticancer drugs, such as cytarabine, which inhibits DNA polymerase.

Some anti-infective agents act by inhibiting bacterial or viral enzymes. For example, trimethoprim inhibits bacterial dihydrofolate reductase, the quinolones inhibit bacterial DNA gyrase, and zidovudine and didanosine inhibit the reverse transcriptase of the human immunodeficiency virus (HIV).

(g) Adverse effects

In some cases the adverse effects of a drug may occur via enzyme inhibition. For example, procaine inhibits pseudocholinesterase and may thus enhance the actions of the depolarizing muscle relaxant succinylcholine. Metronidazole inhibits alcohol dehydrogenase and can thus cause a disulfiram-like reaction to alcohol (see p. 128).

4.1.6 Drug action via direct enzymatic activity or the activation of enzymes

Just as some drugs may act by inhibiting enzymes so some drugs may activate enzymes or may themselves act as enzymes.

(a) Enzyme replacement in genetic and acquired enzyme deficiencies

Genetic diseases which are due to enzyme deficiencies should theoretically be susceptible to treatment by replacement therapy, although treatment of this kind is limited by the difficulty of delivering enzymes to their sites of action. However, clotting factor deficiencies can be treated in this way, the best examples being the parenteral use of factor VIII in patients with haemophilia and of fresh frozen plasma in treating overdose with warfarin. Another example is the oral use of pancreatic enzymes in treating malabsorption in patients with chronic pancreatic insufficiency.

(b) Drugs acting on the clotting system

The clotting and fibrinolytic factors are enzymes, and certain drugs which act on clotting and fibrinolysis do so by increasing their activity.

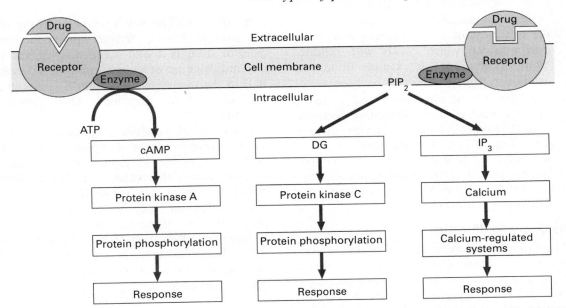

■ **Fig. 4.1** A schematic representation of the second messenger systems which mediate the effects of drugs acting at receptors. When an agonist combines with its receptor it stimulates the activity of an enzyme or enzymes. This leads to a series of events which culminate in the response of the cell to the drug. In one of the messenger systems (left-hand side) the enzyme is adenylate cyclase and this stimulates the production by the cell of cyclic AMP; this stimulates protein kinase A, which leads to protein phosphorylation and hence the response. In the other system (right-hand side) the enzyme is phospholipase C. Stimulation of the phosphoinositide (PI) cycle leads to the response via two mechanisms, increased protein phosphorylation via stimulation of protein kinase C by diacylglycerol (DG) and the activation of calcium-regulated systems in the cell.

Heparin acts as an anticoagulant by activating antithrombin III. Streptokinase, urokinase, alteplase, and anistreplase are activators of plasminogen and thus cause clot lysis. Snake venoms, such as ancrod (Malayan pit viper venom), have thrombin-like activity and thus activate clotting.

(c) Cancer chemotherapy

L-asparaginase is an enzyme which hydrolyses asparagine, the consequent depletion of which in leukaemic cells may be of therapeutic benefit in some patients with acute lymphoblastic leukaemia. Other enzymes which act on amino acids, folate, or RNA are also under study.

(d) Other examples

Other examples of drugs which activate or replace enzymes include pralidoxime, which activates cholinesterase in poisoning with organophosphorus insecticides, and danazol and stanozolol, which increase the activity of the C_1 esterase inhibitor in patients with hereditary angio-oedema. The enzyme superoxide dismutase has been used in the treatment of paraquat poisoning, and it may also eventually prove useful in treating inflammatory conditions.

4.1.7 Drug action via other miscellaneous effects

(a) Chelating agents

Drugs which chelate metals can be used to hasten the removal of those metals from the body, as the following examples show:

(1) calcium sodium edetate (ethylene diamine tetra-acetate or EDTA) chelates many divalent and trivalent metals and is used in the treatment of poisoning, particularly with lead;

(2) dimercaprol chelates certain heavy metals and is used in the treatment of mercury poisoning;

(3) desferrioxamine chelates iron and is used in the treatment of iron poisoning and in the iron overload which occurs with repeated blood transfusion (for example in thalass-aemia);

(4) penicillamine chelates copper and is used in the treatment of hepatolenticular degeneration (Wilson's disease), in which there is deposition of copper in the basal ganglia of the brain due to a deficiency of the copper-binding protein caeruloplasmin; it is also used to chelate cystine and thus prevent renal damage in cystinuria.

(b) Osmotic diuretics

Mannitol is a hexahydric alcohol related to mannose, and an isomer of sorbitol. It is freely filtered at the glomerulus but is reabsorbed to only a small extent by the renal tubules. It therefore increases the concentration of osmotically active particles in the tubular fluid and takes water with it, thus increasing urine volume. It has no other pharmacological effects. Mannitol is used to produce a diuresis in the treatment of some acute poisonings and in cerebral oedema. It has sometimes been used to restore renal tubular function and urinary output in shock. Urea has a similar action to mannitol and has similarly been used in the treatment of cerebral oedema.

(c) Volatile general anaesthetics

These agents lack any obvious molecular feature in common. They form a diverse group of agents, such as the halogenated hydrocarbons (for example halothane, methoxyflurane, enflurane, and trichloroethylene), and non-halogenated agents (for example nitrous oxide, ether, and cyclopropane), which produce very similar effects on the brain. The usual drug–receptor and allied models of drug action do not readily accommodate this group of drugs. It is generally thought that their primary action is on the lipid matrix of the biological membrane, that the biophysical properties of the membrane are thereby changed, and that this results in changes in ion fluxes or other functions which are crucial for the normal operation of neuronal excitability.

(d) Replacement drugs

This is a rather artificial sub-heading pharmacologically, but one which is useful from the clinical point of view. The best examples are the oral and parenteral use of ferrous salts in the treatment of anaemia due to iron deficiency, and the intramuscular use of hydroxocobalamin (vitamin B_{12}) in the treatment of vitamin B_{12} deficiency, particularly that associated with pernicious anaemia.

One could also include under this heading the use of hormones as replacement therapy (for example thyroxine to replace natural thyroid hormone in hypothyroidism), but these are better included under the heading of drugs acting via a direct action on receptors (see section 4.1.1), which is how hormones act. Similarly, the replacement of clotting factors, such as factor VIII in haemophilia, is better classified under the heading of actions via direct enzymatic activity (see section 4.1.5).

4.2 Stereoisomerism and drug action

The phenomenon of stereoisomerism of organic compounds was discovered by Louis Pasteur, following the observation of Jean Baptiste Biot that when one shines polarized light through solutions of certain substances the light may be twisted in one direction or another. This phenomenon is known as optical activity, and Pasteur showed that tartaric acid existed in two forms with different optical activities: one form rotated polarized light to the left and the other rotated it to the right. This difference in the activity of two substances with exactly the same chemical composition is due to an asymmetry in one of the carbon atoms of tartaric acid, which results in two structures which cannot be superimposed on top of one another (in the way that our two hands cannot – try putting your left hand into a right-hand glove).

The terminology used to describe stereoisomers is complex. If a substance rotates polarized light to the right it is called dextrorotatory and is designated by the letter d or by the symbol ($+$). If a substance rotates polarized light to the left it is called laevorotatory and is designated by the letter l or by the symbol ($-$). However, these designations do not tell one anything about the actual spatial configuration of the molecules themselves. If the actual spatial arrangement of the molecules is known then the right- and left-handedness of the configuration about an asymmetric atom are designated by alternative symbols, either R and S (from the Latin 'rectus' = right and 'sinister' = left) or D and L (from the Latin 'dexter' = right and 'laevus' = left). Furthermore, a molecule which is so designated may be either (+) or (−) depending on its milieu, since changes in such factors as pH, temperature, and the wavelength of the light used can affect the direction in which the light is rotated. Even under standard conditions the direction of rotation may differ from compound to compound. For example, although all naturally-occurring amino acids are of the l form some are dextrorotatory and some laevorotatory.

Stereoisomers can be of two types, enantiomers and diastereomers (or 'epimers'). In enantiomers asymmetry occurs either at a single centre of potential asymmetry (or 'chiral' centre) if only one such centre exists in the molecule, or at more than one if more than one exists (in which case there will be more than two enantiomers). In diastereomers asymmetry occurs at only one of the chiral centres, although the molecule has more than one chiral centre, and in such cases the isomers are not mirror images of each other. Enantiomers have similar physicochemical properties to each other while diastereomers do not. Chiral asymmetry is usually due to a carbon atom, but not in all cases, the asymmetrical phosphorus atom in cyclophosphamide being a case in point.

Examples of drug enantiomers are d-propranolol and l-propranolol, R-warfarin and s-warfarin, and L-glucose (laevulose) and D-glucose (dextrose). Quinine and quinidine are diastereomers.

Of all synthetic drugs used in clinical practice about 40 per cent are chiral and about 90 per cent of those are marketed in the racemic form (i.e. as an equal mixture of the two enantiomers). Examples include d,l-propranolol and R, s-warfarin. Naproxen is one of the few examples of a synthetic compound which is marketed as one of its enantiomers. In contrast, naturally-occurring and semi-synthetic compounds are almost all chiral and almost all are marketed as a single isomer. Examples include the naturally-occurring amino acids (for example L-dopa) and D-glucose (dextrose).

The centre of asymmetry of a compound need not be in a part of the molecule which is important for the action of the drug, but if it is there will be pharmacological differences between the different stereoisomers, and these differences may be of clinical relevance. The following examples illustrate some of these differences.

4.2.1 Pharmacokinetic differences between stereoisomers

(a) Absorption

Both D-methotrexate and L-methotrexate are passively absorbed, but only to a small extent. However, L-methotrexate is also transported actively across the gut, while D-methotrexate is not. Thus, L-methotrexate is better absorbed than D-methotrexate.

(b) Distribution

The binding of d-propranolol to plasma albumin is more extensive than that of d-propranolol. The binding of s-disopyramide to α_1-acid glycoprotein is more extensive than that of R-disopyramide. s-warfarin is more highly bound to albumin than R-warfarin, but R-warfarin is more highly protein bound overall than s-warfarin. These differences lead to differences in the distribution and rates of clearance of the different enantiomers.

(c) Elimination

Numerous enantiomeric differences in drug elimination have been described. For example, the first-pass hepatic metabolism of s-metoprolol is less than that of R-metoprolol. However, this is only the case in extensive hydroxylators of the debrisoquine type (see Chapter 8, p. 95), and in poor metabolizers the first-pass metabolism of metoprolol is not affected by stereoisomerism. Both the rates and the routes of metabolism of the enantiomers of warfarin are different. The half-times of s-warfarin and R-warfarin are 32 h and 54 h respectively, and the routes of metabolism are to 7-hydroxywarfarin for s-warfarin and to warfarin alcohols for R-warfarin. The secretion of tocainide into the saliva is greater for R-tocainide than for s-tocainide.

4.2.2 Pharmacodynamic differences between stereoisomers

Enantiomers are sometimes described as being active or inactive (the terms 'eutomer' and 'distomer' have also been used). For example, one might describe the β-adrenoceptor antagonist l-propranolol as the active enantiomer and d-propranolol, which is not a β-blocker, as the inactive enantiomer. However, to do so would be inaccurate, since d-propranolol has membrane stabilizing activity like that of local anaesthetics. There are many other examples of enantiomers which have different pharmacological actions to each other and sometimes this is of clinical importance.

In some cases differences between enantiomers are limited to differences in potency. For example, s-warfarin is about five times more potent as an anticoagulant than R-warfarin. In other cases the differences are differences in pharmacological and therapeutic actions. For example, l-sotalol is a β-adrenoceptor antagonist while d-sotalol is a class III antiarrhythmic drug like amiodarone.

Sometimes the difference between enantiomers is a difference between therapeutic and adverse effects. Nowhere is this more dramatically seen than in the example of thalidomide, whose R-enantiomer is hypnotic but whose adverse effects seem to be due to the s-enantiomer.

Sometimes enantiomeric differences tell one something about the mechanism of action of a drug. For example, s-timolol is a more potent β-adrenoceptor antagonist than R-timolol, but both are equally effective in reducing intraocular pressure in patients with glaucoma. This suggests that the mechanism of action whereby timolol lowers the intraocular pressure is not related to β-blockade.

4.2.3 Interactions between enantiomers

Sometimes two enantiomers can interact with one another. For example, two enantiomers may compete for binding to the same receptor, as in the case of methadone, whose s-enantiomer antagonizes the respiratory depressant effect of the R-enantiomer. If two enantiomers have agonist and antagonist actions respectively, the racemic mixture may appear to act as a partial agonist (see above, p. 41).

In some cases two enantiomers may be metabolically interconverted. This is not uncommon with the arylalkanoic acids, such as ibuprofen, most of whose R-enantiomer is converted to the s-enantiomer after administration.

4.2.4 Drug interactions and enantiomers

Some drug interactions are stereoselective. For example, some drugs, such as metronidazole, sulphinpyrazone, and phenylbutazone, which inhibit the metabolism of warfarin, primarily affect the more potent enantiomer, s-warfarin.

Similarly, enzyme induction may affect one enantiomer more than another. For example, the barbiturate-induced increase in the activity of the glucuronyl transferase of oxazepam affects the (+) enantiomer more than the (−) enantiomer.

Protein binding displacement may be stereoselective, as in the case of the displacement of warfarin from albumin by phenylbutazone, which affects the R-enantiomer more than the s-enantiomer.

4.2.5 The clinical relevance of stereoisomerism

There are no immediate practical consequences for routine drug therapy as a result of these observations, since the pharmacology and clinical pharmacology of drugs which are given as racemic mixtures have been worked out for the racemic mixtures. However, that is not to say that there are not important clinical consequences of the pharmacological differences between stereoisomers.

Firstly, to neglect to study the pharmacology and clinical pharmacology of stereoisomers may be to miss some important facet of their clinical effects. This is exemplified by the elucidation of the complex interaction of phenylbutazone with warfarin. Phenylbutazone inhibits the metabolism of s-warfarin but induces the metabolism of R-warfarin. Thus, the clearance of the racemic mixture is unaffected, and this obscures the nature of the interaction. Further complication comes from the fact that the protein binding displacement effect of phenylbutazone is also different for the two enantiomers. Other warfarin interactions have similar stereoselectivity (e.g. metronidazole, see p. 712).

Secondly, it is clear that the use of pure enantiomers might in some cases improve the quality of drug therapy, by more specific drug action and the avoidance of adverse drug reactions and interactions. For example, R-timolol may have an advantage over s-timolol in the treatment of glaucoma, since it would be less likely to cause systemic β-blockade. Of course, such advantages would be offset in the cases of enantiomers which are subject to metabolic interconversion, but that is by no means a universal phenomenon.

Until recently the synthesis of pure enantiomers has been prohibitively costly. However, new techniques may reduce the costs considerably and we may soon be seeing the emergence of more formulations of pure enantiomers for clinical use.

4.3 Graded responses to drugs: the dose–response curve in drug therapy

The pharmacological effect of a drug is related to the concentration of the drug at its site of action. This means that within certain limits the higher the concentration the greater the pharmacological effect. The relation between the concentration of a drug at its site of action and the intensity of its pharmacological effect is called its dose–response curve, and this often takes the shape illustrated in Fig. 4.2. Note that when the intensity of response is plotted against drug concentration on a linear scale (Fig. 4.2(a)) the shape of the curve is that of a rectangular hyperbola, and when it is plotted against the logarithm of the drug concentration (Fig. 4.2(b)) it is sigmoid. The latter is known as the log dose–response curve. An understanding of the dose–response curve lies at the heart of successful therapeutic practice.

4.3.1 The mathematics of the dose–response curve

In the following discussion we shall analyse dose-responsiveness in terms of the interaction of a drug with its receptor and the translation of that interaction into a pharmacological effect. However, the analysis could equally well be adapted to fit other modes of action of drugs, such as enzyme inhibition, enzyme activation, alterations in ion transport, and indirect actions mediated via receptors. In all cases the final equations and dose–response curves would be identical in form, allowing for differences in symbols. Let us suppose that a drug molecule combines with its receptor to produce a pharmacological effect. We shall make three simple assumptions to help us to derive some equations which describe this interaction: (1) that one molecule of the drug (D) combines with one molecule of receptor (R) to produce a drug–receptor complex (DR); (2) that the association of the drug with its receptor is reversible; and (3) that the pharmacological effect depends on the presence of the drug on the receptor. We can represent the interaction of drug with receptor as follows:

$$D + R \underset{k_{\text{diss}}}{\overset{k_{\text{ass}}}{\rightleftharpoons}} DR \tag{4.1}$$

where k_{ass} and k_{diss} are expressions (rate constants) of the relative rates of association and of dissociation respectively of drug and receptor. If we let [DR] be the concentration of receptors occupied by the drug and [R] be the concentration of receptors unoccupied, then at equilibrium the rate at which receptors are being occupied must be the same as the rate at which new drug–receptor complexes are being formed. Or to put it mathematically:

$$[D][R]k_{\text{ass}} = [DR]k_{\text{diss}} \tag{4.2}$$

Rearranging eqn (4.2) we get:

$$[D][R]/[DR] = k_{\text{diss}}/k_{\text{ass}} \tag{4.3}$$

The ratio of the two rate constants, $k_{\text{diss}}/k_{\text{ass}}$, is obviously itself a constant and can be replaced by a new constant, K_D, which is known as the apparent dissociation constant. We shall shortly see what K_D represents in terms of the drug concentration/effect relation. If the total concentration of receptors available for binding the drug is [R_{tot}], then:

$$[R_{\text{tot}}] = [R] + [DR] \tag{4.4}$$

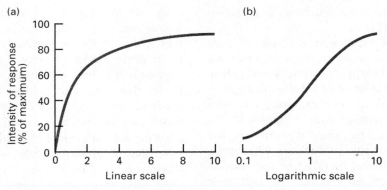

■ **Fig. 4.2** Dose–response curves. (a) When the intensity of the effect a drug produces is plotted against the drug concentration the curve takes the form of a rectangular hyperbola. (b) When it is plotted against the logarithm of the drug concentration the shape is sigmoid the log dose–response curve).

Substituting for [R] in eqn (4.3) we find that:

$$[D][R_{tot} - DR]/[DR] = k_{diss}/k_{ass} = K_D \quad (4.5)$$

and that therefore:

$$[DR]/[R_{tot}] = [D]/(K_D + [D]) \quad (4.6)$$

Let us assume that the intensity of the effect (E) is proportional to the number of receptors occupied by the drug [DR]. Then

$$E = k[DR] \quad (4.7)$$

The maximum possible effect, E_{max}, will occur when all the receptors are occupied, and so:

$$E_{max} = k[R_{tot}] \quad (4.8)$$

Dividing eqn (4.7) by eqn (4.8) we find that:

$$E/E_{max} = [DR]/[R_{tot}] \quad (4.9)$$

If we now substitute eqn (4.9) in eqn (4.6) we find that:

$$E/E_{max} = [D]/(K_D + [D]) \quad (4.10)$$

or, rearranging:

$$E = E_{max}[D]/(K_D + [D]) \quad (4.11)$$

Equation (4.11) is identical in form to the equation we have already seen in relation to the non-linear kinetics of drugs such as phenytoin and alcohol (Chapter 3, eqn (3.39), p. 38) and also to the Michaelis–Menten equation for rates of enzyme reactions.

4.3.2 Properties of the dose–response curve

It may not be immediately obvious that equation (4.11) defines the shape of the dose–response curve, as shown in Fig. 4.2. However, we shall see that that is so if we examine the properties of the equation:

1. When the effect is half-maximal, $E = E_{max}/2$. Substituting this in eqn (4.11) we find that $K_D = [D]$. In other words, K_D is the concentration of drug required to produce a half-maximal effect.

2. When [D] = 0, $E = 0$. In other words when there is no drug there is no effect.

3. When [D] is very low, [D] ≪ K_D and thus:

$$E \approx [D] \times E_{max}/K_D \quad (4.12)$$

In other words, at low concentrations of the drug the response is directly proportional to the drug concentration.

4. When [D] is very high, [D] ≫ K_D and thus:

$$E \Rightarrow E_{max} \quad (4.13)$$

In other words, high concentrations of the drug produce effects which are near maximal This means that further increases in concentration produce only small increases in effect. We can now see why the relation between the concentration of a drug and the intensity of its pharmacological effect has the shape it has (Fig. 4.2(a)). At

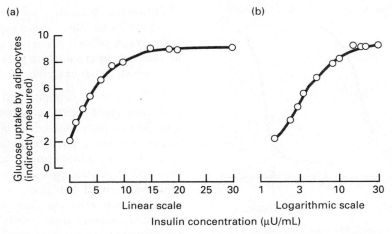

Fig. 4.3 The relation between the concentration of insulin and its effect on glucose uptake by human adipocytes *in vitro*. (Adapted from Cuatrecasas (1969) *Proc. Nat. Acad. Sci.* **63**, 450–7, with permission.)

drug concentrations below the K_D the relation is approximately linear. When the concentrations are increased to above the K_D the increase in effect becomes progressively smaller and smaller until a plateau is reached at the maximum effect. Dose–response curves of the kind shown in Fig. 4.2 are often found in experiments using human tissues *in vitro* or in animals. An example is given in Fig. 4.3, which shows the relation between the concentration of insulin and its effect on glucose uptake in human adipocytes *in vitro*.

In humans it is not usual to be able to define the dose–response curve in full: it is usually too difficult to measure the small effects produced by low doses or concentrations of drugs, and measurements cannot be made at high doses or concentrations because of toxicity. It is therefore more usual to measure drug effects which occur in the middle of the curve. Thus, log-dose–response curves will sometimes be presented as being linear rather than sigmoid, since the middle part of a sigmoid curve is approximately linear. This is demonstrated in the example given in Fig. 4.4, which shows the relation between the plasma concentration of propranolol in man and its effect in reducing exercise-induced tachycardia.

An example of a dose–response curve which can be completely delineated *in vivo* in humans is given in Fig. 4.5, which shows the relations between the urinary concentrations of the loop diuretics bumetanide and frusemide and their

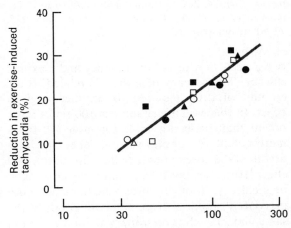

Fig. 4.4 The relation between plasma propranolol concentrations in humans and the effect of propranolol in reducing exercise-induced tachycardia. (Adapted from McDevitt and Shand (1975) *Clin. Pharmacol. Ther.* **18**, 708–13, with permission.)

diuretic effects. The *urinary* concentrations are shown because the site of action of these diuretics is on the luminal side of the renal tubule. This example is also an illustration of the fact that the dose–response relations which result when drugs inhibit ion transport are the same as those which result from drug/receptor interactions.

This comparison of the dose–response curves for bumetanide and frusemide clearly illustrates

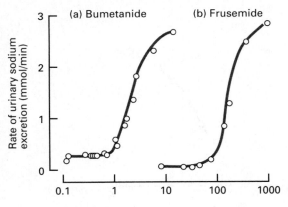

■ Fig. 4.5 The relations between the urinary excretion rates of (a) bumetanide and (b) frusemide and their effects on the rate of sodium excretion in the urine. (Redrawn from Brater *et al.* (1983) *Clin. Pharmacol. Ther.* **34**, 207-13 (bumetanide) and from Chennavasin *et al.* (1980) *J. Pharmacol. Exp. Ther.* **215**, 77–81 (frusemide), with permission.)

two aspects of drug action: potency and maximal efficacy. The potency of a drug is related to the amount of drug required to produce a given effect. In this case bumetanide is 100 times more potent than frusemide mole for mole (70 times more potent mg for mg) since it takes one hundredth of the dose to produce the same natriuretic effect. However, both drugs have the same maximal efficacy; in other words a high enough dose or concentration of frusemide will produce the same maximal effect on urinary sodium excretion as bumetanide, despite the difference in potency. When comparing drugs with each other maximal efficacy is usually a more important criterion to consider than potency. If two drugs have different potencies one simply gives a larger dose of the less potent drug, as in the case of bumetanide and frusemide. However, if two drugs have different maximal efficacies then the drug with the lower maximal efficacy will always produce a smaller maximal effect no matter how large the dose. For example, insulin has a much higher maximal efficacy than the oral hypoglycaemic drugs, whose effects in lowering blood glucose are relatively limited. The term 'high ceiling diuretics' has been applied to the loop diuretics to indicate that they have a higher maximal efficacy than other diuretics, such as the thiazides.

However, sometimes relative potencies may also be of importance. This happens, for example, if the doses of two drugs which are equipotent on one system are not equipotent on another, as the following two examples illustrate.

1. Doses of bumetanide and frusemide which have equivalent effects on urinary sodium excretion do not have equivalent effects on the ear, bumetanide being less ototoxic. This is important when choosing a loop diuretic to use in combination with the aminoglycoside antibiotics, such as gentamicin, since frusemide is more likely than bumetanide to enhance their ototoxic effects. In these circumstance bumetanide is the loop diuretic of choice.

2. Some β-adrenoceptor antagonists have different potencies in their actions on different subtypes of adrenoceptors. For example, atenolol is more potent as an antagonist at β_1-adrenoceptors than at β_2-adrenoceptors (i.e. it is a more selective β-blocker). This makes atenolol less likely than a non-selective drug, such as propranolol, to cause bronchospasm in a susceptible individual.

The concept of the therapeutic index of a drug, that is the toxic:therapeutic dose ratio, relies in part upon differential dose–response curves for therapeutic and toxic effects, as illustrated by these examples. The principles of the dose–response curve are at the core of accurate drug therapy, as the above observations illustrate, although at the clinical level all the details are sometimes hard to appreciate. On the one hand, everyone can see that increasing doses of insulin produce increasing hypoglycaemia (i.e. insulin has high maximal efficacy) and that the dose–response relation changes with so-called insulin resistance (i.e. reduced potency) in the obese. On the other hand, it is not immediately apparent that the effectiveness of aspirin in the secondary prevention of myocardial infarction is rooted in dose-responsiveness. None the less dose-responsiveness is important here too, since this action of aspirin is likely to be related, at least in part, to the extent to which it reduces platelet aggregation, an effect which is related to the dose-dependent inhibitory effect of aspirin on cyclo-oxygenase. All of these examples illustrate only a few of the areas in which dose-responsiveness can be seen to be of clinical relevance.

5 The therapeutic process

Is the pharmacological effect being translated into an appropriate therapeutic effect?

We have seen how the pharmaceutical process, involving the formulation of a drug, can affect the systemic availability of the drug, how the pharmacokinetic process determines the concentrations of the drug at its sites of action, and how in the pharmacodynamic process a pharmacological effect occurs. We must now examine how this pharmacological effect is translated into a therapeutic effect.

5.1 Translation of the pharmacological effect of a drug into a therapeutic effect during short-term drug therapy

The short-term therapeutic and toxic effects of drugs occur as a result of the pharmacological actions discussed in Chapter 4. However, the translation of molecular and cellular pharmacological effects into the therapeutic or toxic effect is not a simple process, but one which involves several translational stages at different pharmacological and physiological levels.

Take, for example, the action of salbutamol, a β_2-adrenoceptor agonist, in the treatment of asthma (Fig. 5.1).

1. Salbutamol stimulates bronchial β_2-adrenoceptors, and so increases the activity of adenylate cyclase (Fig. 4.2); this is its pharmacological effect at the molecular level.
2. The increase in adenylate cyclase activity leads to an increase in the intracellular concentration of cyclic AMP, a pharmacological effect at the cellular level.
3. The increase in cyclic AMP in some way alters the function of bronchial smooth muscle cells, and results in an inhibition of the release of inflammatory mediators from bronchial mast cells, effects on cell physiology.
4. All this in turn results in bronchodilatation, an effect on tissue physiology.
5. Bronchodilatation causes improved lung function, an effect on organ physiology.
6. Finally, the patient is able to breathe more easily, the desired clinical effect.

This analysis of the short-term effects of drugs teaches us several things about drug action. We shall discuss these under the following headings:

(1) how drug action may be modified;
(2) how therapeutic and adverse effects may be mediated via different pharmacological effects;
(3) the relation between the pharmacological effects of a drug and the rate of onset or duration of its action;
(4) drug/disease interactions.

5.1.1 How drug action may be modified

There are often ways in which the action of a drug may be beneficially or adversely modified. For example, the action of salbutamol would be expected to be potentiated at stage 2 above by a xanthine derivative, such as theophylline, which increases cellular cyclic AMP concentrations by the inhibition of phosphodiesterase. This is both

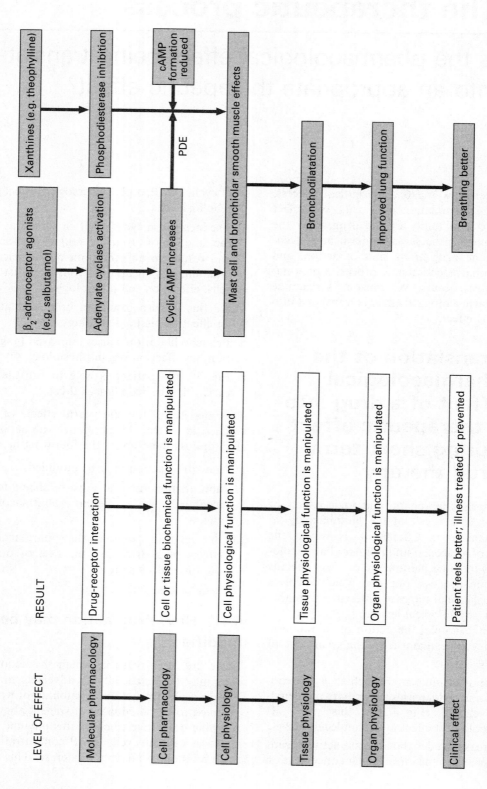

■ **Fig. 5.1.** The chain of effects linking the pharmacological effects of a drug to its clinical effects. The links between the pharmacological effects of a drug at the molecular, cellular, and tissue levels, its physiological effects on cells and organs, and its final clinical (therapeutic or adverse) effects can be considered at the different levels shown in the left-hand and middle columns. The example of the effects of salbutamol and theophylline in asthma is shown in the right-hand column. The way in which this scheme fits into drug therapy overall is shown in Fig. 6.2.

a beneficial and an adverse clinical interaction, beneficial because theophylline enhances the therapeutic action of salbutamol, adverse because it also enhances the hypokalaemia which salbutamol may cause by stimulation of $Na^+ K^+$ ATPase. Conversely, inadvertent co-prescription of propanolol would prevent the action of salbutamol on its receptor, i.e. at stage 1.

5.1.2 How therapeutic and adverse or other effects may be mediated via different pharmacological effects

There is a tendency to consider only that pharmacological effect of a drug which results directly in the therapeutic effect. However, this narrow viewpoint is wrong, since some drugs have more than one molecular mechanism of action. Thus, two different therapeutic effects of a drug may be brought about by two different actions. For example, tetracycline acts as an antibacterial agent by interfering with bacterial protein synthesis, but its therapeutic effect in acne is due to interference with the production of sebum in facial sweat glands.

Alternatively, a therapeutic effect may be brought about by one pharmacological action and an adverse effect by another. For example, the therapeutic effect of salbutamol is brought about by its action on β_2-adrenoceptors, but its main adverse effects (tachycardia and tremor) are due to stimulation of β_1-adrenoceptors.

Commonly, various different therapeutic or adverse effects may be produced by the actions of a single drug on the same or a similar molecular mechanism in different tissues. For example, the inhibition of β_2-adrenoceptors produces bronchoconstriction in the lungs of susceptible individuals and impairs glycogenolysis in the liver. The antihypertensive action of α-methyldopa is mediated by its chief metabolite, α-methylnoradrenaline, which is an agonist at α_2-adrenoceptors in areas of the brain controlling sympathetic nervous system activity, and therefore peripheral resistance; α-adrenoceptor activation elsewhere in the brain may cause drowsiness, lethargy, and depression, which are not uncommon adverse effects of methyldopa.

It is important to remember peripheral or non-therapeutic effects of drugs, since they can be of clinical importance in several ways. For example, the effect of phenobarbitone in inducing hepatic microsomal enzyme activity is peripheral to its anticonvulsant effect, but can cause difficult problems with drug interactions, for example with warfarin (see Chapter 10). Aminoglycoside antibiotics (for example gentamicin, amikacin) can all cause damage to the middle ear, leading to impaired hearing or loss of balance; these effects are quite separate from the antibiotic activity of these drugs but profoundly influence their therapeutic index and have to be taken into account when choosing dosage regimens; this leads to the requirement of plasma concentration monitoring (see Chapter 7).

5.1.3 The relation between the pharmacological effects of a drug and the rate of onset or duration of its action

It can be seen from the pharmacodynamic sequence of events outlined above for salbutamol that the rate of onset of action of a drug is related not only to its pharmacokinetics (i.e. the time it takes for the appropriate amount of drug to build up at the site of action, see pp. 23–5), but also to the time it takes for the full pharmacodynamic sequence of events to take place.

In the case of salbutamol the time between β_2-adrenoceptor stimulation and bronchodilatation is of the order of a few minutes. However, for other drugs the sequence of events takes much longer. For example, corticosteroids react with a receptor protein in the cytoplasm of certain sensitive cells to form a steroid–receptor complex (molecular pharmacology). This complex enters the cell nucleus, where it binds to chromatin and directs the genetic apparatus to transcribe RNA (cellular pharmacology). This leads, for instance in liver cells, to the *de novo* production of several enzymes involved in gluconeogenesis and amino acid metabolism (cellular physiology). Once the steroid has bound to its intracellular receptor it sets off a sequence of reactions which then has its own time-scale, independent of the quantity of steroid either in the blood or combined with the receptor. The induction of protein synthesis by RNA transcription takes several hours and each new protein will have its own biological lifespan. Thus, the eventual therapeutic outcome may take several hours or days to occur.

Similarly, the duration of action of a drug is related not only to its pharmacokinetics (i.e. the time it takes for the drug to be cleared from the body, see pp. 23 and 27), but also to the duration of its pharmacological actions. For example, aspirin inhibits cyclo-oxygenase by acetylating a serine moiety at the active site of the enzyme. In platelets this leads to inhibition of prostaglandin synthesis for the lifetime of the platelet. Thus, although aspirin is cleared from the body within a few hours, its effects on platelets last for days and can be detected by decreased platelet aggregation.

5.1.4 Drug/disease interactions

Because of the many links between the pharmacological effects of a drug and its therapeutic or adverse effects there are many ways in which the pathophysiology of the disease being treated or of other incidental diseases can alter the way in which the pharmacological effect is translated into a therapeutic effect. Interactions of this kind are known as drug/disease interactions, to distinguish them from drug/drug interactions (discussed in Chapter 10).

To consider the ways in which drug/disease interactions may influence drug therapy consider the use of digoxin in the treatment of cardiac failure (Fig. 5.2).

1. Digoxin inhibits the activity of the membrane-bound Na^+/K^+ pump enzyme, sodium-potassium adenosine triphosphatase ($Na^+ K^+$ ATPase). This is its pharmacological effect at the molecular level.

2. This inhibition of transmembrane sodium and potassium transport causes an increase in the intracellular concentration of sodium, which in turn results in an alteration in the intracellular disposition of calcium (a pharmacological effect at the cellular level).

3. The altered disposition of intracellular calcium leads to an alteration in the action potential of cardiac muscle (a physiological effect at the cellular level).

4. This in turn causes an increase in the rate of contractility of the myocardial fibres (a physiological effect at the tissue level).

5. There is a consequent increase in cardiac output (a physiological effect at the level of the whole organ).

If this chain of events occurs without interruption the clinical result will be relief of the signs and symptoms of heart failure. However, there are drug/disease interactions which may alter the therapeutic outcome at the different stages in the chain.

At stages 1 and 2 potassium depletion enhances the binding of digoxin to the $Na^+ K^+$ ATPase and this results in an increase in the extent of inhibition of sodium transport, which can in turn lead to digoxin toxicity. In this case a lower dose of digoxin may produce a satisfactory therapeutic response. Conversely, in hyperthyroidism there is an alteration in the nature of the interaction between digoxin and $Na^+ K^+$ ATPase, which results in resistance to the inhibitory effects of digoxin. However, in hyperthyroidism, increasing the dose in order to try to obtain a therapeutic effect may merely result in digoxin toxicity without ever producing a therapeutic effect.

At stage 4, in patients with chronic cor pulmonale, digoxin may inhibit the $Na^+ K^+$ ATPase and may even cause cardiac arrhythmias without ever causing an increase in the rate of myocardial contractility. The reasons for this are not clear, but they may be related to the occurrence of tissue hypoxia and acidosis in cor pulmonale. Tissue hypoxia and acidosis in patients with cardiac failure after an acute myocardial infarction may also contribute to an increased risk of digoxin-induced cardiac arrhythmias without therapeutic benefit.

At stage 5 an increased rate of myocardial contractility is not translated into an increase in cardiac output in patients with hypertrophic obstructive cardiomyopathy, since there is a fixed obstruction in the left ventricular outflow tract.

This example illustrates the ways in which resistance or increased sensitivity to the effects of a drug can be caused by drug/disease interactions. It is therefore well to remember that simply because one can sometimes demonstrate that a

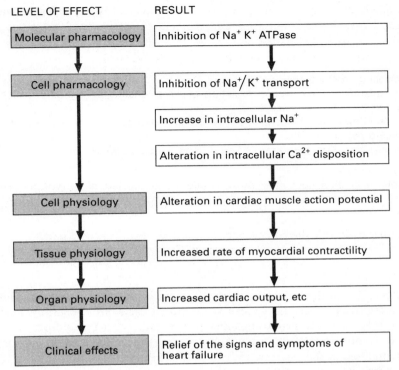

LEVEL OF EFFECT   RESULT

Molecular pharmacology	Inhibition of Na^+ K^+ ATPase
Cell pharmacology	Inhibition of Na^+/K^+ transport
	Increase in intracellular Na^+
	Alteration in intracellular Ca^{2+} disposition
Cell physiology	Alteration in cardiac muscle action potential
Tissue physiology	Increased rate of myocardial contractility
Organ physiology	Increased cardiac output, etc
Clinical effects	Relief of the signs and symptoms of heart failure

■ **Fig. 5.2.** The chain of events linking the pharmacological effects of digoxin to its therapeutic effects.

drug is having its expected action at a particular pharmacological or physiological level, one cannot automatically assume that it will have a consequent therapeutic effect.

5.2 Translation of the pharmacological effect of a drug into a therapeutic effect during long-term drug therapy

Some drugs are used in single doses to deal with an acute problem, for example intramuscular adrenaline in the treatment of anaphylactic shock. In contrast, other drugs may have to be taken for life, for example insulin in the treatment of diabetes mellitus. Between these extremes lie drug courses which vary widely in duration. For example, antibiotics are taken for days or weeks,

anticoagulants in the treatment of deep venous thrombosis for weeks or months, and antidepressants for months or years.

However, prolonged drug therapy may bring with it the phenomenon of adaptation to the short-term pharmacological effects of the drug. The clinical results of adaptation are summarized under four headings in Table 5.1, and we shall discuss them here under those headings.

5.2.1 Therapeutic effects through adaptation

(a) Immunization and vaccination

By adaptation to an initial immunological challenge the immune system develops the ability to respond to a subsequent similar challenge (for example, tetanus immunization).

(b) Tricyclic antidepressants

Although tricyclic antidepressants very quickly produce inhibition of re-uptake of noradrenaline

■ **Table 5.1**   The different ways in which adaptation to drug effects may become apparent clinically

---

1. Therapeutic effects through adaptation
   for example immunization and vaccination, tricyclic antidepressants

2. Tolerance: increasing ineffectiveness of therapy
   (a) Target cell tolerance, for example depletion of noradrenaline by ephedrine; change in sulphydryl function by nitrates; opioid tolerance
   (b) Physiological homoeostatic mechanisms, for example hydralazine (reflex tachycardia), acetazolamide (acidosis reversing hypokalaemia)
   (c) Metabolic autoinduction, for example barbiturates, carbamazepine

3. Withdrawal syndromes
   for example opiates, alcohol, benzodiazepines, clonidine, corticosteroids, enzyme inducers, β-adrenoceptor antagonists

4. Adverse effects directly due to adaptation
   for example tardive dyskinesia due to dopamine antagonists

---

and 5-hydroxytryptamine in the brain, the therapeutic effect of these drugs takes 1–2 weeks to become evident. It is known that the brain adapts to the increased concentrations of noradrenaline and 5-hydroxytryptamine in the synaptic cleft in certain areas, where the sensitivity of certain responses to neurotransmitters is decreased by 'down-regulation'. It could be that some part of this adaptive effect is the pharmacological action through which the antidepressant drugs produce their therapeutic effects.

It is not known to what extent the therapeutic effects of other drugs may be mediated through adaptive responses, but questions can be raised in regard to the therapeutic actions of β-adrenoceptor antagonists and thiazide diuretics in essential hypertension.

5.2.2 Tolerance: increasing ineffectiveness of therapy

Drug tolerance is a state of decreased responsiveness to a drug, brought about by previous exposure to that drug, or to a drug with similar short-term effects. It may occur in several ways.

(a) Pharmacological tolerance at the level of the target cell

(i) Ephedrine

Tolerance may develop to the vasoconstricting effects of ephedrine nose-drops, used in the treatment of vasomotor rhinitis. This is because ephedrine acts by releasing noradrenaline from sympathetic nerve-endings, and when the noradrenaline is depleted the ephedrine can no longer be effective.

(ii) Organic nitrates

Tolerance to organic nitrates has been described in workers handling nitroglycerine (glyceryl trinitrate) in munitions factories. When they first handle nitroglycerine they develop headaches, due to the vasodilatory effects of nitroglycerine on the extracranial arteries. As exposure continues the headaches wear off. When they stop work at the weekend the tolerance disappears, and on returning to work on Monday morning they once more experience headaches which wear off again as the week progresses. Patients who take long-term glyceryl trinitrate, particularly slow-release formulations such as transdermal patches, may also develop tolerance to its effects and may not respond to the acute effects of glyceryl trinitrate.

With the discovery that endothelium-derived relaxing factor is nitric oxide or an organic derivative thereof, it appears likely that the mode of action of the organic nitrates is via the liberation of NO_2^-, from which nitric oxide is produced. In other words the organic nitrates mimic the action of the endogenous relaxing factor. The formation of NO_2^-, and hence of nitric oxide, from organic nitrates requires the oxidation of tissue sulphydryl groups to disulphide groups. When there are no longer sulphydryl groups available to provide this reaction the tissue becomes unresponsive to nitrates. Tissue responsiveness can be restored *in vitro* by the addition of dithiothreitol, which regenerates the sulphydryl groups. This hypothesis for the mechanism of tolerance to organic nitrates is illustrated in Fig. 5.3.

(iii) Opiates

In the treatment of severe chronic pain, for example in malignant disease, tolerance may occur to the analgesic effect of morphine and other narcotic analgesics, and increasing doses may be required to alleviate the pain. However, tolerance does not occur to other effects of morphine (for example miosis of the pupils and decreased gastrointestinal motility). Despite the discovery of opioid receptors and their subtypes, of endogenous opioid peptides (enkephalins and endorphins), and of the interrelation between endogenous opioid functions and neurotransmitters, such as acetylcholine, 5-hydroxytryptamine, noradrenaline, and dopamine, the precise mechanism of morphine tolerance (and addiction withdrawal) is still not understood. However, it is generally agreed that it is at the neuronal level.

(b) Physiological tolerance by homoeostatic mechanisms

(i) Hydralazine

Hydralazine was introduced in the 1950s for the treatment of hypertension. When used alone its efficacy was not impressive, because the short-term fall in blood pressure, which it causes by peripheral vasodilatation, also causes reflex activation of the sympathetic nervous system, resulting in a tachycardia and increased cardiac output. This homoeostatic response reduces the

effectiveness of hydralazine. The problem can be overcome by the concurrent use of β-adrenoceptor antagonists, which prevent the reflex tachycardia and which increase the effectiveness of hydralazine as an antihypertensive agent. Although this interaction also reduces the risk of the hydralazine-induced lupus-like syndrome, this risk is now considered too high to warrant the use of even low doses of hydralazine as a first- or second-line treatment in most cases of hypertension.

(ii) Diuretics

Secondary hyperaldosteronism occurs as a physiological response to the sodium loss produced by loop or thiazide diuretics. The enhanced potassium excretion which this causes may be obviated by the use of a potassium-sparing diuretic (for example amiloride or the aldosterone antagonist spironolactone).

A different type of physiological tolerance occurs in patients given the diuretic acetazolamide. Acetazolamide is a very powerful kaliuretic and can cause severe potassium depletion when it is first given. However, because it inhibits carbonic anhydrase activity in the kidney it causes bicarbonate depletion, and the resulting acidosis causes retention of potassium. Thus, potassium depletion due to acetazolamide lasts only for a few days or weeks.

(c) Metabolic tolerance

Metabolic tolerance to the effects of a drug results from an increased rate of metabolism of the drug. The commonest cause of metabolic tolerance is induction of hepatic microsomal drug-metabolizing enzymes by drugs such as the barbiturates, phenytoin, carbamazepine, and griseofulvin. For example, the hepatic inactivation of the barbiturates is increased after long-term exposure to any of these drugs, so that a given dose of barbiturate produces a reduced effect, although there is also undoubtedly some cellular adaptation to the effects of the barbiturates. If this induction is caused by the barbiturates themselves the phenomenon is called 'autoinduction' (see Chapter 10, p. 127). Induction of drug metabolism in this way also forms the basis of potential adverse drug reactions (see below).

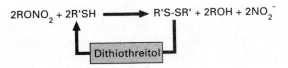

$$2RONO_2 + 2R'SH \longrightarrow R'S\text{-}SR' + 2ROH + 2NO_2^-$$

Dithiothreitol

■ **Fig. 5.3.** A proposed mechanism for tolerance to the effects of nitrates.

5.2.3 Withdrawal syndromes

A common, though not inevitable, outcome of an adaptive response to long-term drug use is the occurrence of a withdrawal response, which occurs either when the drug is withdrawn or when an antagonist is given, and which usually takes the form of some sort of adverse reaction.

(a) Opiates

A withdrawal syndrome occurs in opiate addicts when the opiate is withdrawn or when an antagonist, such as naloxone, is given. The symptoms consist of yawning, rhinorrhoea, and sweating, followed by the so-called 'cold turkey', in which there is shivering and goose flesh. Later nausea, vomiting, diarrhoea, and hypertension may occur. The acute syndrome subsides within a week, but the addict may have anxiety and sleep disturbances for several weeks or months after. This syndrome can be avoided by introducing increasing doses of methadone as the opiate is withdrawn, since withdrawal of methadone at a later stage may not result in this syndrome.

(b) Alcohol

Delirium tremens may occur on withdrawal of alcohol from chronic alcoholics. This syndrome consists of disorientation and visual hallucinations (see p. 483).

(c) Benzodiazepines

Withdrawal of benzodiazepines after long-term therapy may result in a disturbance of sleep pattern (rebound insomnia associated with abnormal sleep patterns), agitation, restlessness, and occasionally epileptic convulsions (see p. 484).

(d) Organic nitrates

Workers handling nitroglycerine have been reported in some cases to have developed acute episodes of angina pectoris and myocardial infarction on Sundays and on Monday mornings before work. This has been attributed to rebound coronary artery spasm after nitrate withdrawal (see also tolerance above).

(e) Clonidine

Sudden withdrawal of clonidine after long-term therapy commonly results in a severe and acute rise in blood pressure, accompanied by nervousness, headache, abdominal pain, sweating, and tachycardia, occurring 8–12 h after the last dose. The mechanism of this syndrome is not known, but it should be treated with α- and β-adrenoceptor antagonists (for example phentolamine and propranolol). Hypertension has also been reported after the withdrawal of another α_2-adrenoceptor agonist, methyldopa, but much less commonly than with clonidine.

(f) β-Adrenoceptor antagonists

There is an increased risk of angina pectoris and myocardial infarction in patients with ischaemic heart disease when β-adrenoceptor antagonists are withdrawn after long-term use. This may be because of an increase in the numbers of tissue β-adrenoceptors (as has been shown to occur in lymphocytes). If there is an increased number of β-adrenoceptors in the heart then when the β-adrenoceptor antagonist is withdrawn the heart might be supersensitive to the β-adrenergic effects of the sympathetic nervous system.

(g) Corticosteroids

Long-term therapy with corticosteroids suppresses pituitary adrenocorticotrophic hormone (ACTH) secretion, leading to 'wasting' of the adrenal cortex and a diminution in the degree of its immediate steroidogenic response to ACTH. When long-term steroid therapy is suddenly withdrawn, ACTH secretion by the pituitary may take several weeks or months to recover (Fig. 5.4). Since the adrenal cortex has to increase in size again in order to become normally responsive to ACTH the patient is at great risk of an Addisonian crisis if stressed.

(h) Inducers of hepatic microsomal drug-metabolizing enzymes

The withdrawal of drugs, such as the barbiturates, phenytoin, or carbamazepine, which induce hepatic microsomal drug-metabolizing enzymes, may cause a metabolic withdrawal syndrome in a patient taking a drug the metabolism of which has been reduced by the induction. The most common problem of this type involves warfarin, and the sequence of events is as follows:

(1) warfarin clearance is increased by hepatic enzyme induction;

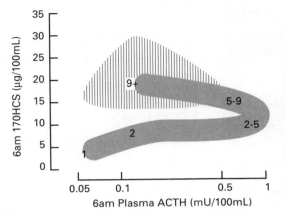

■ **Fig. 5.4.** The recovery of adrenal function after its suppression by long-term corticosteroid therapy. The numbers in the shaded area indicate the numbers of months after the withdrawal of the corticosteroid. The vertically hatched region bounds the reference values. During long-term corticosteroid therapy plasma endogenous corticosteroid and ACTH concentrations are both reduced. After withdrawal there is a gradual increase in the secretion of ACTH by the pituitary over the succeeding weeks and months. However, only much later does the adrenal gland become responsive to the increase in ACTH. When there is an eventual increase in plasma endogenous corticosteroid concentrations the secretion of ACTH by the pituitary gradually returns to normal. (Adapted from the data of Gruber *et al.* (1965). *J. Clin. Endocrinol.* **25**, 11–16, with permission.)

(2) the dose of warfarin is increased to produce a measurable pharmacological effect on clotting;

(3) withdrawal of the inducing agent leads to a decreased clearance of warfarin, which then accumulates;

(4) bleeding occurs.

5.2.4 Adverse effects directly due to adaptation

(a) Drug-induced dyskinesias

Patients taking neuroleptic drugs, such as chlorpromazine, fluphenazine, and haloperidol, continuously for long periods of time commonly develop abnormal movements. Because these abnormal movements come on late during drug use they are known collectively as tardive dyski-

nesia. The face, mouth, and tongue are most commonly affected, causing stereotyped sucking and smacking of the lips, lateral jaw movements, and fly-catching-like darting movements of the tongue. Occasionally the dyskinesia may be more widespread and may resemble choreoathetosis. It is thought that the continuous long-term blockade of brain dopamine function with neuroleptic drugs leads to increased sensitivity to the effects of dopamine in certain areas of the brain (perhaps by an increase in dopamine receptor numbers), and that tardive dyskinesia is an expression of that increased sensitivity in extrapyramidal areas of the brain.

5.3 The aims of drug therapy

In order to understand the various aims of drug therapy we must first understand the pathophysiology of disease. The processes involved in the pathophysiology of disease are illustrated in Fig. 5.5. and their relevance to drug therapy can be illustrated in the light of an example: pneumococcal pneumonia.

Every disease has a cause, which results, sometimes via contributory factors, in the primary pathology. The primary pathology in turn leads to secondary pathology and complications. The signs and symptoms of the disease may be due to the primary pathology, the secondary pathology, or the complications.

In the case of pneumococcal pneumonia the cause is infection with the pneumococcus (*Streptococcus pneumoniae*), and there may be contributory factors, such as impairment of host defence mechanisms. The primary pathology is the inflammatory response, which results in the pneumonic change. This results in abnormalities in lung function, which result in secondary pathology, including hypoxia. Whether one calls pleurisy and pleural effusion secondary pathology or complications is a matter of choice. Metastatic pneumococcal infection (for example cerebral abscess) would be regarded as a complication. Each of these, the primary pathology, the secondary pathology, and the complications, produces its own signs and symptoms (for example breathlessness, pain, cough).

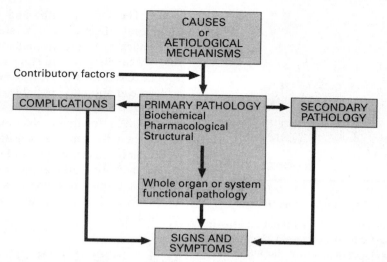

■ **Fig. 5.5.** The pathophysiological processes involved in disease. Drug therapy may be aimed at any or all of the different processes.

The point of this type of analysis of the pathophysiology of disease is that it enables one to analyse as far as possible those processes which one hopes to manipulate with drug therapy, and to define the scope of individual modes of treatment and their overall therapeutic impact. We shall take this one step further with a more detailed example.

5.3.1 The pathophysiology and treatment of bronchial asthma

The main pathophysiological features of bronchial asthma are set out in Fig. 5.6, and alongside each feature is shown the appropriate therapy.

The causes of asthma are many, since the bronchi may be hyperreactive to a number of different stimuli. Hypersensitivity reactions due to external allergens in the inspired air are responsible for so-called 'extrinsic' asthma. These allergens may be pollens, mite protein in house-dust, feathers, fungal spores, or animal dander. The hypersensitivity reactions are usually of type I and are mediated by IgE; the antigen–antibody reaction occurs on the cell membrane of the bronchial mast cell. Occasionally a type III, IgG-mediated reaction may occur (for example in allergic aspergillosis). These reactions cause the release of pharmacologically active substances, such as histamine, leukotrienes, 5-hydroxytrypta-mine, bradykinin, and perhaps other peptides, which promote the contraction of bronchial smooth muscle, leading to bronchoconstriction and an inflammatory reaction in the bronchial mucosa. In certain sensitive individuals bronchial infections may lead to a similar set of reactions. Irritants, such as tobacco smoke, cold air, and acid fumes, may trigger bronchoconstriction. Certain drugs, such as aspirin and β-adrenoceptor antagonists, may be responsible. Emotional stress may trigger attacks of bronchial asthma.

The release of inflammatory mediators results in the primary pathology, consisting of broncho-constriction, oedema of the bronchial mucosa, and the production of bronchial mucus. All these result in airways obstruction, which causes the signs and symptoms of breathlessness, wheezing, cough, fatigue, and anxiety.

Airways obstruction leads to the secondary pathology of hypoxia, and if alveolar ventilation is very poor and the residual volume greatly increased, hypercapnia may result. Emphysema may also occur because of hyperinflation.

Complications of airways obstruction are pneumothorax, bronchial infection, and acute severe asthma ('status asthmaticus'), in which airways obstruction is prolonged and unre-mitting.

As shown in Fig. 5.6 therapy can be aimed at various points in this sequence of pathological

PATHOPHYSIOLOGY	THERAPEUTIC MEASURES
1. Aetiological mechanisms	
Hypersensitivity reactions (Types I and III)	Avoidance of provocative factors; corticosteroids; ?desensitization
Bronchial infection	Antibiotics (early treatment)
Irritants	Identification and avoidance
Exercise	(Cromoglycate, β_2-adrenoceptor agonists)
Drugs	Recognition and avoidance
Psychological stress	Psychosocial management
2. Primary pathology	
Release of inflammatory mediators	Cromoglycate; β_2-adrenoceptor agonists; corticosteroids
Increased vagal tone	Ipratropium
↓	
Bronchoconstriction	β_2-adrenoceptor agonists; theophylline
Oedema of bronchial mucosa	Corticosteroids
Mucus obstruction of bronchi	
↓	
Airways obstruction	
3. Secondary pathology	
Hypoxia	Oxygen
Emphysema	
4. Complications	
Pneumothorax	Drainage
Bronchial infection	Antibiotics
Status asthmaticus	

■ **Fig. 5.6.** The pathophysiology of bronchial asthma and the corresponding therapeutic measures available.

events. Several options are available for attacking the causative mechanisms.

1. Hypersensitivity reactions may theoretically be avoided by the avoidance of provocative factors, and this requires the identification of allergens. Only occasionally is desensitization to an identified allergen successful in preventing asthma, because individuals may be sensitive to a wide range of allergens. It is possible that immune suppression is one of the mechanisms of action of systemically-administered corticosteroids in bronchial asthma.

2. For patients in whom bronchial infections trigger asthmatic attacks, early treatment of upper and lower respiratory tract infections may be effective.

3. Irritants, such as cigarette smoke, should obviously be avoided, as should precipitant drugs.

4. Exercise-induced asthma can be prevented in many patients by the prophylactic use of sodium cromoglycate or a β_2-adrenoceptor agonist, such as salbutamol, by inhalation.

5. When emotional stress seems to be involved psychotherapy and appropriate psychosocial management may seem indicated, but this is very difficult to carry out in practice.

Many of the most effective therapeutic alternatives available are aimed at the primary pathology.

1. Sodium cromoglycate and corticosteroids are given by inhalation to prevent attacks. They both probably act by preventing the release of inflammatory mediators, although cromoglycate may act by inhibiting local axon reflexes in the lungs. Salbutamol and other β_2-adrenoceptor agonists stimulate mast cell adenylate cyclase, raise cellular cyclic AMP concentrations, and thus inhibit the release of inflammatory mediators. They may therefore also be of use in prophylactic therapy.

2. Whether or not there is increased vagal tone in patients with chronic bronchitis accompan-

ied by bronchial asthma is uncertain, but it does seem that anticholinergic drugs, such as ipratropium, might be particularly effective in these patients.

3. Bronchoconstriction may be relieved by β_2-adrenoceptor agonists, which relax bronchial smooth muscle, possibly by the stimulation of adenylate cyclase and a consequent rise in intracellular cyclic AMP concentrations. Theophylline also acts as a bronchodilator by mechanisms which are not understood, but which may be related to its action as a phosphodiesterase inhibitor.

4. Corticosteroids have anti-inflammatory effects, and prevent or reduce oedema of the bronchial mucosa and the degree of mucus secretion. Breathing exercises and coughing during aerosol bronchodilator administration may be effective in removing obstruction by mucus, thus allowing easier access to the site of action of inhaled corticosteroids, β_2-adrenoceptor agonists, or ipratropium.

For hypoxia, the secondary pathology, oxygen should be given, although if there is severe airways obstruction with hypercapnia the danger of reducing the hypoxic drive to ventilation by giving oxygen and of inducing carbon dioxide narcosis because of decreased ventilation must be kept in mind.

The complications of pneumothorax and secondary bronchial infection should be treated appropriately, by drainage and antibiotics.

It should be noted that although this analysis shows how the therapeutic aims can be achieved by an understanding of the pathophysiology of the disease and the pharmacology of the drugs used to treat it, it gives no feeling for the precise therapeutic practices required for the management of the different clinical presentations of asthma: chronic asthma with or without episodic exacerbations, acute episodes with relatively normal airways between attacks, and acute severe asthma. Furthermore, the analysis does not deal with the different ways in which drugs may be given (for example orally, rectally, by inhaler, by nebulizer, or parenterally) in order to best achieve their therapeutic effects in specific circumstances.

Nevertheless, this type of analysis is essential for a basic understanding of the broad aims of drug therapy, and we shall emphasize this approach in the later sections of the book in which we shall deal with the ways in which drugs are used to treat disease.

6 Practical applications of the analysis of drug therapy

In this chapter we shall deal with the ways in which the theory outlined in the previous four chapters can be applied to the use of drugs in clinical practice.

6.1 The application of pharmacokinetics to the planning of drug dosage regimens

A drug dosage regimen is, as it were, a recipe for the administration of a drug so as to produce the desired therapeutic effect with the minimum of unwanted effects. A regimen can be described in terms of the dose of drug to be used, the frequency with which it is administered, the route of administration, and the formulation used.

The simplest way of determining a drug dosage regimen for an individual patient is to base it on the published recommended dosage. Recommended dosages can be found in the Pharmacopoeia of this book, or in standard reference texts, such as the *British National Formulary*, the *Physician's Desk Reference*, or manufacturers' data sheets. These recommendations have generally been derived from the results of studies of the pharmacokinetics of the drug and of dose/effect relationships, although in some cases they may have been empirically derived from simple clinical observations of the dosage which produces therapeutic benefit while minimizing unwanted effects.

The general method of using published dosage recommendations is to start at the lower end of the recommended dosage range and monitor for a therapeutic effect. If the desired effect does not occur one can then increase the dose gradually, until one reaches the upper end of the recommended dosage range.

For example, the recommended oral dosage range for frusemide when used as a diuretic is 40–160 mg once daily. One would therefore usually start with an oral dosage of 40 mg daily; if a satisfactory therapeutic effect did not occur one could then increase the dosage to 80 mg daily, then to 120 mg daily, and finally to 160 mg daily. If even then a therapeutic effect was not obtained one could change the route of administration from oral to intravenous, try another drug (such as bumetanide), or revise one's diagnosis. One can work in this way with frusemide in all patients, because it is a drug which has a high toxic:therapeutic ratio, and because it is not subject to drug interactions which might enhance its toxicity.

However, for drugs with a low toxic:therapeutic ratio, dosage regimens are not so simple, since dosage requirements vary widely from individual to individual, may be affected by changes in renal or hepatic function or other disease processes, and may also be affected by drug interactions. For such drugs it is therefore important to understand some of the principles whereby one may alter dosage regimens to suit the individual.

6.1.1 The loading dose

As described in Chapter 3, if one gives a dose of a drug at regular intervals (the so-called maintenance dose) it takes a certain amount of time before the drug accumulates in the body to a satisfactory degree (see Figs 3.9, 3.10, and 3.12). If this delay is unacceptable it may be circumvented by giving a loading dose. The loading dose is the amount of drug which would be present in the body if the relevant maintenance dose were given for long enough to achieve steady state (i.e. 4 or 5 half-times). This principle is illustrated in Fig. 3.13.

The amount of drug in the body at steady state (i.e. the loading dose) is related to the apparent volume of distribution and the steady-state plasma drug concentration thus:

$$\frac{\text{amount}}{\text{in body}} = \text{volume} \times \frac{\text{concentration}}{\text{in plasma}} \qquad (6.1)$$

This relationship allows one, in theory, to calculate the loading dose of drug required to produce a given plasma drug concentration. In most cases, however, one does not know what plasma concentration is appropriate to produce a therapeutic effect or to avoid toxicity, and in such cases one relies upon collective practical experience for guidance. In contrast, in those cases for which a target plasma concentration is known from clinical studies (for example digoxin, gentamicin) and the apparent volume of distribution from pharmacokinetic studies, one can use these factors in designing dosage regimens, and thus improve the precision of one's drug therapy.

Although this may sound over-complicated, in practice it is implicit in one's use of the drug dosages which are recommended in textbooks and manufacturers' literature. Indeed, during modern drug development the pharmacokinetics of all new drugs are worked out and are used in the design of recommended dosage schedules.

The use of the apparent volume of distribution is also implicit in dosages based on body weight or surface area, since the variability of the apparent volume of distribution is less when that volume is expressed in litres per kilogram of body weight or in litres per square metre of body surface area than when expressed without such correction. Examples, whose dosages can be found in the Pharmacopoeia, include the cytotoxic drugs (for example cytarabine, doxorubicin, 5-fluorouracil), antiarrhythmic drugs (for example lignocaine, amiodarone), cardiac glycosides (for example digoxin), and catecholamines (for example dopamine).

It may also be useful to know that in some circumstances the apparent volume of distribution may be altered, and that in those cases the loading dose may have to be altered accordingly. For example, the apparent volume of distribution of digoxin is reduced in severe renal failure and loading doses should therefore be reduced by about a third. The manner in which one gives the loading dose depends on the drug. For a drug with a high toxic:therapeutic ratio the loading dose can be given as a single dose; for example, one might start treatment with amoxycillin with twice the intended maintenance dose. For a drug with a low toxic:therapeutic ratio and a long half-time, one would divide the loading dose into several portions and give them at intervals long enough to allow the detection of adverse effects but short enough to ensure that the loading dose is a true loading dose (i.e. that relatively little is eliminated from the body during the period of loading); this is the basis on which the dosage recommendations for digoxin given in the Pharmacopoeia have been developed (see p. 574).

Drugs which have a low toxic:therapeutic ratio and a short half-time pose a special problem. Take the example of lignocaine. One wants to give an intravenous loading dose which will produce a particular plasma concentration (say 8 µmol/L) and to follow it up with a maintenance infusion which will maintain that concentration at steady state. In other words, the plasma concentration/time curve should be a square wave. It turns out that if the appropriate loading dose is given, followed by the appropriate maintenance dose, the plasma concentration dips for a time after the loading dose and then recovers to the intended steady-state concentration (this is because of the time it take for the drug to be distributed throughout the body after its initial administration). Thus, for a time the patient is being under-treated. However, if one gives a higher loading dose to compensate for this dip one runs the risk of causing toxicity.

The solution to this problem is to give the appropriate loading dose as a single injection (a 'bolus') and to follow it up not with an ordinary infusion but with a loading infusion, which is one which starts higher than appropriate and is gradually reduced to the appropriate maintenance rate. It can be shown from theoretical calculations that the ideal rate at which such an infusion should be reduced is exponential, but since this is difficult to achieve in practice it is possible to compromise by starting with a high rate of infusion and halving the rate at progressively longer intervals. This is illustrated in Fig. 6.1, which shows the plasma lignocaine con-

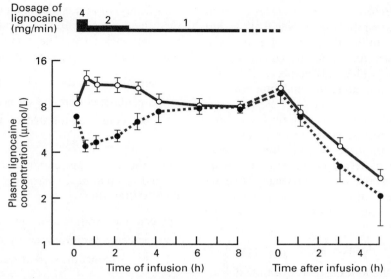

∎ **Fig. 6.1** The plasma lignocaine concentrations resulting from two different intravenous dosage regimens. In both regimens an initial loading bolus dose of 75–100 mg was given. The filled circles show the results of following the bolus with a continuous infusion at a rate of 1 mg/min. The open circles show the results of following the bolus with an intravenous loading infusion, starting at a rate of 4 mg/min for 0.5 h, followed by 2 mg/min for 2 h, and ending up with a maintenance infusion at a rate of 1 mg/min. The second regimen produces a more satisfactory time-course of plasma concentrations. (Adapted from Aps *et al.* (1976) *Br. Med. J.* **i**, 13–15, with permission.)

centrations which result from these two different types of regimen. After an intravenous loading dose of 75–100 mg and a maintenance infusion of 1 mg/min the plasma concentration rises to 7 μmol/L, dips to 4 μmol/L, and then over the next 5 h rises again to 8 μmol/L. In contrast the exponential infusion, mimicked by giving 4 mg/min for 0.5 h followed by 2 mg/min for 2 h, followed by 1 mg/min, produces the desired square wave, maintaining the initial plasma concentration at about 10 mg/L.

6.1.2 The maintenance dose

If one has decided on a particular loading dose, then in most cases the maintenance dose calculation is simple. Since half the total body load will be lost in one half-time, the maintenance dose should be half the loading dose given once every half-time. Take as an example the administration of digoxin (half-time about 40 h if renal function is normal). If the loading dose is 15 micrograms/kg the loading dose for a 60 kg patient will be 0.9 mg (in practice one would give 1.0 mg). The

maintenance dose would be 0.45 mg every 40 h; if one scales this dose down to 24 h by simple proportion one calculates a daily maintenance dose of $(0.45 \times 24)/40 = 0.27$ mg. In practice, one would give 0.25 mg once daily. This proportionality calculation yields a slightly inaccurate answer, since it assumes that the dose–time relationship is arithmetic, whereas it is in fact logarithmic. However, the error in the arithmetic method is so small as to be negligible in practice and the method is easier to remember and the calculation easier to make than with the logarithmic method.

This process can, of course, be carried out in reverse. Having decided on a particular maintenance dose which you think will be suitable you can back-calculate the total body load. Take the example of digoxin again. You decide to give a maintenance dose of 5 micrograms/kg to a 70 kg patient with normal renal function, i.e. 0.35 mg once daily (in practice you would give 0.375 mg, i.e. 0.25 + 0.125 mg). This daily maintenance dose is roughly equivalent (by arithmetical proportionality) to 0.6 mg every 40 h. The appropriate total body load is therefore 2×0.6, i.e. 1.2 mg (given as 1.25 mg). These simple methods will allow you to calculate the total body load for a given maintenance dose, and thus to calculate any alterations in dose which may be necessary if, for example, there is a change in renal function (see below).

These calculations are acceptable for a drug with a long half-time, since the incorrect assumption that the dose–time relationship is linear yields only a small error. However, for a drug with a short half-time (say, less than 24 h) we cannot assume arithmetic proportionality because the error becomes too large. The formula used is:

$$\text{loading dose} = \text{dosage rate} \times t_{1/2}/\log_e 2 \quad (6.2)$$

For instance, in the loading dose example discussed above, if one intends to end up with an infusion rate of lignocaine ($t_{1/2} = 1$ h) of 1 mg/kg/h at steady state in a 70 kg patient (i.e 70 mg/h) the bolus loading dose would be $(70 \times 1)/0.7 = 100$ mg.

6.1.3 Altering the maintenance dose when drug clearance alters

If the clearance of a drug from the body alters, then the maintenance dosage must be changed. For example, in renal impairment the clearance of drugs which are predominantly cleared by the kidneys is reduced. Examples include digoxin, the aminoglycoside antibiotics (for example gentamicin), and lithium.

The total body clearance of a drug and its steady-state plasma concentration are related in the following manner:

Concentration = (fraction of dose absorbed

$\times$ dose)/(total clearance $\times$ dosing interval)

or in symbols:

$$C_{ss} = f.D/CL.\tau \quad (6.3)$$

Thus, in circumstances in which total body clearance is changing one will be able to maintain the same mean steady-state plasma concentration by altering the dose or dosing interval in a way which is proportional to the change in total body clearance (assuming that there is no concomitant change in drug absorption). If the drug is cleared completely, or almost completely, via the kidneys then the dosage should be changed in proportion to renal clearance. The relationship on which one's calculations may be based is:

percentage eliminated in one dosing interval =

percentage eliminated by non-renal routes

+ percentage eliminated by the renal route

$$(6.4)$$

Since the percentage eliminated renally is linearly related to creatinine clearance, this equation can be rewritten thus:

percentage eliminated in one dosing interval =

percentage eliminated by non-renal routes

+ (constant $\times$ creatinine clearance) (6.5)

The percentage eliminated in one dosage interval by non-renal routes is usually constant and known from published data. The constant by which the creatinine clearance must be multiplied to give the percentage excreted in one dosage interval by renal routes will be known from published experiments in patients with different degrees of renal impairment, or can be calculated from the half-time and non-renal clearance.

To illustrate how the calculations are made, take two examples:

(a) Gentamicin

Gentamicin is almost completely cleared unchanged by the kidneys, only about 2 per cent being cleared per day by non-renal mechanisms. Thus, the change in dosage in renal failure is almost exactly proportional to the change in creatinine clearance, although the error one would make in making the assumption that it was exactly proportional becomes greater at very low rates of clearance, when non-renal clearance starts to have a significant effect. The proportionality constant relating renal gentamicin clearance to creatinine clearance is 0.3. Thus, for gentamicin the equation reads:

percentage of total body load eliminated in one

day = 2 per cent + (0.3 $\times$ creatinine clearance)

$$(6.6)$$

From this relationship one can calculate the daily

elimination rate of gentamicin for different values of creatinine clearance, as shown in Table 6.1.

(b) Digoxin

In contrast to gentamicin, a significant proportion of total digoxin clearance is by non-renal mechanisms (about 14 per cent per day). The proportionality constant relating renal digoxin clearance to creatinine clearance is 0.2. Thus, for digoxin the equation reads:

$$\text{percentage of total body load eliminated}$$
$$\text{in one day} = 14 \text{ per cent} +$$
$$(0.2 \times \text{creatinine clearance}) \qquad (6.7)$$

From this relationship one can calculate the daily elimination rate of digoxin for different values of creatinine clearance, as shown in Table 6.1.

In Table 6.2 is a list of drugs for which calculations of this kind may be useful in altering dosage regimens in conditions of changing renal function. Also listed are the percentages eliminated in unit time by non-renal mechanisms and the constant by which creatinine clearance must be multiplied to assess the contribution which the kidneys make to total clearance. This enables one

∎ **Table 6.1** The proportions by which the dosages of gentamicin and digoxin should be reduced in renal failure

Creatinine clearance (mL/min)	Daily elimination rate in per cent (fraction) of total body load	Ratio of renal failure dose: usual dose
(a) Gentamicin		
100	32 (1/3)	32:32 = 1
50	17 (1/6)	17:32 = 1:2
30	11 (1/9)	11:32 = 1:3
20	8 (1/12)	8:32 = 1:4
15	6.5 (1/15)	6.5:32 = 1:5
10	5 (1/20)	5:32 = 1:6
(b) Digoxin		
100	34 (1/3)	34:34 = 1
50	25 (1/4)	25:34 = 3:4
25	19 (1/5)	19:34 = 3:5
10	16 (1/6)	16:34 = 3:6
0	14 (1/7)	14:34 = 3:7

∎ **Table 6.2** Renal and non-renal contributions to the clearance of some drugs whose dosages should be reduced in renal impairment

Drug	NR (% per h)	R (per hour)
Ampicillin	10	0.6
Carbenicillin	6	0.6
Cephalexin	3	0.7
Gentamicin*	2	0.3
Kanamycin*	1	0.25
Lincomycin*	6	0.1
Methyldopa*	3	0.2
Penicillin G	3	1.4
Procainamide*	0.7	0.2
Streptomycin*	1	0.25
Trimethoprim	2	0.04
	NR (% per day)	R (per day)
Digoxin*	14	0.2
Ouabain*	30	0.9

*Drugs with a low toxic:therapeutic ratio.

Instructions: To calculate the per cent of total body drug which is eliminated in one hour or one day (P) calculate:

$$P = NR + (R.CL_{\text{creat}}).$$

Compare the value of P thus obtained using the patient's creatinine clearance in this equation (mL/min) with the value obtained by using a value of 100 mL/min and adjust the dose proportionately. The examples of gentamicin and digoxin are worked out in Table 6.1.

Other drugs whose dosages should be reduced in renal failure include allopurinol, amphotericin, disopyramide, ethambutol, lithium, methotrexate, quinine, and most other penicillins, cephalosporins, and aminoglycosides besides those listed here. For drugs which should be avoided or used with care in patients with renal failure see Table 26.6.

to make the calculations necessary to adjust dosage regimens of these drugs in an analogous way to the calculations for gentamicin and digoxin shown in Table 6.1.

These calculations involve the following assumptions:

(1) that drug elimination follows first-order kinetics (see p. 22);

(2) that the drug's metabolites are inactive;

(3) that absorption, distribution, and metabolism are unchanged in patients with renal failure

(changes in the apparent volume of distribution make no difference to the steady-state plasma concentration);

(4) that there is a linear relationship between the renal clearance of the drug and creatinine clearance;

(5) that renal clearance does not change during dosage;

(6) that there is no change in the response sensitivity to the drug in renal impairment.

In practice most of these assumptions are usually justified, although in cases where renal function is improving with therapy (for example the treatment of an acute septicaemia with gentamicin) it can be very difficult to predict what the correct dose of the drug will be during a given dosage interval. The circumstances in which the response of the tissues changes in renal impairment are discussed in Chapter 26 (p. 355).

In contrast to the relative simplicity of the calculations for altering dosage regimens in renal failure, it is difficult to cope with altered hepatic function, since there is no single test which accurately predicts the way in which metabolism of drugs will change in hepatic impairment in the way that the creatinine clearance predicts the way in which renal excretion will change in renal impairment.

However, if one is in a position to measure the half-time of the drug then dosage calculations may be made on the basis of that measurement, irrespective of the cause of the change in drug disposition (for example renal or hepatic impairment).

Take, for example, the case of digoxin mentioned above. At a loading dose of 15 micrograms/kg in a 60 kg patient (i.e. 0.9 mg), and a half-time of 40 h, the maintenance dose was 0.45 mg every 40 h, i.e. about 0.25 mg daily. If the measured half-time were prolonged to say 96 h, for whatever reason, the maintenance dose would be 0.45 mg every 96 h, i.e. 0.113 mg every 24 h; in this case one would give 0.125 mg daily.

However, as can be seen from Fig. 3.10, changing the maintenance dose to cope with a change in clearance results in an alteration in the degree of fluctuation in plasma concentrations during a dosage interval. This is not so important for digoxin, for which it is the mean steady-state concentration which is important, but it does become important for the aminoglycoside antibiotics, such as gentamicin, for which both peak and trough plasma concentrations are important. In such cases it may be necessary to alter not only the total dose administered in a period of time but also the dosage interval. This is illustrated in Chaper 7 (p. 92), in the various examples of how to change gentamicin dosage regimens based on repeated plasma concentration measurements and can be considered more formally here, at least for the steady-state case.

The general equations which relate the maximum (i.e. peak) and minimum (i.e. trough) plasma concentrations at steady state to the maintenance dose (D_M) and half-time are:

$$C_{ss.max} \times V = [D_M/(1 - e^{-k\tau})] \qquad (6.8)$$

$$C_{ss.min} \times V = [D_M/(1 - e^{-k\tau})] - D_M \qquad (6.9)$$

where $k = \log_e 2/t_{1/2}$ (see eqn 3.11) and $\tau =$ the dosage interval. (In passing, note that eqns 6.1 and 6.8 combine to yield eqn 3.34.) If one knows the half-time at which the original maintenance dosage was appropriate and the new half-time, then the appropriate new maintenance dose or dosage interval can be simply calculated by comparing the values of D_M or τ which will produce the desired values of $C_{ss.max}$ and $C_{ss.min}$ in the two different states.

For example, consider the administration of gentamicin 80 mg 12-hourly to a patient whose gentamicin half-time is prolonged from the normal value of 4 h to 10 h because of renal failure, and whose peak and trough plasma concentrations are 8 mg/L and 1 mg/L. This information can be summarized as shown in Table 6.3.

Fitting the values shown in Table 6.3 into eqn 6.5. we can see that if we keep the dosage interval at 12 h the new maintenance dose which would produce the same peak concentration would be 52 mg. Using eqns 6.8 and 6.9 to calculate the plasma concentrations which would result from a regimen of 50 mg 12-hourly we find them to be 7.8 mg/L (peak) and 3.4 mg/L (trough). The reason that the trough concentration has increased is that the half-time is prolonged and our old dosage interval has not given enough time for the trough concentration to fall as low as it did before. If we wanted to have a lower trough concentration we would have to prolong the dosage interval, and might decide to give twice the

■ **Table 6.3** Pharmacokinetic variables of gentamicin in a case of changing renal function

	Normal	Renal failure
$t_{1/2}$ (h)	4	10
k (h^{-1})	0.173	0.0693
$C_{ss.max}$ (mg/L)	8	5–12 (desired)
$C_{ss.min}$ (mg/L)	1	2 (desired)
D_M (mg)	80	?
τ (h)	12	?
V (L)	11.4	11.4

V is calculated from eqn 6.8 and is assumed to be unaffected by renal failure. For calculation of the required dosage regimen in renal failure see the text.

dose half as often, i.e. 100 mg every 24 h. Now the calculated peak and trough concentrations are 10.8 mg/L and 2.1 mg/L, respectively.

If we were still not satisfied with the trough concentration we might prolong the dosage interval further and think about giving say 150 mg every 36 h. However, the more we spread out the dosages to reduce the trough concentration, the higher the peak concentration becomes (since the area under the curve for a given dose must remain constant at a constant rate of clearance), and so a slight reduction in the administered dose is required to prevent that. A dosage of 120 mg every 36 h would give peak and trough concentrations of 11.5 mg/L and 1 mg/L respectively. This would be a satisfactory regimen.

This was not a straightforward example. It required several calculations before a satisfactory answer was found. However, it does illustrate how it is possible to make rational decisions about drug therapy when the clearance of a drug is altered.

6.2 The application of the processes of drug therapy in analysing failure to respond to treatment

When faced with a problem in drug therapy we can use our understanding of the four processes of drug therapy to help in our analysis of the problem. The previously simplified scheme depicting the four processes (Fig. 1.1) has been elaborated upon in Fig. 6.2.

The main categories of therapeutic problem are:

(1) apparent failure to respond to treatment;

(2) adverse drug effects;

(3) adverse drug interactions.

Beside these 'operational' problems there is also the question of the benefit:risk ratio, which is discussed in Chapter 17. However, that is not specifically a problem involving the analytical approach we have been discussing here.

We shall deal here with the first problem only. Similar principles apply to the first two problems, which are discussed elsewhere, adverse effects of drugs in Chapter 9 and adverse drug interactions in Chapter 10.

If a patient appears not to be responding to treatment with a particular drug we must examine the possible reasons.

6.2.1 The pharmaceutical process (Is the drug getting into the patient?)

(a) Compliance

Is the patient taking the drug? Non-compliance is a common reason for failure to respond to treatment. It is discussed in Chapter 13.

(b) Is the formulation ideal?

There is evidence that the absorption of iron from slow-release iron formulations may be erratic. If a patient is being treated, for convenience, with such a formulation and is not responding it may be worth switching to a simpler formulation (for example ferrous sulphate tablets) before trying more complicated measures, such as intramuscular administration or blood transfusion.

Two other examples of problems arising from formulations occur with formulations of lithium salts and theophylline. In the UK at the time of writing lithium is available as carbonate and citrate salts in different formulations:

(1) Camcolit 250® tablets: 250 mg $Li_2CO_3 =$ 6.8 mmol Li^+;

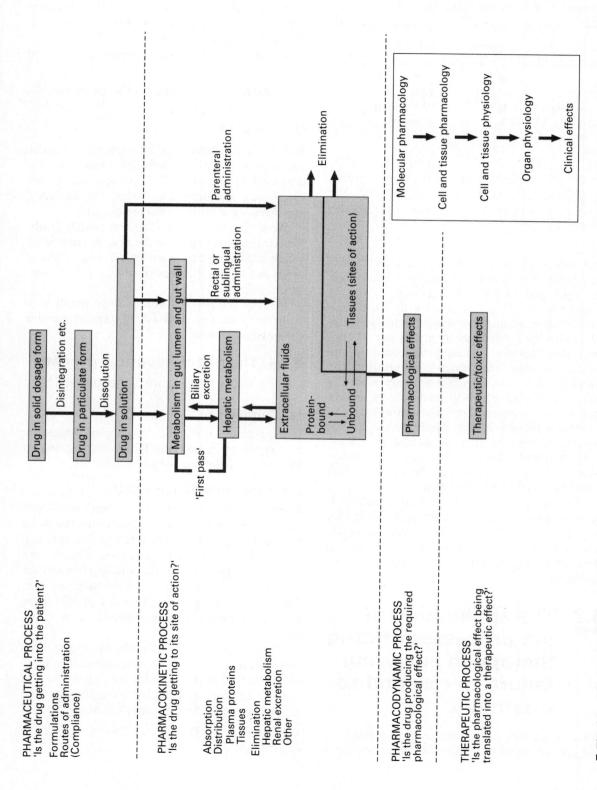

■ **Fig. 6.2** The four main processes involved in drug therapy. This diagram is basically the same as that shown in Fig. 1.1, but more detail is given.

(2) Camcolit 400® tablets: 400 mg $Li_2CO_3 =$ 10.8 mmol Li^+;

(3) Liskonum® sustained-release tablets: 450 mg $Li_2CO_3 = 12.2$ mmol Li^+;

(4) Phasal® sustained-release tablets: 300 mg $Li_2CO_3 = 8.1$ mmol Li^+;

(5) Priadel® sustained-release tablets: 200 mg $Li_2CO_3 = 5.4$ mmol Li^+, and 400 mg $Li_2CO_3 = 10.8$ mmol Li^+;

(6) Litarex® sustained-release tablets: 564 mg lithium citrate = 6 mmol Li^+;

(7) Priadel® liquid: lithium citrate 5.4 mg (= 5.4 mmol) Li^+ in 5 mL.

Similarly, theophylline is currently available in ten different sustained-release formulations containing from 60 mg to 350 mg of theophylline.

The dissolution and absorption characteristics of lithium and theophylline (and aminophylline) formulations may not be suitable for a given patient, and if there is an apparent mismatch between the dose of lithium or theophylline and the plasma lithium or theophylline concentration it may be worth changing formulation. The converse of this principle is that changes in response to treatment may occur if a patient changes from one formulation to another (for example on changing doctors, especially if communication is poor). It is obviously important, therefore, that great care be taken when prescribing lithium salts or theophylline to make sure that the formulation the patient is given is appropriate for that patient. Plasma concentration measurement in monitoring therapy with these drugs is discussed in Chapter 7.

(c) Is the route of administration appropriate?

It is a common clinical observation that patients with oedema in congestive cardiac failure may not respond to oral frusemide in the usual doses, perhaps because of erratic absorption. Such patients may respond to intravenous frusemide.

(d) Is the patient taking the drug properly?

If you ask asthmatics to demonstrate their technique for taking bronchodilators or corticosteroids by inhalation you will be surprised at how many of them use their inhalers incorrectly. The correct technique is described on p. 308.

Occasionally a patient with diabetes mellitus may be injecting insulin intracutaneously rather than subcutaneously. This too can be avoided by careful education.

From time to time patients may make simple errors in regard to other relatively straightforward matters, such as frequency of dosing, timing of dosing, and the actual dose being taken. These can easily be remedied by education.

6.2.2 The pharmacokinetic process (Is the drug getting to its site of action?)

(a) Is the drug being absorbed?

In malabsorption states, or in patients with intestinal resections, the absorption of some drugs may be impaired (for example digoxin, thyroxine). In patients with gastrointestinal hurry the absorption of drugs from slow-release formulations may be impaired. In such cases an alternative should be used (for example effervescent potassium salts rather than slow-release formulations).

(b) Is there altered distribution?

This question of protein binding is discussed in Chapters 3 and 10. The commonly used drugs for which it may be important are warfarin and phenytoin.

(c) Is there an increase in metabolic or renal clearance?

Theophylline clearance is increased in some circumstances, for example in patients who smoke cigarettes (see Table P11). In such cases dosage requirements are increased.

Patients with septicaemic shock and poor renal function may be treated with gentamicin. As their condition improves and renal function returns to normal the dosage of gentamicin may need to be increased to maintain therapeutic efficacy.

In hyperthyroidism the clearance of some drugs may be increased and higher dosages required (see p. 375).

6.2.3 The pharmacodynamic process (Is the drug producing the required pharmacological effect?)

Sometimes there are factors which alter drug effects at the site of action, even when the concentration reaching the site of action is that which one would usually expect to have an appropriate pharmacodynamic effect. For example, bacterial resistance may be the cause of therapeutic failure with antibiotics and there is tissue resistance to the effects of cardiac glycosides in hyperthyroidism.

Progressive tolerance to drugs may reduce their efficacy, as in the case of narcotic analgesics. The subject of drug tolerance is discussed in Chapter 4 and the related topic of drug dependence in Chapter 34. Insulin resistance is common in diabetic ketoacidosis and in certain obese diabetics, particularly if they are also taking glucocorticoids. In these circumstances the need for increased insulin dosages is readily appreciated, because of the ease with which therapy may be monitored by measuring blood glucose concentrations.

Some drugs used in the treatment of hypertension may cause fluid retention (for example ACE inhibitors, minoxidil), and that in turn diminishes their hypotensive actions. Such drugs are therefore more effective when used in combination with a diuretic.

6.2.4 The therapeutic process (Is the pharmacological effect being translated into a therapeutic effect?)

If a drug regimen does not produce therapeutic benefit in a patient, and if pharmaceutical, pharmacokinetic, and pharmacodynamic factors can be ruled out, then clearly the pharmacological effect is not being translated into a therapeutic effect. There may be a number of causes for this.

(a) Inappropriate therapy

Some patients with depression do not respond to antidepressant drug therapy, despite faultless compliance and 'adequate' plasma drug concentrations. There is no way at present of being certain in such circumstances that the drugs are producing an appropriate pharmacodynamic effect, because the precise mechanism by which antidepressants produce their therapeutic effect is not known. However, considering the occurrence of adverse effects with these drugs it would be surprising if they were not having their expected pharmacological effects, even in many

patients in whom the desired therapeutic response, i.e. relief of depression, is not seen. It is interesting, therefore, that some patients who do not respond to antidepressant drugs do benefit from electroconvulsive therapy, which may produce its therapeutic effect in depression by mechanisms different from those of antidepressant drugs. In these cases antidepressant drugs may be looked on as being inappropriate therapy.

Not infrequently, patients with supraventricular and ventricular arrhythmias are unresponsive to antiarrhythmic drug therapy, even when there is every reason to believe that the drug is exerting the pharmacological effect which normally stops or prevents such arrhythmias. For instance, quinidine causes a widening of the QRS complex of the electrocardiogram (ECG) and prolongs the QT_c interval, these effects being concentration-related. In circumstances where ECG changes of this kind are seen but no therapeutic effect occurs it may be helpful to assume that the treatment is inappropriate and to try a drug with a different pharmacological effect on the cardiac conducting system, for example amiodarone.

(b) Variable links between the pharmacodynamic effect and the therapeutic effect

If a drug is to be of use, it must first reach its site of action, and its pharmacodynamic actions there must then be translated into a therapeutic effect. Often there are factors which influence both of these processes. Consider, for example, the action of the diuretic frusemide in the treatment of cardiac failure (Fig. 6.3). Frusemide inhibits sodium and chloride reabsorption by the renal tubules. This effect is probably mediated by inhibition of the $Na^+/K^+/Cl^-$ co-transport system in the renal tubules. To exert this effect, frusemide must first reach the luminal surface of the tubule. In these circumstances the effect of frusemide is dependent on:

(1) renal blood flow (altered in heart failure and hypovolaemia);

(2) glomerular filtration rate (reduced in renal failure);

(3) humoral factors modulating tubular sodium reabsorption (hyperaldosteronism, for example in heart failure, hepatic cirrhosis, the

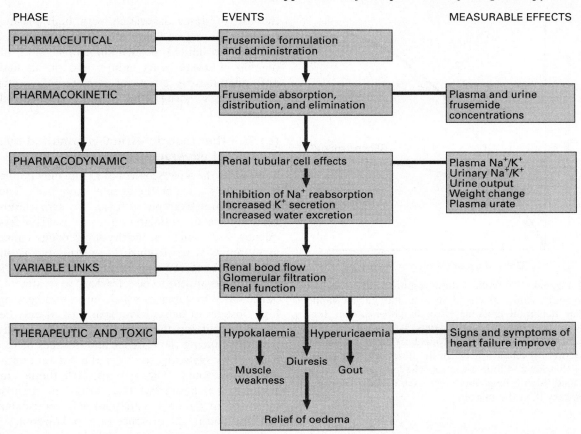

∎ **Fig. 6.3** The chain of events linking the administration of frusemide with its therapeutic or toxic effects. Note the variables which link the pharmacokinetics of frusemide to its pharmacodynamic effects and its pharmacodynamic effects to its therapeutic or toxic effects.

nephrotic syndrome, or as a secondary response to diuretic action).

If renal blood flow is poor, frusemide may not reach the tubular lumen in a concentration sufficient to exert its therapeutic effect. If there is a good intraluminar flow of glomerular filtrate containing sodium and chloride then a diuresis will result. However, if glomerular filtration is poor, and if secondary hyperaldosteronism is increasing sodium reabsorption, frusemide may be less effective.

These are the links which modify the arrival of frusemide at the renal tubular cell, its molecular effects there, and its eventual diuretic effect. If frusemide is ineffective in severe cardiac failure a diuresis may sometimes be produced by the administration of a low dose of dopamine (caus-

ing renal vasodilatation), of a higher dose of dopamine (causing an increase in cardiac output with a consequent increase in renal blood flow), or of spironolactone (inhibiting the effects of aldosterone). In some cases the administration of frusemide by continuous intravenous infusion, rather than by bolus injection, may be effective. It is not known why this should be, but it may be due to improved penetration of the drug into the urine when frusemide is given in this way.

(c) The disease or symptom may be too severe for the drug therapy to be effective

One has to be realistic in drug therapy and understand the limitations to what may be achieved. For instance, oral hypoglycaemic drugs

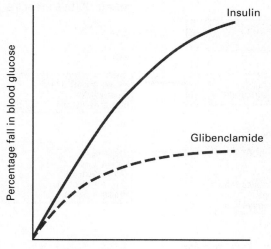

■ Fig. 6.4 Theoretical dose–response curves for the hypoglycaemic effects of insulin and glibenclamide. The maximum possible effect of glibenclamide (and other oral hypoglycaemic drugs) is limited to a level considerably below that of insulin. There is a similar theoretical relation between the dose–response curves of thiazide and loop diuretics. The loop diuretics (also called 'high-ceiling' diuretics) have a higher maximal efficacy than the thiazides.

often do not and cannot produce adequate control of blood glucose in maturity-onset diabetes. In such cases insulin must be given. This difference in maximal efficacy is illustrated schematically in Fig. 6.4.

(d) Toxicity limits the maximum tolerable dose

For some drugs the dose may be limited by adverse effects at high doses. The usual dose may be effective in some patients but not in others, because of interindividual variability in dose-responsiveness. However, in patients in whom the usual doses are ineffective it will not be possible to increase the dose, because of adverse effects. Two examples of this are morphine, whose emetic effect increases in incidence at a dose of about 10 mg, a dose at which the analgesic effect has not reached a maximum, and gentamicin, whose toxicity to the ears and kidneys prevents

the use of doses associated with high plasma concentrations (see Chapter 7). Other examples include the limited positive inotropic effect of digoxin in severe heart failure, and the limited anti-inflammatory effects of non-steroidal anti-inflammatory drugs in severe rheumatoid arthritis.

(e) The therapeutic effect is annulled by incidental adverse effects

Sometimes the adverse effect of a drug may mimic the disease for which the drug is being used. The most common example of this is the arrhythmogenic effects of antiarrhythmic drugs. The frequency with which antiarrhythmic drugs cause arrhythmias varies from drug to drug, but is on average about 10 per cent. If a patient's arrhythmias appear to be refractory to treatment, particularly in cases in which large numbers or high dosages of drugs have been used, it may be worth simplifying the antiarrhythmic drug regimen by reducing the number and dosages of the drugs or by switching to drugs of a different antiarrhythmic class. The risk of arrhythmias in response to antiarrhythmic drugs is greatly increased in patients with poor left ventricular function and in the presence of hypokalaemia.

Less common examples include digoxin toxicity, which can infrequently cause worsening of heart failure or atrial fibrillation, epileptic fits as a manifestation of phenytoin toxicity, and angina pectoris as an adverse effect of nifedipine. In such cases it may appear that therapy has failed, whereas in fact it is toxicity that is preventing the therapeutic response. It should be stressed that these adverse effects are not common, but they can be confusing when they occur.

All of these examples should give a good idea of how the unified scheme outlined in Chapters 2–5 and illustrated in Fig. 1.1 and Fig. 6.2 can be used in formulating questions with which to assess the results of treatment. Sometimes the answers to one's questions will not be known, but one should nevertheless not be inhibited from asking the questions, for it is only by questioning that one can improve one's understanding of the ways in which drug therapy can be optimized.

7 Monitoring drug therapy

In previous chapters we have discussed the ways in which drug therapy can be analysed through its constituent parts, typified by four questions:

1. Is the drug getting into the patient? (The pharmaceutical process.)
2. Is the drug getting to its site of action? (The pharmacokinetic process.)
3. Is the drug producing the required pharmacological effect? (The pharmacodynamic process.)
4. Is the pharmacological effect being translated into a therapeutic effect? (The therapeutic process.)

In this chapter we shall examine the ways in which we can obtain information to help us answer these questions in clinical practice and to help us in rationalizing drug therapy. Questions 1 and 2 can sometimes be answered by measuring drug and metabolite concentrations in body fluids. Question 3 can sometimes be answered by direct measurement of some pharmacological effect of the drug. Question 4 can sometimes be answered by direct measurement of the therapeutic outcome. Not infrequently the answers to questions 3 and 4 may be imprecise, but that should not discourage us from asking the questions. Future research may yield techniques for improving the precision.

Normally one would try to measure the clinical response directly. If that is difficult to measure, or is not related directly in time to a dose of the drug, then some measure of the pharmacological effect of the drug may be required. If measurement of the pharmacological effect of the drug is difficult we may have to resort to measurement of the plasma concentration of the drug.

Because this is the desirable sequence of priorities we shall deal with our questions in reverse order, starting with monitoring of the therapeutic effects of drugs, and continuing with pharmacodynamic and pharmacokinetic monitoring.

7.1 Monitoring the therapeutic effects of drugs

Here we must distinguish between those events which can be directly monitored in the individual patient, and those which are monitored in a population under study. The latter can be applied to the individual only in terms of a statistical probability derived from the observed variability in the population.

7.1.1 Monitoring therapeutic events in the individual

(a) Anticonvulsant drug therapy: seizure frequency

As mentioned below in the section on pharmacokinetic monitoring, knowledge of the plasma concentrations of anticonvulsant drugs can be very useful in the management of epilepsy. However, the end-point of therapy is a decrease in the frequency of seizures, and patients should be encouraged to keep a diary documenting the occurrence of seizures, so that the success of one's treatment or of changes in treatment may be more readily assessed.

(b) Anticholinesterases in myasthenia gravis: improvement in muscle power

The efficacy of cholinesterase inhibitors, such as neostigmine, in myasthenia gravis can be measured by the patients' own assessments of their muscle power and by simple quantitative tests of that power. In cases in which respiratory paralysis might be a problem, tests of pulmonary function, for example vital capacity, may be required.

(c) Drugs for angina pectoris: frequency of attacks

Patients with angina are readily able to tell whether sublingual glyceryl trinitrate prevents an anticipated attack of angina or shortens the duration of pain when an attack occurs. In trials of drugs designed to prevent angina, such as β-adrenoceptor antagonists or calcium channel blockers, the fall in the number of glyceryl trinitrate tablets a patient has to take may be used as a measure of efficacy.

(d) Diuretics in the treatment of oedema: body weight

Various measurements can give information about the efficacy of diuretic therapy in oedema. Urine volume may be used, but is unreliable because of errors in recording or sometimes because of incontinence. Much more reliable is body weight, daily measurement of which gives an accurate assessment of the trend of response to therapy. Assessment of the degree of swelling of the legs in patients with leg oedema gives a more subjective assessment, but should not be neglected. One should also try to make sure that dehydration does not occur, by examining the tongue and skin.

(e) The treatment of ulcerative colitis with glucocorticoids and with 5-aminosalicylic acid (mesalazine) or its derivatives

Besides improvement in the systemic effects of ulcerative colitis during treatment (for example lessening of fever and general malaise and increase of appetite and vigour) there should also be a reduction in the number and severity of attacks of diarrhoea, with a reduction in the amount of blood, mucus, and pus in the stools. These effects are easily measured. Sigmoidoscopy with mucosal biopsy gives an objective measure of therapeutic efficacy.

These examples serve to show how therapy can be objectively assessed. Some effects of therapy are obvious, such as the clearing of psoriatic skin lesions with the use of topical corticosteroids or tar preparations or of acne with retinoids.

Other effects are less obvious. For example, in no area of medicine is it more difficult to gauge the therapeutic effect of treatment than in mental illness, where one has to assess how patients feel and behave. In clinical trials mental symptoms and behavioural signs can be scored and the patient's state quantified. Such an approach is useful in a collective study, but is rarely used in individual routine psychiatric care, when assessment is subjective for both patient and doctor.

7.1.2 Monitoring the effects of drug therapy in the population

With the introduction of public health measures, immunization, and what may be termed 'population therapy', we need to consider what evidence is required to monitor these widely used procedures. The following are examples:

(a) Immunization

Obviously the effects of immunizing the population against diphtheria, tetanus, whooping cough, poliomyelitis, and other infectious diseases can be monitored by surveying the occurrence of those infections in the population.

(b) Currently recommended procedures in preventive medicine

It is hoped that by encouraging people to make changes in their life-style the rates of certain diseases will fall.

1. Stopping smoking – coronary heart disease, peripheral vascular disease, chronic bronchitis, bronchial carcinoma.
2. Losing weight – diabetes mellitus, coronary heart disease, hypertension, osteoarthritis.
3. High-fibre diet – diverticular disease, irritable bowel syndrome.
4. Reducing cholesterol and saturated fats in the diet – coronary heart disease.

(c) Some long-term prophylactic drug therapies widely prescribed

1. Prevention of pregnancy – oral contraceptives.
2. Secondary prevention of myocardial infarction – aspirin, β-adrenoceptor antagonists.

3. Hypertension and its complications – antihypertensive drug therapy.

4. Diabetes mellitus and its complications – diet, insulin, and oral hypoglycaemic drugs.

To discover the efficacy of such measures it is necessary to carry out large-scale studies of comparable groups taking or not taking the treatment (i.e. to carry out a clinical trial). Thereafter one has to rely on the findings of such trials to yield a probability that a treatment will work in an individual, but one will often not know for sure whether or not one's aim was fulfilled in that individual.

Assessment of the efficacy of such measures is a public health matter, no better exemplified than in the assessment of the efficacy of immunization by the compulsory notification of communicable diseases, such as diphtheria, to Government authorities. In the UK the collection of records of births and deaths by the Office of Population Censuses and Surveys can be used to study changes in the patterns of causes of death at a national level, and this can be used as a method of monitoring the efficacy of therapeutic measures, such as immunization.

7.2 Monitoring the pharmacodynamic effects of drugs

In some circumstances the pharmacological effect of a drug can be carefully measured, followed sequentially, and used as a guide to drug therapy, even though it may not be correlated precisely with the therapeutic effect. The following are important examples of commonly used pharmacodynamic measurements used in monitoring drug therapy.

7.2.1 Insulin therapy in diabetes mellitus: effect on blood glucose

There is a tendency to forget how serious a disease diabetes mellitus would be were it not for insulin therapy. The death rate in young diabetics was 614 per 1000 between the years 1897 and 1914 and 411 per 1000 between 1914 and 1922. Insulin was discovered in 1922, and following its introduction there was a dramatic fall in the death rate to 89 per 1000 in 1922–26, since when it has continued to fall.

The management of diabetic ketoacidosis with low-dose continuous intravenous infusion of insulin and frequent monitoring of blood glucose concentrations by simple colorimetric techniques is now accepted practice. Although there are biochemical abnormalities to correct besides the increased blood glucose, lowering of the blood glucose is of prime importance, since the entry of glucose into cells is accompanied to a great extent by resolution of the other abnormalities. In this acute illness the blood glucose is therefore a good guide to a patient's condition and changes in therapy can be guided by it. Of course other measurements must be made, and it is particularly important to ensure that the plasma potassium concentration is kept within normal limits, that the patient's fluid balance is normal, and that the blood pH is not too acidotic.

However, one cannot be so confident about the relationship between the degree of blood glucose control during long-term treatment and the occurrence of the complications of diabetes (retinopathy and cataract, neuropathy, nephropathy, and peripheral vascular disease). Nevertheless, it is generally assumed that good control of the blood glucose concentration is a desirable long-term aim, so much so that patients are now encouraged to measure their own blood glucose concentrations using simple equipment at home. This allows them to alter their doses of insulin to maintain the blood glucose within reasonable limits in order to avoid both hyperglycaemia and hypoglycaemia (10 mmol/L is usually regarded as the maximum and about 4 mmol/L the minimum). For patients who cannot measure their own blood glucose, or for whom such measurement is considered unnecessary, measurement of the urinary concentration of glucose gives a guide to therapy, the aim being to reduce glycosuria to about 0.25–0.5 per cent (i.e. 2.5–5.0 g/L, 14–28 mmol/L). Whether it be blood or urine glucose that is measured it is important that measurements be made regularly to allow careful assessment of day-to-day dosage requirements.

The measurement of the blood glucose concentration gives a momentary indication of how well diabetes is being treated, and one can get some idea of how good overall control has been during a period of weeks or months by looking at serial records of blood glucose concentrations. However, it is also possible to estimate the extent of exposure of the tissues to excess glucose by determining the extent of glycosylation of haemoglobin. This is done by measuring HbA_{1c}, a raised concentration of which suggests poor blood glucose control over the preceding two or three months.

7.2.2 Anticoagulant therapy with warfarin: effect on prothrombin time

The use of the prothrombin time (as the International Normalized Ratio or INR) in monitoring warfarin therapy is discussed in detail in the Pharmacopoeia. The extent to which the INR should be increased during warfarin therapy has been defined on the basis of avoiding spontaneous bleeding and bruising rather than on the basis of any evidence that particular values of the INR are associated with therapeutic benefit.

When one measures the INR in a patient one is measuring the effect of warfarin on the ability of the patient's blood to clot, not, for example, on the likelihood of a pulmonary embolus in a patient with a deep venous thrombosis. However, the accumulated evidence suggests that if one keeps the INR within the generally accepted therapeutic limits one increases the chance of effective treatment.

7.2.3 Bronchodilator therapy in reversible airways obstruction (for example bronchial asthma): effect on FEV_1 and peak flow rate

In asthma, particularly chronic asthma, it can be very difficult to assess the effectiveness of therapy over short periods of time on the basis of symptoms and ordinary physical signs. The effects of bronchodilators, such as salbutamol by inhalation or slow-release theophylline or aminophylline tablets, can be objectively assessed by measuring their effects on the forced expiratory volume in one second (FEV_1), or more simply by measuring the peak flow rate recorded during maximal forced expiration. This is such a simple technique that patients can monitor their own progress at home using simple, cheap equipment.

It is very important to know when after dosing to assess the effectiveness of a bronchodilator. The usual peak effect of a single inhalation of salbutamol from an aerosol occurs 10–15 min after inhalation, and the effect persists for up to an hour; in contrast, the peak effect of ipratropium is at 45–60 min. However, if at these times there is little effect it is as well to test later to see if there is a delayed response.

7.2.4 Allopurinol in gout: effect on blood uric acid

Allopurinol reduces serum uric acid concentrations by inhibiting the conversion of hypoxanthine to uric acid, and the fall in uric acid concentration is used to monitor this pharmacological effect. In this case there is no doubt that the fall in the uric acid concentration is accompanied by a decreased incidence of acute attacks of gouty arthritis and the prevention of gouty renal disease.

7.2.5 Carbimazole in hyperthyroidism: effect on thyroid hormones

In patients with hyperthyroidism physical signs may be difficult to interpret, both in assessing the response to treatment and in preventing overtreatment and resultant hypothyroidism. As an aid to therapy, therefore, one measures the serum concentrations of tri-iodothyronine (T_3) and thyroid stimulating hormone (TSH). The therapeutic effects of carbimazole can be detected by a fall in serum T_3 concentrations. Overtreatment will cause a fall in serum T_3 below normal and an increase in serum TSH above normal.

7.2.6 Cancer chemotherapy: effect on tumour markers

The effectiveness of cytotoxic drug therapy with methotrexate in uterine choriocarcinoma can be monitored by measuring serum concentrations of human chorionic gonadotrophin. Other examples of this are discussed in Chapter 36.

Other obvious examples of pharmacodynamic

monitoring are: the measurement of the reticulo-cyte response and haemoglobin in the treatment of anaemias (for example with ferrous sulphate, vitamin B$_{12}$, or folic acid); the lowering of the blood pressure by antihypertensive drugs; the measurement of intraocular pressure in patients with glaucoma.

7.3 Monitoring drug pharmacokinetics (plasma concentration measurement)

It is obvious that the more information one can gather about drug concentrations in various body tissues, particularly at the site of action, the more likely it is that one will be able to relate those concentrations to the clinical therapeutic response. But one cannot measure the concentration of digoxin in the heart or of phenytoin in the brain, and therefore a great deal of research has been and is being carried out to try to relate plasma drug concentrations to drug effects. In only a few cases has this approach proved itself of value in clinical practice.

In a few additional cases the qualitative detection of drugs in urine is useful in screening for drug abuse (for example cannabis), in drug over-dose (for example paraquat), or for assessing patient compliance (for example salicylates).

Monitoring therapy by the measurement of plasma concentrations of a drug has come to be known as 'therapeutic drug monitoring', or TDM. However, we prefer to avoid this term, since it may be confused with the monitoring of therapy by measuring the therapeutic outcome directly.

It is important to know for which drugs plasma concentration monitoring has been shown to be useful and in what circumstances measurements should be made. It is also important to be able to evaluate the potential usefulness of measuring newer drugs. The uncritical use of plasma drug concentration monitoring can lead to the collection of useless data at the expense of a great deal of money, time, and effort.

There is a combination of criteria which determine whether measuring the plasma concentration of a particular drug may be useful in practice.

These criteria are discussed in the following sections.

7.3.1 Drugs for which the relationship between dose and plasma concentration is unpredictable

If one could predict the effect of a drug simply from its dose then there would be no need to measure its plasma concentration. However, in most cases the absorption, clearance rate, and apparent volume of distribution of a drug vary widely between individuals. Thus, the plasma concentration which will result from a given dose in a given individual is generally unpredictable. In most cases, therefore, the plasma drug concentration will be more closely related to the effect of the drug than the dose. Phenytoin is an important example of this, as can be seen from Fig. 3.5, in which is shown the wide range of dosages required to produce similar steady-state plasma phenytoin concentrations in five different individuals.

There are many factors which may alter the relation between the dose of a drug and its plasma concentration (i.e. which may alter the pharmacokinetics of the drug). These are listed in Table 7.1.

7.3.2 Drugs for which there is a good relationship between plasma concentration and effect

The most important criterion is that there should be a good relationship between the plasma concentration of the drug and its therapeutic or toxic effects. This criterion, combined with the concept of the dose–response curve (see pp. 51–4), leads to the concept of the 'therapeutic range'. If the plasma concentrations of a drug are well related to the therapeutic and toxic effects of the drug then there is likely to be a range of concentrations below which little effect can be expected, within which one can expect a therapeutic effect, and above which one can expect an increased risk of toxicity. This is illustrated diagrammatically in Fig. 7.1. In practice the therapeutic range is derived from plasma concentration measurements in large numbers of patients, and is

▮ **Table 7.1** Factors which may alter the pharmacokinetics or pharmacodynamics of drugs

A. Factors which may alter the pharmacokinetics of drugs, thereby altering the relationship between the amount of drug in the body and the plasma concentration

Factor	Example
Renal failure	Reduced excretion of digoxin, aminoglycoside antibiotics, and lithium
Hepatic failure	Reduced elimination of theophylline
Drug interactions	Reduced elimination of digoxin (verapamil, amiodarone)
	Reduced elimination of theophylline (erythromycin, quinolones)
	Reduced elimination of lithium (diuretics)
	Altered unbound concentration of phenytoin (displacement from albumin)
Thyroid dysfunction	Complex changes in the pharmacokinetics of digoxin
Diarrhoea	Altered absorption of lithium

B. Factors which may alter the pharmacodynamics of drugs, thereby altering the relationship between the amount of drug at the site of action and the effect

Factor	Example
Electrolyte imbalance	Digoxin action enhanced by potassium depletion
Thyroid disease decreased	Digoxin action enhanced (hypothyroidism or hyperthyroidism)
Age	Actions of some drugs enhanced
Drug interactions	Mutual potentiation of the actions of antiepileptic drugs
	Increased ototoxicity of aminoglycoside antibiotics (loop diuretics)

thus a statistical concept (analogous to the normal ranges of concentrations of plasma constituents, such as urea and sodium). However, because of interindividual variability the therapeutic range can be no more than a guide to the plasma concentration that is most likely to be associated with a therapeutic response. Thus, the plasma concentration that is associated with a therapeutic response in one individual may be subtherapeutic or toxic in another. In part this is due to the fact that there are many factors which can alter the relationship between plasma concentration and effect in an individual (i.e. which alter the pharmacodynamic effects of the drug). These are listed in Table 7.1.

7.3.3 Drugs with a low toxic:therapeutic ratio (i.e. therapeutic dose close to toxic dose)

There are many drugs for which the margin between the dose which produces a therapeutic effect and the dose which produces a toxic effect is very narrow. If there is a good relationship between the plasma concentration and the therapeutic or toxic effects of such drugs then measurement of the plasma concentration will allow dosage alterations to be made in order to produce an optimum therapeutic effect or to avoid a toxic effect. Such drugs contrast with drugs for which there is a large margin between the therapeutic and toxic doses (for example penicillin, barring hypersensitivity reactions). With such drugs one can make large changes in dose, ensuring that the amount of drug in the body is sufficient, or more than sufficient, to produce a therapeutic effect, without running into problems with toxicity. In these cases plasma concentration measurement is generally unnecessary.

7.3.4 Drugs which are not metabolized to active metabolites

Some drugs have one or more metabolites which themselves have pharmacological activity, and

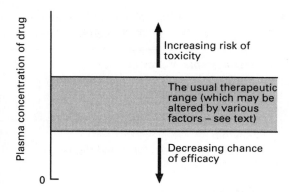

▌ **Fig. 7.1.** A diagrammatic representation of the concept of the 'therapeutic range' in plasma drug concentration monitoring. Within the therapeutic range of plasma concentrations for a particular drug one would expect the majority of patients to have a good therapeutic response, although the precise therapeutic range for an individual may vary according to several factors, individual to each drug (see text and Table 7.1B for examples). At concentrations below the usual therapeutic range one would expect little likelihood of a therapeutic response, although some patients may be adequately treated at these concentrations. At concentrations above the therapeutic range the risk of toxicity will rise with increasing concentrations, although again some patients may be adequately treated without evidence of toxicity at these concentrations.

which can produce either toxic or therapeutic effects. To obtain a comprehensive picture of the relationships between total plasma concentrations of pharmacologically active compounds and clinical effects it would be necessary to measure each active compound separately, or to use an assay which measured the total biological activity of those compounds.

For example, procainamide is metabolized to *N*-acetylprocainamide (acecainide), an antiarrhythmic agent as potent as procainamide. The extent of metabolism varies according to acetylator status (see Chapter 8), and between 10 and 40 per cent of the procainamide administered may be metabolized to acecainide. Thus, measurement of plasma procainamide concentrations alone gives an imprecise guide to therapy.

Chlorpromazine, a neuroleptic drug used in the treatment of psychoses such as schizophrenia, is metabolized to several active metabolites, each

of which has a different degree of neuroleptic activity. It has proved very difficult to relate plasma concentrations of chlorpromazine to its therapeutic effects in psychiatric conditions, and the confounding effects of active metabolites may be the reason. An interesting alternative is to measure all the neuroleptic moieties by using a radioreceptor assay, in which active compounds in the plasma are made to compete with an appropriate radiolabelled ligand for binding sites on a specific receptor. The theory of such an assay is that the extent to which a compound (for example chlorpromazine or one of its metabolites) competes with another ligand (for example ^{3}H-haloperidol) for binding sites on the receptor is proportional to the neuroleptic activity of the compound. Such an assay should measure the total neuroleptic activity of the mixture of chlorpromazine and its metabolites. However, assays of this kind are too specialized to be generally available and their use is limited to research.

7.3.5 Drugs for which there is difficulty in measuring or interpreting the clinical evidence of therapeutic or toxic effects

Some chronic diseases vary naturally in the intensity of their effects from time to time, for example the frequency of depressive episodes in manic–depressive psychosis or of fits in epilepsy. If in careful clinical trials one can demonstrate a relationship between the plasma concentration of a drug and its effects in reducing episodes of illness in a population then that relationship can be a helpful guide to using the drug in individual patients at large, in whom the measurement of effect may not be easy. For example, the measurement of plasma lithium concentrations is of value in two respects: first in helping in an individual case to choose a dosage which one may expect to be of therapeutic benefit in the prevention of manic or depressive episodes, and second in avoiding dosages which may cause short-term or long-term adverse effects.

Adverse effects of drugs sometimes mimic disease. For example, nausea and vomiting occur in both digitalis toxicity and congestive cardiac failure; phenytoin toxicity can occasionally cause an increase rather than a decrease in the frequency of epileptic seizures; renal failure may occur in a patient with Gram-negative septicaemia because of the disease or because of an adverse effect of the gentamicin used to treat it. If one can demonstrate a relationship between the plasma concentration of a drug and its adverse effects then one can use such measurements to distinguish between drug-induced and disease-induced effects, or to prevent the drug-induced effects.

7.3.6 Which drugs fulfil these criteria?

Many drugs fulfil one or even two of these criteria, but only a few drugs fulfil a sufficient number of criteria to make it worth measuring their plasma concentrations in monitoring therapy. They are listed in part A of Table 7.2.

Some drugs fulfil four of these criteria (sections 7.3.1, 7.3.3, 7.3.4, and 7.3.5) but have not been shown conclusively to fulfil the most important criterion (that there should be a good relationship between plasma concentrations and the therapeutic or toxic effects, section 7.3.2). These drugs are listed in part B of Table 7.2. They include antiarrhythmic drugs and tricyclic antidepressants, which warrant some extra discussion.

There has been, and in some centres still is, enthusiasm for monitoring antiarrhythmic drug therapy by plasma concentration measurement. While, in our view, 'routine' monitoring of this group of drugs in this way has not been proven to be very useful, there are undoubtedly some patients with chronic asymptomatic arrhythmias which prove to be very difficult to manage with antiarrhythmic drugs, and in whom it can be very useful to know whether the plasma drug concentration is within an empirical therapeutic range, particularly since antiarrhythmic drug toxicity can itself result in arrhythmias. If the plasma concentration were below the therapeutic range and the arrhythmia is uncontrolled one would be justified in increasing the dose. If the concentration were within or above this range one would be justified in trying another drug. In these circumstances electrophysiological testing may be a helpful adjunct in deciding what plasma concentrations can be deemed 'therapeutic' in an individual patient.

▪ **Table 7.2**   Drugs whose plasma concentrations may provide a guide to monitoring drug therapy

---

A. Measurements of proven value
Aminoglycoside antibiotics (for example gentamicin, kanamycin)
Anticonvulsants
　Carbamazepine
　Phenytoin
Cardiac glycosides (digitoxin and digoxin)
Cyclosporin
Lithium
Theophylline

B. Case not proven
Antiarrhythmic drugs
　Amiodarone
　Disopyramide
　Lignocaine
　Procainamide
　Quinidine
Anticonvulsants other than carbamazepine and phenytoin
Methotrexate
Tricyclic antidepressants

Despite interest in the relationship between the plasma concentrations of antidepressant drugs and their therapeutic effects, there is little case at present for using plasma concentration measurements in the routine monitoring of antidepressant drug therapy. However, one aspect of this subject is particularly interesting. In patients treated with nortriptyline there appears to be what is called an 'inverted U' effect relating plasma concentrations to therapeutic effects (Fig. 7.2). This phenomenon is explained on the basis that above a certain plasma concentration (about 110 ng/mL) nortriptyline somehow negates its own therapeutic effect. This is not seen with other tricyclic antidepressants.

7.3.7 Indications for measuring plasma drug concentrations

We have seen that there are certain criteria which must be fulfilled before a drug becomes eligible as one whose plasma concentration measurement may prove useful in clinical practice. We must

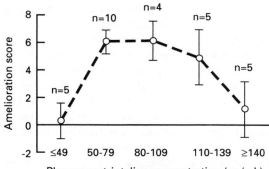

■ **Fig. 7.2.** The relation between plasma concentrations of nortriptyline and its antidepressant effect. Improvement is seen when plasma concentrations increase to between 50 and 110 ng/mL, but above 110 ng/mL the clinical response is less good. (Adapted from Asberg *et al.* (1971). *Br. Med. J.* **iii**, 331–4, with permission.)

now consider when in practice such measurement is likely to contribute significantly to patient care.

(a) In individualizing therapy

For reasons discussed above it may be desirable to aim for a particular range of plasma drug concentrations within which a therapeutic effect is likely to occur and toxic effects are likely to be minimized. This may be particularly useful:

(1) at the start of therapy when the relationship between dose and plasma concentration in the individual is uncertain;

(2) when rapid changes in renal function alter the relationship between dose and plasma concentration: this is particularly important for digoxin, lithium, and the aminoglycoside antibiotics (for example gentamicin);

(3) when another drug alters the relationship between dose and plasma concentration: for example, plasma concentrations of lithium are increased by thiazide diuretics, those of digoxin by quinidine and amiodarone, and those of phenytoin by valproate.

However, it is important to remember never to use the plasma concentration in isolation as a guide to therapy, but to interpret it in the light of the patient's clinical condition. Since the therapeutic range is a statistical concept based on observations of populations of patients, a plasma concentration below the lower end of this range or above its upper end may merely represent values at the extremes of the distribution and in an individual may be associated with a therapeutic response. In a patient who has definitely responded to treatment, but who nevertheless has a plasma concentration below the therapeutic range it might be wrong to adjust the dose simply to engineer a plasma concentration within the therapeutic range, and in some cases the finding of a plasma concentration below the therapeutic range may be an indication for withdrawal of therapy.

(b) In the diagnosis of suspected toxicity

If one has a clinical suspicion of toxicity then a plasma concentration above the therapeutic range will undoubtedly reinforce one's suspicions. However, it must be remembered that toxicity can occur even when the plasma concentration is within the therapeutic range, particularly if any of the factors listed in Table 7.1 has altered the relationship between the plasma concentration of a drug and its effect.

(c) Measuring compliance

This is discussed in Chapter 13.

7.3.8. The importance of steady-state concentrations

If plasma drug concentrations are measured before a steady state has been reached (i.e. before about four half-times of repeated administration) one may be misled into misinterpreting the relationship between dose and the true steady-state plasma concentration. Remember that if you measure the plasma concentration on a day when a steady state has not yet been reached the plasma concentration you measure will underestimate the eventual steady-state concentration. This may happen either during the early stages of therapy, or when the clearance of the drug is decreasing (for example in renal failure) and the half-time of the drug is consequently lengthening. Conversely, if you measure plasma drug concentrations too soon after a reduction in dosage you may overestimate the new eventual steady-state concentration.

7.3.9 The timing of blood sampling in relation to dose

The importance of the blood sampling time in relation to the time of dosing can be seen in the case of digoxin illustrated in Fig. 7.3. After oral administration the plasma concentration changes within quite a wide range before complete tissue distribution has occurred, even during steady-state administration. One may therefore be misled about the true steady-state plasma concentration if the sample is taken before distribution is complete. It is generally simplest to take the blood sample just before the next dose is due, when one will measure the minimum steady-state concentration. However, in the case of the aminoglycoside antibiotics (see gentamicin below) one should also measure the 'peak' concentration. Specific guidelines are given below for individual drugs.

7.3.10 The practical use of specific plasma drug concentration measurements

(a) Phenytoin

The therapeutic range for phenytoin is 40–80 μmol/L. Above 80 μmol/L the incidence of toxicity rises. However, patients with concentrations above this range may not be toxic, and patients with concentrations below the range may

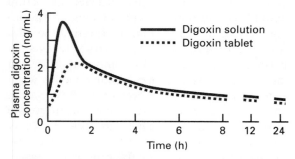

▮ **Fig. 7.3.** Plasma digoxin concentrations during the 24 h after a single dose during daily maintenance therapy. In the 6 h after administration the plasma digoxin concentration is a poor guide to the mean steady-state plasma concentration. (Adapted from Lloyd *et al.* (1978). *Am. J. Cardiol.* **42**, 129–36, with permission.)

not be undertreated. Although plasma concentrations of phenytoin in the toxic range are quite well related to its acute toxic effects (see Fig. 7.4) they are not well related to its long-term adverse effects, such as gingival hyperplasia, hirsutism and acne, and folate and vitamin D deficiencies.

Because of the non-linearity of phenytoin kinetics it is unwise, when an increase in dose is thought necessary, to increase the dose by increments of daily dose of more than 25–50 mg every two weeks or so, from say 300 mg/d to 350 mg/d (see the Pharmacopoeia and Chapter 3, p. 22). When the plasma phenytoin concentration is below 60 μmol/L an increase in daily dose of 50 mg is acceptable; if the concentration is above 60 μmol/L the increase should be no more than 25 mg.

Steady state takes about two weeks of maintenance therapy to occur after a change in dose at low dosages, and the higher the plasma concentration the longer it takes (up to three weeks or longer in some patients). For this reason one should not make changes in dosage too frequently.

Provided the sample is not taken too soon after a dose (i.e. within 1–2 h) the time of sampling is probably of little importance for phenytoin, since plasma concentrations fluctuate very little during a dosage interval.

Alterations in phenytoin plasma protein binding (usually about 90 per cent) set in train a sequence of events which can further complicate plasma concentration interpretation (see Chapter 10 and Fig. 10.1).

1. Displacement of phenytoin from plasma protein binding sites results in an increase in free concentration, without a change in total concentration. Toxicity may then occur if displacement has occurred rapidly enough.

2. Because phenytoin has a low hepatic extraction ratio its total body clearance is proportional to the fraction of unbound drug in the plasma (see Chapter 3). With the increase in unbound fraction its total body clearance increases proportionately, and within a few days the total concentration falls. However, since the unbound fraction remains increased the unbound concentration returns to what it was before the displacement. Toxicity then resolves.

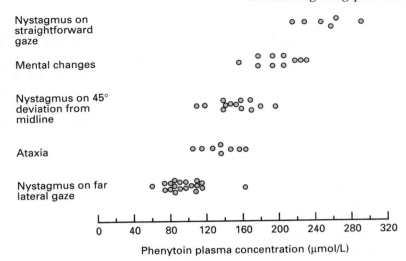

■ **Fig. 7.4.** The relation between plasma concentrations of phenytoin and its acute adverse effects. (Adapted from Kutt *et al.* (1964). *Arch. Neurol. (Chicago)* **11**, 642–8, with permission. Copyright 1967, American Medical Association.)

3. The doctor measures the total plasma concentration, thinks it is inadequate, and increases the dose. Toxicity results.

The main circumstances in which decreased phenytoin plasma protein binding may occur are:

(1) renal failure;

(2) severe hypoalbuminaemia (25 g/L or less);

(3) the third trimester of pregnancy (possibly because of hypoalbuminaemia);

(4) displacement by other drugs (see Chapter 10).

(b) Other anti-epileptic drugs

(i) Carbamazepine

The therapeutic plasma concentration range is 17–42 μmol/L (4–10 μg/mL). Carbamazepine induces its own metabolism, and its half-time is therefore shortened during long-term therapy. Thus, after an initial apparent steady state has been reached three or four days after starting therapy, a new steady state occurs at a lower concentration a few weeks later. Blood samples should be taken immediately before a dose. Plasma carbamazepine concentrations may be increased by dextropropoxyphene and decreased by phenytoin and barbiturates.

(ii) Other anticonvulsants

The value of measuring the plasma concentrations of other anticonvulsants has not been clearly established. Rough guides to the sort of plasma concentration ranges encountered during therapy are given in the section on the treatment of epilepsy (p. 434).

(c) Digitalis

The therapeutic range for digoxin is 1.0–2.6 nmol/L (0.8–2.0 ng/mL). Below 1.0 nmol/L there is little likelihood of therapeutic benefit, and in patients who are clinically well digoxin may be withdrawn, usually without subsequent deterioration. Above 2.6 nmol/L the risk of toxicity rises, and toxicity is highly likely above 3.8 nmol/L. The therapeutic range for digitoxin is 20–35 nmol/L (15–27 ng/mL) and toxicity is highly likely above 40 nmol/L (30 ng/mL).

The time of blood sampling should be at least 6 h after the previous dose, and 12 h is the best time in patients taking once daily treatment (Fig. 7.3). During regular maintenance dosage without a loading dose steady state will be reached after about 7 days (digoxin, normal renal function), 18 days (digoxin, functionally anephric), or 25 days (digitoxin).

There are several factors which alter the relationship between dose and plasma digitalis concentrations. The most important are:

(i) Renal impairment

Renal impairment causes decreased clearance of digoxin, and thus increases the plasma digoxin concentration at a given dose.

(ii) Drug interactions

Certain drugs cause decreased renal clearance of digoxin, notably quinidine, verapamil, and amiodarone. Thus, digoxin plasma concentrations are increased at a given dose. Plasma digitoxin concentrations may be reduced at a given dose by enzyme-inducing drugs such as rifampicin, and by drugs which impair its absorption, such as cholestyramine and colestipol.

There are also several factors which alter the link between the pharmacokinetic and pharmacodynamic phases of drug therapy with both digoxin and digitoxin. In such circumstances the plasma concentration can be difficult to interpret.

(i) Potassium depletion

A low extracellular potassium concentration increases the affinity of digitalis for the $Na^+ K^+$ ATPase and increases the pharmacodynamic effect of a given concentration of digoxin or digitoxin. For this reason one should never try to interpret the plasma digitalis concentration without also knowing the plasma potassium concentration. In circumstances in which digitalis toxicity is suspected a low plasma potassium concentration (i.e. below 3.5 mmol/L) is sufficient to warrant withdrawal of digitalis on the assumption that toxicity has occurred.

(ii) Thyroid disease

Hyperthyroidism causes both a decrease in plasma digitalis concentrations at a given dose and a decrease in pharmacodynamic responsiveness. Hypothyroidism causes the opposite effects. There are no guidelines to the interpretation of plasma digitalis concentrations in these circumstances. However, plasma concentration measurement is sometimes worth while simply to demonstrate the presence of the drug.

(iii) Age

Children under 6 months of age have lower plasma digoxin concentrations at a given dose than older children and adults. They are also more resistant to the pharmacodynamic actions of digitalis, and it is not possible to interpret plasma digitalis concentrations clearly in these circumstances. However, plasma concentration measurement is sometimes worth while simply to demonstrate the presence of the drug.

(d) Lithium

The therapeutic range is 0.4–0.8 mmol/L. At 1.0–1.5 mmol/L there is an increase in the incidence of both acute toxicity and long-term adverse effects. Concentrations above 1.5 mmol/L should be avoided.

Blood samples should be taken at exactly 12 h after the previous dose, or as near to that as possible, since all the work on the relation between the plasma concentrations of lithium and its therapeutic effect has been carried out with that sampling time. It takes about 3 d for steady state to be reached during regular maintenance therapy, but there is wide variability, and in some patients it may take a week before steady state is reached.

Regular plasma lithium concentration monitoring is necessary for several reasons.

1. Lithium is nephrotoxic and is excreted by the kidneys. Toxicity is thus self-perpetuating, since toxicity causes renal damage, further retention of lithium, and further toxicity.

2. Systemic availability varies from individual to individual, is altered by diarrhoea, and varies from formulation to formulation (see p. 73 and the Pharmacopoeia).

3. Changes in sodium balance alter the renal excretion of lithium. For example, renal sodium loss induced by diuretics leads to lithium retention.

(e) Aminoglycoside antibiotics

The same principles apply to all the aminoglycoside antibiotics and we shall illustrate them here with the example of gentamicin. The corresponding concentrations for other aminoglycosides are given in Table 7.3.

∎ **Table 7.3**   Usual therapeutic and toxic plasma concentrations of commonly measured drugs

Drug	Concentration below which a therapeutic effect is unlikely	Concentration above which a toxic effect is more likely
A. Concentrations in mass units		
Aminoglycosides		
Amikacin	20 µg/mL (at peak) 10 µg/mL (at trough)	32 µg/mL (at peak)
Gentamicin	5 µg/mL (at peak) 2 µg/mL (at trough)	12 µg/mL (at peak)
Kanamycin	25 µg/mL (at peak) 10 µg/mL (at trough)	40 µg/mL (at peak)
Aspirin (salicylate)		
Analgesic:	20 µg/mL	300 µg/mL
Anti-inflammatory:	150 µg/mL	
Carbamazepine	4 µg/mL	10 µg/mL
Cardiac glycosides		
Digitoxin	15 ng/mL	30 ng/mL
Digoxin	0.8 ng/mL	3 ng/mL
Lithium	see part B	see part B
Paracetamol		see Fig. 35.2
Phenytoin	10 µg/mL	20 µg/mL
Theophylline	10 µg/mL	20 µg/mL
B. Concentrations in molar units		
Aminoglycosides		
Amikacin	34 µmol/L (at peak) 17 µmol/L (at trough)	55 µmol/L (at peak)
Kanamycin	50 µmol/L (at peak) 20 µmol/L (at trough)	80 µmol/L (at peak)
Aspirin (salicylate)		
Analgesic:	0.15 mmol/L	2.2 mmol/L
Anti-inflammatory:	1.1 mmol/L	
Carbamazepine	17 µmol/L	42 µmol/L
Cardiac glycosides		
Digitoxin	20 nmol/L	39 nmol/L
Digoxin	1.0 nmol/L	3.8 nmol/L
Lithium	0.4 mmol/L	1.0 mmol/L
Paracetamol		see Fig. 35.2
Phenytoin	40 µmol/L	80 µmol/L
Theophylline	55 µmol/L	110 µmol/L

The relation between the plasma concentration of gentamicin and its therapeutic efficacy is complicated by the fact that different organisms have different sensitivities to the antibiotic. A peak plasma concentration of 5–9 µg/mL is generally considered to be necessary, but when gentamicin is used in combination with benzylpenicillin in the treatment of bacterial endocarditis lower plasma gentamicin concentrations may be effective. Measurement of the *in vitro* minimum inhibitory concentration (MIC, see p. 230) by the bacteriologist will help to guide therapy.

The relationship between the plasma concentration of gentamicin and its toxic effects on the ears and kidneys is of great importance. To understand this relationship we must first define 'peak' and 'trough' concentrations. The 'peak' concentration is the highest concentration measured after an intramuscular dose, and usually occurs at about 45–60 min after injection; its equivalent after intravenous administration (which should be by infusion over about 20 min) is the concentration measured about 15 min after the end of the infusion. The 'trough' concentration is the concentration measured just before the next dose is due; at steady state the trough concentration would be equivalent to the minimum steady-state concentration.

Ototoxicity is thought to be related to the trough concentration, but its relationship to the peak concentration is not clear. The relationship between plasma concentration and nephrotoxicity is not clear, and is complicated by the fact that renal damage will itself alter the plasma concentration. It is recommended that peak plasma gentamicin concentrations should be below 12 µg/mL at peak and below 2 µg/mL at trough if toxicity is to be avoided. The corresponding values for amikacin and kanamycin are given in Table 7.3.

Since aminoglycoside toxicity may be related to both peak and trough concentrations it may be necessary to change both the size of the dose and the timing of administration if target plasma concentrations at both peak and trough are to be achieved. This principle is illustrated here for gentamicin in three different cases, as shown in Fig. 7.5. In each case the patient is being given 80 mg at 8 hourly intervals.

Case A

Peak concentration too high (16 µg/mL), trough concentration acceptable (1 µg/mL).

Because the peak is too high the dose must be reduced. If it is halved the peak will be approximately halved (i.e. from 16 µg/mL to 8 µg/mL). The concentration will then fall to a safe concentration (say 1 µg/mL) in 3 half-times (1 half-time to fall from 8 to 4, another to fall from 4 to 2 and a third to fall from 2 to 1). Since the concentration fell from 16 µg/mL to 1 µg/mL in 8 h the half-time must be 2 h and the new dosage interval should therefore be 6 h. So the dosage should be changed from 80 mg 8 hourly to 40 mg 6 hourly.

Case B

Peak concentration too low (5 µg/mL), trough concentration acceptable (1.25 µg/mL).

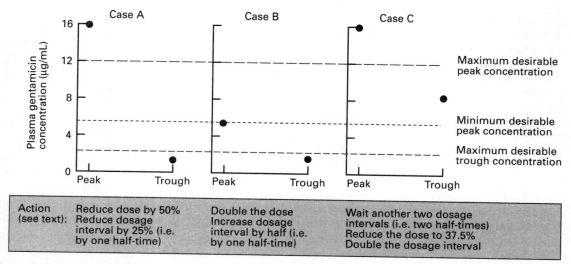

■ **Fig. 7.5.** Some theoretical problems in gentamicin therapy in relation to peak and trough plasma gentamicin concentrations (see text for discussion).

Because the peak is too low the dose must be increased. If it is doubled the peak concentration will be approximately doubled (i.e. from 5 µg/mL to 10 µg/mL). The concentration will then fall to a safe concentration (say 1.25 µg/mL) in 3 half-times (1 half-time to fall from 10 to 5, another to fall from 5 to 2.5 and a third to fall from 2.5 to 1.25). Since the concentration fell from 5 µg/mL to 1.25 µg/mL in 8 h the half-time must be 4 h and the new dosage interval should therefore be 12 h. So the dosage should be changed from 80 mg 8 hourly to 160 mg 12 hourly.

Case C

Peak concentration too high (16 µg/mL), trough concentration too high (8 µg/mL).

This case is more complicated. First, because the trough is too high the next dose must be delayed until the concentration falls to a safe concentration (say 1 µg/mL). It has just fallen from 16 µg/mL to 8 µg/mL in 8 h, so it will take another 24 h to fall to 1 µg/mL. If one then gives half the dose the peak concentration will be about 8 µg/mL and one will have to wait 24 h before it falls to 1 µg/mL. So, after waiting 24 h one should change the dosage from 80 mg 8 hourly to 40 mg daily.

We must stress that these are purely theoretical examples, designed to demonstrate the principles involved. In practice things are never so easy, for several reasons:

1. Estimates of the half-time from only two measurements are very inaccurate.

2. Plasma aminoglycoside concentration measurements take several hours to carry out and one cannot make decisions about dosages immediately after taking the plasma samples.

3. Renal function may be changing, and often is changing more quickly than dosage alterations can be made on the basis of delayed measurements (see the example calculated in Chapter 6).

Despite these problems an understanding of the principles involved will be of some help in these difficult circumstances.

(f) Theophylline

Therapeutic plasma concentrations vary between 10 and 20 µg/mL and the incidence of toxicity rises at above 20 µg/mL. For routine plasma theophylline concentration measurements to be of value in the treatment of acute asthma they must be available very quickly to allow rapid adjustments in dose. In practice this means the use of fast immunoassay techniques. For long-term therapy plasma concentration measurement can help and speed of assay is less important.

The time to steady state is usually less than a day, but the half-time varies from patient to patient because of numerous factors which may alter the pharmacokinetics of theophylline (see the Pharmacopoeia, p. 716). If the half-time is prolonged the time to steady state may be as long as 2–3 days.

Blood samples are best taken just before a dose, and because of diurnal variations in trough concentration should ideally be taken at the same time of day in an individual.

(g) Cyclosporin

Cyclosporin is generally measured in whole blood because of technical problems in separating the plasma or serum without allowing cyclosporin in erythrocytes to leak out. Furthermore, the result of the assay depends on whether the measurement technique is by immunoassay or high-performance liquid chromatography (HPLC). The therapeutic range in whole blood by immunoassay is about 800–1000 ng/mL and by HPLC 100–300 ng/mL. Renal toxicity is related to the trough concentration, and it is usual to keep the trough concentration at around 100 ng/mL (HPLC). When cyclosporin is used in combination with other immunosuppressant drugs it may be possible to achieve a therapeutic effect with a lower risk of toxicity if the trough concentration is kept at 50 ng/mL.

8 ▪ Pharmacogenetics

Pharmacogenetics is the study of the influence of heredity on both the pharmacokinetics of drugs and the pharmacodynamic responses to them.

8.1 Pharmacokinetic defects

The extent to which an individual metabolizes a drug is, at least in part, genetically determined. This fact has emerged from studies on monozygotic (i.e. identical) and dizygotic (i.e. non-identical) twins. Monozygotic twins metabolize drugs similarly, while dizygotic twins often do not (Fig. 8.1). For most drugs the variability in drug metabolism shows a normal (unimodal) distribution. This is illustrated in Fig. 8.2 for sodium salicylate. Sodium salicylate is conjugated in the liver to a glucuronide, an acylphenolic conjugate, and a glycine conjugate, and some is oxidized to gentisic acid. This metabolism accounts for about 90 per cent of its elimination at low doses. The plasma salicylate concentrations 3 h after the administration of the same therapeutic dose of aspirin to a population of subjects show a unimodal distribution, suggesting that the rates of metabolism of sodium salicylate within the population have a continuous distribution of variability.

However, for some drugs the distribution is bimodal or trimodal, indicating the existence of separate populations of subjects capable of metabolizing those drugs at discretely different rates. The important pathways of drug metabolism subject to pharmacokinetic variability are detailed below.

8.1.1 Acetylation

Several drugs are acetylated by the hepatic enzyme N-acetyltransferase, and the distribution of rates of acetylation in the population is bimodal (Fig. 8.3). The difference between fast and slow acetylators depends on the amount of hepatic N-acetyltransferase, rather than a change in its properties. It is known that fast acetylation is inherited as an autosomal dominant character, while slow acetylation is thought to be recessive. The ratio of fast:slow acetylators is racially determined, being, for example, 40:60 in Europe, 85:15 in Japan, and 95:5 in the Inuit.

Drugs whose acetylation is genetically determined in this way are isoniazid, hydralazine, procainamide, phenelzine, dapsone, and some sulphonamides (for example sulphamethoxypyridazine and sulphapyridine). However, not all drugs which are acetylated are affected, since some are acetylated by a different enzyme outside the liver. The exceptions include sulphanilamide, p-aminobenzoic acid, and p-aminosalicylic acid.

The clinical consequences of these differences are that in slow acetylators there may be an enhanced response to treatment, but also an increased risk of drug toxicity. Thus, slow acetylators have been reported to require lower doses of isoniazid and hydralazine than fast acetylators in the treatment of tuberculosis and hypertension respectively. They are also more likely to develop the lupus erythematosus-like syndrome caused by isoniazid, hydralazine, and procainamide, and the peripheral neuropathy caused by isoniazid (which can be prevented or treated with pyridoxine). The interaction between isoniazid and phenytoin, in which phenytoin metabolism is inhibited by isoniazid, resulting in phenytoin toxicity, occurs more frequently among slow acetylators.

The acetylator status of an individual may be easily assessed by giving a sulphonamide, such as sulphadimidine or sulphapyridine, orally and measuring the relative proportions of acetylated and total sulphonamide in a sample of urine passed 5–6 h later.

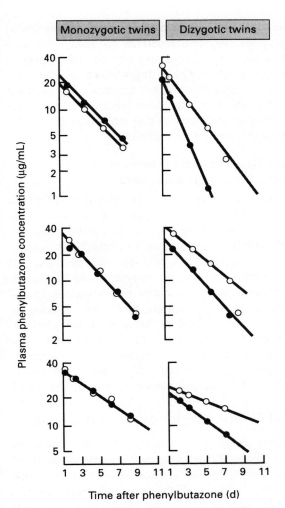

Fig. 8.1. Plasma concentrations of phenylbutazone after its administration to three pairs of monozygotic twins (left-hand panels) and three pairs of dizygotic twins (right-hand panels). The monozygotic twins show virtually identical kinetics while the dizygotic twins differ. (Adapted from Vesell and Page (1968). *Science* **159**, 1479–80, with permission. Copyright 1968, The American Association for the Advancement of Science.)

8.1.2 Oxidation

In the same way that *N*-acetylation is bimodally distributed in the population, so are certain varieties of oxidation. However, in contrast to acetylation, this is a heterogeneous group of defects, and they are not all uniformly due to decreased amounts of enzyme. Thus, individuals with impaired and normal oxidation are classified

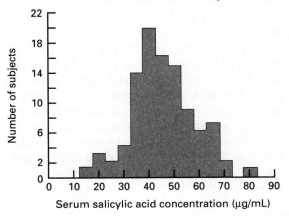

Fig. 8.2. Unimodal drug metabolism, illustrated by the frequency distribution of serum salicylic acid concentrations 3 h after the administration of the same dose of aspirin to 100 individuals. (Adapted from Evans and Clarke (1961). *Br. Med. Bull.* **17**, 234–40, with permission.)

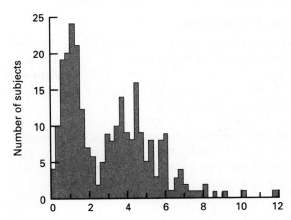

Fig. 8.3. Polymorphic acetylation, illustrated by the bimodal frequency distribution of plasma concentrations of isoniazid 6 h after the oral administration of 9.7 mg/kg to 267 individuals of 53 families. Those with lower plasma isoniazid concentrations are fast acetylators, those with higher plasma isoniazid concentrations are slow acetylators. (Adapted from Evans *et al.* (1960). *Br. Med. J.* **ii**, 485–91, with permission.)

as poor and extensive metabolizers respectively, rather than as fast and slow metabolizers.

(a) Debrisoquine type

Debrisoquine hydroxylation is carried out by the cytochrome P450 known as IID6. Impaired hydroxylation of debrisoquine is an autosomal recessive defect of this cytochrome, the gene being located on chromosome 22. It occurs in about 9 per cent of Caucasians (Fig. 8.4), but has a lower prevalence in other racial types. Drugs which are affected besides debrisoquine include captopril, codeine, flecainide, metoprolol, nortriptyline, perhexiline, phenacetin, phenformin, propafenone, sparteine, and timolol. The dose-related adverse effects of these drugs (for example lactic acidosis with phenformin, peripheral neuropathy with perhexiline, and central nervous system toxicity with nortriptyline) are more likely in poor hydroxylators. In the case of a toxic metabolite one would expect a greater risk in extensive metabolizers, and this may be the case for neutropenia due to carbimazole.

Quinidine inhibits some oxidative reactions and may turn an extensive metabolizer of the debrisoquine type into a poor metabolizer.

(b) Other types

Impaired mephenytoin hydroxylation is a clearly described defect with autosomal recessive inheritance. It occurs in 5 per cent of Caucasians and 20 per cent of Japanese and its clinical consequences are not clear.

Penicillamine is structurally similar to carbocisteine, whose sulphoxidation is polymorphic. Poor sulphoxidation of carbocisteine has been associated with a four-fold increase in the risk of adverse effects with penicillamine in rheumatoid arthritis. Adverse reactions to gold salts containing a thiol group may also be linked to poor sulphoxidation. Other drugs which may be oxidized polymorphically, but for which the evidence is not yet clear, include nifedipine and some sex steroids, which may be polymorphically dehydrogenated, and tolbutamide.

(d) Disease associations with polymorphic metabolism

Since some diseases may be related to the effects of environmental chemicals, it is of interest that polymorphic acetylation, hydroxylation, and sulphoxidation may have other clinical associations. For example, there may be increased risks of bladder cancer in slow acetylators, of Parkinsonism in poor debrisoquine hydroxylators and of bronchogenic carcinoma in extensive hydroxylators, and of primary biliary cirrhosis in poor sulphoxidizers. It may be that these diseases are due to impaired metabolism or excessive production of toxic compounds, although the associations remain to be confirmed.

8.1.3 Succinylcholine hydrolysis

Succinylcholine is metabolized in the plasma by a non-specific esterase called pseudocholinesterase. Normally this metabolism is fast, the blood is quickly cleared of the drug, and neuromuscular

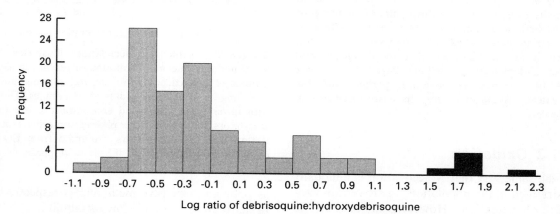

■ **Fig. 8.4.** Polymorphic oxidation, illustrated by the bimodal frequency distribution of urinary debrisoquine:4-hydroxydebrisoquine ratios in the 8 h after a 10 mg oral dose of debrisoquine in 100 Caucasian individuals. Those with a lower ratio are extensive hydroxylators, those with a higher ratio are poor hydroxylators. (Adapted from Peart *et al.* (1986). *Br. J. Clin. Pharmacol.* **21**, 465–71, with permission.)

blockade thus lasts only a few minutes. However, in some individuals the pseudocholinesterase is abnormal and does not metabolize the succinylcholine so rapidly. In these individuals the drug persists in the blood and continues to produce neuromuscular blockade for several hours. This results in respiratory paralysis (sometimes called 'scoline apnoea'), which requires prolonged ventilation until the succinylcholine is cleared from the blood.

In this enzyme abnormality the affinity of the enzyme for its metabolic substrate is decreased and the amount of normal enzyme is also reduced. The abnormalities of pseudocholinesterase are of three main types, each of which is inherited in autosomal recessive fashion. Succinylcholine resistance is discussed later.

(a) Dibucaine-resistant type (Fig. 8.5)

The normal pseudocholinesterase is about 80 per cent inhibited by the local anaesthetic dibucaine at a concentration of 10^{-5} mol/L (10 μmol/L). The percentage inhibition of an individual's enzyme by dibucaine is called the 'dibucaine number'. In some people there is a homozygous defect which results in the production of an abnormal enzyme with a reduced affinity for succinylcholine. This variant is resistant to inhibition by dibucaine. These individuals have low dibucaine numbers (about 15) and are at risk of succinylcholine apnoea.

(b) Fluoride-resistant type

This is a rare variant of pseudocholinesterase abnormality in which the enzyme has a variable response to dibucaine but is resistant to inhibition by fluoride. Homozygotes are at risk of succinylcholine apnoea.

(c) 'Silent' gene type

This is another rare variant in which homozygotes have little or no enzyme activity at all and cannot hydrolyse succinylcholine.

8.1.4 Vitamin D dependency (type I)

This is discussed under the heading vitamin D resistant rickets below.

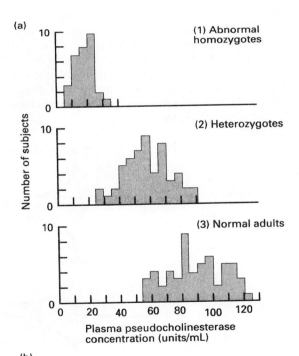

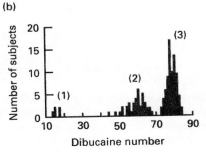

■ **Fig. 8.5.** Pseudocholinesterase deficiency (dibucaine-resistant variety). (a) The frequency distribution of plasma pseudocholinesterase concentrations is trimodal, homozygotes and heterozygotes having lower concentrations than unaffected individuals. (Adapted from Lehmann and Silk (1961). *Br. Med. Bull.* **17**, 230–3, with permission). (b) The frequency distribution of dibucaine numbers (a measure of the affinity of the inhibitor dibucaine for the enzyme) is also trimodal, but the dibucaine number differentiates the groups from each other more clearly than the plasma pseudocholinesterase concentrations. (Adapted from Kalow and Staron (1957). *Can. J. Biochem. Physiol.* **35**, 1305–17, with permission.)

8.2 Pharmacodynamic defects

Some individuals have biochemical abnormalities which make them peculiarly sensitive or resistant to the effects of certain drugs.

8.2.1 Red cell enzyme defects

Unusual drug reactions may occur in individuals whose erythrocytes are deficient in any one of three different but functionally related enzymes:

(1) glucose-6-phosphate dehydrogenase (G6PD);

(2) glutathione reductase;

(3) methaemoglobin reductase.

The metabolic inter-relations of the reactions catalysed by these enzymes are shown in Fig. 8.6. G6PD catalyses the oxidation of glucose-6-phosphate to phosphogluconate, from which pentose-5-monophosphate is eventually generated. Although this phosphogluconate pathway is relatively unimportant as a route of glycolysis, it is important as a source of reduced NADP (i.e. NADPH). NADPH in turn is an important electron donor in the reaction catalysed by glutathione reductase, in which oxidized glutathione is converted to reduced glutathione, which in turn is necessary for the prevention of the oxidation of various cell proteins. Although NADPH also acts as an electron donor for the reduction of methaemoglobin by one of the enzymes in the methaemoglobin reductase complex, this is a relatively unimportant pathway for methaemoglobin reduction, and the enzyme for which NADH acts as an electron donor is more important (see below).

(a) Glucose-6-phosphate dehydrogenase deficiency

There are many variants of G6PD, not all of which are associated with G6PD deficiency and haemolysis in response to drugs. Lack of G6PD in erythrocytes results in diminished production of NADPH. Consequently oxidized glutathione (and, to a lesser and insignificant extent, methaemoglobin) accumulates. If the erythrocyte is then exposed to oxidizing agents haemolysis occurs, probably because of unopposed oxidation of sulphydryl groups in the cell membrane, which are normally kept in reduced form by the continuous availability of reduced glutathione.

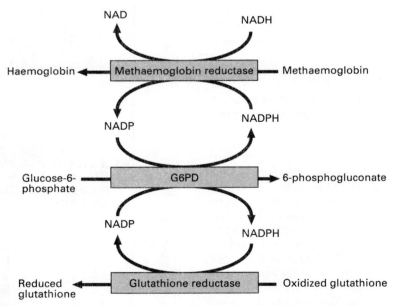

■ **Fig. 8.6.** The reactions catalysed by glucose-6-phosphate dehydrogenase (G6PD), methaemoglobin reductases, and glutathione reductase in red cells, and their metabolic inter-relations. Deficiency of G6PD or of glutathione reductase may result in haemolysis on exposure to certain drugs (see Table 8.1 and the text). Deficiency of methaemoglobin reductase may result in methaemoglobinaemia on exposure to these drugs.

The prevalence of this defect varies with race. It is rare among Caucasians, and occurs most frequently among Sephardic Jews of Asiatic origin, of whom 50 per cent or more are affected. It also occurs in about 10–20 per cent of Blacks.

Inheritance of the defect is sex-linked but complex, the enzyme being heterogeneous. There are broadly speaking two varieties of deficiency, the Black variety and the Mediterranean variety. In the variety which affects Blacks (but is not confined to them) G6PD production is probably normal, but its degradation is accelerated, so that only old red cells (those older than about 55 days) are affected. In this form acute haemolysis occurs on first administration of the drug and lasts for only a few days. Thereafter continued administration causes chronic mild haemolysis (Fig. 8.7). In the Mediterranean variety the enzyme is abnormal, and both young and old cells are affected. In this form severe haemolysis occurs on first administration and is maintained with continued administration.

The commonly used drugs which may cause haemolysis in susceptible individuals are listed in Table 8.1. The reaction is sometimes called 'favism', because it may result from eating broad beans (*Vicia faba*), which contain an oxidant alkaloid.

(b) Glutathione reductase deficiency

This enzyme deficiency may directly cause a deficiency of reduced glutathione (see Fig. 8.6), and haemolysis will then result from the effects of the oxidizing agents listed in Table 8.1. In addition warfarin and phenylbutazone have also been implicated. The defect has autosomal dominant inheritance.

(c) Methaemoglobin reductase deficiency

Although there are several mechanisms for preventing the accumulation of methaemoglobin in the red cell, the methaemoglobin reductase complex of enzymes, and particularly the NADH-dependent enzyme, are the most important. In normal individuals methaemoglobin is continuously being reduced to haemoglobin, and forms only 1 per cent of the total red cell haemoglobin.

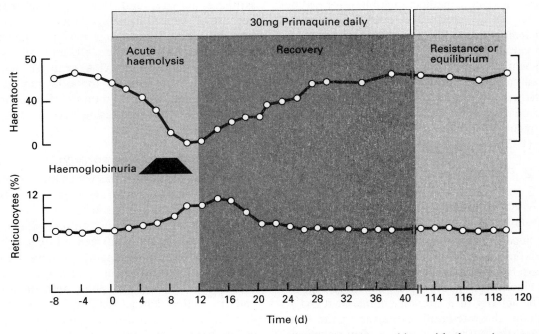

▮ **Fig. 8.7.** The time-course of haemolysis on exposure to primaquine in a subject with the variety of G6PD deficiency which affects Blacks. The abnormality in this variety is accelerated degradation of G6PD. (Adapted from Alving *et al.* (1960). *Bull. Wld. Hlth. Org.* **22**, 621–31, with the permission of the WHO.)

■ **Table 8.1** Drugs which may precipitate haemolysis in subjects with G6PD deficiency

Drugs with the most marked effect	Drugs with possible risk in some individuals
Acetanilid	Analgesics
Doxorubicin	antipyrine
Dapsone and other sulphones	Antimalarials
Furazolidone	chloroquine, mepacrine,
Methylene blue	quinidine, quinine
Nalidixic acid	Sulphonamides other than
Niridazole	those listed in the left-hand column
Nitrofurantoin	Others
Pamaquine	chloramphenicol, dimercaprol,
Phenazopyridine	probenecid, vitamin K
Primaquine	
Sulphonamides	
sulphafurazole	
sulphamethoxazole	
sulphanilamide	
sulphapyridine	
sulphasalazine	

On exposure to the oxidant drugs listed in Table 8.1 (or to glyceryl trinitrate and related compounds) more methaemoglobin is formed but can be rapidly reduced. However, if there is methaemoglobin reductase deficiency this reduction cannot be carried out so efficiently, and methaemoglobin accumulates. Since methaemoglobin causes impairment of oxygen delivery to the tissues this causes tissue hypoxaemia. Inheritance of the defect is autosomal recessive and treatment is with the reducing agent methylene blue (1–2 mg/kg body weight).

8.2.2 Porphyria

(a) Mechanisms of drug-induced attacks of porphyria

The hepatic porphyrias, acute intermittent porphyria and porphyria cutanea tarda, are characterized by abnormalities of haem biosynthesis. The biochemical pathways are shown in Fig. 8.8.

The activity of δ-aminolaevulinic acid (ALA) synthase, the rate-limiting enzyme in the haem biosynthetic pathway, is increased in porphyria, resulting in excess production of ALA and porphobilinogen (PBG), and of the porphyrins down the pathway alternative to haem biosynthesis. Haem normally acts as a repressor of ALA synthase activity, and this action is reduced because of reduced haem synthesis. The mechanisms by which some drugs may precipitate an attack of porphyria are not fully understood, but involve an increase in ALA synthase activity. Drugs which are enzyme inducers may act by diverting haem to the synthesis of cytochrome P450, thereby derepressing ALA synthase activity.

(b) Drugs to avoid in porphyria

In Table 8.2 are listed drugs which are considered unsafe in porphyria and drugs which are probably safe. Although the drugs listed there as being unsafe have all been reported to precipitate acute attacks of porphyria in affected subjects, in some cases (for example diazepam) the data are conflicting and controversial. Furthermore, these drugs do not always precipitate an acute attack, and drug-induced attacks of porphyria are unpredictable. In addition there are many other drugs which have been implicated as being possibly dangerous, but only on the basis of *in vivo* experiments in rats or *in vitro* experiments on

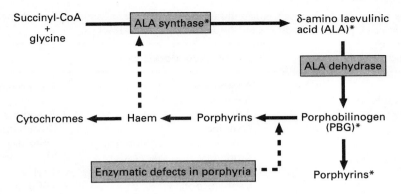

*Increased in hepatic porphyria

■ **Fig. 8.8.** The abnormalities of haem biosynthesis in patients with porphyria.

chick embryo liver cell cultures. If there is any doubt about the safety of an individual drug in a patient with porphyria it would be wise to consult the specialist literature.

(c) Management of an acute attack of porphyria

There are no specific measures of clearly proven value in the management of an acute attack of porphyria. However, it is thought that a high intake of carbohydrate inhibits ALA synthase activity, and a high carbohydrate diet (200 g per day) is unlikely to do any harm. Other measures which are under review include the administration of haematin and large doses of propranolol, both of which may reduce ALA synthase activity.

Because of the lack of specific therapy, the management of an acute attack of porphyria is largely symptomatic. The drugs listed in the right-hand part of Table 8.2. may be used for this purpose, e.g aspirin, paracetamol, or opiates for the treatment of pain, chlorpromazine or promazine for the treatment of vomiting or as tranquilizers, and β-adrenoceptor antagonists for tachycardia and hypertension.

8.2.3 Malignant hyperthermia

This is a serious, potentially fatal complication of general anaesthesia with halothane, methoxyflurane, and succinylcholine. It occurs in about 1 in 20 000 anaesthetized patients and is inherited in autosomal dominant fashion. It is characterized by an acute rise in body temperature to 40–41°C, muscle stiffness, tachycardia, sweating, cyanosis, and tachypnoea. Those affected may have an increase in the plasma activity of skeletal muscle-derived creatine kinase. However, the diagnosis is more readily made by the demonstration of abnormalities in the *in vitro* responses to caffeine and halothane of the muscles of affected individuals. The cause is not fully known, but the defect may involve abnormalities in the compartmentation of sarcoplasmic calcium. Dantrolene, which decreases the amount of calcium released from sarcoplasmic reticulum, is an effective treatment. It is given intravenously in an initial dose of 1 mg/kg, repeated as necessary to a total of 10 mg/kg.

8.2.4 Corticosteroid glaucoma

Intraocular pressure rises during daily use of corticosteroid eyedrops, and the rise is trimodally distributed, 65 per cent, 30 per cent, and 5 per cent of individuals having small, medium, and large increases in pressure respectively. Those who have a large increase in pressure are at increased risk of glaucoma. Inheritance of the abnormal allele is autosomal recessive.

8.2.5 Resistance to drug effects

(a) Vitamin D resistant rickets

There are three varieties of rickets in which the disease is resistant to the effects of vitamin D (cholecalciferol).

∎ **Table 8.2** Drugs which are considered either unsafe or safe to use in individuals with porphyria (adapted from Moore and Disler (1984). *Adv. Drug React. Ac. Pois. Rev.* **2**, 149–189.)

Drugs considered unsafe	Drugs considered safe	
Alcohol (ethanol)	Adrenaline	Prostigmine
Alphaxalone/alphadolone	Aminoglycosides	Quinine
Antipyrine and related drugs	Aspirin	Reserpine
Barbiturates	Atropine	Suxamethonium
Carbamazepine	β-Adrenoceptor antagonists	Thiazides
Chloramphenicol	Bromides	Thioureas
Chlordiazepoxide	Bumetanide	Thyroxine
Colistin	Cephalosporins	Trifluoperazine
Dapsone	Chloral hydrate	Tubocurarine
Diazepam	Chlorpheniramine	Vitamins A, B, C, D, E, K
Dichloralphenazone	Chlorpromazine	
Diclofenac	Colchicine	
Diethylpropion	Cyclizine	
Dimenhydrinate	Dicoumarol	
Ergot preparations	Diethyl ether	
Eucalyptol	Digitalis	
Female sex hormones	Diphenhydramine	
Flufenamic acid	Droperidol	
Flunitrazepam	EDTA	
Frusemide	Flurbiprofen	
Glutethimide	Fusidic acid	
Griseofulvin	Guanethidine	
Hydantoins (for example phenytoin)	Heparin	
Hyoscine butylbromide	Ibuprofen	
Imipramine	Indomethacin	
Isoniazid	Insulin	
Ketoprofen	Labetalol	
Meprobamate	Lithium	
Methyldopa	Meclozine	
Methyprylone	Methadone	
Metoclopramide	Naproxen	
Nalidixic acid	Neostigmine	
Nitrazepam	Nitrous oxide	
Novobiocin	Nortriptyline	
Pancuronium	Opiates	
Pentazocine	Paracetamol	
Phenylbutazone	Penicillamine	
Pyrazinamide	Penicillins	
Ranitidine	Pethidine	
Rifampicin	Prilocaine	
Succinimides (for example ethosuximide)	Primaquine	
Sulphonamides	Procaine	
Sulphonylureas (for example tolbutamide)	Prochlorperazine	
Sulthiame	Promazine	
Theophylline	Promethazine	
Trimethadione	Propantheline	
Troxidone	Propoxyphene	

(i) Familial hypophosphataemic rickets

This is inherited as a sex-linked dominant characteristic. The primary abnormality is probably one of impaired phosphate reabsorption in the kidney, and although the rickets does respond to vitamin D the response is incomplete and the doses required are very large.

(ii) Vitamin D dependency

This is of two types, both inherited as autosomal recessive characteristics. Type I is probably due to decreased 1α-hydroxylation of vitamin D in the kidney (see p. 706), and is therefore strictly speaking a pharmacokinetic abnormality. It responds to high doses of vitamin D and to low doses of 1α-hydroxycholecalciferol and 1α,25-dihydroxycholecalciferol. In contrast, type II is a true pharmacodynamic abnormality, with impaired tissue sensitivity to vitamin D and decreased receptor binding.

(iii) Fanconi syndrome

Rickets in the Fanconi syndrome is due to a failure of tubular reabsorption of phosphate as part of the widespread abnormalities of tubular reabsorption in the syndrome. The syndrome can occur as a result of a variety of hereditary disorders. The rickets responds incompletely to high doses of vitamin D, but can be treated with low doses of 1α-hydroxycholecalciferol or 1α,25-dihydroxycholecalciferol.

(b) Coumarin resistance

There is a wide range of dosage requirements of coumarin anticoagulants in the general population, partly because of genetic variability in both the metabolism of the drugs and the synthesis of clotting factors. However, there is also a very rare type of resistance to the effects of these drugs, in which 20 times the usual dose may be required to produce satisfactory anticoagulation. In affected subjects both the metabolism of the drug and the availability of vitamin K are normal. The mechanism may be resistance of the vitamin K epoxide reductase to inhibition by warfarin. The defect has autosomal dominant inheritance.

(c) Succinylcholine resistance

In some individuals there is a twofold or threefold increase in the concentration of pseudocholinesterase in the plasma, with concomitant resistance to the effects of succinylcholine. The prevalence may be as high as 1 in 1000.

9 Adverse reactions to drugs

9.1 History

From the earliest times pharmaceutical formulations have been recognized as being potentially dangerous. Indeed, it is a truism that unless a drug is capable of doing some harm it is unlikely to do much good.

Public and professional concern about these matters first arose in the late nineteenth century. Between 1870 and 1890 committees and commissions were established in order to investigate sudden deaths occurring during chloroform anaesthesia, now known to be probably due to the effect of chloroform in sensitizing the myocardium to the arrhythmogenic effects of catecholamines. In 1922 there was an inquiry into the jaundice associated with the use of salvarsan, an organic arsenical used in the treatment of syphilis. In 1937 in the USA 107 people died as a result of taking an elixir of sulphanilamide which contained as a solvent diethylene glycol. Although the toxic effects of the solvent were known they were not known to the manufacturer. This led to the establishment in the USA of the Food and Drug Administration (FDA), which was given the task of enquiring into the safety of new drugs before allowing them to be marketed.

These and other examples are listed in Table 9.1, including the major modern catastrophe which changed professional and public opinion toward modern medicines, the thalidomide incident. In 1961 it was reported in West Germany that there was an outbreak in newborn babies of phocomelia (hypoplastic or aplastic limb deformities, so called from the Greek words for seal's limbs). It was subsequently shown that thalidomide, a non-barbiturate hypnotic, was to blame. The crucial period of pregnancy during which thalidomide is teratogenic is the first three months. Of course, not all pregnant women who took thalidomide gave birth to deformed babies, but it is estimated that in West Germany about 10 000 children were born deformed, of whom 5000 survived (the high mortality being due to deformities other than phocomelia). In the UK 600 children were born deformed and 400 survived. In the USA the FDA held up marketing of the drug, because of evidence that it caused hypothyroidism and a peripheral neuropathy, and there were only a few cases of phocomelia in the children of women who took part in clinical trials. At that time teratogenicity testing was not routinely undertaken. It was later confirmed that thalidomide was teratogenic in experimental animals if given early in pregnancy.

The thalidomide incident led to a public outcry, to the institution all round the world of drug regulatory authorities, to the development of a much more sophisticated approach to the preclinical testing and clinical evaluation of drugs before marketing, and to a greatly increased awareness of adverse effects of drugs and methods of detecting them.

None the less, from time to time events occur which result in further modifications of drug regulatory habits. For example, in 1982 a novel anti-inflammatory drug, benoxaprofen, was marketed. Within a year or two there were reports that it could cause liver damage in old people, in some cases severe enough to be fatal. Further investigation suggested that part of the problem was that the doses recommended had been based on studies in young healthy volunteers, while the drug was mainly for use in old people, who metabolized the drug differently. This event led to an increased awareness of the need for pre-marketing testing in subjects (especially the elderly) representative of those who are going to receive the drug in regular therapy. This incident also increased the sensitivity of pharmaceutical manufacturers to the need for the removal of drugs from the market at the first evidence of important adverse effects. Subsequently several

■ **Table 9.1** Drugs of note in the history of adverse reactions

Drug	Date	Adverse reaction	Outcome
Sulphanilamide	1937	Liver damage	Solvent changed FDA established
Diododiethyl tin	1954	Cerebral oedema	Withdrawn
Thalidomide	1961	Congenital malformations	Withdrawn Dunlop Committee (later the CSM) established
Chloramphenicol	1966	Blood dyscrasias	Uses restricted
Clioquinol	1975	Subacute myelo-optic neuropathy	Withdrawn
Practolol	1977	Oculomucocutaneous syndrome	Uses restricted
Benoxaprofen	1982	Liver damage	Withdrawn
Etomidate	1983	Adrenal suppression	Uses restricted
Zimeldine	1983	Hypersensitivity	Withdrawn
Zomepirac	1983	Anaphylaxis	Withdrawn
Indoprofen	1984	Gastrointestinal bleeding and perforation	Withdrawn
Osmosin®	1984	Gastrointestinal ulceration and perforation	Withdrawn
Phenylbutazone	1984	Blood dyscrasias	Uses restricted
Aspirin	1986	Reye's syndrome (children)	Uses restricted
Bupropion	1986	Seizures	Not marketed
Nomifensine	1986	Haemolytic anaemia	Withdrawn
Tocainide	1986	Neutropenia	Uses restricted
Suprofen	1987	Renal impairment	Withdrawn
Spironolactone	1988	Animal carcinomas	Uses restricted
Flecainide	1989	Cardiac arrhythmias	Uses restricted
L-Tryptophan	1990	Eosinophilia–myalgia syndrome	Withdrawn from foodstuffs
Metipranolol 0.6% eyedrops	1990	Anterior uveitis	Withdrawn
Xamoterol	1990	Worse heart failure in some patients	Uses restricted
Noscapine	1991	Gene toxicity	Withdrawn
Terodiline	1991	Cardiac arrhythmias	Withdrawn

drugs have been removed from the market relatively soon after their introduction and very soon after the first reports of adverse effects attributed to them. Non-steroidal anti-inflammatory drugs have been particularly affected (see Table 9.1).

9.2 Incidence of adverse drug reactions

Many different figures have been published on the incidence of adverse drug reactions. In fact, it is very difficult both to be certain how commonly adverse reactions occur overall, and to know what proportion of those which do occur are trivial on the one hand or serious on the other. The following are representative figures:

(1) hospital in-patients – 10–20 per cent suffer an adverse drug reaction;

(2) deaths in hospital in-patients – 0.24–2.9 per cent are due to adverse drug reactions;

(3) hospital admissions – 0.3–5.0 per cent of hospital admissions are due to adverse reactions.

Thus, there is a considerable problem with adverse reactions to drugs, although its precise quantitative nature is unclear.

9.3 Classification of adverse drug reactions

No classification of adverse drug reactions is entirely satisfactory. However, it has been suggested that adverse drug reactions should be classified into two types:

(1) dose-related (so-called type A, or augmented);

(2) non-dose-related (so-called type B, or bizarre).

Since some adverse reactions do not fit neatly into this classification we have added two further groups:

(3) long-term effects;

(4) delayed effects.

Even then, not all adverse drug reactions can be neatly classified, but that is in the nature of classification.

The various subdivisions of these four categories are shown in Table 9.2, and we shall deal with them in the order shown there. We shall deal mainly with the principles underlying the mechanisms involved, giving appropriate examples. Discussions of drugs which cause damage to particular organs are included in the therapeutics section (for example hepatotoxic drugs in the chapter on drugs and the liver, nephrotoxic drugs in the chapter on drugs and the kidney, and so on).

9.4 Dose-related adverse reactions

These are usually due to a pharmacokinetic or pharmacodynamic abnormality producing an excess of a known pharmacological effect of the drug, resulting in an adverse effect. The pharmacological effect which proves adverse may be that through which one hopes to achieve the thera-

■ **Table 9.2** Classification of adverse drug reactions

1. *Dose-related*
   - (a) Pharmaceutical variation
   - (b) Pharmacokinetic variation
     - (i) Pharmacogenetic variation
     - (ii) Hepatic disease
     - (iii) Renal disease
     - (iv) Cardiac disease
     - (v) Thyroid disease
     - (vi) Drug interactions
   - (c) Pharmacodynamic variation
     - (i) Hepatic disease
     - (ii) Altered fluid and electrolyte balance
     - (iii) Drug interactions

2. *Non-dose-related*
   - (a) Immunological reactions
   - (b) Pseudo-allergic reactions
   - (c) Pharmacogenetic variation

3. *Long-term effects*
   - (a) Adaptive changes
   - (b) Rebound phenomena
   - (c) Other long-term effects

4. *Delayed effects*
   - (a) Carcinogenesis
   - (b) Effects concerned with reproduction
     - (i) Impaired fertility
     - (ii) Teratogenesis: adverse effects on the fetus during the early stages of pregnancy
     - (iii) Adverse effects on the fetus during the later stages of pregnancy
     - (iv) Drugs in breast milk

peutic effect (for example hypoglycaemia due to insulin), or to some other effect occurring in parallel with the therapeutic effect (for example the anticholinergic action of tricyclic antidepressants, producing a dry mouth or urinary retention).

Dose-related adverse reactions have led to the concept of the therapeutic index, or the toxic:therapeutic ratio. This indicates the margin between the therapeutic dose and the toxic dose. The bigger the ratio the better. For example, if a patient is not hypersensitive to penicillins then for that patient penicillins will have a high therapeutic index, or a high toxic:therapeutic ratio, since one can safely use much higher doses than one needs to treat the patient effectively. Some examples of commonly used drugs with a low toxic:therapeutic ratio (i.e. for which a small increase in dose beyond the therapeutic dose may result in toxicity) are:

anticoagulants (for example warfarin, heparin);

hypoglycaemic drugs (for example insulin, sulphonylureas);

antiarrhythmic drugs (for example lignocaine, amiodarone);

cardiac glycosides (for example digoxin, digitoxin);

aminoglycoside antibiotics (for example gentamicin, netilmicin);

oral contraceptives;

cytotoxic and immunosuppressive drugs (for example cyclosporin, methotrexate, azathioprine);

antihypertensive drugs (for example β-adrenoceptor antagonists, ACE inhibitors).

Dose-related adverse reactions may occur because of variations in the pharmaceutical, pharmacokinetic, or pharmacodynamic properties of a drug, often due to some disease or pharmacogenetic characteristic of the patient. The following are examples of such mechanisms.

9.4.1 Pharmaceutical variation

From time to time adverse drug reactions can occur because of alterations in the systemic availability of a formulation (see p. 13). The most dramatic example was the outbreak of phenytoin intoxication among epileptic patients in Australia in the late 1960s. This was found to be due to a change in one of the excipients in the phenytoin capsules from calcium sulphate to lactose. This caused an increase in the systemic availability of phenytoin.

Sometimes an adverse reaction can occur because of the presence of a contaminant, for example pyrogens or even bacteria in intravenous formulations, if quality control breaks down. If a febrile reaction occurs in a patient being given an infusion the drip should be taken down and all its components should be sent for bacteriological investigation. The manufacturer should be

urgently notified if ever this sort of contamination is suspected.

Out-of-date formulations may sometimes cause adverse reactions, because of degradation products. For example, out-dated tetracycline may cause Fanconi's syndrome, because it is degraded to anhydrotetracycline and epiandrotetracycline. The omission of the preservative citric acid from tetracycline formulations has reduced the risk of this effect, but has not removed it completely. Paraldehyde which has sat on the shelf for 6 months degrades to acetaldehyde, which is then oxidized to the toxic product acetic acid. In general avoid using out-of-date formulations.

9.4.2 Pharmacokinetic variation

There is a great deal of variation among normal individuals in the rate of elimination of drugs. This variation is most marked for drugs which are cleared by hepatic metabolism and is determined by several factors which may be genetic, environmental (for example diet, smoking, and alcohol), or hepatic (blood flow and intrinsic drug metabolizing capacity). On top of this normal variation there may occur specific pharmacogenetic or hepatic abnormalities which may be associated with adverse reactions. In addition renal and cardiac disease can cause alterations in drug pharmacokinetics.

(a) Pharmacogenetic variation

Pharmacogenetic abnormalities are discussed in detail in Chapter 8. Examples of the pharmacokinetic kind associated with adverse reactions include the increased incidence of peripheral neuropathy in slow acetylators treated with isoniazid, and the prolongation of apnoea following succinylcholine administration to patients with pseudocholinesterase deficiency.

(b) Hepatic disease

Considering the central role of hepatic metabolism in the pharmacokinetic behaviour of many drugs, it might be expected that hepatic disease would frequently be associated with impaired drug elimination. However, such is the reserve of the liver parenchyma that in practice adverse reactions due to impaired hepatic metabolism are not all that common. Nevertheless, in the presence of severe liver disease care must be taken, particularly with drugs with a low toxic:therapeutic ratio and those which are subject to extensive first-pass elimination.

Theoretically, liver dysfunction can affect drug disposition and elimination in several ways, and the outcome in an individual case may be complex and difficult to predict.

1. Hepatocellular dysfunction, as in severe hepatitis or advanced cirrhosis, may reduce the clearance of drugs for which the capacity of the liver is limited, for example phenytoin, theophylline, and warfarin.

2. Portosystemic shunting in portal hypertension, associated with cirrhosis, reduces the clearance of drugs normally cleared by the liver, for example morphine and other narcotic analgesics, propranolol, labetalol, and chlorpromazine.

3. A reduction in hepatic blood flow, as in heart failure, can reduce the hepatic clearance of drugs which have a high extraction ratio (see Chapter 3). Such drugs include lignocaine, propranolol, morphine, and pethidine.

4. Decreased production of plasma proteins (for example albumin) by the liver in cirrhosis may lead to reduced protein binding of drugs. The clinical significance of this effect is discussed in Chapter 10.

5. Drugs which are hepatotoxic may cause reduced clearance of other drugs, even in patients with previously normal liver function. Such drugs need to be used with caution or avoided in patients with liver disease (see pp. 335–9).

(c) Renal disease

If a drug or active metabolite is excreted by glomerular filtration or tubular secretion it will accumulate in renal failure and toxicity will occur. Examples of drugs which may accumulate in renal failure are given in Table 3.7, along with guidance to how dosages should be reduced in those circumstances. Certain pharmacokinetic principles apply in choosing drug dosages in renal failure:

1. The loading dose is not changed, unless the apparent volume of distribution is also altered by renal failure (as in the case of digoxin, whose apparent volume of distribution is lowered by about one-third).

2. Because less drug is cleared per unit time from the body, maintenance dosages should be reduced, either by reducing the size of individual doses, or by reducing their frequency of administration, or by a combination of the two (see, for example, pp. 70–3).

3. The time it takes to reach steady state during repeated dosage will be longer than expected, since the half-time will be prolonged.

4. Protein binding of drugs may be reduced in severe renal failure because of physicochemical changes in plasma albumin (see Chapter 10 for a discussion of the clinical relevance of this effect).

There are some drugs which are nephrotoxic and which should be avoided or used with caution in patients with renal impairment (see p. 361).

(d) Cardiac disease

Cardiac failure, particularly congestive cardiac failure, can alter the pharmacokinetic properties of drugs by several mechanisms:

1. Impaired absorption, due to intestinal mucosal oedema and a poor splanchnic circulation, can alter the efficacy of some oral diuretics, such as frusemide.

2. Hepatic congestion and reduced liver blood flow may impair the metabolism of some drugs (for example lignocaine).

3. Poor renal perfusion may result in decreased renal elimination (for example procainamide).

4. Reductions in the apparent volumes of distribution of some cardioactive drugs, by mechanisms which are not understood, cause reduced loading dose requirements (for example procainamide, lignocaine, and quinidine).

(e) Thyroid disease

The hepatic metabolism of some drugs is increased in hyperthyroidism and decreased in hypothyroidism, but it is not possible to make general statements about all drugs which are metabolized. Drugs reportedly affected are methimazole (the active metabolite of carbimazole), propranolol, practolol, tolbutamide, and hydrocortisone.

Plasma digoxin concentrations are increased in hypothyroidism and decreased in hyperthyroidism, partly because of changes in the apparent volume of distribution, and partly because of changes in renal clearance. In addition there are changes in the pharmacodynamic effects of cardiac glycosides in thyroid disease (decreased in hyperthyroidism, increased in hypothyroidism), and finding the optimum therapeutic dose while avoiding toxicity can be very difficult.

9.4.3 Pharmacodynamic variation

As with pharmacokinetic variability there is a great deal of pharmacodynamic variability within the general population, and that variability may be compounded by the effects of disease, as the following examples show.

(a) Hepatic disease

There are several mechanisms whereby hepatic disease may influence the pharmacodynamic responses to certain drugs.

1. Reduced blood clotting. In cirrhosis and acute hepatitis production of clotting factors may be impaired and patients may bleed more readily. There is also a bleeding hazard in patients with oesophageal and gastric varices caused by portal hypertension in cirrhosis. Drugs which impair clotting, which may impair haemostasis, or which may predispose to bleeding by causing gastric ulceration should be avoided. These include anticoagulants and non-steroidal anti-inflammatory drugs (for example aspirin, indomethacin, and ibuprofen).

2. Hepatic encephalopathy. In patients with, or on the borderline of, hepatic encephalopathy (hepatic coma or pre-coma), the brain appears to be more sensitive to the effects of drugs with sedative actions. If such drugs are used coma may result. It is therefore wise to avoid opioid and other narcotic analgesics and barbiturates. Doses of chlorpromazine should be reduced. Chlormethiazole or short-acting benzodiazepines may be used cautiously as tranquillizers. However, remember that the systemic availability of

chlormethiazole is reduced in hepatic cirrhosis and that oral dosages should be reduced; this stricture does not apply to intravenous dosages (see p. 15).

Diuretics used for the treatment of ascites and peripheral oedema may precipitate hepatic encephalopathy, particularly if there is too rapid a diuresis. This seems to be associated with the production of a hypokalaemic alkalosis, which in turn causes renal ammonia synthesis, resulting in ammonia retention, one of the factors which contributes to hepatic encephalopathy.

3. Sodium and water retention. In hepatic cirrhosis sodium and water retention may be exacerbated by certain drugs. Drugs which should be avoided or used with care include indomethacin and phenylbutazone, corticosteroids, carbamazepine, carbenoxolone, and preparations containing large amounts of sodium, for example some antacid mixtures and sodium salts of penicillins.

Of course, all of these problems may also be exacerbated by drug-induced liver damage (see pp. 335–9).

(b) Altered fluid and electrolyte balance

The pharmacodynamic effects of some drugs may be altered by changes in fluid and electrolyte balance. For example, the toxic effects of cardiac glycosides are potentiated by both hypokalaemia and hypercalcaemia. The class I antiarrhythmic drugs, such as quinidine, procainamide, and disopyramide, may be more arrhythmogenic if there is hypokalaemia, and this combination causes a particular increase in the risk of the polymorphous ventricular tachycardia known as *torsade de pointes*; amiodarone is also subject to this effect. Hypocalcaemia prolongs the action of skeletal muscle relaxants such as tubocurarine, and fluid depletion enhances the hypotensive effects of antihypertensive drugs.

9.5 Non-dose-related adverse reactions

Under this heading we shall deal with immunological and pharmacogenetic mechanisms of adverse reactions.

9.5.1 Immunological reactions (drug allergy or hypersensitivity reactions)

The following are the features of allergic drug reactions:

(1) there is no relation to the usual pharmacological effects of the drug;

(2) there is often a delay between the first exposure to the drug and the occurrence of the subsequent adverse reaction;

(3) there is no formal dose–response curve, and very small doses of the drug may elicit the reaction once allergy is established; the reaction disappears on discontinuation of the drug;

(4) the illness is often recognizable as a form of immunological reaction, for example rash, serum sickness, anaphylaxis, asthma, urticaria, angio-oedema, etc.

The factors involved in drug allergy concern the drug and the patient.

(a) The drug

Macromolecules such as proteins (for example vaccines), polypeptides (for example insulin), and dextrans can themselves be immunogenic. Smaller molecules may act as haptens and combine with body proteins to form antigens. Little is known about the exact nature of many of the haptens (drugs or their metabolites) involved in immunological reactions to drugs. One exception is penicillin, for which the major antigenic determinant is the penicilloyl group which is formed after the splitting of the β-lactam ring (see p. 658).

(b) The patient

There are genetic factors which make some patients more likely to develop allergic drug reactions than others.

(i) A history of allergic disorders

Patients with a history of atopic disease (eczema, asthma, or hay fever) and those with hereditary angio-oedema are more likely to have allergic reactions to drugs.

(ii) HLA status

Antigens on human lymphocytes (HLA) are important in the function of T lymphocytes, which they stimulate in association with foreign antigens. They are controlled by a cluster of genes on the short arm of chromosome 6, the so-called major histocompatibility complex. Several different antigens are expressed by this complex, and some of these have been associated with an increased risk of adverse effects to certain drugs, suggesting genetic mechanisms, although the exact pathology of these reactions has not been elucidated.

For example, the risk of nephrotoxicity from penicillamine is increased in patients with the HLA types B8 and DR3 while patients with HLA-DR7 may be protected. The risk of skin reactions with penicillamine is associated with HLA-DRw6 and the risk of thrombocytopenia is associated with HLA-DR4. Patients with HLA-DR4 also have a greater risk of the lupus-like syndrome (see below) when it is associated with hydralazine. Slow acetylators (see Chapter 8) are also more prone to this reaction. Levamisole toxicity is associated with HLA-B27.

9.5.2 Drug allergy: a mechanistic approach

Theoretically drug allergy and its manifestations should be classifiable according to the classification of hypersensitivity reactions, i.e. into four types, types I to IV. In practice, however, it is not easy to classify allergic drug reactions in this fashion, because they present as clinical syndromes. We shall therefore start by giving examples which do fit this classification, and continue with examples based on the clinical presentation.

(a) Type I reactions (anaphylaxis; immediate hypersensitivity)

In this type of reaction the drug or metabolite interacts with IgE molecules fixed to cells, particularly tissue mast cells and basophil leucocytes. This triggers a process which leads to the release of pharmacological mediators (histamine, 5-hydroxytryptamine, kinins, and arachidonic acid derivatives) which cause the allergic response.

Clinically, type I reactions manifest as urticaria, rhinitis, bronchial asthma, angio-oedema, and anaphylactic shock.

Drugs likely to cause anaphylactic shock include penicillins, streptomycin, local anaesthetics, and radio-opaque iodide-containing X-ray contrast media.

(b) Type II reactions (cytotoxic reactions)

In type II reactions a circulating antibody of the IgG, IgM, or IgA class interacts with a hapten (drug) combined with a cell membrane constituent (protein), to form a hapten–protein/antigen–antibody complex. Complement is then activated and cell lysis occurs. Most examples are haematological: thrombocytopenia associated with quinidine or quinine ('gin and tonic purpura'), digitoxin, and occasionally rifampicin; 'immune' neutropenia can be difficult to distinguish from neutropenia occurring as a direct toxic effect on the bone-marrow, but phenylbutazone, carbimazole, tolbutamide, anticonvulsants, chlorpropamide, and metronidazole have all been incriminated; haemolytic anaemias can also be produced by this mechanism by penicillins, cephalosporins, rifampicin, quinine, and quinidine.

(c) Type III reactions (immune-complex reactions)

In type III reactions antibody (IgG) combines with antigen, i.e. the hapten–protein complex, in the circulation. The complex thus formed is deposited in the tissues, complement is activated, and damage to capillary endothelium results.

Serum sickness is the typical drug reaction of this type and is manifested most commonly by fever, arthritis, enlarged lymph nodes, urticaria, and maculopapular rashes. Penicillins, streptomycin, sulphonamides, and antithyroid drugs may be responsible. This reaction is called 'serum sickness' because it used to occur most commonly as a reaction to injection of foreign serum (for example antitetanus serum). Another example of a type III reaction is the acute interstitial nephritis which may be caused by penicillins and some non-steroidal anti-inflammatory drugs.

(d) Type IV reactions (cell-mediated or delayed hypersensitivity reactions)

In type IV reactions T lymphocytes are 'sensitized' by a hapten–protein antigenic complex. When the lymphocytes come into contact with the antigen an inflammatory response ensues. Type IV reactions are exemplified by the contact dermatitis caused by local anaesthetic creams, antihistamine creams, and topical antibiotics and antifungal drugs.

(e) Pseudo-allergic reactions

We include these reactions here for convenience. 'Pseudo-allergy' is a term applied to reactions which resemble allergic reactions clinically but for which no immunological basis can be found.

For example, asthma and skin rashes caused by aspirin are pseudo-allergic reactions. In a proportion of asthmatics aspirin may trigger an attack of asthma. In cases of extrinsic asthma this may be associated with nasal polyposis and in intrinsic asthma with sinusitis.

Aspirin-sensitive asthmatics are often sensitive to other salicylates and to other non-steroidal anti-inflammatory drugs, such as indomethacin and ibuprofen. In addition, about 50 per cent of aspirin-sensitive asthmatics are also sensitive to tartrazine (E102), a yellow dye used as a colouring agent in some drug formulations and foodstuffs. The prevalence of pseudo-allergic reactions to other food additives is very low (less than half a per cent); agents which have been implicated include quinoline yellow (E104), sunset yellow (E110), carmoisine (E122), amaranth (E123), indigo carmine (E132), green S (E142), annatto (E160(b)), benzoates (E210–E219), sodium metabisulphite (E223), BHA (E320), and BHT (E321). In about a third of patients with chronic urticaria aspirin may make the rash worse.

In some patients the administration of ampicillin or amoxycillin causes a maculopapular erythematous skin rash which resembles the toxic erythema which can occur in penicillin hypersensitivity. However, there is no evidence that the ampicillin rash, as it is called, is immunological in origin. It can be distinguished from true penicillin hypersensitivity on the basis of two features. Firstly, it has a later onset after the first time of administration (typically 10–14 days compared with 7–10 days in penicillin hypersensitivity, although there is some overlap). Secondly, the ampicillin rash does not necessarily recur following re-exposure to ampicillin or amoxycillin, and it is not associated with an increased risk of a serious allergic response to other penicillins. This is contrast to penicillin hypersensitivity, in which further exposure to any member of the penicillin group is contra-indicated because of the high risk of a fatal allergic reaction. The ampicillin rash occurs in about 1 per cent of the normal population, but its incidence is greatly increased in some groups of patients, and it occurs almost invariably in patients with some viral infections (for example infectious mononucleosis, cytomegalovirus infection, measles), lymphomas, and leukaemias. It is also more common in patients who are also taking allopurinol; the reason for this is not known. Of course ampicillin and amoxycillin can also cause allergic reactions in patients with true penicillin hypersensitivity, and if there is any doubt about the nature of a rash which occurs after exposure to ampicillin or amoxycillin it should always be assumed to be a hypersensitivity rash rather than an ampicillin rash, since one should not take the risk of a serious allergic reaction following further exposure to a penicillin.

9.5.3 Drug allergy: a clinical approach

As mentioned above the mechanistic approach does not always fit the clinical presentation. The following are the syndromes with which one is usually faced in clinical practice.

(a) Fever

Drug fever as an isolated phenomenon may occur with penicillins, phenytoin, hydralazine, and quinidine. Such fevers are usually of low grade and the patient is generally not very ill. The fever subsides within a few days of stopping the drug. In the case of the penicillins it can sometimes be difficult to distinguish drug fever from a fever which persists because of resistant infection.

(b) Rashes

These are of several types.

(i) Toxic erythema

This is the commonest skin reaction to drugs. The lesions are macular or maculopapular and can look like those of measles or scarlet fever; sometimes they are more like erythema multiforme; occasionally an urticarial element is present. Antibiotics (for example penicillins), sulphonamides, thiazide diuretics, frusemide, sulphonylureas, and phenylbutazone are commonly implicated.

(ii) Urticaria

Urticarial rashes occur sometimes in response to penicillins, codeine, dextrans, and X-ray contrast media. In some patients with chronic urticaria the rash may be worsened by aspirin.

(iii) Erythema multiforme

In this form of rash target-like lesions often occur on the extensor surfaces of the limbs, and vesicles and bullae may form. In severe cases the mucous membranes of the mouth, throat, eyes, urethra, and vagina may also be involved (Stevens–Johnson syndrome). Penicillins, sulphonamides, barbiturates, and phenylbutazone may be responsible.

(iv) Erythema nodosum

This may be produced by sulphonamides and occasionally oral contraceptives.

(v) Cutaneous vasculitis

Here palpable purpura, vesicles, pustules, and necrotic ulcers may occur. Sulphonamides, phenylbutazone, thiazide diuretics, allopurinol, indomethacin, phenytoin, and alclofenac have all been implicated.

(vi) Purpura

Drugs which produce thrombocytopenia may produce purpura (see type II reactions above and Table 28.8). Non-thrombocytopenic purpura may result from capillary damage or fragility caused by drugs such as corticosteroids, thiazide diuretics, and meprobamate.

(vii) Exfoliative dermatitis and erythroderma

Red, scaly, and exfoliative lesions, which may on occasion involve extensive areas of skin, may be caused by gold salts, phenylbutazone, isoniazid, and carbamazepine.

(viii) Photosensitivity

Increased sensitivity to sunlight (ultraviolet light) may be produced by sulphonamides, thiazide diuretics, sulphonylureas, tetracyclines, phenothiazines, and nalidixic acid.

(ix) Fixed eruptions

These are round, well-circumscribed, erythematous plaques, which are associated with local pigmentation. If they recur they do so at the same site. They may be caused by phenolphthalein, barbiturates, sulphonamides, and tetracyclines.

(x) Toxic epidermal necrolysis (Lyell's syndrome)

This severe eruption is characterized by the shearing of sheets of epidermis, giving the skin the appearance of having been scalded. It may occur with phenytoin, sulphonamides, gold salts, tetracyclines, allopurinol, and phenylbutazone.

(c) Connective tissue disease

A syndrome mimicking systemic lupus erythematosus, often with joint involvement, may result from treatment with hydralazine, procainamide, phenytoin, or ethosuximide. Although this reaction is conveniently discussed here it is to some extent dose-dependent, since the risk is increased at higher drug doses, and in the cases of hydralazine and procainamide it is more common among slow acetylators (see Chapter 8). The features which distinguish this syndrome from the idiopathic form of lupus erythematosus are listed in Table 9.3.

It is possible that sulphonamides may on rare occasions cause polyarteritis nodosa.

(d) Blood disorders

Thrombocytopenia, neutropenia, haemolytic anaemia, and aplastic anaemia may all occur as adverse drug reactions (see above and Chapter 28).

(e) Respiratory disorders

Asthma occurring as a pseudo-allergic reaction to aspirin, other non-steroidal anti-inflammatory drugs, and tartrazine has been mentioned above. Other adverse drug reactions in the lung include pneumonitis associated with the lupus-like syndrome (see above), pulmonary eosinophilia, and fibrosing alveolitis.

9.5.4 Pharmacogenetic variation causing non-dose-related reactions

Pharmacogenetic abnormalities are discussed in Chapter 8. The pharmacodynamic abnormalities cause reactions which are generally not dose-related. They include haemolysis in patients with glucose-6-phosphate dehydrogenase (G6PD) deficiency (see Table 8.1) and acute attacks of porphyria (see Table 8.2) in susceptible patients.

<u>9.6</u> Long-term effects causing adverse reactions

Adverse effects listed under this heading are related to the duration of treatment as well as to dose, and may be regarded as being related to some function of the two.

■ **Table 9.3** Features distinguishing drug-induced from idiopathic lupus erythematosus (LE)

Feature	Idiopathic LE	Drug-induced LE
Age and sex	Usually young women	Any (depends on treatment)
Renal involvement	Common	Rare
Serum complement	Often low	Usually normal
DNA antibodies	Common (native DNA)	Uncommon

9.6.1 Adaptive changes

Adaptive changes which can occur in response to drug therapy have been discussed in detail in Chapter 4. Sometimes such changes can form the basis of an adverse reaction. Examples include the development of tolerance to and physical dependence on the narcotic analgesics (see p. 61) and the occurrence of tardive dyskinesia in some patients receiving long-term neuroleptic therapy for schizophrenia (see p. 63).

9.6.2 Rebound phenomena

When adaptive changes occur during long-term therapy sudden withdrawal of the drug may result in rebound reactions (see also Chapter 4). Examples include the typical syndromes which occur after the sudden withdrawal of narcotic analgesics (see p. 62) or of alcohol (delirium tremens). Sudden withdrawal of barbiturates may result in restlessness, mental confusion, and convulsions. A similar syndrome in which anxiety features prominently may occur after the sudden withdrawal of benzodiazepines. Sleeplessness may also be a feature of the sudden withdrawal of these and a variety of other hypnotic drugs. Sudden withdrawal of some antihypertensive drugs may result in rebound hypertension; this is particularly common with clonidine, which should always be withdrawn slowly. Sudden withdrawal of β-adrenoceptor antagonists may result in rebound tachycardia, which may precipitate myocardial ischaemia.

In a separate category is the effect of the sudden withdrawal of corticosteroids. During long-term treatment with a corticosteroid there is interference with the normal feedback system involving the hypothalamus, pituitary gland, and adrenal gland. As a result, the hypothalamus and pituitary become unable to react normally to the stimulus of low circulating corticosteroid concentrations and adrenocorticotrophin (ACTH) is not produced. The adrenal gland thus atrophies. After sudden withdrawal of the corticosteroid the syndrome of acute adrenal insufficiency occurs. The extent to which this effect occurs depends on both the daily dose and the duration of treatment, and it can to some extent be minimized by giving twice the usual dose but on alternate days. If a corticosteroid has to be given every day, in cases where the therapeutic response is poor with alternate-day therapy, hypothalamic–pituitary–adrenal axis suppression can be reduced by giving the dose in the morning. Withdrawal of corticosteroids should be very slow after long-term administration, for example for prednisolone reduce the daily dose by only 1 mg at intervals of no less than a month.

Reversal of the effects of heparin with protamine sulphate may be associated with rebound hypercoagulability and an increased risk of thromboembolism. However, this risk may have to be taken when there is life-threatening bleeding due to heparin overdosage. In contrast, the withdrawal of oral anticoagulants, such as warfarin, is not accompanied by rebound hypercoagulability. There is therefore no need to tail off oral anticoagulation, which can be stopped abruptly when indicated. Subsequent thromboembolism, if it occurs, will be due to the natural history of the pathology and not to rebound hypercoagulation.

9.6.3 Other long-term effects

Chloroquine, which has a particular affinity for melanin, may accumulate in the corneal epithelium, causing a keratopathy, and in the retina, causing a pigmentary retinopathy and blindness. The former occurs in about 30–70 per cent of patients after 1–2 months of therapy, but although the latter is less common it is more serious. The risk increases with daily doses of over 500 mg and in patients also taking probenecid.

Chronic ingestion of analgesic mixtures, particularly those containing phenacetin, causes papillary and medullary necrosis in the kidney, accompanied by renal tubular atrophy. Later the degenerative and fibrotic changes may extend into the cortex and produce glomerular damage and an overall interstitial nephritis. Clinically these changes can result in renal pain, haematuria, and ureteric obstruction. Eventually chronic renal failure may occur. There is still some confusion about the precise type of analgesic responsible for analgesic nephropathy. Undoubtedly phenacetin was the main culprit in the past, and for this reason it has been taken off the market in the UK and other countries and replaced by its active metabolite paracetamol. However, some have suggested that the nephropathy associated with phenacetin was due to the combination of phenacetin with aspirin, and it is possible that phenacetin metabolites are concentrated in the renal medulla, and that the normal tissue response there to oxidative damage is impaired by aspirin. This hypothesis is unproven, but what is certain is that analgesic abuse must be prolonged and heavy for renal damage to occur, for example six or more tablets per day of a combined analgesic formulation containing phenacetin for 3 y or more. It is still not absolutely certain that chronic ingestion of large doses of aspirin cannot by itself cause analgesic nephropathy, but paracetamol seems to be safe.

Some of the long-term adverse effects of amiodarone are caused by the deposition in the tissues of lipofucsin, and some of these adverse effects may mimic the appearances of Fabry's disease or other systemic lipoidoses. These include a neuropathy, pulmonary alveolitis, liver damage, microdeposits in the cornea, and an increased sensitivity of the skin to sunlight.

9.7 Delayed effects causing adverse reactions

A simple example of a delayed adverse drug effect is that of hypothyroidism occurring years after the treatment of hyperthyroidism with radioactive iodine, ^{131}I. However, this is a recognized and acceptable risk of this form of treatment, whereas our other examples are adverse effects which are highly unacceptable.

9.7.1 Carcinogenesis

The subject of the production of tumours in humans through the actions of drugs is a confused and difficult one. The causes and mechanisms of cancers are, in the majority of cases, still unknown. It is seldom possible, on clinical and pathological grounds, to distinguish a 'naturally-occurring' tumour from one produced by an identifiable chemical carcinogen. One therefore has to rely on statistical associations, and these are not easy to observe in a condition whose pathogenesis involves an indefinite period of exposure to a carcinogen (and possibly other chemical substances) and a latent period for its development.

Much time, effort, and money is expended in testing drugs for carcinogenic potential, and it is likely that the incidence of cancer produced by drugs is low, although precise numerical estimates are hard to come by.

There are three major mechanisms which are currently considered to be important in carcinogenesis.

(a) Hormonal

The incidence of vaginal adenocarcinoma is clearly increased in the daughters of women who have taken stilboestrol during pregnancy for the treatment of threatened abortion. The extent to which there are changes in the incidences of various tumours in women taking oestrogens, and in particular oral contraceptives, is not settled. However, there is probably an increase in the incidence of uterine endometrial carcinoma in women taking oestrogen replacement therapy for menopausal symptoms, and oral contraceptives increase the incidence of benign liver tumours.

(b) 'Gene toxicity'

This term is used to cloak the mystery of what happens when certain molecules bind to nuclear DNA and produce changes in gene expression, leading to abnormalities of cell growth and the production of tumours. In humans it is sometimes difficult to divorce this mechanism from suppression of the immune response (discussed below). There are some examples of drug-induced tumours which might fall into this class:

(1) the increased risk of bladder cancer in patients taking long-term cyclophosphamide;
(2) carcinomas of the renal pelvis associated with phenacetin abuse;
(3) the occurrence of non-lymphocytic leukaemias in patients receiving alkylating agents, such as melphalan, cyclophosphamide, and chlorambucil.

(c) Suppression of immune responses

Patients taking immunosuppressive drug regimens, such as azathioprine with corticosteroids, have a greatly increased risk of developing lymphomas. This has mainly been noted after renal transplantation, but has also been seen in other patients. In immunosuppressed patients there also seems to be an increased risk of cancers of the liver, biliary tree, and bladder, of soft tissue sarcomas, bronchial adenocarcinoma, squamous carcinoma of the skin, and malignant melanoma.

There is probably an association between the occurrence of lymphoma and the long-term use of phenytoin, although at present this does not influence the prescribing of phenytoin for the treatment of epilepsy.

9.7.2 Adverse effects associated with reproduction

(a) Impaired fertility

While impaired fertility due to drugs in women is usually a desired effect in the case of oral contraceptives, it may be an unwanted effect of other drugs. For example, cytotoxic drugs may cause female infertility through ovarian failure with amenorrhoea.

Impairment of male fertility can be caused by impairment of spermatozoal production or function and may be either reversible or irreversible:

(i) reversible impairment may be caused by sulphasalazine, nitrofurantoin, monoamine oxidase (MAO) inhibitors, and antimalarials;

(ii) irreversible impairment, due to azoospermia, can be caused by cytotoxic drugs, such as the alkylating agents cyclophosphamide and chlorambucil. In such cases the impairment may be reversible initially, before complete azoospermia has occurred.

(b) Teratogenesis: adverse effects on the fetus during the early stages of pregnancy

Teratogenesis occurs when a drug taken during the early stages of pregnancy causes a developmental abnormality in a fetus. This is dealt with in detail in Chapter 12.

(c) Adverse effects on the fetus during the later stages of pregnancy

Sometimes a drug taken by the mother during the later stages of pregnancy causes adverse effects in the fetus. This is dealt with in detail in Chapter 12.

(d) Adverse reactions to drugs in breast milk

Certain drugs are excreted in breast milk to an extent which is likely to affect the infant, while others are known to be safe. This is dealt with in detail in Chapter 12.

9.8 Surveillance methods used in detecting adverse reactions

During the period of clinical trial which a drug undergoes before its general release none but the most frequent of adverse reactions will be picked up, despite meticulous monitoring, because so few patients are studied.

In Table 9.4 are shown the numbers of patients usually studied during the various stages of the development of a drug before it is marketed for sale or prescription. The total is usually below 2500. In contrast, in Table 9.5 are shown the numbers of patients one would have to study in order to detect only one, two, or three adverse events for given risks of adverse reactions in the treated population. On this basis only adverse reactions with a relatively high incidence will be picked up before marketing. Note, however, that the numbers in Table 9.5 refer to an adverse event which has no background incidence, i.e. which does not occur either as a natural disease or in response to something other than a drug. However, not many adverse drug reactions are like that: they tend to mimic the signs and symptoms of non-drug-induced diseases. In these circumstances it becomes even more difficult to detect an adverse drug reaction. This is illustrated in Fig. 9.1, in which are contrasted the numbers of individuals who need to be studied to detect an adverse event when there is no background incidence (Fig 9.1a) with the greater numbers required

■ **Table 9.4** Numbers of patients usually recruited in pre-marketing studies

Phase I	Volunteer or very early patient studies	25–50
Phase II	Clinical pharmacology in patients	50–100
Phase II	Dose-finding and early efficacy studies	100–250
Phase IV	Extended clinical studies leading to marketing	250–1000 (rarely >2000)
	Total	Usually <2500

■ **Table 9.5** Numbers of patients one would need to observe to have a 95 per cent chance of detecting 1, 2, or 3 cases of an adverse reaction at a given incidence of the reaction

Expected incidence of adverse reaction	Numbers of patients to be observed to detect one, two, or three events		
	1	2	3
1 in 100	300	480	650
1 in 200	600	960	1300
1 in 1000	3000	4800	6500
1 in 2000	6000	9600	13000
1 in 10000	30000	48000	65000

(a)

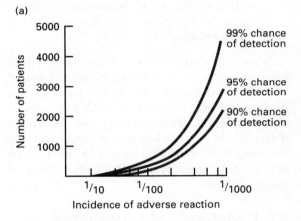

(b)

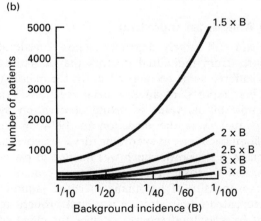

■ **Fig. 9.1** The contrast between the number of individuals who need to be studied to detect an adverse event (a) when there is no background incidence and (b) the greater numbers required when there is a background incidence of varying degrees. (Adapted from Newbould (1981) In Cavalla (ed.) *Risk-Benefit Analysis in Drug Research*, p. 22, MTP Press, Lancaster, with permission.)

when there is a background incidence of varying degrees (Fig 9.1b).

With these considerations in mind adverse reactions can be classified as follows:

1. The drug commonly produces an otherwise rare illness. An example is phocomelia due to thalidomide. Such an event is relatively easily detected by clinical observation.

2. The drug uncommonly produces an otherwise uncommon illness. Aplastic anaemia due to phenylbutazone is an example, again detectable by clinical observation, but with more difficulty than phocomelia.

3. The drug commonly produces an otherwise common illness. It has been suggested that tolbutamide may cause an increased incidence of myocardial ischaemic damage in diabetics. There is, in fact, evidence that that is not the case, but were it so it would be detectable only

by large formal studies. The controversy which surrounded the first publication of this suggestion underlines the difficulty of proving such associations; the results of a large study of the outcome of treating patients with maturity-onset diabetes are awaited.

4. The drug sometimes induces an illness which itself has a moderate incidence. An example of this is the production of endometrial carcinoma by oestrogens. Such an occurrence can be detected only by large formal epidemiological studies.

5. The drug rarely produces an otherwise common illness. This would be extremely difficult to detect by any means, as evidenced by the lack of good examples.

If only the most common of adverse reactions are going to be detected during the pre-marketing stage it is important to devise methods for detecting adverse reactions as quickly as possible after marketing, for confirming that the events detected are truly adverse reactions, and for assessing their overall incidence, in order to be able to make some evaluation of the balance of benefit and risk.

9.8.1 Methods of surveillance

(a) Anecdotal reporting

We are still largely dependent upon anecdotal reports from individual doctors that a patient has suffered some peculiar effect for the majority of 'first reports' of adverse drug reactions. An example of the value of astute observation by individuals was the detection in 1974 of the oculomucocutaneous syndrome (dry eyes, corneal damage, a skin rash which was likened to psoriasis, and sclerosing peritonitis) due to practolol. The propensity of halothane to cause jaundice on repeated administration was first brought to light by anecdotal reports, as was the effect of chloramphenicol in causing neutropenia.

Of course, such anecdotal reports need to be verified by further studies, and these sometimes fail to confirm a problem. Nevertheless, the skill of individual observant clinicians is still a valuable force in the detection of adverse drug reactions.

(b) Voluntary but organized reporting

In Fig. 9.2 is shown the 'yellow card' used in the UK for voluntary reporting of suspected adverse drug reactions to the Committee on Safety of Medicines (CSM). If a doctor sees what is suspected to be an adverse drug reaction he or she should complete one of these cards (they are to be found as detachable pages in the back of the *British National Formulary*) and send it to the CSM. At a later date the doctor may receive a follow-up request for more information.

Every doctor is urged to report a suspected adverse reaction to the CSM on a yellow card as soon as possible after detection. At that stage it does not matter whether the suspected reaction can be fully validated, since the system is geared to detecting patterns of reporting which may implicate a particular drug from the conjunction of a handful of similar reports. Although doctors are asked to report adverse reactions to any therapeutic agent, the CSM is particularly interested in reports on the following types of reactions.

1. Reactions to drugs which are marked with the symbol of a black inverted triangle in the *British National Formulary*. These are usually drugs which have not been on the market for very long. From time to time the CSM issues a list of such drugs, entitled 'New drugs under intensive surveillance'. Doctors are asked to report all suspected reactions to black triangle drugs.

2. Reactions to any drug when the suspected adverse reaction is serious. This includes reactions which are fatal, life-threatening, disabling, or incapacitating, or which result in a prolonged stay in hospital.

3. Reactions which may represent delayed drug effects (see p. 115).

4. Congenital abnormalities.

5. Reactions to all vaccines.

Doctors are also asked to pay special attention to suspected adverse reactions in elderly people.

This system suffers from various problems. For example, it is difficult to be ingenious enough to spot an adverse effect which you do not know exists. Furthermore, there is a natural desire to report an adverse reaction that one has just heard about, and not to report those about which

```
IN CONFIDENCE — COMMITTEE ON SAFETY OF MEDICINES      (For advice on reporting reactions see
REPORT ON SUSPECTED ADVERSE DRUG REACTIONS            Adverse Reactions to Drugs section of BNF)

PATIENT'S DETAILS SURNAME_____ OTHER NAMES _____
DATE OF BIRTH (OR AGE) _____  SEX:  M ☐  F ☐     WEIGHT (kg) [_____]
Hospital if relevant _____ Hospital Number _____ Consultant in charge/GP Principal_____

SUSPECTED DRUG (Give brand name of drug and batch number if   ROUTE _____ DAILY DOSE _____
known) _____
DATE STARTED _____ DATE STOPPED _____   THERAPEUTIC INDICATION _____

SUSPECTED REACTIONS                              REPORTING DOCTOR
_____           Name _____
_____           Address _____
DATE REACTION STARTED____ DATE REACTION ENDED ____        _____
OUTCOME (e.g. fatal, recovered, continuing)_____    _____

SEND TO CSM, FREEPOST, London SW8 5BR                    _____
OR if you are in one of the following NHS regions:   Telephone _____ Specialty _____
TO CSM Mersey, FREEPOST, Liverpool L3 3AB            Signature _____ Date
OR CSM West Midlands, FREEPOST, Birmingham B15 1BR
OR CSM Northern, FREEPOST 1085, Newcastle upon Tyne NE1 1BR   If you would like information about
OR CSM Wales, FREEPOST, Cardiff CF4 1ZZ             other reports associated with the
                                                    suspected drug, tick here ☐        PTO
```

OTHER DRUGS TAKEN IN THE LAST 3 MONTHS INCLUDING SELF-MEDICATION **Give brand name if known** Write **none** if no other drug has been taken	ROUTE	DAILY DOSE	DATE DRUG STARTED	DATE DRUG STOPPED	THERAPEUTIC INDICATION

Additional information including medical history, investigations, known allergies, suspected drug interactions relevant to the reaction and LMP for drugs taken during pregnancy. _____

_____

_____

■ Fig. 9.2 The 'Yellow card' used to report suspected adverse reactions to the Committee on Safety of Medicines. (Reproduced by the permission of the CSM.)

everybody already knows; this introduces an element of bias into the system. Finally, there is a tendency to under-report, mainly because of indolence.

Despite these difficulties this organized voluntary system of reporting in the UK has provided extremely useful information on the occurrence of adverse reactions in the national community. Coupling these occurrence figures with the figures on the numbers of prescriptions issued (information which is available from the Prescription Pricing Authority) the incidence of a given adverse drug reaction can be very roughly calculated.

Although the system has not often been responsible for the initial detection of an adverse reaction, it has been helpful in monitoring adverse reactions in the national community, in validating adverse reactions, and in assessing in a large population the risk of an adverse reaction relative to the potential benefit of treatment. This in turn has led to the formulation of specific advice to doctors about prescribing or warnings not to prescribe a drug in particular circumstances. In serious cases a drug may be taken off the market because of this kind of monitoring, as happened with practolol and benoxaprofen. In those cases the risk of adverse reactions was thought to be greater than the potential benefits.

(c) Other systems of post-marketing surveillance

Because of the imperfections of voluntary reporting systems other surveillance methods have been tried or considered, but for various reasons none has yet proved completely satisfactory. What one needs is speed of detection, an estimate of the incidence or prevalence of the reaction in the population taking the drug, and clues to the factors involved (for example age, sex, concurrent diseases, concurrent drug therapy). From information of this kind one may be able to estimate the benefit:risk ratio and even be able to give advice which will allow the prescriber to prevent the adverse reaction.

(i) Intensive event recording

The aims of certain hospital-based adverse reaction reporting schemes have been to designate a group of individuals to screen a defined population specifically to detect adverse reactions and then to relate them to specific drugs. Such schemes (for example the Boston Collaborative Surveillance Program) have provided interesting statistics on the occurrence of adverse reactions in hospitals around the world, but have not generally been effective in detecting anything new. That is partly because the population studied in such schemes is relatively small and, more importantly, each patient is studied for only a short period of time.

(ii) Cohort studies (prospective studies)

In a cohort study, patients taking a particular drug are identified and events are then recorded. The weakness of this method is the relatively small number of patients likely to be studied, and the lack of a suitable control group in which to assess the background incidence of any apparent adverse reactions noted. Such studies are also very expensive and it would be difficult to justify and organize such a study for every newly marketed drug.

(iii) Case-control studies (retrospective studies)

In a cohort study one starts with the drug and looks for an effect; in a case-control study one starts with the effect and looks for the drug. In a case-control study patients who present with symptoms or an illness which could be due to an adverse drug reaction are screened to see if they have taken the drug. The prevalence of drug-taking in this group is then compared with the prevalence in a reference population who do not have the symptoms or illness. The case-control study is thus suitable for determining whether a drug causes a given adverse effect once there is some initial indication that it might. However, it is not a method for detecting completely new adverse reactions. The relationship between maternal stilboestrol ingestion and vaginal adenocarcinoma was confirmed by this method.

(iv) Use of population statistics

Registers of causes of death and of congenital malformations are held in the UK by the Office of Population Censuses and Surveys, and other information may be available from other sources (for example hospital and other records, see the next item). A change in the pattern of deaths (as happened, for example, among young asthmatics in the early 1960s and again more recently) might stimulate an investigation of a possible drug-related cause. In the case of the young asthmatics it was subsequently shown that the increase in deaths was attributable to the increased use of bronchodilator aerosols containing non-selective (i.e. β_1 and β_2) adrenoceptor agonists. More recently a similar increase in deaths in young asthmatics, particularly in New Zealand, has been attributed to the chronic use of β_2-adrenoceptor agonists, particularly fenoterol. Following the suggestion that Debendox® (Bendectin®) was teratogenic a study was made of congenital malformation data in Northern Ireland. No association was found, and in this case it was possible to provide reassurance that the formulation was probably safe. It was none the less withdrawn from the market.

(v) Record linkage

The idea here is to bring together a variety of patient records:

> general practice records of illness events;
> general practice records of prescriptions;
> hospital records of illness events;

hospital records of prescriptions.

In this way it may be possible to match illness events with drugs prescribed. Particularly interesting are studies in which general practice prescribing is related to hospital admissions and diagnoses. One such analysis suggested a link between antihistamine prescribing and motorcycle accidents. Retrospective linkage of drugs prescribed in general practice with illness events noted in hospital confirmed the association between practolol and eye complaints.

A specific example of the use of record linkage is the so-called Prescription-Event Monitoring Scheme, in which all the prescriptions issued by selected practitioners for a particular drug are obtained from the Prescription Pricing Authority. The prescribers are then asked to inform those running the scheme of any events (whether attributable to adverse reactions or not) in the patients taking the drug. This scheme is less expensive and time-consuming than other surveillance methods. The debate on how best to monitor adverse drug reactions continues, and no system is perfect. The various advantages and disadvantages of the different schemes are outlined in Table 9.6.

■ **Table 9.6** Advantages and disadvantages of various post-marketing surveillance schemes

Scheme	Advantages	Disadvantages
Anecdotal reports	Simple; cheap	Rely on individual vigilance and astuteness; only detect relatively common effects
Voluntary organized	Simple	Under-reporting; reporting bias by 'bandwagon' effect
Intensive event monitoring	Easily organized	Selected population studied for a short time
Cohort studies	Can be prospective; good at detecting effects	Very large numbers required; very expensive
Case-control studies	Excellent for validation and assessment	Will not detect new effects; expensive
Population statistics	Large numbers can be studied	Difficult to co-ordinate; quality of information may be poor; too coarse
Record linkage	Excellent if comprehensive	Time-consuming; expensive; retrospective; relies on accurate records

10 Drug interactions

A drug interaction occurs when the effects of one drug are altered by the effects of another drug. Usually this results in an adverse drug reaction, but in a few cases a drug interaction may prove beneficial.

For clarity of discussion we shall call the drug which precipitates an interaction the *precipitant* drug and the drug whose action is affected the *object* drug. Occasionally in an interaction the effects of both drugs may be altered, as, for example, in the complex interaction of phenytoin with phenobarbitone. In such cases our nomenclature does not apply.

10.1 Incidence of significant drug interactions

Hundreds of interactions have been described. However, relatively few are of clinical importance, and it is those with which we shall deal here. The incidence of such reactions is hard to gauge, since there are certain distinctions which are difficult to make: the distinction between the frequency with which two potentially interacting drugs are prescribed together and the frequency with which clinically important interactions occur as a result of such prescriptions; the distinction between events which occur spontaneously and events which occur as a result of adverse drug effects; and the distinction between adverse drug effects which occur as a result of misuse of the drug causing the adverse effect and those which occur as the result of a drug interaction.

Clearly there will be problems in collecting incidence figures of this kind. In regard to the general incidence of drug interactions of clinical importance a further difficulty is created by geographical differences in drug prescribing habits. For example, in the USA the number of drugs being taken by patients on admission to hospital is nearly twice that in the UK, and the more drugs a patient is taking the greater the chance of an interaction.

Despite these problems incidence figures are available. It has been estimated that interactions form about 7 per cent of all adverse drug reactions, and that among the few patients who die from adverse drug reactions (about 4 per cent of all deaths) about a third are due to interactions.

10.2 Drugs likely to be involved in interactions

Although it is not always possible to be sure about the clinical importance of a reported drug interaction, it is possible to predict which types of drugs are likely to be involved in important reactions. The following are examples.

10.2.1 Drugs which are likely to precipitate drug interactions

1. Drugs which are highly protein bound, and are therefore likely to displace object drugs from protein binding sites. Such drugs include aspirin, phenylbutazone, sulphonamides, and trichloracetic acid (a metabolite of chloral hydrate and its congeners).

2. Drugs which alter (stimulate or inhibit) the metabolism of other drugs. Examples of drugs which may stimulate drug metabolism include various anticonvulsants (phenytoin, carbamazepine, and phenobarbitone), rifampicin, dichloralphenazone (because it contains antipyrine), and griseofulvin. Examples of drugs which may inhibit drug metabolism include allopurinol, chloramphenicol, cimetidine, metronidazole and other imidazoles (for

example ketoconazole), monoamine oxidase inhibitors, phenylbutazone and related drugs (for example azapropazone and sulphinpyrazone), and quinolone antibiotics (for example ciprofloxacin).

3. Drugs which affect renal function and alter the renal clearance of object drugs (for example diuretics, probenecid).

10.2.2 Drugs which are likely to be the objects of drug interactions

The drugs which are most likely to be the object drugs in interactions are those which have a steep dose–response curve (i.e. drugs for which a small change in dose results in a relatively large change in therapeutic effect, important in interactions causing decreased efficacy of the object drug) and drugs which have a low toxic:therapeutic ratio (i.e. drugs for which the dose at which toxic effects start to occur is little more than the therapeutic dose, important in interactions causing toxic effects of the object drug). These two criteria are two sides of the same coin and they are fulfilled by aminoglycoside antibiotics, anticoagulants, anticonvulsants, antihypertensive drugs, cardiac glycosides, cytotoxic and immunosuppressant drugs, oral contraceptives, and drugs acting on the central nervous system.

10.3 Pharmaceutical interactions

Pharmaceutical interactions are physicochemical interactions, either of a drug with an intravenous infusion solution, or of two drugs in the same solution. Such interactions result in the loss of activity of the object drug.

Pharmaceutical interactions are too numerous to remember in detail. However, they can be simply avoided by adhering to the following principles.

1. Give intravenous drugs by bolus injection if possible or via an infusion burette.

2. Do not add drugs to infusion solutions other than dextrose or saline. Even in those solutions some drugs are unstable, while others are light-sensitive and must be protected from the light to prevent rapid loss of activity. These drugs are listed in Table 10.1.

3. Avoid mixing drugs in the same infusion solution, unless you know the mixture to be safe (for example potassium chloride with insulin).

4. Read the manufacturer's literature to look for specific warnings and to check that the drug is suitable for intravenous administration. For example, the data sheets for dopamine and dobutamine warn against mixing these drugs with alkaline solutions such as bicarbonate, a procedure which would also be avoided by following principle 2 above. The *British National Formulary* also contains information about the intravenous administration of a large range of drugs.

5. Mix the drug thoroughly in the infusion solution and check both soon after and later during the infusion for visible changes (turbidity,

■ **Table 10.1** Stability of drugs in saline and dextrose solutions

1. Unstable: infuse within 2–4 h
   Ampicillin (dextrose only; stable in saline for 12 h)
   Erythromycin

2. Stable for 6–8 h
   Benzylpenicillin
   Dacarbazine
   Diazepam
   Frusemide (use only in saline)
   Tetracosactrin

3. Stable for 12 h
   Flucloxacillin
   Oxytetracycline
   Tetracycline

4. Photosensitive drugs
   Amphotericin
   Dacarbazine
   Sodium nitroprusside

5. Drugs which must not be infused after 6 h in solution
   Cephaloridine
   Colistin

precipitation, or colour change). However, the absence of such changes does not guarantee the absence of an interaction.

6. Prepare solutions only when needed. The exceptions to this rule are those drugs which are available in prepacked infusion solutions, for example potassium chloride, lignocaine, metronidazole, and chlormethiazole.

7. Label all infusion bottles clearly with the name and dose of drug added and the times of starting and ending the infusion.

8. Use two separate infusion sites if you must infuse two drugs simultaneously, unless you are sure that there is no interaction.

9. Consult your local hospital pharmacist if in doubt.

10.4 Pharmacokinetic interactions

Pharmacokinetic interactions occur when the absorption, distribution, or elimination (metabolism or excretion) of the object drug is altered by the precipitant drug.

10.4.1 Absorption interactions

Although there are several mechanisms whereby the absorption of a drug may be altered by another drug (for example, the decrease in gastrointestinal motility caused by morphine-like drugs and drugs with anticholinergic effects, such as the tricyclic antidepressants; chelation of calcium, aluminium, magnesium, and iron salts by tetracyclines), such effects are rarely of clinical importance. Among the exceptions are the interactions of cholestyramine with warfarin and digitoxin, whose initial absorption and reabsorption after biliary excretion are reduced, resulting in increased dosage requirements.

There are two important examples of beneficial absorption interactions. Metoclopramide increases the rate of gastric emptying and this hastens the absorption of analgesics in the treatment of an acute attack of migraine (Fig. 10.1). Charcoal binds certain drugs in the gut and thus prevents their initial absorption or their reabsorption after biliary excretion or intestinal secretion.

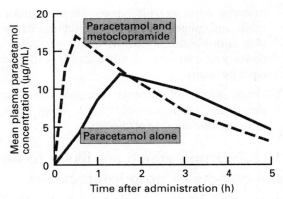

■ **Fig. 10.1** The effect of metoclopramide on the absorption of paracetamol. When metoclopramide (10 mg i.v.) was given with paracetamol (1.5 g orally) the rate of paracetamol absorption was increased, as evidenced by a higher and earlier peak paracetamol plasma concentration. However, the extent of absorption of paracetamol was not changed, since the area under the plasma concentration versus time curve was unaffected (see p. 13). (Adapted from Nimmo *et al.* (1973) *Br. Med. J.* **i**, 587–9, with permission.)

This principle is of value in the treatment of self-poisoning with drugs such as phenobarbitone and the tricyclic antidepressants (see Chapter 35, pp. 490–1).

10.4.2 Protein-binding displacement interactions

Displacement of one drug by another from its sites of binding to plasma proteins will cause an increase in the circulating concentration of unbound drug, and thus the potential for an increased effect of the displaced drug. If the precipitant drug is withdrawn the reverse will occur. However, such interactions are only likely to be of importance if two criteria are fulfilled: the object drug must be highly protein bound (greater than 90 per cent) and must have a low apparent volume of distribution (see Chapter 3, p. 15). If the object drug is less highly bound the amount displaced (which is usually of the order of a few per cent) will make little impact on the circulating unbound concentration, and if it is widely distributed to the tissues any increase in unbound concentration will be diluted by further distribution.

The important drugs which fulfil the criteria of high protein binding and a low apparent volume of distribution (V), and which may therefore be object drugs in protein-binding displacement interactions, are warfarin (99 per cent bound, $V=9$ L), phenytoin (90 per cent bound, $V=35$ L), and tolbutamide (96 per cent bound, $V=10$ L).

The commonest precipitant drugs involved in protein-binding displacement interactions are the sulphonamides, the salicylates, chloral hydrate and some of its congeners (because of their metabolite trichloracetic acid), and phenylbutazone and related drugs (oxyphenbutazone and azapropazone). In addition, valproate specifically displaces phenytoin.

However, the importance of protein-binding displacement interactions has been exaggerated, and such interactions are often of no clinical importance. The reason is that drugs such as warfarin, phenytoin, and tolbutamide have a low hepatic extraction ratio (see Chapter 3, p. 31 and Table 3.5), and for such drugs the rate of total clearance from the body is proportional to the fraction of unbound drug in the plasma. Thus, when the object drug is displaced its rate of clearance increases in proportion to the degree of displacement. This means that at steady state the total concentration of drug in the plasma will have fallen to a new equilibrium value, such that the free concentration is the same as it was before the precipitant drug was introduced, in spite of an increase in the free fraction. This is illustrated in Fig. 10.2. In some cases the change in free fraction occurs so slowly that the compensatory increase in clearance reduces the transient increases in free concentration of the object drug to negligible proportions. Provided the patient can 'weather' the increase, if any, in free concentration of the object drug for as long as it takes to reach the new steady state such an interaction will not be of clinical importance. This implies that such interactions can be mitigated by the slow introduction of the precipitant drug. An example of a protein-binding displacement interaction is shown in Fig. 10.3.

However, there is another consideration which must be taken into account when interpreting the plasma concentration of the object drug in these circumstances, and it is of importance for the

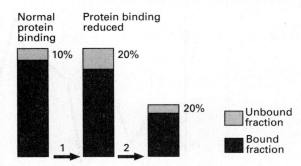

■ **Fig. 10.2** The events following displacement of a drug from its binding sites on plasma proteins. (1) Displacement of the drug leads to an increase in unbound fraction from 10 per cent to 20 per cent. This leads to an increase in the unbound concentration and therefore to increased effects of the drug. (2) If the drug has a low extraction ratio (see p. 31) its total clearance is proportional to the unbound fraction, and the clearance increases. Eventually the total concentration falls, so that although the unbound fraction is still increased, the unbound concentration is the same as it was before displacement occurred.

monitoring of therapy with phenytoin. The principle can be understood by reference to Fig. 10.2. Suppose that a patient has a therapeutically effective total plasma phenytoin concentration of 60 µmol/L (usual 'therapeutic' range 40–80 µmol/L) of which 10 per cent is unbound (i.e. unbound concentration 6 µmol/L). If the unbound fraction is increased to 20 per cent very rapidly, the unbound concentration will double to 12 µmol/L. However, the clearance rate of total phenytoin will also double and at the new equilibrium the total phenytoin concentration will fall to 30 µmol/L, of which 20 per cent will be unbound (i.e. an unbound concentration of 6 µmol/L). From the point of view of how the patient feels (which is determined by the concentration of unbound drug in the plasma) the new equilibrium is no different from the old, but it is clear that the 'therapeutic' plasma concentration range (measured as total drug) is now lower than before the interaction. In other words, for this patient the 'therapeutic' range is reduced. This emphasizes the importance of interpreting the plasma concentration of a drug in terms of the patient's clinical condition and of not treating the patient according to the plasma concentration.

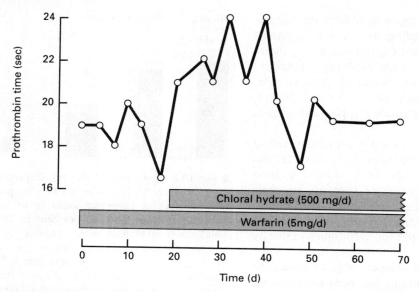

■ **Fig. 10.3**   An example of an interaction involving the displacement of a drug from its binding sites on plasma proteins. This patient had a stable prothrombin time while taking warfarin 5 mg daily. When chloral hydrate was given in a dose of 500 mg daily it displaced warfarin from its albumin binding sites and the plasma concentration of unbound warfarin rose, with a consequent increase in prothrombin time. However, as described in theory in Fig. 10.2, this effect was transient, since the rate of clearance of warfarin increased in proportion to the increase in unbound fraction. Thus, the unbound concentration of warfarin returned to its previous value, as did the prothrombin time, within 30 days, despite continuing administration of chloral hydrate. (Adapted from Weiner (1971) *Ann. N. Y. Acad. Sci.* **179**, 226–33.)

10.4.3 Cellular distribution interactions

Rifampicin may reduce the effects of warfarin by inhibiting its uptake by hepatocytes. However, it also induces warfarin metabolism and reduces its effects principally by that mechanism (see below).

The active transport of some antihypertensive drugs (bethanidine, guanethidine, debrisoquine) into sympathetic nerve-endings, where they have their therapeutic effects, is inhibited by tricyclic antidepressants (and perhaps also by some phenothiazines), with resultant loss of blood pressure control. This may also be the basis for the similar interaction of the tricyclic antidepressants with clonidine and α-methyldopa.

10.4.4 Metabolism interactions

Drug interactions involving metabolism occur when the metabolism of an object drug is either inhibited or increased by a precipitant drug. Of the different metabolic pathways (see Chapter 3)

it is Phase I oxidation which is usually affected. 'Oxidation' is a term which embraces several different metabolic transformations, all of which involve oxidation by the so-called 'mixed function' oxidase system. Such transformations include hydroxylation (for example phenytoin, debrisoquine), deamination (for example amphetamine), dealkylation (for example morphine, azathioprine), sulphoxidation (for example chlorpromazine, penicillamine), desulphuration (for example thiopentone), and dehalogenation (for example DDT, halogenated anaesthetics). The hallmark of these reactions is their dependence on the presence of both NADPH and a haem-containing protein called cytochrome P450. The biochemical processes involved in these reactions, which occur in hepatic microsomes, are shown in Fig. 10.4.

First the drug combines with oxidized cytochrome P450. This combination is reduced by the oxidation of a flavoprotein, cytochrome c, and the flavoprotein is returned to the reduced

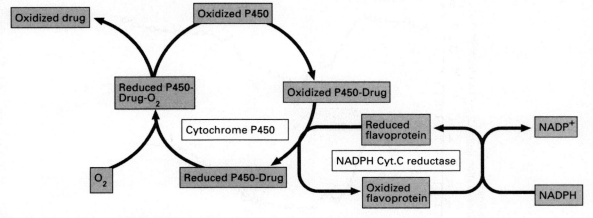

∎ **Fig. 10.4** The role of cytochrome P450 in hepatic microsomal drug oxidation.

state by cytochrome c reductase, NADPH being the electron donor. The reduced P450–drug complex is then oxidized, with the formation of oxidized drug and the regeneration of oxidized P450.

(a) Induction of drug metabolism

Drugs which increase ('induce') drug metabolism do so by increasing the amount of endoplasmic reticulum in hepatocytes and by increasing the content of cytochrome P450 and cytochrome c reductase. The mechanisms whereby these changes occur are not fully understood.

The important interactions of this type are listed in Table 10.2, and an illustrative example is shown in Fig. 10.5. The result of induction of the metabolism of an object drug by a precipitant drug will be a reduction in the plasma concentration of the object drug, and therefore a reduction in its effects (for example epileptic fits while on phenytoin, pregnancy while on an oral contraceptive). If such failure of treatment occasions an increase in dose of the object drug, subsequent withdrawal of the precipitant drug may lead to an enhanced effect of the object drug (for example bleeding after barbiturate withdrawal from a patient otherwise well-controlled on warfarin).

(b) Inhibition of drug metabolism

Interactions involving inhibition of drug metabolism fall, broadly speaking, into two types: those in which the precipitant drug is an inhibitor of mixed function oxidase reactions and those in

∎ **Table 10.2** Drug interactions due to induction of drug metabolism

Precipitant drug(s)	Object drug(s)
Alcohol	Coumarin anticoagulants, phenytoin
Barbiturates	Chlorpromazine, corticosteroids, coumarin anticoagulants, doxycycline, oral contraceptives, phenytoin
Carbamazepine	Phenytoin
Dichloralphenazone	Warfarin
Glutethimide	Coumarin anticoagulants
Griseofulvin	Warfarin
Orphenadrine	Chlorpromazine
Phenylbutazone	Corticosteroids
Phenytoin	Corticosteroids, coumarin anticoagulants, oral contraceptives, tolbutamide
Rifampicin	Coumarin anticoagulants, oral contraceptives, tolbutamide

which other specific metabolic pathways are involved. Important examples of interactions involving inhibition of drug metabolism are listed in Table 10.3, and illustrative examples, one of each type, are shown in Figs. 10.6 and 10.7.

Important examples of inhibition of drug metabolism by inhibition of the mixed function

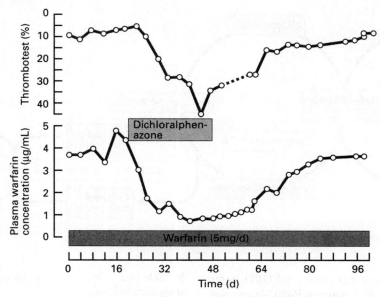

■ **Fig. 10.5** An example of an interaction involving enzyme induction. Although dichloralphenazone contains chloral hydrate, and would be expected to displace warfarin from its binding sites on plasma albumin, it also contains phenazone (antipyrine), which is a powerful enzyme inducer. The result of this interaction is that the metabolism of warfarin is increased and plasma warfarin concentrations fall. In consequence there is a reduction in the prothrombin time (indicated in this case by an increase in the per cent value of the thrombotest). Note that the effect in this case was not complete until 24 days, the time it takes for enzyme induction to occur; after the withdrawal of dichloralphenazone the effect took a similar time to wear off. (Adapted from Breckenridge and Orme (1971). *Ann. N. Y. Acad. Sci.* **179**, 421–31, with permission.)

oxidase are the inhibition of warfarin metabolism by cimetidine, metronidazole, chloramphenicol, norfloxacin and other quinolones, phenylbutazone, and sulphinpyrazone, inhibition of phenytoin metabolism by isoniazid (particularly in slow acetylators, see Chapter 8, p. 94), inhibition of tolbutamide metabolism by phenylbutazone, and inhibition of theophylline metabolism by quinolone and macrolide antibiotics.

The metabolism interaction of phenylbutazone with warfarin is complicated by the fact that it is stereoselective (see also p. 48). Phenylbutazone inhibits the metabolism of the s(−) stereoisomer and thus reduces its clearance. However, it enhances the clearance of the R(+) stereoisomer by protein binding displacement (see above). Thus, although there is no overall effect on the clearance of the racemic mixture, the clinical result is one of increased anticoagulant effect, since the s(−) stereoisomer is about five times more potent than the R(+) stereoisomer. The interactions of metronidazole and

sulphinpyrazone with warfarin are also stereoselective.

The interaction of allopurinol with azathioprine and 6-mercaptopurine is an important example of the effect of inhibition of a specific metabolic pathway distinct from the mixed function oxidase system. During allopurinol therapy xanthine oxidase activity is inhibited. Both 6-mercaptopurine and azathioprine (which is metabolized to 6-mercaptopurine) are metabolized by xanthine oxidase. Thus, their metabolism is inhibited by allopurinol and their dosage requirements are reduced (see Pharmacopoeia). This is of practical importance in the treatment of leukaemia, when allopurinol is given to prevent the hyperuricaemia which results from increased cell turnover induced by cytotoxic drugs such as 6-mercaptopurine.

An inhibitory interaction which has been put to therapeutic use is that of disufiram with alcohol. Alcohol is metabolized to acetaldehyde, which is in turn metabolized to carbon dioxide

▌ **Table 10.3** Drug interactions due to inhibition of drug metabolism

1. Inhibition of the mixed function oxidases

Precipitant drug(s)	Object drug(s)
Azapropazone	Phenytoin
Chloramphenicol	Phenytoin, tolbutamide, warfarin
Cimetidine	Diazepam, propranolol, warfarin
Macrolides	Theophylline
Isoniazid (slow acetylators)	Phenytoin
Metronidazole	Alcohol, S(−)warfarin
Phenylbutazone	Chlorpropamide, phenytoin, tolbutamide, S(−)warfarin
Quinolones	Theophylline, warfarin
Sulphinpyrazone	Warfarin

2. Inhibition of specific metabolic enzymes

Precipitant drug(s)	Enzyme	Object drug(s)
Allopurinol	Xanthine oxidase	Azathioprine
Carbidopa and benserazide	Dopa decarboxylase	L-dopa
Disulfiram	Alcohol dehydrogenase	Alcohol
MAO inhibitors	Monoamine oxidase	Amine-containing foods (see below), amphetamine

3. Amine-containing foods which may interact with MAO inhibitors

Cheese (matured, especially Cheddar; cream and cottage cheeses are safe.)
Meat and yeast extracts
Some red wines
Unfresh protein (especially hung game or poultry; canned or frozen foods are safe if eaten immediately after opening or thawing.)

and water (see Fig. P2). Disulfiram inhibits the metabolism of acetaldehyde, which accumulates and causes an unpleasant reaction, which includes abdominal colic, flushing, dizziness, breathlessness, tachycardia, and vomiting. Disulfiram has therefore been used to try to break the drinking habit in alcoholics.

An example of a therapeutically beneficial interaction involving inhibition of a specific enzyme is that of L-dopa with the dopa decarboxylase inhibitors benserazide and carbidopa. L-dopa is decarboxylated to dopamine by dopa decarboxylase. In the brain this leads to a therapeutic increase in dopamine concentrations, but peripheral decarboxylase activity diverts much of the administered L-dopa to dopamine, which cannot itself enter the brain. Dopa decarboxylase inhibitors decrease this peripheral metabolism and do not themselves enter the brain, where dopamine formation can continue uninhibited. The therapeutically effective dose of L-dopa can therefore be reduced and its peripheral adverse effects, such as hypotension, minimized.

The interaction of monoamine oxidase (MAO) inhibitors with dietary tyramine (Fig. 10.7) results in severe hypertension, which may be fatal. The sequence of events is complex.

1. Inhibition of MAO results in an increase in the noradrenaline content of sympathetic nerve-endings.

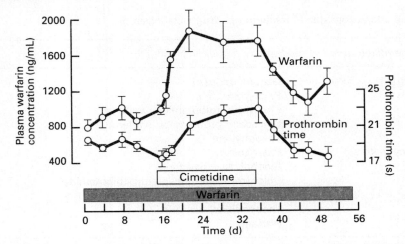

■ Fig. 10.6 An example of an interaction involving inhibition of drug microsomal oxidation. Plasma warfarin concentrations and the prothrombin time both rose after cimetidine (200 mg t.d.s.) was introduced in volunteers taking daily maintenance doses of warfarin. Note that the effect occurred almost immediately, in contrast to the effect of enzyme induction (Fig. 10.5). (Adapted from Serlin *et al.* (1979). *Lancet* **ii**, 317–19, with permission.)

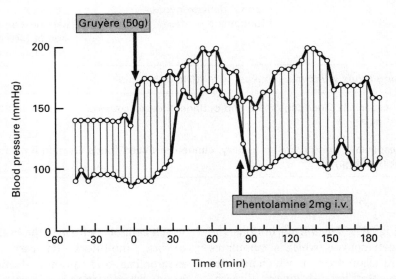

■ Fig. 10.7 An example of an interaction involving the inhibition of a specific drug metabolizing enzyme. In this case the metabolism of tyramine in Gruyère cheese by monoamine oxidase (MAO) was inhibited by debrisoquine, one of whose actions is the inhibition of MAO. As a result, tyramine was absorbed from the gut, and displaced noradrenaline from nerve-endings. Because the noradrenaline was not then metabolized by MAO it caused acute hypertension. This was reversed by the α-adrenoceptor antagonist phentolamine. (Adapted from Amery and DeLoof (1970). *Lancet* **ii**, 613, with permission.)

2. When tyramine is ingested it is normally metabolized by MAO in the gut wall. However, when MAO is inhibited tyramine passes through the gut wall and liver and reaches the systemic circulation.

3. Tyramine releases noradrenaline from its increased stores in nerve-endings and a hypertensive crisis results.

Because it is due to excess noradrenaline the hypertension due to this interaction can be effectively treated with the α-adrenoceptor antagonist phentolamine (Fig. 10.7). Since there are two types of MAO, types A and B, only one of which (MAO A) is responsible for the metabolism of dietary tyramine, this interaction does not occur with the MAO B-selective inhibitor selegiline.

10.4.5 Excretion interactions

Most interactions involving drug excretion occur in the kidneys. The important interactions are listed in Table 10.4 and an illustrative example is shown in Fig. 10.8.

Competition for renal tubular secretion is an important mechanism in excretion interactions. For example, probenecid inhibits the tubular secretion of penicillin so that the blood concentration of penicillin is increased and its therapeutic effects are prolonged; this is a beneficial interaction. A similar effect may underlie the enhanced ocular toxicity of chloroquine in patients also taking probenecid. Quinidine inhibits the tubular secretion of digoxin, and the consequent rise in plasma digoxin concentrations (on average twofold) may be associated with toxicity. The tubular secretion of digoxin is also inhibited by verapamil. Salicyl-

∎ **Table 10.4**   Drug interactions involving altered drug excretion

Precipitant drug(s)	Object drug(s)	Result
Activated charcoal	Tricyclic antidepressants, phenobarbitone	Enhanced excretion rate of object drug
Diuretics	Lithium	Lithium retention
Loop diuretics	Gentamicin	Nephrotoxicity
Phenylbutazone	Acetoheximide, chlorpropamide	Hypoglycaemia
Probenecid	Penicillin	Penicillin retention
Quinidine	Digoxin	Digoxin toxicity

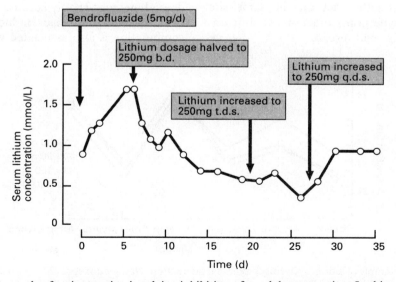

∎ **Fig. 10.8.**   An example of an interaction involving inhibition of renal drug excretion. In this case bendrofluazide (5 mg daily) inhibited the renal elimination of lithium, causing an acute increase in plasma lithium concentrations. The subsequent events suggest that tolerance to this effect may have developed, but this has not been clearly demonstrated. (Adapted from Chambers *et al.* (1977). *Br. med. J.* **iv**, 805–6, with permission.)

ates inhibit the active secretion of methotrexate, thereby potentiating its toxic effects.

An interesting example of a pharmacokinetic interaction which results from a pharmacodynamic effect is that of lithium with frusemide and thiazide diuretics. By their effects on renal tubular sodium transport diuretics cause retention of lithium with consequent toxicity. If diuretics and lithium are used concurrently lithium doses should be reduced, using plasma concentration measurements as a guide.

10.5 Pharmacodynamic interactions

Pharmacodynamic interactions are those in which the precipitant drug alters the effect of the object drug at its site of action. Such interactions may be either direct or indirect. The important examples are listed in Table 10.5 and illustrative examples of the two types are shown in Figs. 10.9 and 10.10.

10.5.1 Direct pharmacodynamic interactions

Direct pharmacodynamic interactions occur when two drugs either act on the same site (antagonism or synergism) or act on two different sites with a similar end result.

(a) Antagonism at the same site

There are numerous examples of such interactions, some of which are therapeutically beneficial. They include the reversal of the effects of opiates with naloxone and the reversal of the actions of warfarin by vitamin K.

(b) Synergism at the same site

The effects of warfarin may be increased or decreased in direct synergistic interactions. The precise mechanisms of these interactions are not clear, but they may involve changes in the affinity of warfarin for vitamin K epoxide reductase (clofibrate, D-thyroxine, anabolic steroids), alterations in the synthesis rate of clotting factors (anabolic steroids), changes in the activity of clotting factors (tetracyclines), or decreased availability of vitamin K secondary to decreased plasma lipids (D-thyroxine, anabolic steroids).

The effects of depolarizing skeletal muscle relaxants are potentiated by some antibiotics (for example aminoglycosides, polymixin B, and colistin) and by quinidine and quinine. These interactions are due to the curare-like effects of the precipitant drugs on the motor end-plate of skeletal muscle.

Verapamil and β-adrenoceptor antagonists cause a higher frequency of cardiac arrhythmias when they are used in combination than either does alone, presumably because of an interaction in the specialized cardiac conducting tissues. This combination is also associated with an increased

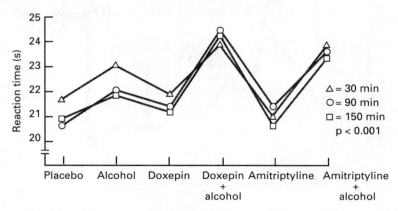

■ **Fig. 10.9** An example of a direct pharmacodynamic interaction. Neither doxepin (20 mg t.d.s.) nor amitriptyline (20 mg t.d.s.) alone altered the reaction time. Alcohol alone prolonged the reaction time slightly. However, the combination of alcohol with either doxepin or amitriptyline prolonged the reaction time by much more than one would expect from the separate effects of each component of the combination. (Adapted from Seppala *et al.* (1975) *Clin. Pharmacol. Ther.* **17**, 515–21, with permission.)

■ Table 10.5   Pharmacodynamic drug interactions

Precipitant drug(s)	Object drug(s)	Result
1. *Direct*		
Aminoglycosides, quinidine, quinine	Depolarizing muscle relaxants	Enhanced skeletal muscle relaxation
Centrally-acting drugs	Centrally-acting drugs	Potentiation
β-Adrenoceptor antagonists	Verapamil	Arrhythmias, asystole, heart failure
Physostigmine	Tricyclic antidepressants	Reversal of anticholinergic effects
Naloxone	Opiate analgesics	Reversal of opiate effects
Vitamin K_1	Coumarin anticoagulants	Diminished anticoagulation
Anabolic steroids Clofibrate Corticosteroids Oestrogens Tetracyclines	Warfarin	Increased anticoagulation
2. *Indirect*		
Class I antiarrhythmic drugs and amiodarone	Class I antiarrhythmic drugs and amiodarone	Increased risk of cardiac arrhythmias
Drugs affecting platelet adhesiveness*	Anticoagulants	Impaired haemostasis
Drugs causing gastrointestinal ulceration*	Anticoagulants	Increased chance of bleeding
Drugs causing fibrinolysis*	Anticoagulants	Impaired haemostasis
Drugs causing potassium loss*	Cardiac glycosides	Increased effects
	Antiarrhythmic drugs	Increased risk of arrhythmias
	Sulphonylureas	Decreased effects
Drugs causing hypercalcaemia	Cardiac glycosides	Increased effects (for example calcium salts, vitamin D)
Drugs causing fluid retention*	Diuretics	Decreased effects
Vasodilators	β-Adrenoceptor antagonists	Improved control of hypertension or angina

* See text for examples.

risk of heart failure, since both have negative inotropic effects on cardiac muscle.

(c) Summation or synergism of similar effects at different sites

Any drug which has a depressant action on central nervous function may potentiate the effect of another such drug, whether or not the two drugs have effects on the same receptors. The most common example is that of alcohol with any centrally-acting drug, but any two such drugs may participate in such an interaction.

Other examples include the numerous combinations of cytotoxic drugs used in the treatment of lymphomas and leukaemias, and the use of combinations of antibiotics in the treatment of some infections, even when only one organism is implicated (for example in infective endocarditis and tuberculosis).

10.5.2 Indirect pharmacodynamic interactions

In indirect pharmacodynamic interactions a pharmacological, therapeutic, or toxic effect of the precipitant drug in some way alters

∎ **Table 10.6** Clinically important drug-drug interactions
In the three parts of this table the interactions discussed in Chapter 10 and listed in Tables 10.2 to 10.5 are iterated and supplemented. However, here they are classified not according to mechanism but according to whether the effect of the object drug is increased (part 1) or decreased (part 2). Interactions which affect both drugs are listed in part 3.

1. *Interactions in which the effects of the object drug are increased*

Object drug(s)	Precipitant drug(s)
Acetoheximide	β-Adrenoceptor antagonists, phenylbutazone
Alcohol	Disulfiram, metronidazole
Amines in foods	MAO inhibitors
Amphetamines	MAO inhibitors
Azathioprine	Allopurinol
Cardiac glycosides	Hypokalaemia (diuretics, purgatives, corticosteroids, amphotericin B), hypercalcaemia (calcium salts, vitamin D), quinidine, spironolactone, verapamil, amiodarone
Cefoxitin	Probenecid
Cephaloridine	Ethacrynic acid, frusemide
Chlorpropamide	β-Adrenoceptor antagonists, phenylbutazone
Coumarin anticoagulants	Amiodarone, anabolic steroids, chloral hydrate, chloramphenicol, cimetidine, clofibrate, dipyridamole, disulfiram, D-thyroxine, indomethacin, ketoconazole, mefenamic acid, metronidazole, neomycin, oxyphenbutazone, phenylbutazone, quinolones, salicylates, sulphinpyrazone, tetracyclines
Gentamicin	Ethacrynic acid, frusemide
Hypoglycaemic drugs (see also individual names)	β-Adrenoceptor antagonists
L-Dopa	Dopa decarboxylase inhibitors (benserazide, carbidopa)
Lithium	Diuretics
Local anaesthetics	Adrenaline
Mercaptopurine	Allopurinol
Penicillin	Probenecid
Pethidine	MAO inhibitors
Phenytoin	Azapropazone, chloramphenicol, coumarin anticoagulants, disulfiram, isoniazid, phenylbutazone
Theophylline	Macrolides, quinolones
Tolbutamide	Chloramphenicol, clofibrate, coumarin anticoagulants, phenylbutazone, salicylates, sulphonamides

2. *Interactions in which the effects of the object drug are decreased*

Object drug(s)	Precipitant drug(s)
Anticholinergic drugs	Cholinesterase inhibitors, cholinoceptor agonists
Bethanidine	Tricyclic antidepressants
Chlorpromazine	Barbiturates, orphenadrine
Hydrocortisone	Barbiturates, phenylbutazone, phenytoin
Clonidine	Tricyclic antidepressants
Coumarin anticoagulants	Alcohol, barbiturates, carbamazepine, cholestyramine, dichloralphenazone, glutethimide, griseofulvin, hydrocortisone, nortriptyline, phenytoin, rifampicin, vitamin K_1
Debrisoquine	Tricyclic antidepressants
Guanethidine	Tricyclic antidepressants

Methyldopa	Tricyclic antidepressants
Opiates	Naloxone
Oral contraceptives	Barbiturates, carbamazepine, phenytoin, rifampicin
Tolbutamide	Rifampicin

3. *Interactions in which the effects of both drugs are increased (↑), decreased (↓), or unpredictable (?)*

↑ ACE inhibitors	Potassium-sparing diuretics
↑ Alcohol	Centrally-acting drugs
↑ B-adrenoceptor antagonists	Verapamil
↑ Barbiturates	Phenytoin
↑ Centrally-acting drugs	Centrally-acting drugs
↑ Class I antiarrhythmics and amiodarone	Class I antiarrhythmics and amiodarone
↓ Salicylates	Sulphinpyrazone
? β-adrenoceptor antagonists	Vasodilators

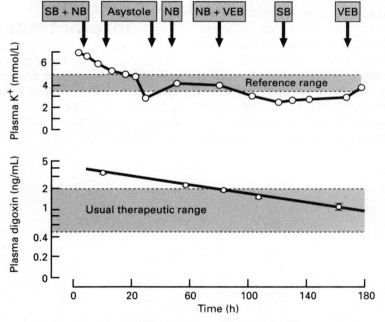

■ **Fig. 10.10** An example of an indirect pharmacodynamic interaction. When this patient's plasma digoxin concentration was high (lower panel) she had frequent cardiac arrhythmias. When the plasma digoxin concentration fell to within the therapeutic range she had no arrhythmias, except when her plasma potassium concentration fell below the reference range, during vigorous haemodialysis (upper panel). (Adapted from Aronson and Grahame-Smith (1977). *Br. J. clin. Pharmacol.* **3**, 1045–51, with permission.)

the therapeutic or toxic effect of the object drug, but the two effects are not themselves related and do not themselves interact.

Warfarin and other anticoagulants may be involved in indirect interactions in three ways:

(a) Platelet aggregation

Some drugs decrease the ability of platelets to aggregate (for example salicylates, dipyridamole, sulphinpyrazone, mefenamic acid, phenylbutazone, and other non-steroidal anti-inflammatory drugs). They therefore impair haemostasis if warfarin-induced bleeding occurs. Thrombocytopenia caused by the precipitant drug would have a similar effect.

(b) Gastrointestinal ulceration

If a drug causes gastrointestinal ulceration it provides a site for bleeding in patients on anticoagulants (for example aspirin, phenylbutazone, indomethacin, and other non-steroidal anti-inflammatory drugs).

(c) Fibrinolysis

Drugs which are fibrinolytic (for example the biguanides) may enhance the effect of warfarin.

Alterations in fluid and electrolyte balance may secondarily alter the effects of some drugs. The effects of cardiac glycosides are enhanced by potassium depletion, while the effects of some antiarrhythmic drugs (for example lignocaine, quinidine, procainamide, phenytoin) are decreased. The common precipitant drugs in such interactions are potassium-wasting diuretics, corticosteroids, and purgatives. The thiazide diuretics may attenuate the hypoglycaemic effects of the sulphonylureas. Although the mechanism of this interaction is not known it has been suggested that it is due to impairment of insulin secretion secondary to potassium depletion. However, the fact that the effect of frusemide and bumetanide in this respect is less marked is evidence against that hypothesis, and a direct interaction at the site of insulin secretion (for example at potassium channels) cannot be ruled out, particularly in view of the similarity in structure between these diuretics and the sulphonylureas.

Finally, the effects of diuretics themselves may be attenuated by fluid-retaining drugs such as carbamazepine, indomethacin, and phenylbutazone.

10.6 Lists of clinically important interactions

In the previous Tables in this chapter drug interactions have been listed according to their mechanism. In Table 10.6 these interactions are listed according to whether the effects of the object drugs are potentiated (Table 10.6.1) or diminished (Table 10.6.2).

11 Drug therapy in young and old people

11.1 Drug therapy in young people

Paediatricians tell us that neonates, infants, and children are not just little adults, and this is certainly true of the ways in which they absorb, distribute, eliminate, and respond to drugs.

Although some dosage schedules for children have already been determined by clinical trial or experience, most are based on some formula relating body weight, age, or body surface area, of the child to the adult dose. Probably the best way to scale down dosages from adult dosages is in proportion to the body surface area:

Dose = (Patient's body surface area/adult body

surface area) × adult dose

The infant's body surface area can be calculated from tables or a nomogram, if one knows its height (length) and weight (see *Martindale's Extra Pharmacopoeia*). Adult body surface area is taken to be 1.73 m^2. The dose calculated in this way is only approximate and is not reliable for preterm neonates and infants, and in some cases for other ages, as illustrated in some of the examples below.

This way of determining a dosage regimen is better than nothing, but it will become apparent that there can never be a simple all-embracing formula relating the dose for a child to the dose for an adult, because of the variability of drug kinetics at various ages, the variability of responses at various ages, and the variability in the properties of individual drugs. It follows that there can be no substitute for carefully executed clinical studies and trials in which optimal paediatric regimens are defined, followed by the intelligent use of those regimens in the individual case. Yet because of the ethical constraints placed upon such investigations in children it often happens that drugs which might be useful in children come on to the market without proper information on dosage regimens in children.

Of course dosage regimens have been developed for paediatric practice, and if you find it necessary to prescribe for a child, and if you are not certain of the correct dosage, or indeed whether the drug can be used in children at all, look it up in the *British National Formulary*, *Martindale's Extra Pharmacopoeia*, a paediatric source book (such as the *Paediatric Vade-mecum*), or the manufacturer's data sheet. If still in doubt consult an experienced paediatrician.

We shall discuss here the general principles underlying the problems of drug therapy in children. Differences among neonates, infants, toddlers, older children, and adults occur in respect to:

(1) pharmaceutical factors – mode of administration;

(2) pharmacokinetic factors – absorption, distribution, metabolism, and excretion;

(3) pharmacodynamic factors – different pharmacological sensitivity to drug effects;

(4) therapeutic and toxic effects peculiar to children – differences in the disease process and its interaction with drugs;

(5) practical matters – compliance, dosage schedules, behavioural problems, and problems with school.

11.1.1 Pharmaceutical factors

Children do not like injections, so oral formulations are preferable. However, vomiting is a common occurrence with febrile illnesses in children, and antibiotics may have to be given parenterally. Small children find swallowing tablets and capsules difficult, so liquid medicines are preferable. However, in practice it is less easy to be precise about dosages when using a 5 mL teaspoon, particularly when unpleasant-tasting medicine is spat out or drooled down the lower lip. On the other hand, the use of pleasant-tasting medicines incurs the risk of self-poisoning and sweetened medicines may contribute to dental caries.

All these common-sense factors have to be taken into account when deciding upon the formulation and route of administration.

11.1.2 Pharmacokinetic factors

(a) Absorption

Although there is reduced gastric acid secretion in the neonate, the practical importance of this in regard to the absorption of drugs and the efficacy of oral therapy has not been well documented.

Oral absorption of drugs in older infants and children is similar to that in adults.

Percutaneous absorption is generally enhanced in neonates, infants, and children, particularly if the skin is excoriated or burnt, and several cases of toxicity due to excessive percutaneous absorption have been recorded. Examples include corticosteroid excess from ointments and creams, boric acid toxicity (diarrhoea, vomiting, convulsions, and occasionally death in infants) from boric acid lotion and ointment, and deafness from aminoglycoside/polymixin antibacterial sprays on burns.

(b) Distribution

Premature babies, neonates, infants, and young children differ from adults in the distribution of their body water and fat, as is shown in Table 11.1. The extent to which a drug distributes between water and fat is related to its physico-chemical characteristics, and it would be expected that the distribution between various body compartments would be different in children, particularly neonates. This difference would be most evident for those water-soluble drugs which are mainly distributed within the extracellular space. Indeed, this has been documented for sulphonamides, whose apparent volume of distribution

in the neonate is about twice that in the adult. However, the overall effect of any changes in distribution of such drugs is usually confounded by concomitant changes in elimination, and well-documented examples of how this theory affects practice are not available.

Plasma protein binding of drugs is reduced in the neonate, but increases with age and reaches adult values by about one year. This is because of lower concentrations of plasma albumin and a lower capacity of that albumin to bind drugs. This is particularly important in the infant with malnutrition and hypoalbuminaemia. It is thought that lowered plasma protein binding is one factor causing the increased apparent volume of distribution of phenytoin in the neonate (1.3 L/kg in neonates compared with 0.6 L/kg in adults).

The interaction of drugs with the binding of bilirubin to plasma proteins in neonates is important, since unconjugated non-protein bound bilirubin can cross the blood–brain barrier and cause kernicterus (see p. 155). Many sulphonamides, aspirin, novobiocin, diazoxide, and vitamin K analogues can displace bilirubin from plasma albumin binding sites, and if the hepatic conjugating mechanisms for bilirubin are immature the concentration of unconjugated bilirubin in the blood may rise and predispose to kernicterus.

The blood–brain barrier is less efficient in neonatal animals, and is thought to be so in neonatal humans. This may be one of the reasons why neonates are sensitive to the effects of centrally-active drugs, such as morphine, but other factors may be involved, and the exact role of an immature blood–brain barrier in the neonatal response to drugs remains undefined.

(c) Metabolism

In general hepatic oxidative metabolism and glucuronide conjugation are deficient in the newborn, and the maturation of these drug-metabolizing systems is variable. The following are examples of changed drug metabolism in the young.

(i) Diazepam

The hydroxylation of diazepam is related to age and is particularly poor in neonates. The half-times of diazepam at different ages are listed in Table 11.2.

▌ **Table 11.1**   Relative amounts of body water and fat at different ages

	Total body water (% of weight)	Extracellular fluid (% of weight)	Intracellular fluid (% of weight)	Fat (% of weight)
Premature baby	85	50	35	1
Full-term neonate	70	40	30	15
Infant (6 months)	70	35	35	15
Child	65	25	40	15
Young adult	60	15	45	20
Elderly adult	45	10	35	10

▌ **Table 11.2**   The half-times of diazepam and phenytoin at different ages

Age group	Half-time of diazepam
Premature neonates	38–120 h
Full-term neonates	22–46 h
Infants of one month	10–12 h
Children of 1–15 y	15–21 h
Adults	24–48 h

Age group	Half-time of phenytoin
Neonates	30–60 h
Infants of one month	2–7 h (NB shorter than in adults)
Children of 1–15 y	2–20 h
Adults	20–30 h

(ii) Phenytoin

Phenytoin is normally hydroxylated. Its elimination is related to age and is particularly poor in the newborn. The half-times of phenytoin at different ages are listed in Table 11.2. Remember that the apparent half-time of phenytoin is also dose-dependent, being longer at higher doses. Phenytoin, in common with phenobarbitone, theophylline, carbamazepine, ethosuximide, and some sulphonamides, has a shorter half-time in young children than in neonates and adults, and children of this age may therefore require different dosage intervals. This illustrates the dangers of global assumptions about drug regimens in children.

(iii) Theophylline

Theophylline is an important drug in this context, because of its use in the treatment of apnoea of the newborn. The half-time of theophylline in the neonate is 14–58 h; in adults it is 3–8 h. The advocated aminophylline intravenous infusion dosage protocols for the treatment of adult asthma and those for the treatment of apnoea of preterm neonates are shown in Table 11.3. Note that the weight-related loading dose is the same in neonates as in adults, but that the maintenance infusion dose is several-fold lower, because of decreased clearance of the drug in the neonate. In the neonate monitoring of the plasma concentration is advisable (see Chapter 7).

(iv) Chloramphenicol

Chloramphenicol may be indicated in the treatment of *Haemophilus influenzae* meningitis in the newborn. However, great care should be taken, because of the occurrence of the 'grey syndrome', which is a toxic effect due to the accumulation of chloramphenicol. Chloramphenicol is norm-

▌ **Table 11.3**   Dosage regimens of aminophylline in adults and preterm neonates

	Loading dose (mg/kg)	Infusion dose (mg/kg/h)
Adults (asthma)	5–6	0.9
Preterm neonate (apnoea)	5–6	0.1–0.2

ally conjugated with glucuronide by glucuronyl transferase in the liver. However, this enzyme has inadequate activity during the first month of life, and in addition the neonate is unable to excrete unconjugated chloramphenicol adequately in the urine. Thus, chloramphenicol accumulates and causes vomiting, difficulty in feeding, failure to suck, poor and rapid respiration, cyanosis, and loose green stools. The child becomes ashen-grey (hence the name of the syndrome), flaccid, and hypothermic, and may die.

Because of this toxicity infants less than one month old should not be given more than 25 mg/kg daily in four divided doses at six-hourly intervals. In older infants and children doses of 50 mg/kg daily in four divided doses may be given.

(d) Renal excretion

In the neonate both the glomerular filtration rate (GFR) and renal tubular function are immature and take about 6 months to reach adult levels. For example, the GFR in the neonate is about 30–40 per cent of that in the adult (corrected for body surface area).

Thus, drugs and active metabolites which are excreted in the urine tend to accumulate in neonates and young infants. Examples include gentamicin and the penicillins, the dosages of which need adjustment, particularly in premature neonates. Because the urinary excretion of gentamicin improves markedly over the first weeks of life a dose which was safe and effective initially can become inadequate as therapy proceeds, and plasma concentration monitoring is important (see Chapter 7).

Digoxin dosages in children are very complicated and are discussed below.

11.1.3 Pharmacodynamic factors

There is some evidence that the responsiveness of the tissues to digoxin is reduced in children, and that this may be related to an increase in the amount of the pharmacological receptor for cardiac glycosides, the Na^+K^+ ATPase. However, dosage regimens for digoxin in the young are complicated by the fact that its pharmacokinetics are also altered. For example, GFR is reduced in neonates, particularly in premature

neonates, and since digoxin is cleared principally by renal excretion its half-time is prolonged to twice or three times the adult value. Some studies have also shown an increased apparent volume of distribution in neonates. In the end with digoxin one relies upon long-established empirical dosage regimens. The sort of dosage regimens which have been found to be suitable in the neonate, infant, child, and adult are shown in Fig. 11.1, along with the therapeutic serum concentrations with which they are associated. This illustrates how complex drug therapy can be in children.

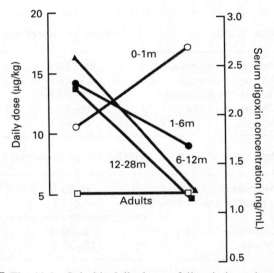

■ **Fig. 11.1** Suitable daily doses of digoxin in patients of different ages and the therapeutic steady-state serum digoxin concentrations with which they are usually associated. Note that neonates (0–1 month) and young infants (1–6 months) are relatively resistant to the effects of digoxin and require higher serum digoxin concentrations (right-hand axis) than older children and adults for a therapeutic effect. However, there is the additional complication that the pharmacokinetics of digoxin are different at different ages, and there is therefore variability in the daily doses required (left-hand axis) to produce the same steady-state serum digoxin concentration (right-hand axis). The axes have been positioned so that the line joining the usual daily dose of digoxin in an adult with the corresponding steady-state serum digoxin concentration is horizontal. (Adapted from Iisalo *et al.* (1973). *Int. J. Clin. Pharmacol.* **7**, 219–22.)

Neonates have increased sensitivity to non-depolarizing neuromuscular blocking agents, such as tubocurarine, while neonates and children seem less sensitive to depolarizing neuromuscular blocking agents, such as succinylcholine, independent of genetic abnormalities in its metabolism (see Chapter 8).

11.1.4 Therapeutic and toxic effects peculiar to children

In adults amphetamine increases motor and behavioural activity. However, in so-called 'hyperkinetic' or 'hyperactive' children it increases attention span and decreases disruptive social behaviour. This may be related to the well-known effect of amphetamine in inducing stereotyped behaviour in animals, i.e. in reducing the numbers of behavioural responses the animal needs to make at any time. Thus, a child who will not pay attention, and who disrupts a school class, may be made to pay attention and to concentrate on the task in hand. It is beyond our scope to discuss whether or not such behavioural control is desirable.

Systemic corticosteroid therapy in children is particularly dangerous, because it may result in stunted growth. The use of inhaled corticosteroids and disodium cromoglycate in the treatment of childhood asthma have been particularly important in avoiding this complication.

11.1.5 Practical matters

There is good advice on prescribing for children in the *British National Formulary*, and you should read the relevant section. We shall mention here some obvious problems.

1. Dosage difficulties with teaspoons and liquids.
2. Children do not like injections, and tablets can be difficult to swallow.
3. Children vomit readily.
4. Parents give in to fractious children, so that compliance can be bad, and the duration of antibiotic and other therapy curtailed, since it no longer seems necessary to continue the treatment when the child seems better.
5. Young children will try anything, and will poison themselves with their own pleasant-tasting medicines or anyone else's drugs. Keep medicines out of their way.
6. Nursing staff responsible for children (and casualty staff may be forgotten in this) need to be reminded from time to time about drug and drug dosage problems in children.

11.2 Drug therapy in old people

The importance of considering drug therapy in old people as a specific group is illustrated by the following facts.

1. In most developed countries old people constitute about 12 per cent of the population, but they consume 25–30 per cent of health service expenditure on drugs.
2. Adverse drug reactions are two to three times more common in old people than in young and middle-aged adults.
3. Polypharmacy in old people is common. In one survey 34 per cent of patients over 75 years of age in a general practice were taking three to four different drugs. The scope for drug interactions is therefore large.
4. The error rate in taking drugs is about 60 per cent in patients over 60 years of age, and the rate of error increases markedly if more than three drugs are prescribed. More of these errors are potentially serious in old people than in young and middle-aged people.

It is easy to understand why there are high prescribing rates and polypharmacy in old people. Old people get ill and often have multiple diseases and symptoms requiring treatment; our task is to learn how best to use drugs to treat them in order to maximize efficacy and minimize adverse reactions.

The term 'old people' implies a homogeneous group, and the first thing to understand is that this is not so as far as drug therapy is concerned. In this respect, at least, old people are like younger individuals: they are very variable in their handling of and responses to drugs. Indeed, the degree of biological variability gets greater as people age, because ageing occurs at different rates in different people.

There are several factors in old people which signal potential trouble, and difficulties in drug therapy increase with an increasing prevalence of these factors. The important factors are: frailty, severe illness, poor appetite and nutrition, poor fluid intake, immobility, multiple diseases, confusion and forgetfulness, an inability for self-care, and lack of supervision. Some of these factors lead to problems with compliance, confusion over treatment, and the use of wrong dosages and wrong drugs (for example from hoarded past prescriptions). Other factors impinge on drug handling and action and it is these factors which we shall discuss here. As in the discussion of drug therapy in young people the problem can be considered according to the all-pervading themes of clinical pharmacology.

1. Pharmaceutical factors – mode of administration.
2. Pharmacokinetic factors –absorption, distribution, metabolism, and excretion.
3. Pharmacodynamic factors – different pharmacological sensitivity to drug effects.
4. Therapeutic and toxic effects peculiar to old people – differences in the disease process and its interaction with drugs.
5. Practical matters – compliance, understanding, dosage schedules, physical problems.

11.2.1 Pharmaceutical factors

Many old people find it difficult to swallow tablets, and the more frail, the more ill, the more dehydrated, and the more confused they are the more difficult it becomes. For example, many potassium tablets are quite large and can cause difficulty, particularly as the diuretic they are given with may be causing dehydration. Some tablets or capsules may adhere to the oesophageal mucosa and dissolve there. Thus, oesophageal ulceration has been attributed to emepromium bromide in the 200 mg tablet strength. The currently available formulation of emepromium bromide, 100 mg, is said not to produce this effect, but to avoid hold-up in the oesophagus the tablets should be swilled down with at least 60 mL of water.

The use of elixirs may help, but not all drugs are available as elixirs, and they may have their own problems. For example, effervescent potassium tablets have to be allowed to dissolve completely in water, and instructions for their use (and for that matter the use of any medicines) are particularly important for old people. Even if they are prepared properly the taste of potassium chloride solution may not be acceptable. The problem of measuring out an exact volume of a preformulated elixir may be particularly difficult for old people with arthritis or other manipulative problems.

11.2.2 Pharmacokinetic factors

(a) Absorption

There are no well-documented examples to show that this is an problem of specific importance in old people.

(b) Distribution

It is important to adjust dosages for body weight in old people, particularly for drugs with a low therapeutic index. There are reductions in plasma protein binding of some drugs in old people (for example phenytoin), the fall being accounted for by the fall in plasma albumin concentration with age.

The distribution of body water and fat is altered in old people (see Table 11.1) and lipid-soluble drugs tend to accumulate to a greater extent than in younger patients because of an increased proportion of fat in the elderly.

Because of different sources of variability it is exceedingly difficult to predict what might happen to the apparent volume of distribution of a drug in old people. For instance, the apparent volume of distribution of diazepam is increased while that of nitrazepam is not.

(c) Metabolism

The elucidation of the ways in which increasing age affects drug metabolism in old people and of the ways in which any changes may affect clinical practice is very difficult, and there are many pitfalls. The following questions will illustrate the problems.

Do you compare healthy old people (and if so how old) with healthy young people (and if so how young)? Do you compare ill old people with ill young people? Do you study smokers or non-smokers (smoking may affect drug metabolism)? Do you control comparisons for nutrition (diet may affect drug metabolism)? Do you compare old patients taking other drugs with young patients not taking other drugs (because so few old patients are taking one drug only and some drugs may alter the metabolism of others)?

When one examines the literature on the subject of drug metabolism in old people the subject becomes confusing, because there are so many variables to take into account. For example, the rates of clearance of warfarin, indomethacin, phenylbutazone, and ethanol are reportedly unaffected by age.

However, there are some clear-cut examples of reduced drug metabolism in old people, and these include propranolol, lignocaine, chlormethiazole, theophylline, phenobarbitone, and paracetamol. The example of nifedipine is shown in Fig. 11.2. Plasma nifedipine concentrations after an intravenous dose of nifedipine are higher in old people than in the young, and this difference is entirely attributable to reduced metabolism of nifedipine to its metabolite nitropyridine, the apparent volume of distribution of nifedipine being unaltered in old people. As a result the half-time of nifedipine is prolonged.

(d) Renal excretion

There is a well-documented decrease in glomerular filtration rate with age, such that by the age of 80 y it may have fallen to 60–70 mL/min. Tubular function also declines with age. Therefore, drugs which are mainly excreted in the urine, or which have active metabolites which are so excreted, may require reductions in dosage. Examples include digoxin, gentamicin and other aminoglycosides, lithium, and procainamide (see Table 3.5). The reduction in the renal excretion of frusemide which occurs in old people is shown in Fig. 11.3.

Some drugs are best avoided in old people. For example, tetracyclines accumulate when renal function is poor and cause nausea and vomiting, which in turn causes dehydration, which may cause further deterioration in renal function. In addition tetracyclines have an antianabolic action which worsens uraemia and promotes muscle wasting. All of these adverse effects are particularly hazardous in old people.

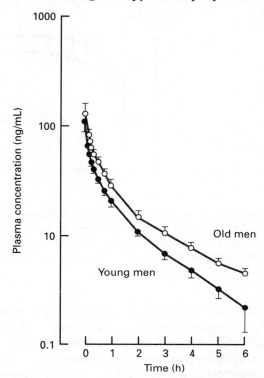

■ Fig. 11.2 Plasma concentrations of nifedipine after the intravenous administration of 2.5 mg of nifedipine to six healthy old men (open circles) and to 11 healthy young men (closed circles). The rate of fall of plasma concentrations of nifedipine was slower in the old men than in the young, and this was entirely attributable to a reduction in the rate of metabolic clearance of nifedipine. (Adapted from Robertson *et al.* (1988). *Br. J. Clin. Pharmacol.* **25**, 297–305, with permission.)

11.2.3 Pharmacodynamic factors

For various reasons drug sensitivity (independent of pharmacokinetics) may be altered in old age, and in many cases this results in increased sensitivity to drugs.

In some cases, altered sensitivity to drugs in old people is due to an alteration in the response of their pharmacological receptors. For example, old people are more sensitive to the effects of digoxin, probably because of increased sensitivity of their Na^+K^+ ATPase. This, combined with their increased susceptibility to potassium loss due to diuretics and their decreased renal function, makes them more liable to digitalis toxicity.

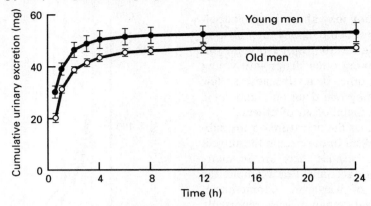

■ **Fig. 11.3** Urinary concentrations of frusemide after the intravenous administration of 80 mg of frusemide to 8 healthy old men (open circles) and to ten healthy young men (closed circles). The old men excreted less frusemide in their urine than the young men, and this was attributable to a reduction in the rate of renal tubular secretion of frusemide (Adapted from Andreasen *et al.* (1983). *Br. J. Clin. Pharmacol.* **16**, 391–7, with permission.)

Another example of this is the decreased sensitivity of β-adrenoceptors in old people, and this may reduce some of the pharmacological effects of β-adrenoceptor agonists and antagonists. An example of this is shown in Fig. 11.4. The increase in heart rate which occurs in response to the β₂-adrenoceptor agonist terbutaline is less in old people than in the young. However, it should also be noted that this difference does not extend to the effect of terbutaline on plasma potassium concentrations, which fall equally in both the young and the elderly. This effect is probably due to adrenoceptor-mediated stimulation of the Na^+K^+ pump in skeletal muscle, and this suggests that adrenoceptors in skeletal muscle and in cardiac muscle may be subject to different forms of regulation in old people.

In other cases altered sensitivity to drugs in old people may be due to altered physiological responses. For example, there is evidence of reduced baroreceptor function in old people, and this can lead to increased hypotension after the administration of antihypertensive drugs. This is illustrated in the case of the calcium antagonist nifedipine in Fig. 11.5.

Other examples of altered pharmacodynamic sensitivity in old people include increased sensitivity to the anticoagulant effects of warfarin and increased responsiveness of the brain to centrally-active drugs, for example hypnotics, sedatives, tranquillizers, antidepressants, and neuroleptics.

11.2.4 Therapeutic and toxic factors peculiar to old people

There are all sorts of practical problems which arise in old people, due to the interaction of drugs with diseases or with aged physiology. Take the treatment of hypertension. The cerebral circulation in old people does not auto-regulate efficiently. Old patients easily become hypovolaemic with diuretics (or even without, if not eating and drinking normally). Peripheral autonomic responses may be sluggish in response to hypotension. All these factors accumulate to make the treatment of hypertension in old people a matter to be cautious about, as it is often very easy to inadvertently produce hypotension, causing syncope, which results in a fall, injury (for example fractured femur, subdural haematoma), immobilization, and all the consequent complications, such as hypostatic pneumonia and pulmonary emboli, which can be fatal. Currently it is believed that treatment of hypertension in old people may be associated with a reduced risk of some of its complications. None the less, hypotensive therapy should be undertaken with caution in old people, because of these other problems.

Then take diuretic therapy. Old people are particularly prone to diuretic-induced hypokalaemia, which may increase the effects of digoxin and cause digitalis toxicity. A brisk diuresis in

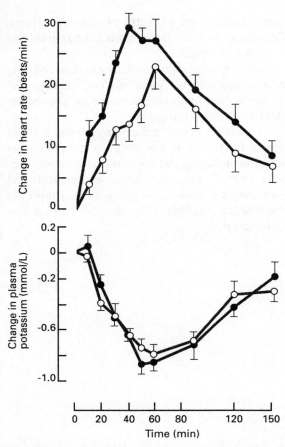

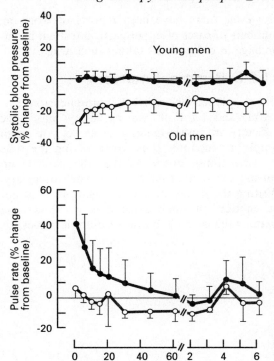

■ **Fig. 11.4** Changes in heart rate (upper panel) and plasma potassium concentrations (lower panel) after the intravenous administration over 60 min of 6 mg/kg of the β-adrenoceptor agonist terbutaline to eight healthy old women (open circles) and to eight healthy young women (closed circles). In the old women the heart rate rose during terbutaline infusion less than it did in the young women. However, the falls in plasma potassium concentrations were the same in the two groups, as were changes in blood glucose concentration (not shown). This difference was attributed to decreased adrenoceptor responsiveness in the old women in the heart but not elsewhere. (Adapted from Kendall *et al.* (1982) *Br. J. clin. Pharmacol.* **14**, 821–26, with permission.)

■ **Fig. 11.5** Changes in systolic blood pressures (upper panel) and pulse rates (lower panel) after the intravenous administration of 2.5 mg of nifedipine to six healthy old men (open circles) and to 11 healthy young men (closed circles). In the old men the systolic blood pressure fell significantly, while there was no effect in the young men. This difference was attributed in part to the difference in plasma concentrations in the two groups (see Fig. 11.2) but mostly to a reduction in baroreceptor function in the old men, since the young men were able to increase their pulse rates in order to maintain blood pressure after nifedipine, while the old men were not. (Adapted from Robertson *et al.* (1988) *Br. J. clin. Pharmacol.* **25**, 297–305, with permission.)

an old man with prostatic enlargement can cause acute urinary retention and diuretics may also cause urinary incontinence in women. Old people, who are at an increased risk of gout anyway, may have gout more easily precipitated by diuretics.

Confusion and hyperactivity in an old person is often treated with a neuroleptic agent, such as chlorpromazine or haloperidol, and this can result in severe Parkinsonism, to which old people are more prone. It is not certain whether or not the clearance rates of non-steroidal anti-inflammatory drugs are decreased in old people, and whether or not the stomach in old people is more prone to peptic erosion or ulceration.

However, there have been reports of worrying numbers of cases of upper gastrointestinal haemorrhage in old patients taking such drugs.

11.2.5 Practical matters

Old people may be slow of comprehension, forgetful, and hard of hearing. They may have difficulty in understanding what to you seem simple instructions. It is worth taking the time to write things down, so that the patient can consult the written instructions when necessary. Writing the names of drugs on bottles may not be enough; in some cases it is worth writing 'water tablets' on a bottle of diuretic tables, or 'heart tablets' on a bottle of digoxin tablets. Remember to write large, since old patients may have poor eyesight.

Old people may have difficulty in manipulating bottles and tablets. Some modern 'child-proof' medicine containers are more easily opened by children than by old people.

In general, when prescribing drugs for old people try to use as few drugs as possible, start with low dosages, and increase the dosages carefully only if required. Choose easily-swallowed formulations, and keep therapy as simple as possible (for example with once-a-day drugs and formulations).

12 Drug therapy and reproduction

12.1 Hormonal contraception

Contraceptive methods can be divided into two broad categories: mechanical methods (condoms, diaphragms, caps, and intrauterine devices, all of which may be combined with chemical spermicides) and hormonal methods. We shall deal here only with the hormonal methods.

Until very recently, hormonal contraception in women has been achieved by the daily oral administration of either progestogens alone or a combination of progestogens with oestrogens. However, other modes of administration are now being investigated. For example, 'morning after' contraception can be achieved with a high dose of oestrogen and progestogen. The frequency of administration of progestogens alone can be reduced by the use of long-acting formulations, for example by depot intramuscular injection, intrauterine inserts, vaginal rings, and subdermal implants. Other types of hormonal manipulation have also become possible, such as the use of antiprogestogens and luteinizing hormone releasing hormone (LHRH) analogues. However, none of these methods is yet in regular use, and virtually all hormonal contraception in the UK is currently achieved by conventional oral formulations.

Hormonal contraception in men is still at the experimental stage, and involves the use of combined formulations of androgens and progestogens. Other drugs which alter sperm function, such as gossypol and d-propranolol, have also been studied.

12.1.1 Mechanisms of action of sex hormones as contraceptives

The mechanisms whereby a progestogen alone or a progestogen plus an oestrogen act as contraceptives are not completely understood, although some of their actions are known. The oestrogens suppress ovulation by inhibiting gonadotrophin release. The progestogens cause changes in the endometrium similar to those found during pregnancy (thus discouraging implantation) and changes in cervical mucus (decreasing its penetrability by spermatozoa). Some progestogens, such as norethisterone and norgestrel, are partly metabolized to oestrogen-related compounds which may have some anti-ovulatory effects.

Oestrogen/progestogen combinations are very effective contraceptives, with a failure rate of around 5 per 1000 woman years of administration. The oral progestogen-only contraceptives have a failure rate of around 25 per 1000 woman years, but the failure rates of the progestogen intrauterine inserts and subdermal implants may be lower, and in the case of the latter the failure rate is said to be similar to that of the combined oestrogen/progestogen formulations.

12.1.2 Hormonal contraceptive formulations and their use

Combination formulations intended for use as oral contraceptives can be classified according to their oestrogen content, since the most important adverse effects are caused by the oestrogen and are dose-related (see Pharmacopoeia). The formulations available in the UK for use as oral contraceptives at the time of writing are listed in Table 12.1. Note that there are some other formulations, not listed in Table 12.1, which contain a combination of oestrogen and progestogen but which are not licensed for use as oral contraceptives. Before prescribing a combination as a contraceptive check the Data Sheet or the manufacturer's literature carefully.

The dosage of oral contraceptive formulations in most cases is one tablet orally daily, starting on the first or fifth day of the cycle and continuing

■ **Table 12.1** Oestrogen/progestogen combination formulations marketed in the UK for oral contraception at the time of writing

Oestrogen	Progestogen	Brand name(s)
Ethinyloestradiol 20 μg	Norethisterone 1 mg	Loestrin-20
Ethinyloestradiol 20 μg	Desogestrel 150 μg	Mercilon
Ethinyloestradiol 30 μg	Desogestrel 150 μg	Marvelon
	Ethynodiol 2 mg	Conova-30
	Gestodene 75 μg	Femodene, Minulet
	Levonorgestrel 150 μg	Ovranette,
Microgynon-30	Levonorgestrel 250 μg	Ovran-30, Eugynon-30
	Norethisterone 1.5 mg	Loestrin 30
Ethinyloestradiol 35 μg	Norethisterone 0.5 mg	Brevinor, Ovysmen
	Norethisterone 0.5/1 mg	BiNovum*, Synphase*
	Norethisterone 0.5/0.75/1 mg	TriNovum*
	Norethisterone 1 mg	Norimin, Neocon 1/35
Ethinyloestradiol 50 μg	Levonorgestrel 250 μg	Ovran, Schering PC4†
Mestranol 50 μg	Norethisterone 1 mg	Norinyl-1, Ortho-Novin 1/50
Ethinyloestradiol 30/40/30 μg	Levonorgestrel 50/75/125 μg	Logynon*, Trinordiol*

*Phased formulations (see text). †Postcoital contraceptive.

for 21 d, followed by a 7-day interval of no treatment, during which menstruation should occur. In order to aid compliance and to make administration easier manufacturers package 21 tablets into a blister pack (see Fig. 12.1), and some include seven dummy tablets to make up the four-week course.

Some formulations are described as 'phased' (see Table 12.1). In these cases the dose of oestrogen and/or progestogen is varied through the cycle. For example, in one such regimen (Logynon® and Trinordiol®) ethinyloestradiol and levonorgestrel are taken in respective doses of 30 and 50 micrograms (for 6 d), followed by 40 and 75 micrograms (for 5 d), and finally by 30 and 125 micrograms (for 10 d). After 7 d of no treatment the cycle is repeated.

For progestogens the usual oral dose is one tablet daily (350 micrograms in the case of norethisterone) in a cycle similar to that for the combined oral contraceptive.

It is important that oral formulations of hormonal contraceptives should be taken regularly (i.e. once a day) if efficacy is to be maintained. The time of day at which combined formulations are taken is unimportant to within about 12 h (see below). However, for progestogen-only formulations the time of administration is crucial: they should be taken at the same time of day to within no more than 3 h and preferably near the usual time of sexual intercourse.

Thus, if a tablet is forgotten the correct course of action depends on both the type of formulation and the time since the last dose. A woman who

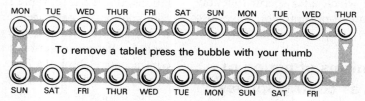

■ **Fig. 12.1** An example of a 'blister pack' for an oral contraceptive. (Reproduced by permission of the manufacturers, Syntex Pharmaceuticals Ltd.)

has missed a tablet should be given the following advice where appropriate.

(a) Combined oestrogen/progestogen formulations

(i) A delay of less than 12 h

Take a tablet immediately and take the next tablet at the usual time.

(ii) A delay of more than 12 h

Take a tablet immediately and then continue as before. If the 21-day cycle ends before seven days are up start the next cycle immediately (i.e. no treatment-free period; in the case of blister packs which contain seven dummy tablets the dummies should be omitted). During the first seven days after resuming treatment another method of contraception should be used.

(b) Progestogen-only formulations

If there has been a delay of more than 3 h (i.e. more than 27 h after the last dose) contraception is lost and the next tablet should be considered as the first of a new regimen. In that case another method of contraception should be used for the next two days.

In an emergency, contraception may be obtained after unprotected intercourse by taking a combination of ethinyloestradiol 50 micrograms and levonorgestrel 250 micrograms, 2 tablets within 72 h of intercourse and another 2 tablets 12 h later. This method should not be used in a woman whose menstrual period is overdue. In women who become pregnant despite this type of contraception there may be an increased likelihood of ectopic pregnancy, which is not prevented by this method.

12.1.3 Adverse effects of oral contraceptives

The adverse effects of oral contraceptives are discussed in detail in the Pharmacopoeia (p. 683).

12.1.4 Drug interactions with oral contraceptives

Drug interactions with oral contraceptives are discussed in detail in the Pharmacopoeia (p. 683).

12.2 The treatment of infertility

The treatment of infertility is a specialist problem. Here we shall merely outline the principles involved in drug therapy. About 33 per cent of cases of infertility are due to an identifiable abnormality of spermatozoa, about 20 per cent to failure of ovulation, and 20 per cent to disease of the Fallopian tubes, often in association with pelvic inflammation. The rest have causes which cannot be discovered.

12.2.1 The treatment of male infertility

If there is an identifiable cause of abnormalities of spermatozoa they should be treated. These include surgical correction of varicocele and of obstruction of the vas deferens or epididymis, hormonal replacement in patients with hypogonadism (see p. 365), and the use of corticosteroids and immunosuppressants in men with antisperm antibodies. Apart from hormone replacement therapy in hypogonadism none of these measures is very satisfactory in restoring fertility.

Anti-oestrogens (clomiphene and tamoxifen) and androgens (mestrolone) have been used to remove the negative feedback to the secretion of gonadotrophin-releasing hormone and gonadotrophins in cases in which no identifiable cause of infertility has been found, but the results are not good.

Artificial insemination using the husband's sperm may be used if there is a mechanical problem, but is of no value if there is oligospermia. However, in such cases *in vitro* fertilization may be used, since very few sperm are required.

12.2.2 The treatment of female infertility

In contrast to male infertility, female infertility responds relatively easily to treatment, except in women with ovarian disease.

Failure of ovulation can be treated by treating identifiable causes. These include prolactin-secreting adenomas (see p. 366), hypothyroidism (see p. 371), drugs which cause hyperprolactinaemia (see Table 27.1), tubal disease, pelvic infection (for example due to *Chlamydia* or *Mycobacterium tuberculosis*), weight loss, and anorexia nervosa.

Endometriosis is sometimes associated with infertility. It generally responds to the progestogen dydrogesterone (10 mg t.d.s. either continuously or from the 5th to the 25th day of the cycle for 3 cycles). Danazol is an alternative (400 mg daily in up to four divided doses for 6 cycles).

The anti-oestrogen clomiphene is used in treating female infertility in cases due to anovulation (for example in anorexia nervosa and polycystic ovarian disease) and when the cause of infertility is unknown. It acts as an antagonist at oestrogen receptors in the hypothalamus, where it prevents the inhibitory effect of circulating oestrogens on the release of gonadotrophin-releasing hormone. Clomiphene is given in a dose of 50 mg daily for 5 d, starting on the 2nd to 5th day of menstruation. In some cases further courses may be tried (100 mg daily for 5 days in the 3rd and 4th cycles). Women who are not menstruating may start clomiphene therapy at any time.

The adverse effects of clomiphene include flushing (an anti-oestrogenic effect), nausea, vomiting, abdominal discomfort, breast discomfort, and weight gain. Multiple pregnancies (mostly twins) occur in about 8 per cent of cases. In women with polycystic ovaries clomiphene may cause enlargement of ovarian cysts. If it causes ovarian hyperstimulation or visual disturbances it should be withdrawn. Clomiphene should not be used until other treatable causes of infertility, such as hypothyroidism and hyperprolactinaemia, have been excluded. Since it is metabolized in the liver and excreted in the bile, care should be taken in patients with diseases of the liver or biliary tract.

If clomiphene does not work in anovulatory infertility gonadorelin (LHRH) may be used. It is given in a pulsatile fashion in order to mimic the normal secretory pattern. This involves the insertion of a portable infusion pump programmed to give a subcutaneous or intravenous infusion of 10–20 micrograms every 90 min continually for up to 6 months. If ovulation occurs the gonadorelin should be withdrawn and an intramuscular injection of human chorionic gonadotrophin (10 000 units) should be given to support the corpus luteum.

The adverse effects of gonadorelin include nausea, abdominal discomfort, headaches, lightheadedness, and flushing. Local pain and swelling may occur at the subcutaneous injection site and thrombophlebitis if the intravenous route is used. Rarely hypersensitivity reactions may occur.

In some cases intrauterine insemination may increase the chance of pregnancy after gonadotrophin-induced ovulation. If other methods fail *in vitro* fertilization or gamete intrafallopian transfer (GIFT) may be used.

12.3 Drug therapy during pregnancy

The potential for doing harm to the fetus by prescribing drugs for the mother during pregnancy is considerable, as was emphasized by the thalidomide disaster (see Chapter 9). It is thought that about 35 per cent of women take drug therapy at least once during pregnancy and that 6 per cent take drug therapy during the first trimester (this excludes iron, folic acid, and vitamins). The most commonly used drugs are simple analgesics, antibacterial drugs, and antacids. However, drugs should only be given to pregnant women if the likely benefit to the mother outweighs the risk to the fetus. In general only those drugs should be prescribed of which there is extensive experience in human pregnancy. This is usually not the case with newly-introduced drugs. Rarely a drug may be given to the mother for a specific therapeutic effect on the fetus.

12.3.1 Altered pharmacokinetics in pregnancy

(a) Absorption

The extent of absorption of drugs is generally unaltered in pregnancy, although the rate of absorption may be reduced because of a reduced rate of gastric emptying. Vomiting is common in pregnancy and may affect drug administration.

(b) Distribution

Plasma volume increases by about 50 per cent and total body water by about 20 per cent during later pregnancy. Thus, if the apparent volume of distribution of a drug is normally low it will increase significantly. However, this is generally not of great clinical importance, firstly because steady-state plasma concentrations are independent of the apparent volume of distribution, and secondly because although an increase in volume causes an increase in half-time, this is usually more than offset by an increase in clearance, due to decreased protein binding and increased metabolism. For example, the apparent volume of distribution of phenytoin is increased in pregnancy, but clearance increases and protein binding decreases. As a result plasma concentrations of total phenytoin, and to a slightly lesser extent, free phenytoin fall (Fig. 12.2).

Plasma protein binding of drugs may fall during pregnancy because plasma albumin concentrations fall by up to 10 g/L. There may therefore be a fall in the bound fraction of drugs

normally extensively bound to plasma albumin. For example, there is an increase in the unbound fraction of phenytoin in the plasma during pregnancy, and as a result total plasma phenytoin concentrations fall because of increased clearance (see p. 124). However, the concentration of free phenytoin does not fall to the same extent, and great care must be taken in adjusting dosages and in interpreting plasma concentration measurements (Fig. 12.2).

(c) Metabolism

Because of the ethical problems of doing drug studies in pregnant women there is not much information about drug-metabolizing capacity in pregnancy. Indirect evidence, such as liver histology and urinary excretion of D-glucaric acid and 6-β-hydroxycortisol, suggests that drug-metabolizing activity may be increased in pregnancy, and this is consistent with the observed

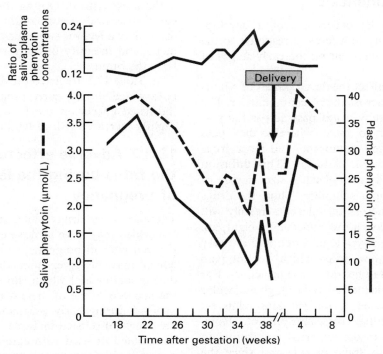

■ **Fig. 12.2** The changes in plasma and salivary phenytoin concentrations during and after pregnancy. The salivary concentration is used as an indirect measure of the unbound concentration of phenytoin in the plasma. Note that both the total and the unbound phenytoin concentrations fall during pregnancy, but that the fall in the unbound concentration is less than that in the total concentration, since the ratio of the two rises. Thus, the fall in the total concentration is due to both decreased protein binding and an increased rate of clearance of phenytoin. (Adapted from Knott *et al.* (1986). *Br. J. Obst. Gynaecol.* **93**, 1030–7, with permission.)

increase in the clearance rate of theophylline during pregnancy. The rate of clearance of phenytoin is also increased in pregnancy, and this is due partly to increased metabolism and partly to decreased protein binding (Fig. 12.2). In contrast, there is no change in liver blood flow during pregnancy, and the clearance of drugs whose hepatic extraction ratio is high (see Table 3.5) does not change.

(d) Excretion

In pregnancy the glomerular filtration rate increases by about 70 per cent. Thus, drugs which are mainly eliminated by renal excretion will be cleared more quickly. The dosage requirements of lithium and digoxin may therefore increase during pregnancy, and plasma concentration monitoring will help to guide therapy (see Chapter 7). Ampicillin clearance is increased during pregnancy and increased dosages are required.

12.3.2 Teratogenesis

Teratogenesis is the occurrence of a developmental abnormality in a fetus in response to the effect of a drug taken during the early stages of pregnancy.

For a drug to affect the development of a fetus it must first pass across the placental barrier. The mechanisms whereby drugs pass across the placenta are similar to those whereby they pass across any lipid cell membrane, and most drugs pass across by simple diffusion. This diffusion depends in part upon molecular size, degree of ionization, and lipid solubility. Thus, the drugs which will pass across the placenta readily will be those which have a low molecular weight, are poorly ionized at physiological pH, and are very fat soluble. The few drugs which do not pass across the placenta illustrate these principles. For example, heparin is ionized and of high molecular weight; tubocurarine is ionized and relatively lipid insoluble; neither crosses the placenta. However, most drugs in the maternal circulation do reach the fetus to some extent, and since the thalidomide incident (see p. 104) great care has been taken about prescribing drugs during pregnancy, particularly during the early stages (i.e. the first trimester). Furthermore, during the development of a drug its potential for teratogen-

esis has to be explored if there is any likelihood of its being promoted for use in women of child-bearing age.

If a drug is known to be teratogenic in humans or animals then the Data Sheet will say so. However, if a drug is not known to be teratogenic in humans a lack of evidence of teratogenicity in animals cannot be taken as evidence that the drug is not teratogenic in humans, and a warning such as the following may be given: 'This drug has not been shown to be teratogenic in animals, and so far there is no evidence that it is teratogenic in humans. However, it should not be used in pregnant women if possible.' If one is tempted to prescribe a drug in a pregnant woman, especially during the first trimester, it is very important to be aware of the current trend of opinion about its safety (see Chapter 20 on sources of information).

The first trimester of pregnancy, and particularly the period from the second to the eighth weeks of gestation, the period of organogenesis, is the most critical. During this time drugs may cause structural abnormalities. Later in fetal life drugs may affect the subsequent growth, development, and integrity of body structures, particularly the brain.

In Table 12.2 are listed the drugs which should be avoided during early pregnancy because of the listed effects on the fetus, or because of a slightly increased risk of fetal abnormality.

12.3.3 Adverse effects of drugs on the fetus during the later stages of pregnancy

There are some drugs which are not teratogenic, but which may have adverse effects on the fetus if given later in pregnancy. These include drugs which may be given immediately before and during labour and which can cause problems in the neonate. Some of these drugs should also be avoided during early pregnancy. The following are drugs (also listed in Table 12.3) which should be avoided or used with care during later pregnancy, and in some cases throughout the whole duration of pregnancy.

(a) Aspirin

Aspirin has been suggested to be teratogenic in early pregnancy, but the case has not been

■ **Table 12.2**   Drugs to avoid during early pregnancy

1. *Drugs with a high risk of causing abnormalities (known teratogens) or of inducing abortion*

Drug	Effect
Alcohol	Fetal alcohol syndrome
Androgens	Virilization and multiple congenital defects
Antineoplastic agents, (e.g. methotrexate)	Multiple congenital defects
Carbimazole	Aplasia cutis
Corticosteroids (high dosages)	Cleft palate
Cyproterone	Feminization of male fetus
Diethylstilboestrol	Vaginal adenosis and adenocarcinoma in daughters
Distigmine	Increases uterine tone
Ergotamine	Increases uterine tone
Misoprostol	Increases uterine tone
Fibrinolytic drugs (e.g. streptokinase)	Placental separation
Tetracyclines	Yellow discoloration of teeth, inhibition of bone growth
Valproate	Neural tube defects
Vitamin A analogues (etretinate etc)	Congenital defects
Warfarin	Multiple congenital defects

2. *Drugs under strong suspicion of producing abnormalities (slightly increased risk)*

Drug	Effect
Amiodarone	Goitre
Chloroquine	Deafness (do not withhold in acute malaria)
Lithium	Goitre, cardiovascular defects
Phenytoin	Multiple congenital defects (do not withhold if absolutely necessary for control of epilepsy)

3. *Other drugs to avoid (theoretical risk from animal and other studies)*

ACE inhibitors	Omeprazole
Auranofin	Quinolone antibiotics
Chenodeoxycholic acid	Rifampicin
Desferrioxamine	Spironolactone
Diltiazem and dihydropyridine calcium antagonists	Sulphonylureas
Fibrates (clofibrate etc)	Thiabendazole
Griseofulvin	Tocainide
Idoxuridine	Trimethoprim (and co-trimoxazole)
Ketoconazole	Vaccines (live)
Mebendazole	Vigabatrin
Mefloquine	Xamoterol

■ **Table 12.3** Drugs to be avoided or used with care during later pregnancy (see text for discussion)

Drug(s)	Risk to fetus or neonates
Aspirin	Kernicterus, haemorrhage (also maternal)
Aminoglycoside antibiotics	Eighth nerve damage
Antithyroid drugs	Goitre and hypothyroidism
Benzodiazepines	'Floppy infant syndrome'
Chloramphenicol	Peripheral vascular collapse
Disopyramide	May induce labour
Fibrinolytic drugs	Fetal/maternal haemorrhage
Misoprostol	May induce labour
Narcotic analgesics	Respiratory depression; opiate withdrawal syndrome if mother dependent
Nitrofurantoin	Haemolysis
Non-steroidal anti-inflammatory drugs	Closure of the ductus arteriosus; delayed and prolonged labour
Oral anticoagulants	Fetal or retroplacental haemorrhage, microcephaly
Sulphonylureas	Hypoglycaemia
Pethidine	Respiratory depression
Reserpine	Bradycardia, hypothermia, nasal congestion with respiratory distress
Sulphonamides and novobiocin	Kernicterus
Tetracyclines	See Table 12.2
Thiazide diuretics	Thrombocytopenia

proven. However, in high doses in late pregnancy it may displace fetal bilirubin from plasma proteins and thus cause kernicterus (see sulphonamides below). Furthermore, if it is taken within about one week of delivery it can cause impaired haemostasis in the mother at the time of delivery and haemorrhage in the neonate.

(b) Aminoglycoside antibiotics

Aminoglycoside antibiotics should be used in pregnancy only if absolutely essential, because of their effects on the eighth nerve.

(c) Antithyroid drugs

Antithyroid drugs may be used during pregnancy, but at the minimum dosage necessary to control maternal hyperthyroidism. Some recommend using half the usual doses during pregnancy.

(d) Benzodiazepines

Benzodiazepines given at around the time of labour may cause the 'floppy infant syndrome' with muscular hypotonia, hypothermia, respiratory difficulties, and difficulty with sucking.

(e) Chloramphenicol

Chloramphenicol is poorly metabolized by the immature liver and can cause peripheral vascular collapse if given to neonates in weight-corrected adult doses (see Chapter 11, p. 139). It should therefore not be used at all during pregnancy.

(f) Oral anticoagulants

Oral anticoagulants are not only teratogenic during the first trimester, but if given later in pregnancy may also cause microcephaly or fetal or retroplacental haemorrhage. They should be avoided altogether during early and late pregnancy. *Heparin* does not cross the placenta and may be used with relative safely at those times, although it occasionally causes reversible osteoporosis and frequently causes subclinical bone demineralization (see the section on anticoagulation in pregnancy below).

(g) Oral sulphonylurea hypoglycaemic drugs

The sulphonylureas may cause fetal and neonatal hypoglycaemia. *Insulin* should be used to control diabetes mellitus during pregnancy.

(h) Pethidine

The effects of pethidine on the neonate after its administration to the mother as an analgesic during labour do not constitute a contra-indication to its use. However, care should be taken not to give too high a dose. Neonatal respiratory depression due to pethidine can be reversed by naloxone. In this context it should be noted that babies born to mothers who are dependent on narcotic analgesics may have a narcotic withdrawal syndrome after delivery, especially if they are given naloxone.

(i) Sulphonamides and novobiocin

Most sulphonamides and novobiocin should be avoided completely during the third trimester. They displace bilirubin in the fetal circulation from plasma proteins, and the free bilirubin enters the brain and is deposited in the basal ganglia, causing the condition known as kernict-erus, in which there may be any of a variety of neurological abnormalities, including lethargy, muscular hypotonia, and poor feeding, pro-gressing to spasticity and convulsions, with extra-pyramidal movement disorders later on in those who survive. Of course, different sulphonamides have different affinities for the bilirubin binding protein, and sulphasalazine, which has a relatively low affinity, may be safe in pregnancy, in contrast to most other sulphonamides. This distinction is important, since ulcerative colitis may get worse in pregnancy and prevention of an acute attack is greatly desirable.

(j) Tetracyclines

Tetracyclines should not be used at any time during pregnancy because of their effects on growing teeth and bones (see Table 12.2 and the Pharmacopoeia).

(k) Thiazide diuretics

Thiazide diuretics may cause thrombocytopenia in the neonate, probably by a direct toxic effect on the marrow, and should be avoided in late pregnancy.

12.3.4 Drugs which are safe in pregnancy

There are certain drugs which may be safely prescribed during pregnancy. Iron and folic acid are routinely given to all pregnant women to prevent deficiency. Because of the frequency of nausea and vomiting early in pregnancy it is often necessary to prescribe an antiemetic; meclo-zine and cyclizine are almost certainly safe and may be prescribed when necessary. As a mild analgesic paracetamol is recommended; the case against aspirin as a teratogen is undecided and its adverse effects in late pregnancy are detailed above. In the cases of antibiotics the penicillins are safe in the absence of hypersensitivity. No tranquillizers or hypnotics can be said to be completely safe (see, for example, the benzodiaz-epines above) and all should be avoided. The use of insulin in the treatment of diabetes and of heparin as an anticoagulant have been mentioned above. For the treatment of hypertension in pregnancy see pp. 157 and 264.

12.3.5 Management of the pregnant woman who has taken a possible teratogen

The problem sometimes occurs that a woman of child-bearing potential is given a drug, and then finds out days or weeks later that she is pregnant. The precise course of action to be taken in such a case rests on a careful history and, if necessary, investigation.

First one should identify the drug and the exact time of exposure to it. If it is a known or a likely teratogen one should try to determine the relation between the time of exposure and the likely time of conception. It is sometimes possible to identify the precise date of conception, but if that is not possible one should try to estimate the gestational age by carefully docu-menting the recent menstrual history and, if necessary, carrying out an ultrasound scan, which can date a pregnancy to within one week of gestation. If there has been exposure to a known teratogen during the first eight weeks of preg-nancy then further investigation may be necessary to identify precise fetal abnormalities. For example, many structural abnormalities can be detected by ultrasound, and neural tube defects may be diagnosed by measurement of serum and amniotic α-fetoprotein concentrations.

Any decision to advise termination of a preg-nancy in such circumstances should be based on a careful consideration of the risk of fetal abnormality from both published information and investigation of the individual case.

12.3.6 Common practical problems of drug therapy during pregnancy

(a) Anaemia

Iron supplements are routinely given to pregnant women, and because the need for folic acid doubles during pregnancy formulations containing both iron and folic acid are usually given as prophylaxis against both iron deficiency anaemia and the megaloblastic anaemia of pregnancy. There are numerous iron and folic acid formulations available (see Table 27.2), but the aim should be to provide a minimum daily dose of 30 mg of iron in the form of a ferrous salt, and of between 200 and 500 micrograms of folic acid. The use of high dosages of folic acid in preventing neural tube defects in the babies of women who have previously given birth to an affected child is discussed below.

(b) Antibiotic therapy

Antibiotic therapy is commonly indicated for urinary tract infection during pregnancy. However, the antibiotics listed in Table 12.4 should not be given unless absolutely necessary, because of the risks indicated.

Ampicillin, amoxycillin, and the cephalosporins appear to be safe to both mother and baby, if penicillin hypersensitivity is not a problem.

(c) Hyperthyroidism

If it becomes necessary to treat maternal hyperthyroidism with drugs then carbimazole or methimazole or propylthiouracil are indicated, and treatment carries about a 10 per cent risk of fetal hypothyroidism with goitre. Because of this one should use the lowest dose of anti-thyroid drug which will control maternal hyperthyroidism, particularly during late pregnancy.

(d) Diabetes mellitus

Because of the potential complications to mother and child of badly controlled diabetes during pregnancy careful management is very important.

(i) Pre-existing diabetes

Oral hypoglycaemic drugs should not be used during pregnancy, because of the risk of teratogenesis and prolonged neonatal hypoglycaemia. Treatment should therefore be with insulin in all cases. Short- and intermediate-acting highly purified insulins are the types usually used.

Maternal insulin requirements reach their maximum during the third trimester of pregnancy, and patients may require from two-thirds more insulin to three times as much as usual. The insulin should be given in a twice daily regimen, and this should be instituted before the second half of the pregnancy. If possible, diabetic control should be monitored using blood glucose measurements rather than the less accurate urinary glucose measurements, particularly since the renal threshold for glucose rises during pregnancy, and pregnant women should learn how to measure the blood glucose themselves. The blood glucose concentration should be kept at or below 7 mmol/L.

The complexities of diet and of the overall management of diabetes in pregnancy are beyond

■ **Table 12.4** Antibiotics to be avoided in pregnancy unless absolutely necessary

Antibiotic	Risk to fetus or neonate
Aminoglycoside	Ototoxicity
Chloramphenicol	Infant 'grey syndrome' (see text)
Co-trimoxazole	Kernicterus (sulphonamide); folate antagonist (?significant); teratogenesis
Quinolones	Arthropathy (animal studies)
Rifampicin	Possible teratogenicity; neonatal bleeding
Sulphonamides	Kernicterus
Tetracyclines	Tooth discolouration (Acute hepatic toxicity in mother)

our scope. Suffice it to say that this is a most important subject, requiring the careful attention of physicians and obstetricians, and the organization of careful and skilled antenatal care.

(ii) Gestational diabetes

Gestational diabetes is diabetes diagnosed for the first time during pregnancy (sometimes called chemical diabetes of pregnancy). It is usually mild and management consists of diet, with insulin if necessary. In this case once-daily insulin may be enough.

(iii) Treatment during labour

During labour the continuous intravenous regimen described for use during operations (p. 390) can be used to control blood glucose satisfactorily. After delivery insulin requirements fall rapidly and dosage regimens can be further complicated by breast feeding.

(e) Hypertension in pregnancy

(i) Pre-eclampsia

Hypertension due to pre-eclampsia occurs during the third trimester, and delivery produces a rapid and complete cure (although the risk of hypertension in later life is increased). However, drug therapy can be used to protect the mother from eclamptic complications if the rise in blood pressure occurs too soon in the third trimester for delivery to be suitable. Even so, drug therapy has not been shown to improve fetal prognosis.

Oral therapy with α-methyldopa 0.5–1 g t.d.s. is usually effective in lowering the blood pressure, and has not been shown to be harmful to either the fetus or the infant on long-term follow-up. Methyldopa may be given intravenously if it cannot be taken by mouth. A calcium antagonist is a suitable alternative if methyldopa is not well tolerated, e.g. nifedipine 5–20 mg t.d.s. Fears about the adverse effects of β-blockers on the neonate, based on anecdotal reports, have been shown in large studies to have been ill-founded, and atenolol may be used in patients in whom a β-blocker is not contra-indicated.

Occasionally it is necessary to lower the blood pressure more rapidly, when termination of the pregnancy is the treatment of choice. If drug therapy is required hydralazine by intravenous infusion is often effective. Alternatively, oral infedipine can quickly lower the b.p. if the capsule is bitten and the solution it contains is swallowed.

Diuretics are not used in pregnancy because they are not very effective and aggravate the hypovolaemia which occurs in pre-eclampsia. If it is necessary to prevent fits or to treat fits before delivery intravenous diazepam or chlormethiazole may be used (see p. 433).

(ii) Chronic hypertension and pregnancy

Although pre-existing chronic hypertension in pregnancy predisposes to pre-eclampsia, with its consequent risks to mother and child, mild to moderate hypertension without the problem of pre-eclampsia does not in itself appear to be a particular hazard to the fetus. Some believe that chronic hypertension with a blood pressure below 170/110 mmHg may not need treatment during pregnancy, since the duration of pregnancy is short, the blood pressure tends to fall during pregnancy, and pre-eclampsia can be dealt with if it arises (in the third trimester). Others feel that if the pregnant woman is on antihypertensive therapy this should be continued and she should be carefully observed for the occurrence of pre-eclampsia.

Certain points about continuing with antihypertensive drug therapy during pregnancy should be emphasized. Reserpine and angiotensin converting enzyme inhibitors (for example captopril and enalapril) are hazardous and should be withdrawn. Diuretics may exacerbate volume depletion in pregnancy and should be withdrawn if possible. They should certainly be discontinued if pre-eclampsia occurs. The effects of other antihypertensive drugs in pregnancy (for example clonidine, bethanidine, debrisoquine) have not been adequately studied, and these drugs should be withdrawn. If treatment becomes necessary because of the withdrawal of any of these drugs then methyldopa, a calcium antagonist, or a β-adrenoceptor antagonist should be used (see above).

(f) Anticoagulation during pregnancy

The use of warfarin is associated with major hazards to mother and child. They are maternal haemorrhage, fetal haemorrhage (cerebral), and multiple congenital abnormalities (teratogenesis during the first three months of development).

For these reasons it has become common practice to substitute heparin subcutaneously during the first trimester, to use warfarin if necessary from 13 to 36 weeks, and then heparin subcutaneously until it again becomes safe to use warfarin after delivery. However, there is no entirely safe or ideal anticoagulant for use during pregnancy, and the above advice is a compromise.

(g) Epilepsy

The treatment of epilepsy during pregnancy poses the problem of the assessment of the teratogenicity of the anticonvulsant drugs against a background of an increased risk of congenital abnormalities in children born to untreated epileptic mothers. The incidences of congenital abnormalities are 2.4 per cent in non-epileptic mothers, 4.2 per cent in untreated epileptics, and 6 per cent in treated epileptics. There is undoubtedly a risk of teratogenicity from phenytoin. The position with valproate is confusing, and the data are insufficient to exonerate it completely. Although carbamazepine may cause fetal abnormalities, the risk is probably small. Vigabatrin is teratogenic in animals and should be avoided.

For the woman with chronic epilepsy counselling before pregnancy is important, in order to discuss the relative risks. Special advice should also be given about contraception, since phenytoin and carbamazepine may reduce the effectiveness of oestrogen-containing oral contraceptives. If an epileptic woman taking an anticonvulsant intends to become or becomes pregnant and has not had a fit for 2 to 3 years treatment should be withdrawn and her progress should be monitored carefully. Otherwise treatment should be continued and the drug dosage should be altered to cope with the altered drug disposition which occurs during pregnancy. Careful plasma concentration monitoring should be carried out if possible, to avoid toxic plasma concentrations. Remember that because of changes in plasma protein binding during pregnancy the effective plasma concentration of phenytoin is probably in the lower part of the usual therapeutic range, i.e. about 40–60 µmol/L or lower (10–15 µg/mL; see Chapter 7).

In the woman who has her first fit during pregnancy careful elucidation of the type of seizure and of any identifiable cause are of great importance, so that she may be given relevant therapy with minimum risk.

(h) Vomiting

The treatment of vomiting during pregnancy is discussed on p. 323.

(i) Prevention of neural tube defects

There is now good evidence that neural tube defects in the fetus can be prevented if women who have previously given birth to one or more affected children take large dosages of folic acid during pregnancy. The current advice is that for such women folic acid supplementation should start before conception if possible and that they should take a daily dose of 4 mg until the end of the first trimester. (At the time of writing the nearest tablet strength available is 5 mg, and this may be used.)

The usual daily dose of folic acid for the prevention of anaemia of pregnancy is at most 500 micrograms. The question of whether a daily dose of 4 mg should be given to all pregnant women has not been studied, but the current advice is that pregnant women should eat foods rich in folic acid, for example green vegetables, bread, potatoes, fruit, nuts, and fortified breakfast cereals.

12.4 Drug therapy in the termination of pregnancy and in the management of preterm labour and labour

We shall limit ourselves here to a brief discussion of drugs which are used for stimulating or inhibiting uterine contractions. For detailed information on their indications for use consult specialist obstetric texts.

12.4.1 Inhibition of uterine contraction in preterm labour

The neonate born before 30 weeks of maturity is at great risk, particularly from hyaline membrane disease, intraventricular haemorrhage, or infections, and premature birth is directly responsible for 25 per cent of perinatal mortality and an associated factor in another 25 per cent.

Before 34 weeks the risks to the neonate can be reduced if premature labour can be averted and delivery postponed, especially if there is a high risk of hyaline membrane disease, indicated by an immature ratio of lecithin:sphingomyelin in the amniotic fluid. After 34 weeks there may be little advantage in delaying delivery should labour start, except in cases in which the lecithin:sphingomyelin ratio remains immature.

The initial measures used to delay or arrest premature labour are bed rest, sedation, and raising the foot of the bed. In selected cases β-adrenoceptor agonists may be used to relax uterine smooth muscle. Currently the choice lies among isoxsuprine, ritodrine, salbutamol, and terbutaline. For example, in the case of ritodrine one gives an infusion at a rate of 50 micrograms/min, increasing the dose by 50 micrograms/min every 15 min until uterine activity is suppressed or the maternal heart reaches 130/min. This will usually be at a dose of 150–350 micrograms/min, and this upper limit should not be exceeded.

When uterine contractions have been suppressed the dosage of ritodrine may be reduced, but the infusion should be continued for 12–48 h after uterine contractions have stopped. If continued suppression of uterine contractions is required, 10 mg of ritodrine should be given orally before the infusion is stopped and oral ritodrine should be continued in a dose of 10 mg 2-hourly for 24 h and then 10–20 mg every 4–6 h; the total daily dose should not exceed 120 mg.

There are many contra-indications to this type of treatment, including significant uterine bleeding, intrauterine death or infection, a severely deformed fetus, eclampsia and severe pre-eclampsia, maternal cardiac disease (because of the risk of cardiac arrhythmias), diabetes mellitus (since hyperglycaemia is worsened by β-agonists), thyrotoxicosis, hypokalaemia (worsened by β-agonists), and corticosteroid therapy. If the maternal heart rate rises above 130/min or the blood pressure falls below 100 mmHg the dose of β-agonist should be lowered. Other adverse effects which may occur during this type of treatment include palpitation, flushing, headache, sweating, tremor, agitation, nausea, and vomiting.

12.4.2 Stimulation of uterine contraction

(a) Termination of pregnancy

For the precise indications, contra-indications, nationally preferred practices, and dosage regimens of drugs used in the termination of pregnancy, appropriate obstetric texts should be consulted.

The choice of method of termination depends on the stage of pregnancy. Up to 10 weeks surgical evacuation of the uterus is usually carried out. In the middle trimester, prostaglandin E_2 (dinoprostone) or prostaglandin $F_{2\alpha}$ (dinoprost) may be used. Dinoprostone is preferred, and dinoprost is more likely to cause gastrointestinal adverse effects. These drugs are given intravenously, by extra-amniotic injection, or, after 14–16 weeks, by intra-amniotic injection.

Termination in late pregnancy, because of fetal death or serious fetal abnormality, is carried out by extra-amniotic or intravenous infusion of dinoprostone or dinoprost. Sometimes a vaginal pessary of dinoprostone may be sufficient to induce labour in cases of intrauterine death.

(b) Induction of labour

The initial method for inducing labour is low rupture of the fetal membranes. If the cervix is long, firm, and undilated, dinoprostone (prostaglandin E_2) pessaries or gel may be given 12 h before the membranes are ruptured to ripen the cervix; this by itself may cause the onset of labour.

Following rupture of the fetal membranes oxytocin is given by slow intravenous infusion in order to induce or augment labour. It is given in a solution containing 1000 milliunits/L at a rate of 1–3 milliunits/min (i.e. 1–3 mL/min)

Oxytocin should be used with great caution in women with uterine scars and in those who have had many children. Its adverse effects include hypertension and subarachnoid haemorrhage, water intoxication, cardiac arrhythmias, and violent uterine contractions, which can cause fetal asphyxia and uterine rupture.

Oxytocin is also used in the management of uterine inertia and in the management of the third stage of labour. Its use is complex and it is often combined with other drugs and obstetric manoeuvres, for details of which obstetric texts should be consulted.

(c) The third stage of labour

In the UK it is common practice to stimulate uterine contractions and assist the expulsion of the placenta by the use of oxytocic drugs, thereby reducing the risk of postpartum haemorrhage. Ergometrine 500 micrograms with oxytocin 5 units is given by intramuscular injection with or immediately after the delivery of the anterior shoulder.

Ergometrine and oxytocin both stimulate the myometrium directly, oxytocin by its action on

---

■ **Table 12.5** Drugs and breast feeding

1. *Some drugs to be avoided in breast-feeding mothers*

Amiodarone	Colchicine	Nitrofurantoin
Amphetamines	Corticosteroids (high dosages)	Oral contraceptives
Androgens	Co-trimoxazole	Oral hypoglycaemics
Anthraquinones (e.g. cascara)	Cyclosporin	Penicillins
Antineoplastic drugs	Ergot alkaloids	Phenindione
Antipsychotic drugs	Erythromycin	Phenobarbitone
Antithyroid drugs	Ethosuximide	Phenytoin
Aspirin	Immunosuppressive drugs	Radioactive iodine
Atropine	Indomethacin	Streptomycin
Barbiturates	Isoniazid	Sulphonamides
Benzodiazepines	Lithium	Tetracyclines
Bromocriptine	Meprobamate	Trimethoprim
Chloral derivatives	Methysergide	Vitamin A analogues
Chloramphenicol	Metronidazole	Vitamin D (high dosages)
Ciprofloxacin	Nalidixic acid	Xanthines

2. *Some drugs which appear to be safe*

ACE inhibitors	Disopyramide	Non-steroidal anti-inflammatory drugs
Acetazolamide	Ethambutol	
ACTH (corticotrophin)	Frusemide	Nortriptyline
Adrenaline	Heparin	Pyrazinamide
Antiasthmatic drugs (inhalations)	Hydralazine	Pyridostigmine
	Insulin	Rifampicin
Antihistamines (H$_1$ antagonists)	Methyldopa	Terbutaline
Baclofen	Mexiletine	Thyroid hormones (but may alter screening tests for thyroid disease)
β-Adrenoceptor antagonists	Neuroleptics in moderate dosages (for example chlorpromazine, haloperidol) (but monitor neonate for bradycardia and hypoglycaemia)	
Carbamazepine		Tricyclic antidepressants (except doxepin)
Chlormethiazole		
Chloroquine		Valproate
Clavulanic acid		Verapamil
Codeine		Warfarin
Digoxin	Nifedipine	

oxytocin receptors and ergometrine by effects on α-adrenoceptors, 5-HT receptors, or both.

Ergometrine may cause nausea, vomiting, hypertension, and peripheral vasospasm. It should preferably not be given to patients with hypertension, cardiac disease, vascular disease (including Raynaud's disease), and impaired hepatic or renal function. Apart from its use in the third stage of labour, it is also used in postpartum haemorrhage due to uterine atony.

12.5 Drug therapy and breast-feeding

The problem of adverse effects in suckling infants through the passage of drugs into the breast milk is determined by the following factors:

the passage of the drug from the maternal blood into the milk;

the concentration of the drug in the milk;

the volume of milk sucked;

the pharmacokinetics of the drug in the infant, particularly the absorption and clearance of the drug;

the inherent toxicity of the drug.

A list of drugs which may cause adverse effects in a breast-fed infant is given in Table 12.5. This list includes drugs which are excreted in breast milk to an extent likely to cause dose-related adverse effects in the infant, and drugs which do not necessarily enter the milk in large amounts, but whose adverse effects are not dose-related. The latter include drugs which may cause hypersensitivity reactions even in the small quantities excreted in breast milk (for example penicillins and sulphonamides), and drugs which are hazardous to babies with G6PD deficiency (for example nitrofurantoin; see Chapter 8).

Some drugs are hazardous for more than one reason (for example sulphonamides, which can cause kernicterus in any baby and haemolysis in G6PD deficient babies).

Also listed in Table 12.5 are drugs known to be safe in breast feeding. These include drugs which are destroyed in the gut (for example insulin, adrenaline) and drugs whose concentrations in milk have been measured and found to be very low (for example warfarin).

If there is any doubt about the safety of a drug it is best either to choose another drug or, if the drug must be used, to advise the mother not to breast-feed.

13 Patient compliance

Patient compliance with drug therapy may be defined as the extent to which the patient follows a prescribed drug regimen. The extent of non-compliance varies widely, and in different studies has been recorded as low as 10 per cent and as high as 92 per cent.

13.1 Factors which affect compliance

Numerous studies have shown that compliance may be affected by many different factors, which may be considered under the following headings.

1. The nature of the treatment.
2. Characteristics of the patient.
3. The type of illness.
4. The behaviour of the doctor.

13.1.1 The nature of the treatment

Here two factors are important, the complexity of the regimen and adverse effects.

(a) The complexity of the prescribed regimen

This involves two factors: the frequency of administration (the more often during the day patients have to take a drug the less likely they are to take it) and the number of drugs prescribed (the more drug prescribed the less likely is overall compliance).

When several different tablets (or other formulations) have to be taken at different dosages which involve different numbers of tablets and at different times of the day, compliance suffers (see for example the prescription on p. 7).

(b) Adverse effects

If patients experience symptoms which they attribute to adverse drug effects then, unless they can be persuaded that the potential benefits of treatment outweigh the disadvantages, they will stop taking the medicine.

13.1.2 Characteristics of the patient

These are nebulous factors which mostly involve the shortcomings of human nature.

People tend to forget or can't be bothered; they may feel no need for treatment (for example in asymptomatic hypertension); they may be unclear about the prescribing instructions; they may not want to feel dependent or be thought to be dependent on 'drugs'.

In addition there may be social or physical problems about their getting to the chemist's shop, difficulty with paying prescription charges, or everyday inconveniences in carrying and taking the medication.

Some patients, notably children, have problems with certain formulations, for example sickly elixirs or large, dry, bitter tablets.

13.1.3 The type of illness

Compliance is likely to be poor in people who are severely mentally disturbed, for example patients with schizophrenia.

Physical disability may interfere with compliance, despite the patient's desire to comply. It may sound silly, but if patients with rheumatoid arthritis or osteoarthritis cannot get the top off a child-proof container they will not be able to take the tablets.

Dysphagia may make it difficult for a patient to swallow tablets, particularly if the tablets are large.

Some diseases may promote compliance. Patients with insulin-dependent diabetes may easily become very ill quite quickly if they forget to take their insulin, and that is likely to make them comply, although they may not comply precisely as advised. Patients in whom β-blockers or vasodilators have significantly reduced the frequency of anginal attacks will be conditioned to good compliance.

13.1.4 The behaviour of the doctor

The enthusiasm and confidence with which a treatment is prescribed, and the extent to which these attitudes are transmitted to the patient, may influence not only compliance but also the response to therapy (the placebo effect, see Chapter 14).

13.2 Methods of measuring compliance

Measurement of compliance is important both in everyday practice and in research. For example, one needs to know the extent of a patient's compliance before attributing the failure of a particular therapy to incorrect or inappropriate prescribing, while in clinical trials the need to measure compliance is obvious.

13.2.1 Pharmaceutical methods

The fact that patients collect their prescriptions is at least evidence of the first stage of compliance, and can be checked by asking to see the tablets. As a guide to the actual number of tablets which a patient has taken one can count the tablets in the bottle and assume that those missing have been taken. However, this method may be misleading in the case of patients who throw their tablets away without taking them, and tablet counts will therefore tend to lead to an overestimate of the extent of compliance. None the less, this method is better than estimation by the doctor on the basis of the patient's personality, a method which overestimates even more the extent of compliance. The development of the silicon chip has led to the use of recording devices which can be fitted in the caps of medication containers. Such devices have been used in research into compliance. They can record the frequency and exact timing of the opening of the container and although they do not allow for patients who throw away their tablets at regular intervals (an unlikely event) they can provide useful information about compliance.

13.2.2 Pharmacokinetic methods

Measurement of some compounds in the plasma or urine may give a good indication of compliance, although it does not allow for the patients who take their treatment only on the day of visiting the doctor. The compound measured will usually be the drug itself, but it may be a marker of some sort. Examples of the former are the measurement of digoxin, phenytoin, or lithium in the plasma, or of salicylates in the urine. An example of a marker for compliance is riboflavin, which is easily detected in the urine. Riboflavin and other markers have been used in research on compliance and as a means of checking compliance in clinical trials.

13.2.3 Pharmacodynamic methods

If the pharmacological effect of a drug can be measured then that may afford evidence of compliance. Thus, measurement of the response of the heart rate to exercise gives information about β-blockers, measurement of the prothrombin time information about oral anticoagulants, and measurement of the reticulocyte count information about haematinics. Failure to detect the pharmacological effect of a drug implies non-compliance or inadequate dosage.

13.2.4 Therapeutic methods

Obviously, if the desired therapeutic effect occurs then in routine practice the question of compliance is unimportant. However, one should remember that a good therapeutic outcome may occur irrespective of the treatment used. It would be wrong to attribute a good outcome to the effect of a drug which the patient may not have taken, and this principle is important in clinical trials (see Chapter 15).

13.3 Methods of improving compliance

Compliance may be improved by:

(1) administration of the drug by the doctor, nurse, or other attendant;

(2) simplification of the therapeutic regimen;

(3) education of the patient on the need to take the medicine, with reminders when possible.

13.3.1 Supervised administration

Administration of a drug by the doctor or nurse obviously ensures compliance. However, this is only possible when the patient is in hospital, or in some circumstances in which only occasional administration is required. For example, intramuscular injections of vitamin B_{12} in the treatment of pernicious anaemia are required only once every few months, and the injection can easily be given in the doctor's surgery. The use of long-acting depot injections of phenothiazines and thioxanthenes in the treatment of schizophrenia allows the treatment to be given to the patient at special clinics for this purpose. Sometimes compliance may be ensured by giving a single dose of a drug at the time of consultation, rather than a short course of tablets (for example intramuscular antibiotics in the treatment of gonorrhoea, which not only solves the problem of treatment of the individual patient but in this case also prevents the spread of the disease). In some cases compliance may be assured by administration by a relative at home.

13.3.2 Simplification of the therapeutic regimen

Simplification of the therapeutic regimen can be achieved by reducing the number of drugs a patient has to take and by reducing the frequency of administration. The first of these objectives may be achieved by trying to avoid the unnecessary use of a drug or by using acceptable combinations of drugs in single tablet formulations (see p. 11).

A reduction in the frequency of drug administration may be achieved either by using drugs with long durations of action in preference to those with shorter durations (for example chlorpropamide versus tolbutamide) or by using a slow-release formulation in preference to a conventional one (for example aminophylline). The extreme reduction in frequency of administration

allowed by depot injections in patients with schizophrenia is referred to above.

In some cases a single dose of a drug may be used to replace a course of treatment. The example of the intramuscular injection of an antibiotic to treat gonorrhoea (for example penicillin with oral probenecid) was mentioned above. Another example is the use of two large oral doses of amoxycillin (3 g) to treat a urinary tract infection.

13.3.3 Education

Educating the patient undoubtedly improves compliance, but is not often applied properly, partly because it is so time-consuming. However, patients with, for example, asymptomatic hypertension or glaucoma who learn the importance of taking drugs when they are feeling well are more likely to comply than patients who are simply given a prescription without being told the reasons.

Even when patients are well motivated, reminders to take the treatment may improve compliance, since it is easy to forget to take medication. A simple *aide-mémoire* consists of the 'calendar pack', commonly used for dispensing oral contraceptives (see Fig. 12.1).

One imponderable in all this is one's view of who is responsible for ensuring that the patient takes the treatment. It is our view that it is the responsibility of the doctor to educate the patient about the need for therapy and give them encouragement to comply, but that the final responsibility to take the treatment lies with the patient. However, sometimes problems crop up in which the responsibilities of the doctor are more difficult to define. For example, the treatment of tuberculosis or other infections in large populations with a high rate of infection, when poor compliance may make widespread control of the disease difficult; the use of certain immunization procedures (for example against whooping cough); the use of mass sterilization or contraception programmes in over-populated countries; the addition of fluoride to water supplies. Some of these problems are controversial, all are difficult, and there are no simple answers.

14 Placebos

'Placebo' is a Latin word meaning 'I shall please'. Originally a placebo was a formulation of a pharmacologically inactive compound 'adopted to please rather than to benefit the patient' (Oxford English Dictionary), although it could be argued that anything which pleases patients also benefits them. However, in its modern usage the term goes further than that.

Placebos are of two types, those which contain pharmacologically inactive ingredients, and those which contain some compound with pharmacological activity. Although the former are always knowingly used as placebos by physicians, the latter may be given either in the knowledge that their pharmacological action is not appropriate or in the mistaken belief that it is. Some examples are given below.

14.1 Uses and abuses of placebos

14.1.1 Inert placebos

(a) Clinical trials
The commonest use of the inert placebo is as a dummy for the real treatment in clinical trials, in order to reduce the element of subjective bias (see Chapter 16).

(b) The misuse of the placebo as a 'therapeutic test'
Occasionally inert placebos, rather than drugs known to have pharmacological activity, are given to patients who are incessantly complaining of some symptom and who are thought to be exaggerating. Pain is the symptom usually involved. If the pain responds to the placebo then it is often assumed that the patient was making an unnecessary fuss. However, it is quite wrong to assume that because the pain is reported by the patient to have been relieved by an intramuscular injection of saline the symptom did not exist, or was not severe, or that the patient was exaggerating. One-third of all people are placebo reactors, i.e. will report symptomatic relief of real pain after the administration of an inactive compound. It would therefore not be surprising if on occasion, and despite real pain appropriate to real pathology, relief was obtained from a placebo. Placebos should not be used in this way.

14.1.2 'Active' placebos

(a) To terminate a visit
The issue of a prescription is a common way of ending a patient's visit to the doctor, and not infrequently the doctor will prescribe a compound whose pharmacological action is irrelevant to the case. The doctor may be aware of this, as in the prescription of a vitamin preparation, for example, the patient being informed of the nature of the prescription and being told that it is 'a tonic'. On the other hand, the doctor may misunderstand the proven indications for which a drug has been shown to be effective, for example in the case of a prescription of cimetidine for symptoms of acute 'dyspepsia' in the absence of proven peptic ulceration or oesophagitis.

(b) To 'treat' the untreatable
Some doctors find it difficult to accept that there is no effective treatment for their patient and they feel constrained to try something. There are many examples of pseudotherapy, based on apparently good ideas which do not hold up when examined scientifically, for example the use of cerebral vasodilators in the treatment of senile dementia. Some patients cannot believe that there is not a medicine to cure their disease, and sometimes no amount of talk will persuade them otherwise. Often, in exasperation, the doctor

prescribes something which, however tenuously, could be interpreted as being rational treatment, for example the use of diuretics in the treatment of obesity, despite lack of evidence of their long-term efficacy.

14.2 Factors which influence the response to placebos

Certain factors are thought to increase the likelihood of a response to a placebo.

14.2.1 The doctor's attitude

If a placebo is to be prescribed then it should be prescribed with enthusiasm and some show of belief in its efficacy.

14.2.2 The doctor–patient relationship

One would suppose that a placebo is more likely to work if there is a respectful rapport between doctor and patient, although there is no clear proof that that is the case.

14.2.3 The formulation

Several studies have shown that the placebo response may be affected by the presentation or route of administration of the drug. For example, in a study on pain relief different colours of placebo (red, blue, green, and yellow) were compared for their efficacy. The order of decreasing analgesic potency was red blue green yellow (Fig. 14.1). The pain-relieving effect of red placebo was as good as that of white aspirin.

14.3 Mode of action of placebos

The way in which placebos produce symptomatic relief is not known. There has been some interest

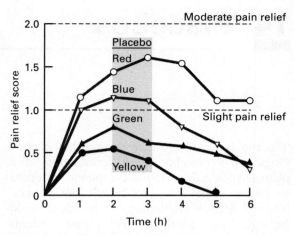

■ **Fig. 14.1** The effect of the colour of a placebo formulation on the analgesic effects of its administration. (Adapted from Huskisson (1974). *Br. med. J.* **iv**, 196–200, with permission.)

in the role which endorphins and enkephalins might have in the placebo response, but at present their relevance is unclear.

14.4 Adverse effects of placebos

If a doctor uses placebos unthinkingly he or she may ignore the patient's real problem, and that may lead to delayed diagnosis of a treatable condition. Delay in diagnosis, and hence in instituting proper treatment, will be prolonged if the patient initially responds to the placebo.

Just as they may relieve real symptoms placebos may cause real adverse effects. For example, in a survey of placebo studies, common symptoms were dry mouth (9 per cent), nausea (10 per cent), fatigue (18 per cent), difficulty in concentrating (15 per cent), and headache (25 per cent).

15 Drug discovery and development: the pharmaceutical industry and the regulatory authorities

Almost all the drugs mentioned in this book have been synthesized and developed by pharmaceutical companies. Doctors and patients are dependent on high and predictable standards of quality of formulation and proper ethical evaluation of the safety and efficacy of drugs, and the standards of the pharmaceutical industry in regard to the development of new drugs are in general high and are regulated by law.

15.1 Drug discovery

Drug discovery comes about in several ways.

15.1.1 As a development from herbal or traditional remedies

Many plants and herbs contain substances which have useful pharmacological actions, and new examples are continually being discovered. Established examples include the isolation of morphine from the opium poppy (*Papaver somniferum*) and the subsequent synthesis of related analgesics, the isolation of atropine from the deadly nightshade (*Atropa belladonna*) and the subsequent development of related anticholinergic drugs, and the isolation of digoxin and digitoxin from foxgloves (*Digitalis lanata* and *Digitalis purpurea*, respectively).

15.1.2 From the study of endogenous agents in animals

The identification of insulin was made from studies of pancreatic function in dogs. The anticoagulant action of the venom of the Malayan pit viper led to the identification of the anticoagulant ancrod. Numerous animal and plant toxins have been identified as modulators of the actions of many endogenous receptors and ion channels in humans. These have been useful in elucidating the mechanisms of drug action, although they have not themselves been used therapeutically. They include tetrodotoxin (which closes sodium channels) and batrachotoxin (which closes potassium channels).

15.1.3 Serendipity

The word 'serendipity' was coined by Horace Walpole from the title of the fairy tale 'The Three Princes of Serendip', who, he said, 'were always making discoveries, by accidents and sagacity, of things they were not in quest of'. Into this category of discoveries comes Alexander Fleming's observation of the effect of *Penicillium* mould on bacterial growth, although his conclusions about his observations went further and revealed the mind of an inquiring man as well as an observant one. The extraction and isolation of penicillin 14 years later by Florey, Chain, and Heatley is an excellent example of applied science at its best.

Another form of serendipity is the discovery of the therapeutic usefulness of a side-effect of a drug, i.e. an effect which is unrelated to the therapeutic effect originally intended. Clonidine was originally tested as a nasal decongestant and was then found to lower the blood pressure. The hypoglycaemic effects of sulphonamides in patients being treated for typhoid fever led to the development of the structurally-related sulphonylureas as oral hypoglycaemic drugs. The observation that isoniazid elevated mood in patients being treated for tuberculosis led to the development of the monoamine oxidase inhibitor iproniazid as an antidepressant.

Sometimes faulty reasoning leads to a lucky discovery. In the early 1940s Nana Svartz in Sweden reasoned that rheumatoid arthritis, which was thought to be an infective disease, would respond to a molecule containing a sulphonamide to combat the infection and a salicylate as an anti-inflammatory agent. She therefore synthesized a new molecule, sulphasalazine, from sulphapyridine and 5-aminosalicylic acid (now called mesalazine), but found that it had no effect in rheumatoid arthritis. However, a rheumatoid type of arthropathy sometimes occurs in patients with ulcerative colitis, and the therapeutic efficacy of sulphasalazine in ulcerative colitis was noted when those patients were given the drug. Further study of sulphasalazine has yielded other safer drugs (see section 15.1.4 below). The wheel has recently come full circle with the use of sulphasalazine in the treatment of rheumatoid arthritis!

15.1.4 Metabolites of existing drugs

Sometimes active metabolites of drugs are found to have therapeutic advantages over the original parent compound. For example, paracetamol is the main metabolite of phenacetin; it is effective as an analgesic but does not cause renal damage. The benzodiazepine chlordiazepoxide is metabolized to a variety of other active benzodiazepines (for example oxazepam) which have shorter durations of action than chlordiazepoxide itself. The main metabolite of procainamide, *N*-acetylprocainamide (acecainide), is an effective anti-arrhythmic drug, but does not cause the lupus-like syndrome which can occur with procainamide. Sulphasalazine is metabolized in the large bowel to sulphapyridine and 5-aminosalicylic acid (mesalazine); the sulphapyridine causes the adverse effects associated with sulphasalazine and the mesalazine is the therapeutically active ingredient. Mesalazine is now used in the treatment of ulcerative colitis. The observation that the actions of morphine, which is mostly metabolized, are none the less enhanced in renal failure was explained by the discovery of an active metabolite, morphine-6-glucuronide, which accumulates when renal function is impaired and

which is currently being studied as a narcotic analgesic.

15.1.5 Empirical chemistry coupled with applied pharmacology

To date, this has been the most productive process of discovery. One takes an active molecule and chemically alters it on the basis of known structure/activity relationships, on an intuitive hunch, or out of curiosity. One then tests the pharmacological activity of the new compound in a number of carefully chosen pharmacological screening tests. If some activity is found the compound will be tested in animals and then perhaps in humans. Subsequent refinement of the molecule may result in a new and better compound. Thousands of compounds are synthesized and screened for every one which appears as a new entity worthy of clinical testing.

15.1.6 Rational molecular design

This is the approach of the future to drug discovery. Take the development of L-dopa (levodopa) and the peripheral dopa decarboxylase inhibitors in the treatment of Parkinson's disease. The sequence was as follows.

1. The discovery of dopamine in the brain and the suggestion that it was a neurotransmitter (1957) (the pathway of its synthesis was already known).
2. The localization of dopamine in the basal ganglia (1958).
3. The discovery that reserpine, which was already known to produce symptoms like those of Parkinson's disease, depletes brain dopamine in animals (1958).
4. The discovery that dopamine was deficient in the brains of patients with Parkinson's disease (1960).
5. The administration of the dopamine precursor, L-dopa, to patients with Parkinson's disease, initially in too low a dose (1962) but later in therapeutic dosages (1967).
6. The recognition that many of the adverse effects of L-dopa were due to its peripheral decarboxylation to dopamine.

7. The use (1967) of already available peripheral dopa decarboxylase inhibitors, which do not enter the brain, thus diminishing the peripheral adverse effects of dopamine and allowing the use of lower dosages with the same effect on the brain as higher dosages without the use of inhibitors.

This example emphasizes the importance of understanding the pathophysiology of a disease in designing appropriate strategies for its treatment.

The understanding of drug/receptor interactions has led to the synthesis of specific receptor agonists and antagonists, based on modifications of the structures of known agonists. Some of these compounds are useful tools in exploring the functions of the receptors and some have therapeutic uses. The best-known examples are the β-blockers, based on the structure of the β-adrenoceptor agonist isoprenaline, and the histamine H_2 antagonists, based on the structure of histamine.

More recently, developments in computer technology have allowed the design of new compounds by an examination of the three-dimensional structures of existing compounds, and this technique, supplemented by a knowledge, when it comes, of the three-dimensional structures of drug receptors and of drug ligand/receptor complexes, delineated by modern biochemical and molecular biological techniques, promises to provide a highly efficient method of designing novel compounds in the future.

15.2 Drug development

Once a new chemical entity has been discovered it has to be put through a strict developmental process which culminates in its being licensed for use and marketed.

15.2.1 Preclinical pharmacology and toxicology

Every new promising compound undergoes extensive pharmacological testing *in vivo* in animals and in *in vitro* preparations, so that as much as possible may be learnt about those of its properties which will be of importance in therapeutic practice and about its dose-related adverse effects. At the same time, studies of its pharmacokinetic properties are carried out in animals. It also undergoes short-term and long-term toxicity testing in animals, so that its toxicological properties may be defined in a rough dose-response fashion. The duration of this toxicological testing is geared to the likely duration of therapeutic use. In addition, at this stage other special tests may be necessary, such as tests of the effects of the compound on fertility and reproduction, teratogenicity testing, and tests for mutagenicity and carcinogenicity.

15.2.2 Clinical testing (volunteer studies)

At some point during the preclinical toxicological testing programme a decision will be made that enough is known about the safety of the drug to allow it to be given to healthy volunteers, if that is appropriate (for example, one would not give a new cytotoxic drug to healthy subjects). The drug's pharmacokinetic behaviour is studied after single and multiple doses, and if it has measurable effects in healthy people its human pharmacology can also be studied. Adverse effects are recorded and clinical, biochemical, and haematological toxicity are assessed.

15.2.3 Phase I clinical studies in patients

The first (phase I) studies in patients are searching and scrupulously monitored. They concentrate on the clinical pharmacology of the drug, its short-term safety, its promise of efficacy, its pharmacological effects, and its pharmacokinetics in disease. These early studies will also provide information as to the likely effective dose.

15.2.4 Phase II clinical studies in patients

Phase II studies are concerned with gathering further evidence of safety and efficacy in larger numbers of patients (see Table 9.7) with further attention to dose-ranging and adverse effects. Although monitoring for safety and efficacy is still important, the intensity of investigation is a little less at this stage, particularly in so far as invasive investigations are concerned.

15.2.5 Phase III clinical studies in patients

Phase III studies are full-scale clinical trials (see Chapter 16), which, if successful in demonstrating safety and efficacy, will lead to marketing of the drug. The numbers of patients studied at this stage are larger than before (see Table 9.7), and although safety and efficacy are still carefully monitored the investigations performed at this stage are fewer in number and less intense than in phases I and II.

15.2.6 Marketing

If all is well and the regulatory authority is convinced about quality, safety, and efficacy, the drug will then receive a product licence and be marketed for approved indications. This is accompanied by advertising to the profession by post and in the medical press, by visits to doctors and pharmacists by the company's representatives, and by promotional meetings for doctors.

15.3 Post-marketing surveillance

In the UK there is now a system whereby the Committee on Safety of Medicines can require post-marketing surveillance studies to be carried out on a defined number of patients, in order to monitor the occurrence of adverse drug reactions. Increasingly, pharmaceutical companies who market a drug likely to have large sales will voluntarily organize post-marketing surveillance studies. Many doctors become involved in studies of this kind, since the numbers of patients studied need to be very large if infrequent adverse effects are to be detected (see Table 9.7). It is therefore important for doctors to decide for themselves whether such studies are really aimed at post-marketing surveillance or are a marketing ploy, as may be the case from time to time.

Whether or not formal post-marketing surveillance occurs, soon after a drug is marketed articles start to appear in scientific journals on various aspects of its use, regulatory authorities and other bodies receive anecdotal notifications of adverse effects, and the profession gradually makes up its corporate mind about the overall safety and efficacy of the drug and its proper place in therapeutic practice. It takes a long time for this to happen, and the full potential of a good drug may not be realised for many years after it has been marketed.

Medical practitioners may be involved in the processes of post-marketing surveillance at different stages. The pharmaceutical industry employs suitably qualified medical practitioners to help plan and execute clinical studies. Clinical pharmacologists in both industry and academic departments are commonly involved in phase I and phase II studies and sometimes in phase III studies as well. Those practitioners who regularly deal with the patients for whom the drug is relevant, whether in hospital or general practice, will often be involved in subsequent early clinical investigations. Later on all medical practitioners who may be in a position to prescribe the drug will have a chance to assess its safety and efficacy in their own patients.

15.4 Advertising

The advertising of a drug plays an important part in disseminating information about it to medical practitioners. Unfortunately, many of the drug advertisements in the medical press are an insult to the knowledge and scientific understanding of their readers. It would be better if they contained more medical and scientific information and fewer slogans, although market research doubtless shows that it is the slogans which sell the drugs. When you see an advertisement for a drug read it critically, question drug representatives carefully about their claims, try to assess the claims of clinical trials (see Chapter 16), and whatever you do do not automatically prescribe the newest drug. Always ask:

Is this drug safe in general?
Will it be safe for this particular patient?
Is it effective, and if so is it more effective than an already available drug about which more is known?
If it is equally effective is it safer?

One of the reasons for scientific training in medicine is to teach doctors to use their critical faculties to make up their own minds about the answers to such questions.

15.5 Regulatory authorities

Throughout the world, and particularly in the developed countries, there are regulatory authorities whose task, to a greater or lesser extent, is to ensure that drugs are of acceptable quality, safety, and efficacy. In the UK the responsibility for ensuring this lies with the Health Ministers responsible for the populations of England and Wales, Scotland, and Northern Ireland. These Ministers constitute the Licensing Authority, and it is this Authority which actually issues the various licences and certificates for drugs, and with whom the statutory legal responsibility rests.

The Licensing Authority is served by the Medicines Control Agency. This Agency is composed of administrative staff, pharmacists, and doctors, to whom all regulatory matters concerning medicines are referred. The Medicines Control Agency is advised by the Committee on Safety of Medicines (CSM). Medical experts who cover a wide spectrum of medical knowledge sit on this Committee and on its expert subcommittees. The CSM advises the Agency on all matters referred to it, and in practice it is the CSM to which the medical profession looks for guidance and assurance about the quality, safety, and efficacy of drugs.

The CSM reviews the evidence supplied to it by the pharmaceutical industry and advises the Licensing Authority on the issuing of certificates and licences. For example, it can advise the Authority that a drug may be licensed for clinical trial (i.e. Clinical Trial Certification or CTC), although the Authority itself can speed up drug development by issuing Clinical Trial Exemption (CTX) certificates for new drugs if there appear to be no problems from the results of preclinical studies.

When a pharmaceutical company feels that it has amassed sufficient information about a drug to warrant its being marketed the CSM is responsible for advising the Licensing Authority whether or not to grant the drug a Product Licence, based on its assessment of the drug's quality, safety, and efficacy. It is this Product Licence which allows the pharmaceutical company to market the drug for the specified indications which are listed on its Data Sheet (the issue of which to all registered practitioners is required by law).

The CSM is responsible for communicating with doctors about current problems in drug therapy. It does this through articles and letters in the medical press, through its Current Problems leaflet, which is issued at regular intervals and sent to all registered practitioners, and occasionally by sending practitioners a letter about a serious urgent problem.

Finally, the CSM is responsible for post-marketing surveillance, through its yellow card reporting system, and for encouraging doctors to look for and to report adverse reactions. Each practitioner is sooner or later going to be in a position to report problems to the CSM through the yellow card system, and it is as well to have some idea of how the system works (see p. 118).

15.6 Local drug and therapeutics committees

Practically all District Health Authorities in the UK have a Drug and Therapeutics Committee consisting of physicians, surgeons, nurses, pharmacists, and administrators. Such committees help to formulate local policies suited to local needs. They advise on local prescribing policies, disseminate information on drug matters, and advise the Health Authority on drug costs and economics. They may also sometimes take responsibility for research into local matters concerning drugs.

15.7 Drug costs

Modern drugs are expensive, and although in the perfect world this would not be taken into account when prescribing, it is in fact an important aspect of drug therapy. In the UK drug costs are monitored by the Prescription Pricing

Authority, which is responsible for monitoring the costs of prescriptions in the community and for providing information about drug costs to doctors, Health Authorities, and the Department of Health. The information system it administers (PACT) is described below.

Drugs cost a lot to prescribe because they cost a lot to develop. At the time of writing (1991) the total cost of discovering, developing, and marketing a new drug which is pharmacologically and therapeutically innovative is in the region of £100 million. Considerable commercial risks are involved, and at any point during the development process the drug may come to grief because of problems with safety, poor efficacy, changes in therapeutic fashion, or a better competitor. The duration of a drug's patent from the time of its registration with the UK Patent Office is 20 years. Seven to nine of those years will be taken up with research and development, so that after marketing there will be about 11 to 13 years left during which the company can recoup its investment and make a profit, some of which will be ploughed back into the research and development of another drug. That is why drugs cost what they do, why pharmaceutical companies are anxious to sell their drugs through various marketing techniques, such as advertising and the activities of drug representatives, and why, when a drug's patent expires and other formulations are marketed by competitors (who have not had to expend so much time and money in the development of the drug), the price often drops considerably. Changes in UK patent law may occur when the European Community is formalized at the end of 1992.

While drugs are expensive, countries' drugs budgets are limited, and in many countries efforts have been made, both locally and nationally, to reduce expenditure on drugs. This has been done in two ways: by informing and educating doctors and patients about drug costs and expenditure, and by formal restriction of prescribing.

(a) Information and education

There are several ways in which doctors and patients can learn about relative drug costs. For example, drug costs are listed in the *British National Formulary*, and the *Drug and Therapeutics Bulletin* makes a point of comparing the costs of different treatments when discussing new drugs.

After the report of the Tricker enquiry in 1976, general practitioners in the UK were enabled to find out about their prescribing habits by applying to the Prescription Pricing Authority for information on their recent prescriptions. The information distributed consisted of an outline of the costs of the drugs which the practitioners had prescribed over a period of a month and a comparison of that expenditure with that of their colleagues both locally and nationally. If a practice was spending too much money on drugs it was visited by the Regional Medical Officer and the problem was discussed.

This type of information scheme has recently been expanded into the PACT (Prescribing Analysis and Cost) information system. PACT reports are issued quarterly and provide three levels of information to doctors.

(i) Level 1

This is a four-page report which is sent quarterly to all general practitioners. It contains information on the number of items prescribed by each practice and by each doctor in the practice, the cost of each item, and the overall cost. Comparisons are made with average expected costs derived from prescribing in comparable practices. Costs are also subdivided according to groups of drugs (for example cardiovascular, respiratory).

(ii) Level 2

This contains more detailed information and emphasizes areas of high cost. It is sent automatically to all practices whose expenditure is more than 25 per cent higher than average, and on request to other practices.

(iii) Level 3

This is available on request and contains full information on all prescriptions, detailing for each drug in each therapeutic category the total number of items prescribed, the total cost, the cost per 1000 patients, and the cost per 1000 prescribing units (a way of counting up prescriptions according to the age of the patient).

It is hoped that the information presented in this way will encourage doctors to prescribe more rationally and perhaps more cheaply, although the two do not necessarily go hand in hand, since effective prescribing is often also expensive. It may also be useful in teaching, in research, and in monitoring patterns of drug use.

In hospitals drug information pharmacists often supply doctors with information on their prescribing costs.

(b) Restriction of prescribing

In the UK many hospitals have an official formulary, which contains lists of the drugs which the hospital pharmacy will stock and which doctors may prescribe. If a doctor wants to prescribe a drug which is not in the formulary he or she must make a case for it. In Australia a similar type of scheme has been implemented nationally. In the UK this trend is being followed by general practitioners, many of whom have devised formularies for use in their own practices. In doing this they are being encouraged partly by the introduction of so-called indicative budgets, which make them responsible for their own drug expenditure.

16 Clinical trials

Medicines should be effective. In other words they should alleviate a symptom or ameliorate or cure a disease. In an individual the efficacy (or benefit of treatment) should outweigh the potential hazard (the risk), and the decision to use a drug depends on assessing the benefit:risk ratio in the individual patient.

Experience has shown that clinical impressions of the efficacy of a drug can be misleading, partly because of bias on the part of both doctors and patients in favour of the treatment, partly because of the placebo response (see Chapter 14), and partly because of the selectivity of doctors' memories. The dangers of having ineffective medicines on the market are that they may be hazardous, that the patient may be denied alternative really effective treatments, and that time and resources may be wasted.

The clinical trial is a means whereby the efficacy of a drug may be tested. It may also give some guidance to the risks involved, although usually this is not the primary consideration.

In general the more predictable and clear-cut the outcome of an illness or disease, and the more efficacious the therapy, the easier it is to demonstrate that efficacy. For example, the effect of benzylpenicillin in the treatment of pneumococcal pneumonia is dramatic and easy to demonstrate. However, dramatic effects of this kind are rare in drug therapy and most treatments require a formal trial of some sort. This is especially important in the treatment of diseases with an uncertain outcome in the individual (for example mild hypertension, myocardial infarction, stroke), and in cases where treatment may improve outcome only slightly (for example the use of β-adrenoceptor antagonists in reducing the incidence of sudden death after myocardial infarction or the use of low-dose subcutaneous heparin to prevent deep venous thrombosis and pulmonary embolism after myocardial infarc-

tion). In such cases the doctor can never be sure that the treatment is doing any good in the individual patient; for example, if the blood pressure is lowered in a patient with essential hypertension there is a chance that the patient's outlook will be improved, but one never knows. In such circumstances the rationale for therapeutic action will depend entirely upon the results of carefully designed and carefully executed clinical trials.

It is also important never to assume that simply because a treatment seems logically right it is therefore either efficacious or safe. An example which underlines this point was the failure of paediatricians to appreciate, until convinced by a clinical trial, that 100 per cent oxygen, used for some years in the treatment of premature infants in incubators, was associated with retrolental fibroplasia.

16.1 Definition of a clinical trial

A clinical trial of a drug in a patient has been defined in the UK Medicines Act of 1968 as an investigation or series of investigations which:

(1) consists of the administration of one or more medicinal products by, or under the direction of, a doctor or dentist to patients, where

(2) there is evidence that the products have effects which may be beneficial to the patients, and

(3) the administration is for the purpose of ascertaining whether, or to what extent, the products have those or any other effects, whether beneficial or harmful (i.e. the assessment of efficacy and risks).

This definition was specifically designed to cover trials of drugs in patients. It could be extended to include, for example, therapeutic procedures (such as a surgical operation) and volunteer trials, in which benefit would not be expected, or indeed required.

16.2 The conduct of a clinical trial

We cannot emphasize too strongly that the reliability of the conclusions based upon the results of a clinical trial depend entirely upon the care with which the trial is designed, carried out, and analysed. Many clinical trials are poorly designed, carried out with insufficient attention to detail, and analysed inappropriately. Publication of the results of a clinical trial in a scientific journal does not necessarily guarantee their validity.

As experience of clinical trials has increased over the last 60 years or so, certain principles have come to be recognized as being important in regard to the conduct of such trials. These principles are related to:

(1) the aims of the trial;

(2) its design;

(3) the drugs to be tested;

(4) the subjects to be studied;

(5) the analysis and interpretation of the results;

(6) ethical considerations.

A checklist of the important facets of each of these considerations is given in Table 16.1, and the conduct of clinical trials will be discussed under those headings.

16.2.1 Aims

Investigators should carefully formulate the aims of their trial before embarking on any other aspect. It is generally best to ask one or two specific questions, and to design the trial in order to answer those questions and those questions only. In a drug trial the main aim is usually to answer the question 'How effective is this therapeutic strategy in this condition, compared with another therapeutic strategy or no therapy at all?' If one tries to answer too many questions in one study then the trial design becomes more and more complex and organization becomes difficult. Even if a complex study is well organized

there may be difficulty in interpreting the data, as happened in the Multiple Risk Factor Intervention Trial, a large and complex study carried out in the USA in order to assess the benefit of a multifactorial therapeutic strategy called 'stepped care' on mortality from coronary artery disease. The study involved 12 866 men and was operationally successful, but no difference was found in mortality in the treated group compared with controls. The trial group concluded that the likeliest explanation for the lack of difference was that some of the measures did reduce mortality but that the benefit was annulled by an increase in mortality from other factors. A trial of a single therapeutic measure would at least have demonstrated the effect of that one measure.

In addition to assessing the efficacy of a particular treatment a drug trial will also be designed to assess, however inadequately, the benefit:risk ratio for the treatment, at least by noting the occurrence of adverse reactions. However, sometimes the aim is more circumscribed, such as the determination of the most appropriate dosage regimen; for example, in the treatment of urinary tract infections one might compare a 10-day course of low-dose antibiotic therapy with two large doses only.

Whatever the aim of a trial, the formulation of that aim will also involve a careful decision about the exact end-points to be measured. It will generally be wise to make the end-point as simple as possible. For example, in a trial of the secondary prevention of myocardial infarction one might simply count the number of deaths in the treated group compared with the untreated group. Of course, aims should not be sacrificed to simplicity, but they should not be unreasonably complex.

Sometimes it is desirable to evaluate the feasibility of a trial by a pilot study before embarking on the full-scale trial. In a pilot study a small number of patients may be studied without recourse to blindness (see below). The main aim of a pilot study should be to pinpoint problems with the trial design and so to help in designing the formal study. A pilot study should never be carried out to determine what the likely result of a full study might be: whatever the result of a pilot study it cannot be used to predict the outcome of a full-scale study and valuable time

■ **Table 16.1** Factors to be considered when designing and evaluating clinical trials

1. *Aims*
   End-point(s)
   Pilot study

2. *Basic design*
   Choice of subjects
   Choice of controls
   Randomization
   Blindness
   Placebos
   One or more centres
   Prospective or retrospective
   Methods of assessment
   Records

3. *Subjects*
   Numbers
   Controls
   Inclusions and exclusions
   Disease characteristics
   In-patients or out-patients
   Age and sex
   Race
   Other diseases or drugs

4. *Drugs*
   Dosage regimens
   Run-in and wash-out periods
   Compliance
   Other therapy

5. *Analysis and interpretation*
   Appropriate statistical tests
   A priori hypotheses
   Exclusions from analysis
   Intermittent analysis
   Statistical versus clinical significance
   Extrapolation to other populations
   Ethics
   Consent
   Permissible techniques
   Placebos
   Children
   Correct design
   Control of ethical problems

and patients may be wasted. Whenever possible, try to randomize the first patient to your full-scale trial.

16.2.2 Basic design

(a) Subjects to be studied

See below, section 16.2.3.

(b) Control subjects

See below, section 16.2.3.

(c) Randomization

The purpose of randomization is to eliminate bias, for example to avoid recruiting patients who are have a particular characteristic to one treatment group and not to the other. Randomization should not be carried out until immediately before the treatment begins. There may therefore be a delay between the time when the patient is approached and asked to take part and the time of randomization. Sometimes this delay can be

useful: it may allow the patient to have second thoughts about taking part, or it may allow the investigator to have second thoughts about admitting the patient to the study (for example if he or she feels that the patient's compliance will be poor); it may also be used as a run-in period with dummy treatment, during which the investigator might, for example, assess a patient's likely compliance, or in some cases to allow the patient's condition to reach a stable state (for example in essential hypertension, in which it is well recognized that the blood pressure may continue to fall for several weeks after the first clinic visit). Once randomization of a patient has occurred the investigator is committed to include that patient's data in the final analysis (see below under analysis of results).

Simple methods of randomization can be designed using, for example, published tables of random numbers, but whatever technique is used certain principles must be observed. Firstly, the order in which the subjects are to be allocated to the different treatment groups when they are recruited should be decided before the trial starts. Code lists should be drawn up so that the main investigators may be kept blind to the treatment an individual is receiving, but so that at the same time the treatment any individual is receiving can be readily discovered at any time by breaking the code. Secondly, the code used to identify treatments should be such that if the code has to be broken the knowledge of what treatment a patient was taking does not yield information about the treatments other patients are taking. For example, if two treatments are coded 'A' and 'B' then as soon as the code is broken for one patient the code for every patient is broken automatically. Thirdly, it is better if the information on which patient is to receive which treatment is left to one person, say the pharmacist holding the tablets. In large multicentre trials it is usual for this to be done by a trial co-ordinator operating from one centre. When randomization is required a telephone call to the co-ordinator will elicit the randomization instructions, for example 'Give this patient treatment number 34.' Only the co-ordinator knows what treatment number 34 is, and his or her choice is randomly predetermined. All this may seem excessively tedious, but the outcome of a trial may depend upon the success with which randomization is carried out and blindness maintained. The use of stratification to minimize chance differences between randomly allocated groups is discussed below in section 16.2.3(b).

(d) Blindness

Blindness in a trial means that the individual (investigator or patient) does not know what treatment is being given. The purpose of blinding (or 'masking') the investigator is to eliminate bias. For example, an investigator who knows what treatment the patient is taking may in some way influence a measurement or an outcome by his or her own actions in a way which shifts the outcome in one direction or another. Such bias may occur both consciously and unconsciously. Only if he or she is blind to the treatment can the investigator have full confidence in his or her own judgement of a patient's progress. The purpose of blinding the patient is to eliminate the differences in responses that can occur because

of differences in the patient's expectation of what a particular treatment, or no treatment, may do. For example, a patient who thinks that he or she is being given a pain-killer and who expects relief may report an effect of pain relief in excess of the true effect.

The ideal trial is double-blind, i.e. neither the patient nor the investigator knows what treatment the patient is taking. However, it may not always be possible to keep both investigator and subject blind, and in that case one may have to settle for a single-blind design, i.e. either the investigator or the subject, but not both, knows what treatment the patient is taking. For example, it is impossible to keep an investigator blind to the obvious clinical effects of a β-adrenoceptor antagonist (for example bradycardia). In such cases it may be possible for the results of some objective measurement (for example a chest X-ray) to be assessed by another investigator who does not see the patient and who can therefore be kept blind to the treatment. By a similar token it may sometimes be difficult to keep the patient blind to the treatment if it has a distinct adverse effect (for example drowsiness with antihistamines, discoloration of the urine by rifampicin). In such cases it may also be difficult to prevent the investigator from finding out that the patient knows what treatment he or she is receiving, and this should be guarded against if possible, say by using several investigators, some to make measurements and others to assess them.

A careful choice of treatment with which the active treatment is to be compared may help to get round this problem. For example, if a drug colours the urine then it may be possible to compare the therapeutic dose of the drug with a subtherapeutic dose which however also colours the urine; this has been done in the case of methylene blue, used as an antioxidant. Alternatively, it may be possible to incorporate in both the active treatment and the dummy some colorant which masks the colour of the active compound.

(e) The use of placebos

Placebos (or 'dummies') are used in order to achieve blindness. It is therefore important that placebos be made to match the active treatment as closely as possible. This means that the placebo formulation should as far as possible be of the same size, shape, colour, texture, weight, taste, and smell as the active formulation.

If two different doses of an active drug are being compared then any differences in the numbers of tablets to be given must be balanced by placebo tablets. If two different formulations, whether of the same drug or of different drugs, are to be compared then each must be given at the same time as the placebo form of its counterpart (the so-called 'double dummy' technique).

(f) Number of centres

Ideally a clinical trial should be carried out in one place only, in order to minimize variations in the population and variations in investigators' techniques, and in order to avoid the problems of communication, collection of data, and follow-up. However, because the need for adequate numbers of patients in a clinical trial overrides everything else except the elimination of bias, it is often necessary to involve more than one centre in order to obtain enough patients. Large numbers, and therefore multicentre trials, may be necessary when studying a rare disease, or when the effect one is looking for is a small one, albeit occurring in many patients, or when the number of patients in whom an effect can be expected is small. As an example of the last problem consider the influence of drugs on the rate of pulmonary embolism due to deep venous thrombosis after myocardial infarction. Although the effect of a treatment (for example low-dose subcutaneous heparin) may be large (say a 50 per cent reduction in incidence) the actual number of patients who have a pulmonary embolism is very small compared with the number who have a myocardial infarction. Thus, very many patients with myocardial infarction must be studied before enough cases of pulmonary embolism will occur for even a large effect to be detectable.

In multicentre trials the desirability of asking only one or two questions and of making those questions simple ones becomes more obvious. For example, in a study of the effects of a β-adrenoceptor antagonist in patients who have had a myocardial infarction one might simply ask the question 'Does treatment with a β-blocker for one year after a myocardial infarction result in a reduced death rate?' With an easily detectable end-point and simple but carefully applied selection criteria such a study could readily be organized among a large number of centres and be expected to produce an answer in a relatively short space of time, even though several thousands of patients might have to be recruited.

(g) Prospective design or not?

Clinical trials designed to evaluate the efficacy of new drugs should always be prospective. In other words, the characteristics of the population to be studied should be identified before the study begins and the results of treatment should be observed thereafter. For example, if one randomized all patients with heart failure to treatment with either digoxin or a new positive inotropic drug, and then studied the outcome over the following 6 months, that would be a prospective trial. It would be wrong to compare the effects of the new drug in the new population with the known effects of digoxin, obtained from studying a previous population (i.e. 'historical controls'; see below).

However, it is possible to study aspects of existing treatments by methods other than that of the prospective clinical trial, for example by a case-control study. In such a study the outcome is first identified and then comparisons are made retrospectively between the characteristics of the patients who did or did not have that outcome. Such studies have, for example, shown that lignocaine is beneficial in the management of ventricular arrhythmias after myocardial infarction and that oral anticoagulants can reduce the incidence of re-infarction in patients who have already had a myocardial infarction. Studies of this kind may be carried out some time after the introduction of a drug therapy in order to get some idea of its place in the overall management of the disease, or to evaluate adverse effects (see Chapter 9).

Case-control studies are cheap and easy to carry out. However, it is not possible to ensure either blindness or random allocation to treatment groups, and the results may be less reliable than those of a randomized prospective trial. None the less, the results of a case-control study may prompt a formal prospective trial in order to confirm the original findings and to extend investigation of the problem.

(h) Methods of assessment

Methods of assessment may be subjective or objective. Investigators often feel that subjective ('soft') data are of less value than objective ('hard') data. However, subjective assessments may be essential (for example, in studies of antidepressants), and if analysed appropriately may provide as much useful information as objective measurements. Although the patient's feelings will always be subjective it is sometimes possible to eliminate the investigator's subjective interpretation of the patient's feelings by the use of visual analogue scales, in which the patient might, for example, mark on a line the extent to which he or she feels happy or sad, tired or energetic (see Fig. 29.2).

Objective measurements, on the other hand, should not necessarily be regarded as incontrovertibly accurate. Assessment criteria should be shown to be reproducible in terms of within-subject, between-observer, day-to-day, diurnal, or other variability.

Of particular importance is the choice of the scale of measurement, since that influences the statistical techniques to be used in later analysis (see below). Scales of measurement are of three kinds.

(i) Nominal scales

A nominal scale is one in which different attributes are codified (or given a name from the Latin *nomen*). For example, one might codify the time of day at which an event occurred as 1 = morning, 2 = afternoon, 3 = evening, and 4 = night (the exact times of each named period being defined). It is then convenient to record the data as frequencies.

(ii) Ordinal scales

Here some form of ranking (or ordering from the Latin *ordo*) is generally involved. For example, one might rank grades of consciousness from 0 to 4 on the basis of a patient's response to stimuli (see the scheme outlined in the chapter on self-poisoning, p. 488).

(iii) Interval scales

Here continuous measurements are possible, for example blood urea concentrations, plasma drug concentrations, or white cell counts.

(i) Records

The importance of keeping careful, simple, accurate records during a trial is obvious. Suitable forms for keeping such records should be compiled before the trial begins and should contain reminders to the investigator of the questions to be asked and the routine to be followed in each case.

16.2.3 Subjects

(a) Numbers

Having enough patients in your study is, after the elimination of bias, the most important consideration in a clinical trial. Before discussing how to decide on the number of patients you will need in a study we must first introduce the statistical concept of the null hypothesis. Although the aim of a drug trial is generally to find out if there is a difference between different treatments, the statistical approach is to assume that there is no difference between the treatments and then to test the validity of that assumption. The assumption that there is no difference is called the null hypothesis. If the statistical analysis of the results of the trial leads one to reject the null hypothesis it is then accepted that there is, or rather that there is likely to be (for one can only demonstrate probability, not certainty), a difference between the treatments. It is important to appreciate this inverted thinking before tackling the question of numbers.

The number of patients necessary for a successful clinical trial depends on four factors. If one wants to predict the number of patients one will need to recruit for a successful trial one must first make some estimate of the size of these factors.

1. The difference in the effect that different treatments will have on whatever measure is being used to assess the effect of the treatments. In other words the difference between the mean value of the measurement in the treated population (m_1) compared with the mean value (m_2) in the reference population. This difference ($|m_1 - m_2|$) is sometimes designated by the symbols δ or θ. For example, if one is studying the effect of a diuretic one might use as an estimate of δ the increase in mean sodium

excretion in the urine which the diuretic is expected to cause.

2. The reliance one can place on the accuracy of a given measurement. This is usually expressed as the standard deviation of the mean of the difference between the two populations.

   (These two factors, i.e. the expected difference between the two populations and the standard deviation of the difference, are sometimes combined into a single factor, called the standardized difference. The standardized difference is the ratio of the expected difference between the populations to the standard deviation of the difference.)

3. The level of chance one will accept for the so-called type I (or α) error. This is the error of rejecting the null hypothesis incorrectly. This chance is set near to zero. For example, if one rejected the null hypothesis because a trial showed that there was likely to be a difference between treatments with a probability value of $\alpha = 0.05$ (on a scale from $0 =$ no likelihood of acceptance of the null hypothesis to $1 =$ complete certainty of acceptance), one would have to accept that there was a 5 per cent (1 in 20 or 0.05) chance that the apparent difference was not a true difference, i.e. that a mistake had been made in rejecting the null hypothesis. This value of 0.05 is, by convention only, the value which is usually taken as the upper limit of chance of a type I error that one is prepared to take when rejecting the null hypothesis. If the value found on comparing results is less than 0.05 (say 0.02), the null hypothesis is rejected, and the difference is regarded as being likely to be a true one.

4. The level of chance one will accept for the so-called type II (or β) error. This is the error of accepting the null hypothesis incorrectly. For instance, let us suppose that because of incorrect trial design too few patients had been recruited, and that the results of the trial showed no apparent difference between treatments, where in fact a difference did exist, the incorrect conclusion that there was no difference would be a type II error. The numbers studied would have been too small to pick up the real difference between treatments. The level of probability for the type II error is set

near to one, but is generally allowed more latitude than that for the type I error and is often arbitrarily set as low as 0.8, accepting that there is a 20 per cent (1 in 5) chance that the type II error has been made.

When reporting trials with negative results it is important to report the power of the trial to detect a difference of a given size and the exact confidence limits of one's measurements, so that a quantitative assessment can be made of the chance that the treatment really does not work, or is not different from the reference treatment.

If one can estimate the size of these four factors in a study, the number of patients required can be estimated using the nomogram shown in Fig. 16.1. In the nomogram factors 1 and 2 (the expected difference between the two populations and the standard deviation of the difference) have been combined as the 'standardized difference', plotted on the line on the left-hand side. Factor 4 (the probability of the type II error) is plotted on the line on the right-hand side, and factor 3 (the probability of the type I error) on the diagonal lines in the middle. To use the nomogram one draws a line between the standardized difference and the level of the type II error one is prepared to accept. The number of patients in each group one would want to recruit is then shown by the intercept of this line on whichever diagonal line represents the value of the type I probability one is prepared to accept. Note that while one can choose a range of values for β, one is restricted here to two values of α (0.05 and 0.01). However, one would rarely, if ever, want to choose other values of α, and if one did one could use the equations on which the nomogram is based, but which are too complicated to discuss here.

In illustration of the use of the nomogram take two practical examples.

(i) Drug versus placebo

Suppose one wanted to compare the blood glucose-lowering effects of a new hypoglycaemic drug with that of a placebo. From preliminary studies the new drug is expected to lower the glucose concentration by a mean of 4.0 mmol/L compared with no effect of a placebo. Thus, the expected difference between treatments is 4.0. The standard deviation of this difference is estim-

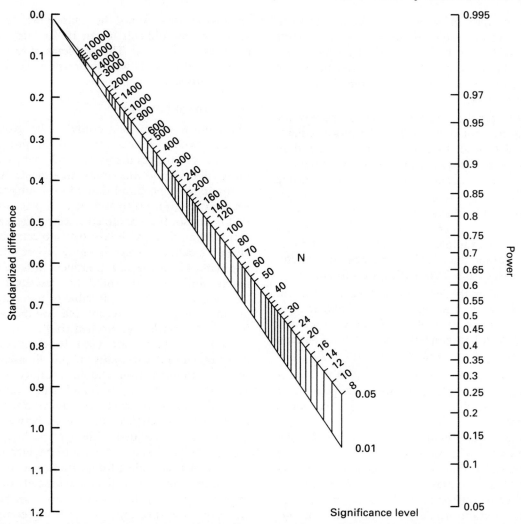

■ **Fig. 16.1** A nomogram for calculating the numbers of subjects required for a clinical trial when the expected standardized difference (the ratio of the expected difference between groups to its standard deviation) is known and the levels of the type I and type II errors have been fixed. (Adapted from Gore and Altman (1982) *Statistics in Practice*, p. 7, British Medical Association, London, with permission.)

ated to be 3.5 mmol/L and the standardized difference is thus 4.0/3.5 or 1.14. Choosing a power of 0.8 one draws the line joining 1.14 on the left to 0.8 on the right. The line cuts the diagonal line for $\alpha = 0.05$ at 24, and that is the number of patients one should try to recruit to each group in such a study.

(ii) Drug versus drug

Now suppose one wanted to compare the new drug with an established drug which was expected

to lower the blood glucose by 3.0 mmol/L on average. The expected difference is now 1.0 mmol/L. If the expected standard deviation of this difference were, say, 1.5 mmol/L the standardized difference would be 1.0/1.5 or 0.67. For $\alpha = 0.05$ and $\beta = 0.8$ one would want to recruit 70 patients to each group.

The ways in which altering the four factors affects the numbers of patients required can be seen from some simple examples using the nomogram.

1. The smaller the expected difference between the results of two treatments, the more patients one will need. In example (i) if the difference is reduced from 4.0 to 3.0 the number of patients required increases from 24 in each group to 44.

2. The larger the variation in the accuracy of the measurement one is using, the more patients one will need. In example (i) if the standard deviation increases from 3.5 to 4.0 the number of patients increases from 24 in each group to 32.

3. The smaller the level of type I error one is prepared to accept, the more patients one will need. In example (i) if one chooses α to be 0.01 rather than 0.05 the number of patients increases from 24 in each group to 36.

4. The higher the level of the type II error one is prepared to accept, the more patients one will need. In example (i) if one chooses β to be 0.09 rather than 0.08 the number of patients increases from 24 in each group to 32.

Of course, the nomogram can also be used in reverse, for example to calculate the power of a completed study to have detected a particular difference.

If one's study involves a measurement which is expressed as a proportion of the population studied, rather than as a continuous variable, one does not need to know the standard deviation of the expected difference, and a different equation and nomogram would be used. We shall not discuss them in detail here, but simply give an example, that of a study of the effect of a new antidepressant. The expected placebo response in depression is 30 per cent (i.e. 30 per cent of the patients will get better spontaneously during the study) and if the expected drug response is 50 per cent the expected difference would be 20 per cent or 0.2. If we set α at 0.05 and β at 0.9 we would need to recruit 127 patients to each group.

If we wanted to compare the new drug with an established drug with a response rate of 40 per cent the expected difference would fall to 0.1 and we would need to study a minimum of 533 patients in each group.

These figures should emphasize firstly how important it is to plan carefully the numbers of patients needed to be reasonably sure of getting an answer that is not by chance wrong, and secondly how difficult it can be to carry out a rigorous clinical trial. The problems of recruiting nearly 1100 patients with depression into a clinical trial would be enormous.

(b) Control subjects

The control group in a study is the group of subjects whose results are used to provide a reference for the results in the study subjects, i.e. those who receive the study treatment. It is a common misconception that control subjects are necessarily given no treatment or a placebo, but that is not so. If there are ethical problems about withholding therapy the control subjects may be given a treatment which is known to be effective and with which the new treatment will be compared. Such a trial would be described as a 'controlled trial'. If it is possible to use a control group of subjects who receive placebo that would be called a 'placebo-controlled trial'.

Control subjects are used to eliminate the effect of natural variability of the disease, since proper randomization should produce similar variability among control and study subjects. However, even the best randomization cannot guarantee that chance differences between the groups will be avoided, although the bigger the groups the less likely there are to be such differences. If it is considered important to match the groups in respect of particular characteristics (for example age, sex) then stratification can be carried out to ensure that like is being compared with like. Stratification can be done either before entry to the trial or retrospectively at the analysis stage.

If the outcome of the trial can be easily measured, and can be expected to occur within a relatively short period of time, then variability can be reduced even further by using a 'cross-over' design. In a cross-over trial of two treatments the subject takes one treatment during the first half of the study and the other during the second half. Subjects are randomized to take one or other treatment first, so that half will receive treatment A followed by treatment B while the other half will receive B then A. A wash-out period between treatments may be necessary to avoid overlap effects. If more than two treatments are to be studied then this cross-over principle can be extended. However, if there are several treatments it becomes too complicated to cater for all possible orders of treatments. Take for example a study of the effects of four different treatments. If using a cross-over design one would ideally want to study the effects of the treatments given in every conceivable order, of which there are 24, i.e. ABCD, ABDC, ACBD, ACDB, ADBC, ADCB, etc. However, to do this is cumbersome and requires more patients. A design based on the so-called Latin square takes care of that. One writes down the treatments in the form of a square in which each treatment is contained once only in each row and column. For example:

1	A	B	C	D
2	C	D	A	B
3	D	C	B	A
4	B	A	D	C

One then allocates patients at random to order 1, 2, 3, or 4. The result of this design is that if the effect of say treatment A when studied in group 1 is consistently greater or smaller than its effect in group 2, even so the difference will not affect the overall mean results. Systematic variation between the groups is thus eliminated.

Occasionally the natural history of a condition is highly predictable, and the effects of a new treatment can be compared with one's knowledge of the natural history. In this case the subjects in the reference group are said to be 'historical controls'. Historical controls can be used when the natural history is known with a high degree of certainty, for example when there is a high rate of fatality, and the result of treatment is fairly large. Since all the control information is available before the study starts fewer subjects are required. However, there are certain disadvantages to the use of historical controls. Firstly, since all the subjects receive the new treatment, blindness is not possible. Secondly, incorrect comparisons may be made if the nature of the disease changes with time (obvious examples are scarlet fever and influenza), or if changes in other forms of management occur between the gathering of the control data and the start of the new treatment (for example changes in the management of cardiac arrhythmias after myocardial infarction). This means that the circumstances in which such studies can be carried out with con-

fidence in obtaining clear-cut results are very few, and restricted to treatments such as the use of penicillin in lobar pneumonia. However, this approach has sometimes been of use, for example because of ethical problems. For example, the effects of cysteamine and acetylcysteine in limiting the extent of liver damage after paracetamol overdose were first compared with the outcome in patients who had been studied before their therapeutic effectiveness was recognized. Although these studies cannot be said to have proved beyond doubt the efficacy of these treatments, the results were good enough to warrant the regular use of acetylcysteine in selected patients after paracetamol overdose (see Chapter 35).

(c) Criteria for selection or exclusion

There are several factors which influence the selection of patients for inclusion in a trial or their exclusion from the trial.

Certain groups of individuals are generally excluded from clinical drug trials, unless the trial is designed specifically to study those individuals. These include pregnant women, children, and seriously ill patients. Patients at particular risk of an adverse reaction would also usually be excluded (for example asthmatic patients in a trial of a β-adrenoceptor antagonist, patients with peptic ulcer in a trial of a non-steroidal anti-inflammatory drug). This principle also applies to the avoidance of drug interactions.

There are specific problems about studying old people. Drug trials are frequently carried out in younger adults, because of the difficulties of studying old people: they are less mobile and easily confused, they may have poor compliance, and they are likely to be on other drugs and to have other diseases, both of which may interact with the treatment being tested. However, it is old people who most often take drugs, and if possible one should therefore try not to exclude old patients from drug trials. Indeed, it is often worth studying the data from old patients separately to try to pick up adverse effects early on, since they are more likely to suffer them. The importance of studying old people early in the development of a drug was highlighted by the case of the non-steroidal anti-inflammatory drug benoxaprofen, which only after it had been marketed was found to be toxic to old people in dosages which were relatively safe in younger individuals. It was widely prescribed among old people before this was realized, and several deaths occurred as a result.

Because poor compliance may reduce the power of a study it is useful to try to identify poor compliers before randomization. This can be done by having a run-in period, during which compliance is specifically studied. Poor compliers may then be excluded before randomization, and this does not introduce bias. A run-in period can also be useful to allow subjects to decide whether or not they want to be included in the study.

It is always important to be sure of the diagnosis before admitting a subject to a trial and one would exclude subjects who did not fulfil certain predetermined criteria of diagnosis. For example, one might define criteria for the diagnosis of myocardial infarction in terms of chest pain and changes in plasma enzyme activities and the electrocardiogram. Patients in whom the preset criteria were not fulfilled would not be admitted to a trial of, say, a new thrombolytic drug.

(d) Disease characteristics

The choice of subjects for a trial may be determined by the characteristics of their disease.

(i) Severity

The value of treating moderate and severe hypertension was clearly demonstrated in early trials. More recently large-scale studies of mild hypertension seem to have demonstrated benefit there too, but the relative benefit:risk ratio has not yet been properly established. In any trial of a new antihypertensive drug, therefore, the severity of the hypertension is an important factor in patient selection.

(ii) Duration

If a disease is self-limiting one might want to choose patients in whom the disease has persisted beyond its usual course. For example, it might be best to study an antidiarrhoeal drug only in patients with diarrhoea of more than a few days duration, in order to eliminate the problem that the majority of acute diarrhoeal illnesses resolve quickly and spontaneously.

(iii) Failure to respond to other treatment

If the risks of treatment with a drug are likely to be considerable at first, and if one therefore wants to proceed cautiously, one might study only those patients in whom other treatment had failed. Examples include the initial introduction of captopril in the treatment of severe, refractory hypertension, or of bromocriptine in patients with Parkinson's disease whose response to L-dopa had been poor.

(e) In-patients or out-patients

Some diseases can be studied only in in-patients (for example the prevention of cerebral arterial vasospasm after subarachnoid haemorrhage), while for others an in-patient study may be impracticable (for example oral hypoglycaemic treatment of maturity-onset diabetes). The choice will usually be straightforward.

(f) Age and sex

Differences in drug handling between the sexes and in different age groups (see Chapter 11) must be taken account of. It is best, if possible, first to establish the efficacy of a treatment in adults and then in older children before trying it in the very young. This does not apply, of course, to the treatment of a disease which is limited to the very young (for example the respiratory distress syndrome).

(g) Race

Occasionally a genetic factor may alter the nature of a disease, the nature of its response to treatment, or the chance of an adverse reaction (see, for example, Chapter 8 on pharmacogenetics).

(h) Complicating diseases or drugs

These are usually factors which lead to the exclusion of patients from trials, as discussed above.

16.2.4 Drugs used

(a) Dosage regimens

The various features of routine dosage must all be carefully considered: they are formulation, dose, frequency of administration, time of administration, and total duration of treatment (see also Chapter 18 on prescribing). At the time the clinical trial is carried out these should be chosen in order to obtain the best possible effect, using the knowledge available at that time.

(b) Run-in and wash-out periods

It is sometimes important to have a run-in period, i.e. to wait some time after deciding that a subject is eligible for a trial before actually starting the formal treatment. One may, for example, want to establish a set of baseline measurements in an individual before the trial and to demonstrate their reproducibility. A run-in period may also be used in conditions which alter spontaneously with the passage of time while under observation; for example, the blood pressure of a subject with apparent hypertension may settle to within the normal range over a few weeks of simple observation and repeated measurement. The use of a run-in period to study compliance has been mentioned above.

In cross-over designs a wash-out phase may be required at the end of one of the treatment periods in order to ensure that the effects of that treatment are not carried over into the next treatment period. For example, if one were studying a drug with a long half-time one might have to wait several days or weeks (four or five half-times) between treatment periods in order to ensure that there was no carry-over effect due to persistence of the drug in the body.

(c) Compliance

The methods used for assessing patient compliance are outlined in Chapter 13. Careful consideration should be given to the best method in individual cases.

(d) Other therapy

The question of avoiding drug interactions has been mentioned above, but one has to consider what other drugs a patient may be allowed to take during a trial, and if possible to control their prescription. If therapy is complex this may be a factor to consider in stratification (for example, separately randomizing all patients taking thiazide diuretics).

16.2.5 Analysis and interpretation

These are complex subjects about which only a few points can be made here.

(a) Choice of statistical tests

All too often data are analysed using the wrong tests, such as parametric tests (for example Student's *t*-test) for discontinuous data (for example ordinal scores, see section 16.2.2(h) above), or *t*-tests for comparing sets of data with different degrees of variability. There are many different ramifications of statistical analysis, and it is wise in the early stages of planning a trial (not after the trial has already started) to consult a statistician for advice on the design of the trial and its later analysis. When approaching the statistician one should be well prepared. He or she will want to know what you want to study, what your intended design is, and above all what the numbers are likely to be: how many patients you will be able to recruit and how many you expect to respond to each treatment (i.e. the likely size of the effect).

(b) *A priori* hypotheses

Before starting a trial one must formally state one's hypothesis. When the trial is over the data will be tested on the basis of that hypothesis. However, during the analysis other questions will often arise, not based on properly formulated *a priori* hypotheses. If many such questions arise and are tested then from time to time statistically significant differences will crop up. This is because the more statistical tests you do the more likely it is that at least one comparison will be found to be statistically significant simply by chance. After all, if a hundred comparisons are made at least five will be statistically significant at the 5 per cent level by chance alone, i.e. even if there is no real difference. If the hypotheses thus tested were not formulated *a priori* (i.e. before the study began) then one would have to be more rigorous about testing them. For example, if one were to analyse a set of data in terms of five different subgroups (for example male versus female, over-60s versus under-60s) one would be wise to reduce the acceptable level of α from 0.05 to say 0.01. One would not then be prepared to accept the hypothesis at a level of significance that was not better than 1 per cent. Methods for interpreting the results of multiple statistical tests have been devised and statistical guidance should be sought. However, it is also wise in these circumstances to be flexible about one's interpretation of the data, since there is always a chance that one might incorrectly reject a correct hypothesis by being too rigorous. One should always therefore be prepared to consider carrying out another trial specifically designed to confirm the new hypotheses that have been generated by apparently significant differences arising from multiple comparisons.

(c) Exclusions from analysis

Once individuals have been randomized to a treatment group in a study then even if they fail to complete the study, for whatever reason, their data should be analysed as if they had continued with the treatment to which they were allocated. This is because one cannot guarantee that the reasons for default will be the same in the different treatment groups, and the analysis of the remaining data may therefore be subject to bias. This is the so-called 'intention to treat' approach. Unfortunately this approach reduces the power of one's study, since one will inevitably have to include in one's analysis of the effects of treatment data from subjects who have not completed the study. However, that is the price one pays for eliminating bias.

Rarely it may be necessary to omit a patient from the analysis if it transpires after randomization that there has been a gross violation of the entry criteria. In such cases careful judgement may be necessary to decide whether the degree of violation of the criteria is sufficient to warrant exclusion from the analysis, and if there is any doubt the data should be included. When the results of the trial are published all such exclusions, with the outcome, should be reported. A simple method for reporting data from clinical trials, including the outcome in subjects who have been withdrawn is shown in Fig. 16.2.

(d) Intermittent analysis

Intermittent analysis of data as they accrue in a clinical trial is sometimes desirable, but great care must be taken in the application of such analyses. The chief purpose of intermittent analysis is to detect any beneficial or adverse effects of treatment as soon as possible, so that the trial may be stopped if indicated. In this way it may be possible to minimize both the number of subjects recruited and the risks of adverse effects. However, it must be remembered that a beneficial effect of a treatment may appear to have occurred at some time during a trial purely by chance and may not be borne out by the final results. For this reason it is important that one's criteria for stopping a trial prematurely on the basis of an apparent interim beneficial effect should be more rigorous than one's criteria for accepting that there is a beneficial effect once the trial is complete. On the other hand, the occurrence of a clear adverse effect during a trial might be grounds for stopping the trial. The value of analysing data from old subjects separately in this respect has been mentioned above.

There is a particular form of intermittent analysis called 'sequential analysis', in which one analyses the result for each subject as the trial progresses. When it becomes clear (and specific statistical tests are available) that there is either a difference or no difference between treatments the trial is stopped. Sequential analysis has the advantage of minimizing the number of subjects studied, but there are also disadvantages: it is easy to miss small differences with this type of design and when a difference is detected the size of the difference tends to be overestimated. Sequential analysis should be reserved for specific cases, particularly when one thinks that a large difference may occur in a short space of time.

(e) Statistical versus clinical significance

In a clinical trial it may be found that although the effect of a drug is statistically significantly better than placebo or the reference treatment, the overall effect is very small and clinically unimportant. For example, paracetamol has been reported to increase the effect of warfarin on clotting time by a second or two; the difference was statistically significant but of no practical relevance. This principle is important to remember when assessing the practical relevance of the results of any clinical study.

(f) Extrapolation

Clinical trials are often carried out on highly selected populations in specially controlled circumstances. No matter what the result it would be wrong to assume that the same result would occur in a less highly selected population, such as one expects to encounter in the uncontrolled conditions of clinical practice. One should there-

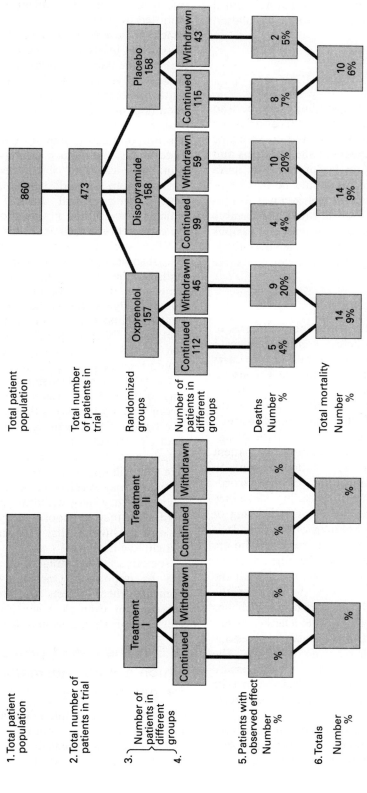

■ **Fig. 16.2** A diagrammatic method for reporting the summary results of clinical trials. On the right is shown an example of the use of the method. (Adapted from Hampton (1981). *Br. Med. J.* **282**, 1371–3, with permission.)

fore be circumspect when extrapolating from a small or select study population to the population at large.

16.3 Ethics

This is a very difficult subject, but everyone who is about to be involved in a clinical trial, or whose patients are to be involved in someone else's trial, should be aware of the problems and be prepared to make up his or her own mind about how those problems should be tackled or avoided. The Declaration of Helsinki was formulated by the Eighteenth World Medical Assembly in 1964 to offer guidelines, and there are various other published codes of conduct (see the Bibliography in Chapter 20). The following are some of the issues involved.

16.3.1 Consent

It is customary nowadays in almost all cases to seek patients' consent before admitting them to a clinical trial and it is usual to talk in such cases of obtaining the patient's 'informed consent' (exceptions would include cases in which the procedure of the trial was trivial, such as the taking of a few extra millilitres of blood to study some effect of a drug which the patient was already taking or as a control sample in a patient having blood taken for some other reason). In fact the close juxtaposition of the words 'informed' and 'consent' is misleading, since they constitute two separate processes: the giving of information and the obtaining of consent. It is an investigator's duty to inform subjects who are being recruited for trials what the purpose of the trial is, how it will be carried out, and what the important risks will be. It is the duty of the subjects to consider the information which has been given to them and to decide whether or not they want to take part in the study, if necessary after consultation with relatives or friends. The investigator should not bring any sort of pressure to bear on the subject, and the decision to take part should be one which the subject has freely taken.

Put like this, informed consent sounds very straightforward, but there are many problem areas. For example, how does one obtain the informed consent of a patient who has just been admitted to the coronary care unit with an acute attack of severe chest pain, perhaps due to a myocardial infarction? Even if the patient's consent to take part in a study of the effects of say an antiarrhythmic drug is obtained after all the acute problems have been dealt with, the obtaining of consent may be influenced by a change in mental state due to the pain-killing injection of diamorphine or by the patient's gratitude to the investigator for having relieved the pain. How can one obtain properly informed consent from an old demented patient, from patients with mental illness, or from other patients who are not in a position to understand the explanations, such as children?

When subjects can be expected to understand at least some of the issues involved it is customary to discuss the trial with them, explaining in simple terms what the purpose of the study is, what it would involve as far as they are concerned, and what the important risks are. If the subjects are unlikely to benefit directly from the trial then that should be clearly explained. The subjects should then be given a brief written explanation of the trial, couched in simple terms, and given time to think it over. Later on they should have an opportunity to discuss the trial again with the investigator if they want to. It should always be made clear to subjects that there is no compulsion to take part in a trial and that a decision not to take part will not alter the quality of any medical care they may receive. It should also be made clear that they may withdraw from the trial at any time if they so choose. One should never try to convince subjects that they ought to take part in a clinical trial.

Sometimes the timing of requesting consent may be important. One should try to avoid moments when subjects are likely to be under pressure, for example when about to have an operation or when a woman is in labour.

16.3.2 The use of procedures which are not normally indicated for patient care

It is important when intending to use any procedure which would not normally be used in the clinical care of a patient to explain to the patient that that is so and what the risks are. In some cases invasive procedures may be risky or uncomfortable, for example cardiac catheterization to determine the haemodynamic effects of a drug; such procedures are generally best limited to those in whom they are indicated as part of their medical care.

16.3.3 Placebos

Although, as we have seen above, placebos can be of value in the design of a clinical trial there are some circumstances in which their use may be considered to be unethical. For example, it would generally be considered unethical to use a placebo for comparison with a new treatment when an established treatment already exists.

16.3.4 Trials in children

The legality and ethics of trials in children (anyone under the age of 18 years) are very difficult. However, ethical guidelines have been formulated by the 1978 Working Party on Ethics of Research in Children and have been accepted by the British Paediatric Association. The guidelines depend on four premises:

1. That research in children is important for their benefit.
2. That research in children should not be carried out if the same investigation could be carried out in adults.
3. That research which involves a child and which is not beneficial to that child is not necessarily unethical or illegal.
4. That the benefit:risk ratio should be estimated.

In the context of the last premise risk is defined as 'negligible' (less than that run in everyday life) and 'more than minimal'. Benefit is defined on the basis of 'therapeutic' research (of potential benefit to the subject) and 'non-therapeutic' research (which may potentially benefit others or add to basic knowledge).

The guidelines are discussed in detail in the *British Medical Journal* 1980;**282**:229–31.

16.3.5 Study design

It is unethical to carry out an improperly designed trial, since it is unethical to subject patients or volunteers to the various hazards and discomforts involved if the trial is too badly designed to yield an answer to one's original question. This again underlines the importance of good design.

16.3.6 The control of ethical problems

Various bodies may exert control of one kind or another on the ethics of a clinical trial:

(a) The Committee on Safety of Medicines

No new drug should be used in a clinical trial in patients in the UK unless it has a Clinical Trials Certificate (CTC) or Exemption Certificate (CTX) issued by the UK Licensing Authority after advice from the CSM (see p. 171).

(b) Ethics committees

All major centres of clinical research and some pharmaceutical companies have independent committees whose job it is to scrutinize clinical research proposals and to advise whether or not they consider them to be ethical. Serving on such committees are lay members of the public as well as doctors (including clinical pharmacologists), nurses, pharmacists, and administrators. While the approval of an ethics committee is not essential and does not carry legal authority, one would be ill-advised to embark on a clinical trial without such approval. Guidelines for such committees are published in a variety of journal articles and books (see the Bibliography in Chapter 19).

(c) Insurers

If a pharmaceutical company commissions a piece of research on one of its products it is important that it provides indemnification in case adverse effects occur during the trial. In other words the company must be prepared to accept responsibility for adverse effects attributable to its drug.

(d) The law

Very little is clear about the influence of British law on clinical trials, since there have been very few cases tested in the courts. However, there are two basic principles involved: consent and negligence. Of these negligence has been the more widely tested, albeit in circumstances other than clinical trials, and the principle that a doctor is expected to exercise 'reasonable care' is well understood.

17 The drug history and the clinical examination and investigation of drug effects

The drug history and the clinical examination and investigation of drug effects are important parts of the general history, examination, and investigation. They should be undertaken with as much care. The importance of doing so is underlined by the following considerations.

1. A knowledge of the drugs a patient has taken in the past or is currently taking is essential in planning future treatment.

2. Drug effects should always be on the list of differential diagnoses, since drugs may be a cause of disease, either directly or as a result of an interaction.

3. Drugs may mask clinical signs. For example, β-adrenoceptor antagonists may prevent the adrenergic signs and symptoms of acute hypoglycaemia or the tachycardia which would normally occur in response to haemorrhage; corticosteroids may prevent the abdominal pain and rigidity which would normally occur in response to a perforated intra-abdominal viscus or the fever which would normally occur in response to an infection.

4. Drugs may alter the results of investigations. For example, if the patient has been taking an antibiotic the chance of culturing an infective bacterium may be reduced; amiodarone inhibits the peripheral conversion of T_4 to T_3, and this results in an increase in the serum concentrations of T_4 and reverse T_3 and a reduction in serum T_3, causing confusion in the diagnosis of thyroid dysfunction when it occurs.

5. The act of taking the drug history may give one an opportunity to educate patients about the drugs they are taking.

17.1 Taking the drug history

There is more to taking a drug history than asking 'What drugs are you taking?' As in all history taking there are many questions, some obvious, some subtle, which can be asked in trying to elicit an accurate history. Most drug histories will be easily and quickly obtained, but in some cases it may be important to spend some time eliciting an accurate and complete history.

In taking the drug history one's aims are to identify any drug or drugs the patient is taking currently or has been taking until recently, and to identify for each drug the original indication for treatment, the formulation, the doses used, the frequency and route of administration, the duration of treatment, and any beneficial or adverse effects the drug may have had. One also wants to find out if the patient is allergic to any drugs, in case one wants to use them at some time in the future.

The simplest way to identify the drugs a patient is taking is to ask to see them. Often one can then identify the medicines from labels on containers, or, in the absence of such labels, by direct recognition of the formulation. In some cases the name of the drug may be written on a tablet. If a formulation cannot be recognized it is worth consulting a pharmacist, who may have access to an identification system, based for example on the colour, shape, and size of a formulation.

Looking at patients' medicines may also be valuable in other ways, as we shall mention below. However, patients do not always bring all, or indeed any, of their drugs with them, and it is important to be able to identify the medicines they are taking without actually seeing them.

The first question to ask is 'What medicines are you taking at present?' Notice the use of the word 'medicines' rather than 'drugs'. Nowadays many people associate the word 'drugs' with drugs of dependence, such as heroin or cocaine, or with drugs taken by athletes to enhance their sporting performances, such as anabolic steroids. It is also wise when asking this question to spread the net as widely as possible by asking about medicines obtained from sources other than a doctor's prescription. For example, many people do not think of medicines they get directly from the chemist's shop or the drug store ('over-the-counter' drugs) as medicines they should bother mentioning; homoeopathic prescriptions, drugs obtained from health food shops, drugs obtained while abroad, and preparations which are peculiar to an ethnic minority may come into this category as well. Occasionally people make their own medicines from herbs they pick in gardens or fields (for example comfrey tea).

Sometimes it is necessary to ask direct questions about specific drugs. For example, a woman will not necessarily think of an oral contraceptive ('the pill') as a medicine, despite the fact that she will have obtained it by prescription.

Having asked about current medicines ask about medicines which may have been taken during the previous few days or weeks, since drugs with long durations of action may still exert effects in the body for some time after treatment has stopped. An extreme example of this is amiodarone, which has a half-time of several weeks, and whose effects may persist for months after the patient has stopped taking it.

Names of drugs may prove problematic. For example, a patient may know a drug by its proprietary name and not by its generic name or vice versa (see p. 210). It is as well for the doctor to know both. Sometimes patients do not know the names of the drugs they are taking, but even in that case one should not give up trying to find out, since they may be able to describe the drugs in other terms. For example, patients may say that they are taking 'water tablets' or 'heart tablets'. From this clue one can proceed to ask questions which may elicit precisely what drug

they are talking about. One might start by hazarding a guess at a likely drug and mentioning its name to the patient. For example, in the case of a 'water tablet' one might name some commonly used diuretics in the hope of stirring the patient's memory. If that failed one would ask for information about the formulation: 'Is it a tablet or a capsule? What colour is it? Are there any distinguishing marks on it?' In order to make use of this information the doctor needs to know what commonly used drugs look like, and one way of learning is always to ask to see any drugs patients have with them. A tray containing a selection of commonly used drugs may help to jog the patient's memory.

Sometimes asking about the route of administration may help to identify a drug. For example, very few drugs are taken sublingually, and if the indication is chest pain then the drug is almost certainly glyceryl trinitrate. Occasionally the frequency or timing of administration may give a clue. For example, if a patient is taking an inhaler for asthma then if it is taken for an acute attack it is likely to be a β-adrenoceptor agonist, such as salbutamol. However, one would not be able to pinpoint the identity of a drug taken by inhalation four times a day, since all inhaled drugs used in the treatment of asthma can be taken in this way.

Having discovered the identity of the drug try to find out the indication for its use. Apart from the possibility that this will yield a clue to the current problem, it may be important in deciding whether or not to continue with treatment. For example, a β-adrenoceptor antagonist may have been given for hypertension, in which case one would generally want to continue to give it; on the other hand, if the indication was acute hyperthyroidism then one would want to withdraw it when the acute problem had resolved. One should also ask whether the patient has benefited from the drug or not. If not, one may want to increase the dose, or withhold the drug and try something else.

The next thing to discover is the dosage regimen, i.e. the daily dose and the frequency of its administration. This is sometimes useful in determining, for example, whether adverse effects may be related to the administration of the drug, or in deciding whether an alternative regimen may be more effective or safer. For example, if a dose of frusemide has been effective, another dose given within 6–8 h is likely to be ineffective; in such a case one would extend the interval between doses or give the total daily dose as a single dose. Similarly, the patient who is suffering from nocturia because of a night-time dose of a diuretic may benefit from a change in timing of dosage.

In discovering the exact dosage regimen it is important to examine the drugs themselves if possible. Firstly, because the exact regimen is likely to be written on the label attached to the bottle or packet in which the drugs are kept. Secondly, because by doing so one sometimes discovers errors in drug administration. Two recent examples in Oxford illustrate the problems that can arise. In the first case the patient's doctor had given her a prescription for digoxin tablets of 0.0625 mg strength but the pharmacist had given her tablets of 0.25 mg strength; she presented with life-threatening digitalis toxicity. In the second case a woman who was taking 100 micrograms of thyroxine a day was given tablets of 50 microgram strength and directed to take two a day; she put them in an old bottle marked 'one tablet a day' and presented some weeks later with the signs and symptoms of hypothyroidism.

Inspection of the drugs a patient is taking may reveal other information about the ways in which patients use their drugs. For example, glyceryl trinitrate is unstable and trinitrate tablets should be kept in a dark bottle with an aluminium foil-lined cap and without cotton wool, which may absorb the drug; inspection of the bottle in which the tablets are kept will reveal any misuse of this kind. Checking the consumption of trinitrate tablets also helps in estimating the frequency of attacks of angina, and in general the tablet count helps in estimating the extent of patient compliance (see Chapter 13).

It is also important in most cases to find out about the duration of treatment. For example, the adverse effects of some drugs are related to the total amount of drug taken over a long period of time. This is particularly the case for the corticosteroids. While one would be prepared to withdraw corticosteroids rapidly after a short course of treatment it would be hazardous to do so after a long course, because of the risk of acute adrenal insufficiency (see Fig. 5.4). In other cases one may want to know whether the drug has been given for long enough to have had a therapeutic effect, for example in the case of an antibiotic; if it has and a therapeutic effect has not occurred one might want to change the drug or reconsider the diagnosis (see Chapter 6).

It is important always to inquire about events which may be attributable to adverse effects of drugs, including adverse drug interactions. One would do this in the way that one would take the rest of the history, avoiding leading questions, at least to start with, and then making direct enquiries about any specific adverse effects of importance. For example, one might ask patients taking amiodarone general questions about how they tolerate the weather before proceeding to ask them more specific questions about symptoms of thyroid disease and the sensitivity of their skin to sunlight.

In asking questions related to possible adverse drug effects it is important to look for information about the timing of the treatment in relation to the supposed adverse effects. For example, an attack of syncope in a patient who has recently started antihypertensive therapy may be due to postural hypotension secondary to treatment. However, some adverse effects take longer to occur. For example, in a patient taking penicillin the typical hypersensitivity rash comes on at 3–10 d after the start of therapy. More strikingly, adverse effects due to corticosteroids or amiodarone may take weeks, months, or even years to occur.

A recent change in the patient's condition may be important in determining adverse effects, as for example in the case of digitalis toxicity in the patient whose renal function has recently begun to deteriorate or who has recently been given a diuretic which has caused acute hypokalaemia.

In elucidating possible drug interactions the timing of drug administration may be important in both diagnosing the interaction and elucidating the mechanism. An adverse interaction which occurs immediately or soon after the introduction of the precipitant drug is likely to be due to inhibition of elimination of the object drug (see Chapter 10) or to a pharmacodynamic interaction. A transient adverse effect following the introduction of a new drug, for example a bout of bleeding in a patient taking warfarin, may be due to a protein binding displacement interaction (see p. 124). An adverse effect which starts to occur only after one or two weeks after the introduction of a new drug may be due to induction of hepatic drug metabolism.

In all cases it is imperative to inquire about a history of drug allergy, particularly if one is intending to prescribe a drug for which the risk of an allergic reaction is high (for example penicillins and sulphonamides). This should at first take the form of a simple question about known allergies, for example 'Are you allergic to any medicines?' If the answer is no, then it is still worth asking about a few specific examples, in particular the drugs you are about to prescribe, if the risk of allergy is high. If the answer is still no, the matter can be left there. However, if the answer is yes, more information must be sought. In particular one should ask about the exact nature of the supposed allergic reaction and its timing in relation to administration of the suspected drug. For example, some patients think that a bout of diarrhoea during a course of an orally-administered penicillin is evidence of penicillin allergy, which it is not. In such a case it would be wrong to deny the patient the benefit of penicillin on the basis of a misleading history. If, after having taken a careful history, one is in any doubt whatsoever about the nature of the supposed allergic reaction, one should assume that the patient is allergic to the drug in question and not use it. A history of hereditary angiooedema (see p. 524) may support a diagnosis of drug allergy.

17.2 Clinical examination and investigation of drug effects

During one's general examination and investigation of the patient one should take the opportunity of looking for evidence of compliance with drug therapy, signs that the drugs used are having therapeutic or toxic effects, and evidence that the patient has been taking drugs of dependence.

17.2.1 Pharmaceutical evidence

The examination of the patient's medicines for evidence of compliance has been mentioned

above. Other pharmaceutical methods of assessing compliance are discussed in Chapter 13.

Under the heading of examining for pharmaceutical evidence one can include examination for evidence of puncture marks in the skin, which may give information about drugs of abuse.

Under this heading one can also consider examination of the techniques patients use to take medicines. For example, when treating asthma with inhaled drugs it is important to ask patients to demonstrate their inhalation technique (see p. 308 for a description of the correct technique). It is surprising how often a patient will be found to be using an inhaler incorrectly. In a patient whose diabetes is responding poorly or irregularly to insulin one might examine the skin, to look for evidence about the adequacy of injection (for example in the patient who is mistakenly giving the drug intradermally instead of subcutaneously). Sometimes patients misunderstand the doctor's instructions and take the wrong dose of a drug; talking about the drug with the patient and looking at the formulation and the way the patient handles it may give useful information about this.

17.2.2 Pharmacokinetic evidence

In some cases it is possible to detect the concentrations of drugs in body fluids, such as urine or plasma, and this may be helpful in determining compliance and in planning drug therapy. The monitoring of drug therapy by measurement of plasma drug concentrations is discussed in Chapter 7.

17.2.3 Pharmacodynamic evidence

In some cases it is possible to look for evidence of pharmacodynamic actions of drugs. For example, one can measure blood pressure and pulse rate after exercise for evidence of the actions of β-adrenoceptor antagonists and the peak expiratory flow rate for evidence of the action of antiasthmatic drugs. Investigation for pharmacodynamic evidence of drug action is also possible, for example in the measurement of plasma uric acid concentrations in patients being treated for gout and measurement of the prothrombin time in patients taking anticoagulants. This aspect of monitoring drug therapy by examination and investigation for the pharmacodynamic actions of drugs is discussed in Chapter 7.

17.2.4 Evidence of therapeutic or toxic effects of drugs

In some cases it is possible to detect clinical evidence of therapeutic or toxic effects of drugs. For example, one can measure the ventricular rate in a patient with atrial fibrillation in assessing the therapeutic effect of digoxin, or look for signs of thyroid function to assess the therapeutic effect of thyroxine. Toxic effects of drugs which can be elicited on clinical examination include nystag-mus in a patient with phenytoin toxicity and pupillary constriction in a patient with opiate toxicity. Looking for signs of adverse drug effects may also sometimes be helpful in making a diagnosis in patients who have taken an overdose (see Chapter 35).

This discussion should have made it clear that the drug history and clinical examination and investigation of drug effects are important parts of the general history, examination, and investigation. If they are carried out carefully they can add much of value to the overall assessment of the patient and repay the time taken over them.

Section II

Practical prescribing

18 Principles of prescribing

Good prescribing is not an easy discipline to master. By good prescribing we mean prescribing the right drug at the right time, in the right dosage of the right formulation, and for the right length of time. Furthermore, this definition includes not prescribing any drug at all if no prescription is called for. To achieve this requires detailed knowledge of the pathophysiology of the diseases one intends to treat and of the clinical pharmacology of the drugs one intends to use, as we shall show here in dealing with the questions one should ask before prescribing. However, we must first consider the benefit:risk ratio in prescribing.

18.1 The benefit:risk ratio in prescribing

One prescribes drugs because of their potential benefit to the patient, but in every case this is accompanied by the risk of adverse effects. Before prescribing one should always try to assess the potential benefits which may accrue from one's treatment and the likelihood of the accompanying risks, in order to decide which outweighs the other. How does one assess the relative benefits and risks of a particular treatment? When possible one relies on published data on efficacy and adverse effects, particularly in regard to the relative efficacy and risks of comparable drugs. In doing this five factors need to be considered.

1. The seriousness of the problem to be treated.
2. The efficacy of the drug you intend to use.
3. The seriousness and frequency of possible adverse effects.
4. The safety of other drugs which might be used instead.
5. The efficacy of other drugs which might be used instead.

At one end of the spectrum the benefit:risk ratio will be high if the disease is life-threatening, the drug highly effective and the only one available, and the risk of serious adverse effects negligible. At the other end of the spectrum the benefit:risk ratio will be low if the disease is trivial, the drug poorly effective with more effective and safer competitors, and the risk of serious adverse effects high. This spectrum is illustrated in Table 18.1, and most cases will lie somewhere between the two extremes. To illustrate the principles involved take the example of phenylbutazone.

Phenylbutazone is a highly effective non-steroidal anti-inflammatory drug, which was used for many years in the treatment of acute and chronic inflammatory conditions, such as acute gout, acute and chronic rheumatoid arthritis, and ankylosing spondylitis. However, the incidence of marrow aplasia in patients taking phenylbutazone is between 1:30 000 and 1:100 000 and is at the higher end of this range in old people and during prolonged therapy. While there were no other non-steroidal anti-inflammatory drugs of equal efficacy available the therapeutic benefit to be had from phenylbutazone was considered large enough to outweigh the relatively high risk of marrow aplasia that its use carried. However, once other equally good drugs became available, drugs which did not carry any risk of marrow damage, or for which the risk was very much smaller, the risk of the adverse effects of phenylbutazone were seen to outweigh whatever benefit its use carried. It was therefore decided that phenylbutazone should no longer be prescribed as a first-choice anti-inflammatory drug and it is now available only for use by specialists in some cases of ankylosing spondylitis.

Note the important features that were considered in making this decision. The benefit of the drug was considered not in terms of its absolute

■ **Table 18.1** A schematic representation of the factors which contribute to an assessment of the benefit:risk ratio in drug therapy. A drug which fulfils the criteria in the top line has a very high benefit:risk ratio, while one which fulfils the criteria in the bottom line has a very low benefit:risk ratio. Most drugs lie somewhere between the two extremes

Seriousness of the indication	Efficacy of the drug	Adverse reactions		Other drugs		Benefit: risk ratio
		Severity	Frequency	Efficacy	Safety	
Life-threatening	High	Trivial	Rare	Poor	Poor	Very high
Trivial	Poor	Serious	Frequent	Good	Good	Very low

benefit, but in relation to the severity of the disease and the benefit available from other drugs: while phenylbutazone was more potent therapeutically than other drugs available it was considered to be highly beneficial, but when equally effective drugs became available its benefit was felt to be reduced, despite the fact that the therapeutic effect of the drug itself had not changed during that time. Even so, in some severe cases of ankylosing spondylitis, which respond poorly to other anti-inflammatory drugs, the benefit of phenylbutazone may still be regarded as outweighing the risk of marrow aplasia. Similarly, the main adverse effect of marrow aplasia was considered not as an absolute risk but in relation to the seriousness of the risk and the risks of other drugs of similar efficacy. While a risk of 1 : 100 000 of a minor adverse effect, such as a headache, would be considered unimportant, a similar risk of a serious adverse effect, such as marrow aplasia, must be considered important. Furthermore, if there are other drugs available which are equally effective but less toxic, they would be preferred to the drug of higher risk.

Of course, it may not always be possible to know what the relative benefits and risks are before giving a patient a drug. For example, there may be no published figures on the size of a particular risk and different patients may be at different risk of the same adverse effect (for example in the case of an adverse effect which is genetically determined). Furthermore, the extent of therapeutic benefit due to a drug, particularly in the case of symptomatic relief, varies widely from patient to patient and often one's appreciation of the potential benefit only comes after

one has tried the treatment and assessed its effects.

None the less, one should always try to assess the likely benefit:risk ratio before instituting therapy, no matter how unsure one may be about the magnitude of the factors which contribute to it. To illustrate some of the difficulties which can arise in assessing the benefit:risk ratio consider the following problems.

1. In a patient with moderate left ventricular failure in sinus rhythm, is the benefit which is likely to accrue from adding digoxin to a diuretic and a vasodilator likely to outweigh the risk of digoxin toxicity engendered by renal impairment secondary to hypertensive renal disease? The answer will depend among other things on the cause of the heart failure, the likelihood of good patient compliance, the ease with which plasma digoxin concentrations can be monitored, and the stability of renal function. A therapeutic trial may answer the question in hospital, but it may be more difficult to avoid digitalis toxicity after discharge.

2. Is the benefit likely to be gained from a course of an antibiotic in treating a urinary tract infection in a woman who is two months pregnant likely to be outweighed by the risk to the fetus? The answer will depend on whatever information is available at the time about the actual risk of teratogenesis compared with the risk to the mother of renal damage due to an untreated infection; added to this will be the relative risks to the fetus of other antibiotics. Since there is scarcely any hard

information on the absolute risks of teratogenesis with many antibiotics this is a virtually insoluble problem. Furthermore, even if quantitative estimates of the benefits and risks were known the problem might still be intractable, because one is comparing the likelihood of benefit to one individual with the risk to another.

3. Is the benefit to be gained from treating an old lady with giant cell arteritis with the corticosteroid prednisolone likely to be greater than the risks of making her osteoporosis worse, of increasing the difficulty of treating her diabetes mellitus, and of exacerbating her hypertensive heart disease because of sodium and water retention? Here, apart from the pain that giant cell arteritis can cause, the main problem is that there is a high risk of blindness from untreated giant cell arteritis affecting the cranial arteries. The decision on whether or not to offer treatment in such a case will depend on the severity of the arteritis, the vessels it is affecting, the severity of the complicating conditions, and the ease with which they too can be treated.

Questions of this kind can be very difficult to answer, because until appropriate studies of benefit and risk are carried out we have no data to go on, and anyway each case has to be decided on its own often complex merits. However, by thoughtful prescribing one may be able to lessen the risks of drug therapy while maintaining a high degree of efficacy. In the rest of this chapter we shall outline the sequence of questions one should ask oneself before writing a prescription. With experience the process of going through this sequence becomes more and more automatic, but whether or not one formally considers each part of the sequence on each occasion of prescribing, it is the answers to the questions in the sequence which determine what is and is not good prescribing.

18.2 Is drug therapy indicated?

This question really has two parts:

(1) Is the intended treatment necessary?

(2) Is the potential benefit likely to be greater than the risk?

Unnecessary prescribing is not uncommon, and the following are examples.

1. The prescription of broad-spectrum antibiotics (for example neomycin) for bacillary dysentery. It has been shown that such treatment confers no benefit and may even prolong diarrhoea.

2. The prescription of cerebral vasodilators for patients with senile dementia. There is very little evidence that this type of drug confers any benefit at all, and there is evidence that they may do harm by diverting blood flow from compromised areas of the brain to areas already quite well perfused.

3. The prescription of vitamin and mineral (for example iron) formulations as 'tonics' in the absence of any evidence of vitamin or mineral deficiency. These formulations act only as placebos in such circumstances, and should be recognized as such by the prescriber (see Chapter 14).

The reasons for unnecessary prescribing are numerous. They include imprecision of diagnosis, the lack of time and resources to deal adequately with the sadnesses and anxieties of life (relevant to the wide prescribing of psychotropic drugs), and the needs patients have for comfort and action.

The main consideration in answering the question of whether drug therapy is necessary is the question of the size of the benefit:risk ratio, as discussed above. However, even if the benefit:risk ratio is high it may be worth waiting before instituting therapy if the disease is likely to be self-limiting (as in the case of acute diarrhoeas, mentioned above), since that eliminates risk altogether.

18.3 Which drug?

If one has decided that drug therapy is indicated then one has to go through the process of deciding which particular drug to use. This involves further detailed questions, relating to the choice from among the classes of drugs available, the appropriate group of drugs within a class, and the particular drug within that group.

18.3.1 Which therapeutic class of drug?

This is sometimes immediately obvious: for example, one would prescribe an antibiotic for an infection, an antidepressant for depression, and a bronchodilator for an acute attack of asthma. However, in other cases the decision can be more complicated: for example, in the treatment of congestive heart failure the choice lies among diuretics, positive inotropic drugs, and vasodilators, and in the treatment of hypertension it lies among diuretics, β-adrenoceptor antagonists, vasodilators, and ACE inhibitors.

18.3.2 Which group of drugs within the class?

Take for example the treatment of an infection. The therapeutic class is the antibiotics, but within that class there will be a choice among several different groups of drug, for example penicillins, cephalosporins, tetracyclines, aminoglycosides, macrolides, and many more. The choice will depend on the sensitivities of the infecting organism, the site of infection, and particular features of the patient which may constitute contra-indications.

18.3.3 Which particular drug in the group?

Finally, the name of an individual drug has to be written on the prescription. To continue with the example of antibiotics, if one chooses to prescribe a tetracycline one has the choice of tetracycline, oxytetracycline, minocycline, doxycycline, and others. Again the choice may depend on numerous different factors.

18.3.4 How to make a rational choice

Is there a rational way of arriving at a best choice of drug? Sometimes it is a choice among equals. For example, there is little to choose among the large variety of thiazide diuretics available (for example, bendrofluazide, cyclopenthiazide,

chlorothiazide, hydrochlorothiazide, polythiazide, and several others). In such cases it is best to choose the drug with which one is most familiar. However, in other cases it may be possible to choose one drug in favour of another. The factors which dictate one's choice are numerous, and the following are examples.

(a) Pharmacokinetic considerations

(i) Absorption

One might choose bumetanide rather than frusemide for a patient with congestive cardiac failure, in which frusemide may be erratically absorbed and bumetanide better absorbed. Of course, as an alternative, one could give frusemide intravenously, thereby circumventing the problem of absorption.

(ii) Distribution

If an antibiotic is well distributed to a particular tissue then that antibiotic may the antibiotic of choice when that tissue is infected. For example, tetracyclines are concentrated in the bile, and lincomycin and clindamycin in bones.

(iii) Metabolism

Drugs which are extensively metabolized may be less useful in patients with severe liver disease. For example, one would generally avoid using opiate analgesics in patients with hepatic cirrhosis (and there are also pharmacodynamic reasons for doing so, see p. 109).

(iv) Excretion

Similar considerations apply in renal failure. One might, for example, avoid the aminoglycoside antibiotics in patients with renal impairment if an alternative group of antibiotics were suitable. If a tetracycline were indicated in a patient with renal impairment then doxycycline would be the drug of choice, since it does not accumulate in renal failure, as other tetracyclines do.

(b) Pharmacodynamic considerations

Sometimes the pharmacological effect of a drug or group of drugs is appreciably greater than that of another. For example, the sulphonylurea drugs as a whole are more potent hypoglycaemic drugs than the biguanides, and are usually used as first-line drug treatment. In patients with an acute myocardial infarction the positive inotropic effects of adrenoceptor agonists, such as dopamine or dobutamine, are likely to be greater than that of the cardiac glycosides, such as digoxin.

(c) Therapeutic considerations

(i) Features of the disease

If one knows, or has good reason to suspect, the identity of an infective organism then one would choose one's antibiotic appropriately. For example, one might choose a penicillin, a tetracycline, or co-trimoxazole for a patient with bronchopneumonia, since the likeliest organisms involved will be the pneumococcus (*Streptococcus pneumoniae*) or *Haemophilus influenzae*, both of which are likely to be sensitive to those antibiotics. Sputum culture, with identification of the organism and of its sensitivity to different antibiotics, will help in making the choice. Other factors may also help: for example, one would avoid most tetracyclines in patients with renal impairment, penicillins in patients with penicillin hypersensitivity, and co-trimoxazole in patients with sulphonamide hypersensitivity.

The severity of the disease may also influence one's choice of drug. For example, mild pain will generally respond to aspirin or paracetamol, while more severe pain may require more potent analgesics, such as codeine phosphate or even morphine. Moderate hypertension often responds to a single drug, such as a diuretic or a β-adrenoceptor antagonist, while more severe hypertension may require treatment with a combination of antihypertensive drugs.

(ii) Co-existing diseases

In the treatment of moderate hypertension one's choice lies between a diuretic, such as bendrofluazide, and a β-adrenoceptor antagonist, such as atenolol. In a patient with left ventricular failure a diuretic would be the logical choice, while one would choose a β-adrenoceptor antagonist for a patient with co-existing angina pectoris. In a patient with asthma one would generally avoid β-adrenoceptor antagonists altogether, while in diabetes mellitus a β-blocker which was selective for β_2-adrenoceptors would be preferred to a non-selective one.

(iii) Avoidance of adverse effects

A short-acting benzodiazepine, such as temazepam, might be preferred as a sedative to a longer-acting compound, such as nitrazepam, in the hope of avoiding excess sedation during the day. In patients with drug hypersensitivity an alternative drug may be necessary. For example, one would use chloramphenicol to treat meningococcal meningitis in a patient with penicillin hypersensitivity, or trimethoprim to treat a urinary tract infection in a patient with sulphonamide hypersensitivity.

(iv) Avoidance of adverse drug interactions

In patients taking warfarin one often needs to be careful in one's choice of other drugs. For example, aspirin and some other non-steroidal anti-inflammatory drugs are to be avoided; barbiturates and chloral derivatives are to be avoided as sedatives; tetracyclines, sulphonamides, and chloramphenicol are to be avoided in the treatment of infections. For a list of drugs which are likely to be safe in patients taking warfarin see the Pharmacopoeia (p. 713).

(d) Patient compliance

Sometimes a drug may be chosen simply because it can be taken once a day, in the hope that by minimizing the frequency of drug administration one may improve patient compliance (see Chapter 13). Thus, one might choose once-daily atenolol in preference to twice-daily propranolol and once-daily chlorpropamide in preference to twice-daily glibenclamide or thrice-daily tolbutamide.

18.4 Which route of administration?

Routes of administration of drugs are dealt with in Chapter 2. The route of administration may be dictated by the drug chosen, in which case the question answers itself; for example, dopamine can only be given intravenously. However, sometimes the prescriber may choose a particular route of administration because it confers some particular therapeutic benefit.

For example, glyceryl trinitrate is usually given sublingually, since it is rapidly absorbed through the oral mucosa straight into the systemic circulation, thus avoiding its first-pass metabolism in the liver, and rapidly relieving angina pectoris during an acute attack. However, it can also be applied as a patch to the skin, through which it is absorbed slowly. In this way it has been used to prevent attacks of angina pectoris (although this route may carry the disadvantage of nitrate tolerance).

The rectal route may be chosen for a direct effect on the large bowel (for example prednisolone in the treatment of ulcerative colitis) or occasionally to circumvent problems in the stomach (for example phenothiazines as antiemetics).

The intramuscular route may sometimes be chosen to ensure compliance, for example, in the single-dose treatment of gonorrhoea with intramuscular penicillin, or in the regular treatment (once every 2–4 weeks) of schizophrenia with depot injections of phenothiazines and thioxanthenes.

The subcutaneous route may be chosen because it allows easy administration of a drug by the patient or a relative (for example insulin and glucagon). The subcutaneous route may also provide a more prolonged effect by slow release of the drug from the site of injection (for example the different formulations of insulin).

The intravenous route may be chosen in order to circumvent problems of systemic availability (for example intravenous frusemide in a patient in whom poor absorption results in a lack of diuresis in congestive heart failure).

18.5 Which formulation?

There is a large number of different drug formulations for different circumstances. For example, oral formulations include tablets, capsules, granules, elixirs, and suspensions. Drugs for injection come as lyophilized powders for reconstitution before injection, or as solutions ready for injection; solutions come in single-dose ampoules, single-dose or multiple-dose vials, and half-litre or litre bottles for infusion.

Where oral administration is concerned drugs usually come in one formulation only and no choice is necessary. However, there are some exceptions, as the following examples show.

Aspirin is available in several different tablet formulations, including soluble, buffered, and enteric-coated. In each case the aim is to avoid the direct gastric irritation caused by using an ordinary formulation. However, for the treatment of acute pain the rapidly acting formulations (i.e. soluble and buffered aspirin) will be preferred, whereas for the treatment of the symptoms of chronic rheumatoid arthritis one might prefer to use an enteric-coated formulation.

Potassium salts are available in either slow-release formulations, or as effervescent tablets which dissolve in water for drinking, or as elixirs immediately ready to drink. One's choice here often depends on patient preference, but one might choose a soluble formulation in a patient with gastrointestinal hurry, in whom the slow-release formulation might pass through the gut unabsorbed.

Lithium salts and theophylline come in several different ordinary and slow-release formulations, each with different absorption characteristics (see p. 73). A formulation which produces adequate plasma lithium or theophylline concentrations in one patient may not be suitable for another, and it is sometimes worth changing the formulation if plasma concentrations are suboptimal.

Iron salts are available as ordinary tablets for twice- or thrice-daily administration or as slow-release formulations for once-daily administration. One would often choose the latter in the hope of improving patient compliance and diminishing the adverse effects that the ordinary formulations may have on the stomach. However, the iron in slow-release formulations is more erratically absorbed, and one might choose the ordinary tablets in a patient whose iron deficiency was not being corrected by a slow-release formulation.

The acceptability of some formulations may influence their use. For example, a child may prefer a pleasant-tasting suspension of paracetamol to a less pleasant elixir, while old people may prefer a tasteless solution of benorylate, which they can add to their tea, rather than tablets, which they may find hard to swallow.

18.6 What dosage regimen?

A dosage regimen has three aspects: the dose of the drug, the frequency of its administration, and the timing of its administration. Usually these can be considered together, although in some cases they may require separate consideration.

There are certain principles governing dosage regimens of drugs, and these principles show how dosage regimens should be altered, depending on the pharmacokinetic and pharmacodynamic characteristics of the prescribed drug, certain characteristics of the patient, and the characteristics of the symptoms or disease being treated.

18.6.1 Pharmacokinetic variability

Variation in absorption, distribution, and elimination of drugs from patient to patient means that one must be flexible in one's approach to dosages. If there is poor absorption one may have to increase the dose or choose another route of administration, or indeed another drug. Dosages may have to be reduced if elimination is impaired (for example in hepatic or renal disease). For drugs which are subject to first-pass metabolism in the liver one may have to use completely different dosage regimens for the intravenous route compared with the oral route. If the pharmacokinetics of the drug are altered by another drug then an alteration in the dosage regimen may be needed.

18.6.2 Pharmacodynamic variability: the dose–response curve

It is often forgotten that one of the fundamental tenets of pharmacology, the dose–response curve, demonstrates how the effect of a drug varies with dose, and that this is as true in the whole patient as it is in an experimental tissue *in vitro* (for example compare the *in vitro* data shown in Fig. 4.3 with the *in vivo* data shown in Fig. 4.5). Because the nature of the dose–response curve varies from patient to patient flexibility in prescribing is necessary, and if a therapeutic effect does not occur with the initial dosage chosen, an effect may be produced by making small dosage increases within a stated therapeutic dosage range. Of course, at the same time increasing the dosage will increase the risk of dose-related adverse effects, and part of the art of drug therapy lies in finding the regimen which produces a beneficial effect while avoiding adverse effects. Remember also that certain diseases can alter a dose–response curve (for example resistance to digoxin in hyperthyroidism) and that if the pharmacodynamics of a drug are altered by another drug an alteration in the dosage regimen may be needed.

18.6.3 Characteristics of the patient

Dosage regimens may be different in old people than in the young (for example see metoclopramide in the Pharmacopoeia). Dosages may have to be related to body weight, in which case heavier patients will need higher dosages than lighter ones. Conversely, if a drug is poorly distributed into body fat a muscular patient may need a higher dosage than a fat patient of the same weight. This applies particularly to digoxin, doses of which should be based on estimated lean body weight.

18.6.4 Characteristics of the disease

Sometimes dosage regimens are different for the same drug in different diseases, because of the nature of the effect required or because of some other aspect of dose-responsiveness. For example, the dosage of bromocriptine required for suppression of lactation is considerably lower than that needed for the relief of symptoms in Parkinson's disease (see the Pharmacopoeia).

18.6.5 Choosing a dosage regimen for the individual patient

While it is true that dosage regimens in clinical practice cannot always be as precise as one would like them in theory to be, it is nevertheless possible to approach the problem of tailoring a dosage regimen for an individual patient in a systematic manner:

1. Look up the dosage regimen recommended in a reliable source of information (see Chapter 20). These have been arrived at through careful study and clinical experience.
2. Consider the dose-related toxicity of the drug, i.e. does it have a low toxic:therapeutic ratio,

the toxic dose being little more than the therapeutic dose? If so (for example digoxin, phenytoin, warfarin, gentamicin, lithium) it will be necessary to be particularly careful not to give too much.

3. Decide on the initial dosage. In general, if there is nothing to guide you to the appropriate dosage from the start, it is best to start with a dose which is at the lower end of the recommended range and to increase it gradually if it appears that a therapeutic effect or the optimal effect has not occurred. For some drugs, this gradual increase in dosage from a small initial dosage is an important strategy in avoiding adverse effects (for example the ACE inhibitors and L-dopa), while for some drugs increasing dosages may be necessary because of tolerance (for example opiate analgesics). However, one needs to be flexible in one's approach to the initial dosage. For example, it may be necessary to start with a loading dose before giving a low maintenance dose (for example warfarin, digoxin), while in a few cases one starts with high dosages and then reduces gradually to a maintenance dosage (for example carbimazole in hyperthyroidism and corticosteroids) .

4. Consider possible pharmacokinetic factors which may alter dosage requirements (for example impaired renal function or drug interactions).

5. Consider the dose–response curve for the patient and whether there are any factors which may alter the pharmacodynamics of the drug. For example, insulin requirements are greater in patients with ketoacidosis and dosages of neuroleptic drugs are lower in previously untreated patients. Drug interactions may alter the pharmacodynamic effects of drugs.

6. Consider other patient characteristics which may influence dosages (for example age and weight).

When one has decided on and instituted one's dosage regimen there may still be room for improvement, and the patient's progress should be monitored carefully (see Chapter 7) for evidence that the treatment regimen is satisfactory (i.e. effective and safe).

18.6.6 Frequency of drug administration

The frequency of drug administration is usually fixed for a given formulation of a given drug and if so there is no need to make a separate decision about that. However, there are sometimes circumstances which lead one to alter the frequency of administration without necessarily altering the total daily dose. The following are examples of this.

1. Although the duration of action of spironolactone is sufficiently long for once-daily administration, some patients complain of gastrointestinal symptoms and benefit from splitting the dose into two parts, one to be taken in the morning and one in the evening.

2. If frusemide produces a satisfactory diuresis then the kidney is refractory to its effects for another six or so hours and the next dose should be withheld for at least that length of time; however, if a first dose has not proved effective then another dose can be given soon after the first.

3. Occasionally the half-time of the drug in the individual may be crucial, as in the case of gentamicin, when doses may have to be given as often as eight-hourly or as infrequently as once every 24 or 36 h; in this case plasma concentration measurements guide one's therapy (see Chapter 7).

4. In cases where symptomatic treatment is being given the frequency of symptoms may regulate the frequency of dosage. For example, patients will take a tablet of glyceryl trinitrate as often as they suffer attacks of angina pectoris, and some patients may need up to 20 or 30 tablets a day.

5. The use of prednisolone in some diseases provides a special case in which the adverse effects of corticosteroids may be diminished by giving twice the usual daily dose but only on alternate days.

6. The use of slow-release formulations to improve compliance and in some cases to reduce adverse effects has already been mentioned in this Chapter and elsewhere. In some cases one may also achieve prolonged action

of a drug overnight by the use of such a formulation (for example slow-release amino-phylline).

18.6.7 Timing of drug administration

The study of the ways in which the pharmacokinetics and pharmacodynamics of drugs vary with time (for example diurnally or seasonally) is called chronopharmacology. Chronopharmacological studies have revealed many such variations, and a few of those are of relevance to the timing of drug therapy. Furthermore, variations with time in the presentation of diseases may affect the timing of drug administration.

In most cases the timing of drug administration is fixed for a given formulation of a given drug, and if so there is no need to make a separate decision about that. However, in some cases timing may be important, as the following examples show.

(a) Minimizing adverse effects

For some drugs adverse effects may be minimized by taking them last thing at night. For example, sleep may mask some of the adverse effects of the tricyclic antidepressants (dry mouth and drowsiness) and of cytotoxic drugs (nausea and vomiting). On the other hand, potent diuretics, such as bumetanide and frusemide, are generally best taken in the morning to avoid the inconvenience of a diuresis later in the day. If one is using corticosteroids as replacement therapy, for example, in Addison's disease, then they should be given in two divided doses during the day, two-thirds in the morning and one-third at night, in order to mimic roughly the normal pattern of endogenous corticosteroid secretion. However, if corticosteroids are to be used for other purposes they are best given as a single dose in the morning, in order to minimize their inhibitory effects on ACTH secretion by the pituitary gland and glucocorticoid secretion by the adrenal glands, which are normally at an ebb overnight.

There is a diurnal variation in the secretion of gastric acid, and it has been found that it is sufficient to give histamine H_2 antagonists, such as cimetidine or ranitidine, only once a day, usually in the evening, in order to maintain remission from peptic ulceration after the initial phase of treatment. This means that gastric acid secretion during the rest of the day is unaffected, and the risk of adverse effects which might occur with prolonged hypochlorhydria is thus reduced.

(b) The timing of symptoms

The occurrence of symptoms often dictates the timing of therapy, as in the treatment of attacks of angina pectoris or in the use of antacids. Although it may be preferable to take non-steroidal anti-inflammatory drugs last thing at night, in order to minimize their adverse effects on the stomach, timing is more often dictated by the timing of symptoms.

(c) Timing in relation to meals

Some drugs are best taken before food (for example most penicillins, whose absorption is delayed by food, and tetracyclines, whose absorption may be impaired by calcium and other salts). Others may be better taken with food (for example aspirin, in order to reduce gastrointestinal adverse effects, and griseofulvin, whose absorption is improved by food).

18.6.8 Nomograms as guides to dosage regimens

A nomogram is a diagram in which the relationship among three or more variables is represented in the form of a number of straight or curved scales, arranged in such a way that the value of one variable corresponding to given values of the others can be read off its scale by drawing straight lines intersecting the other scales at the appropriate values (for an example see Fig. 16.1).

Numerous nomograms have been devised to help decide on dosage regimens of certain drugs (notably digoxin, gentamicin, kanamycin, phenytoin, and theophylline). They have been devised from pharmacokinetic equations using the mean values of variables which have been estimated from studies in patients.

We cannot stress too heavily that while such aids may be useful as guides to the range of dosages likely to be therapeutically effective in an individual patient, or in some cases as an initial guide to dosage adjustments in renal impairment, they should not be depended upon to give accurate predictions. If they are used they should be backed up by appropriate plasma concentration measurement (see Chapter 7).

18.7 For how long should treatment last?

The duration of treatment depends on the nature of the disease or symptoms and to a great extent on collective experience. At one end of the scale a single dose of aspirin may be sufficient to treat a headache, or a single dose of diamorphine sufficient to treat the pain of myocardial infarction. In the latter case further doses may be necessary, but it is not likely that treatment will need to be continued for more than a day. At the other end of the scale chronic therapy for the individual's lifetime is usually required for the treatment of diabetes mellitus, essential hypertension, hypothyroidism, pernicious anaemia, and several other diseases.

Difficulties and controversy often arise in relation to treatments of intermediate duration. For example, in the use of cimetidine, ranitidine, and other histamine (H_2) antagonists in the treatment of peptic ulceration symptoms generally resolve in about a week and healing occurs within about six weeks; however, if treatment is then withheld there is an appreciable rate of recurrence, and it is not clear for how long one should continue treatment thereafter. This is particularly a problem in view of concern about possible long-term adverse effects of the histamine H_2 antagonists. In practice the duration of treatment will depend on factors such as the age of the patient and the severity of the problem. With increasing experience of these drugs over many years the solution to this problem will become clearer.

The duration of treatment of infections with antibiotics varies from infection to infection, and depends on the infecting organism, the site of infection, the response to treatment, and in a few cases the dosage of antibiotic. For example,

streptococcal tonsillitis and pneumococcal pneumonia might require treatment with penicillin for 7–10 d, non-gonococcal urethritis treatment with tetracycline for 10–21 d, and infective endocarditis due to 'viridans' streptococci treatment with intravenous penicillin for up to six weeks. However, in the last case it is not clear what the minimum duration of treatment should be, and it may be that treatment for six weeks is unnecessarily long. In contrast, gentamicin, given in conjunction with penicillin in this infection, is usually continued only for the first 10–14 d. If amoxycillin is used in the treatment of a urinary tract infection two large doses 12 h apart may be sufficient to effect a cure, while treatment for several days may be necessary if conventional doses are used.

Tuberculosis is an example of a disease for which the duration of treatment is complex. Quadruple drug therapy (for example rifampicin, isoniazid, pyrazinamide, and ethambutol) is usually given in the initial phase for eight weeks, or until the organism's sensitivities are known, when a change of drugs may be seen to be necessary. This regimen is used because it takes several weeks to culture the infecting organism and the risk of resistance to therapy is reduced by using several different drugs. Treatment is then continued with three drugs (for example rifampicin, isoniazid, and pyrazinamide) for six months in pulmonary infections or longer in extrapulmonary infections. However, there are many different types of antituberculous regimens in use around the world, taking into account the resistance of *Mycobacteria* to antituberculous drugs, drug costs, patient compliance, and the problems of the delivery of medical care to the population.

As this discussion of the principles underlying drug prescribing will have emphasized, it is not always easy in drug therapy to achieve optimal efficacy while keeping the risks of adverse effects to a minimum. However, thoughtful prescribing along these lines will help one to achieve this aim.

19 How to write a prescription

19.1 Practical prescription writing

There are four common types of prescription.

1. Hospital prescriptions for in-patients.
2. Hospital prescriptions for an 'external' pharmacy.
3. Prescriptions in general practice.
4. Private prescriptions.

In all cases there are certain principles to be followed. A prescription should be a precise, accurate, clear, and readable set of instructions. The instructions should be sufficient for a nurse to administer a drug accurately in hospital, or for a pharmacist to provide a patient with both the correct drug and the instructions on how to take it.

The following information must be given on a prescription:

19.1.1 The date

19.1.2 Identification of the patient

(a) In hospital

Name, initials, and hospital case number. If there are two patients of the same name in the ward this should be clearly stated.

(b) For non-hospital pharmacies

Name, initials, and address. In all cases the age must be given for a child under the age of 12 years. Giving the age of an adult may sometimes be useful (for example if the patient is old) but it is not essential.

19.1.3 The name of the drug

Preferably in capitals. The issue of whether one should use the approved name or a proprietary name is discussed below.

19.1.4 The dose of the drug

The following important points should be noted.

1. Quantities of 1 gram or more should be written in grams. For example write 2 g.
2. Quantities less than 1 gram but more than 1 milligram should be written in milligrams. For example write 100 mg, not 0.1 g.
3. Quantities less than 1 milligram should be written in micrograms or nanograms as appropriate. Do not abbreviate micrograms or nanograms, since this may lead to prescribing errors. For example write 100 micrograms, not 0.1 mg, nor 100 mcg, nor 100 ug, nor 100 µg.
4. If a decimal point cannot be avoided for values less than 1, write a zero before it. For example write 0.5 mL, not .5 mL.
5. Use mL for millilitres.
6. For liquid medicines given orally the dose should be stated as the number of milligrams in either 5 mL or 10 mL, since these are readily measured amounts, and special spoons are given to patients for the measurements. If the dose of a drug is contained in less than 5 mL the pharmacist will dilute the formulation so that the volume to be given will be 5 mL.
7. For some drugs a maximum dose may need to be stated (for example ergotamine in migraine and colchicine in gout). For example: 'Ergotamine 1 mg at onset of attack and repeat every 30 min if necessary. Do not take more than 6 mg in one day or more than 12 mg in one week.'

19.1.5 Frequency of administration

This should be clearly indicated. Accepted abbreviations may be used (see below), although these are becoming less fashionable. For example:

Atenolol 100 mg once daily.
Amoxycillin 250 mg t.d.s.

Generally speaking the simpler the instruction the better. Patients outside of hospital are often unable to follow a rigid six-hourly or eight-hourly regimen and compromises have to be made. Sometimes it is worth telling patients what you mean by 'three times a day'. To most people 'three times a day' would mean 'with or after breakfast, mid-day meal, and evening meal'. Obviously whether or not that is optimal depends on the timing of the meals and the pharmacokinetics of the drug. If it is important that dosage intervals be as near to 6 or 8 h as possible, that should be made clear to the patient.

In hospital the frequency of administration is determined by two factors:

(a) The demands of the treatment

If, for example, you want to give gentamicin eight-hourly, then it must be given eight-hourly, and not as a haphazard three-times-a-day regimen. The times of administration must be clearly stated on the prescription chart, but the times should be chosen for maximum convenience to both the patient and the nursing staff. If intramuscular gentamicin is to be given it may be kinder to the patient to give the night-time dose by intravenous infusion over half an hour instead.

Prescriptions for drugs to be given as required ('p.r.n.') should have exact instructions as to the maximum frequency, for example 'paracetamol tabs 2 p.r.n., not more often than four-hourly'.

(b) The nursing drug round

On most hospital wards some form of drug round is held four-hourly or six-hourly, and treatment should, if possible, be organized to fit in with those times. Remember that a drug round takes time (as much as 1–2 h in some cases) and the actual time at which a patient receives a drug may be different from the notional time of the round.

Every student should take the opportunity of accompanying the nurses on a drug round. To see at first-hand the use of the doctor's prescription, the process of drug administration, the patient's response, and the nurse's problems is very revealing.

19.1.6 Route and method of administration

The route of administration should be clearly indicated (for example oral, sublingual, i.v., i.m., s.c.), unless the route is obvious (for example 'beclomethasone inhaler, 2 puffs four-hourly'). In hospital the method of giving a drug intravenously may need to be indicated separately. For example, one may want to give the contents of a one-dose ampoule as a single undiluted injection, as an infusion in a small volume of saline over a few minutes (for example in an infusion burette), or in a larger volume over a longer period of time. In some cases it may be necessary to indicate the precise rate of flow of a precisely specified solution of drug (for example dopamine).

19.1.7 Amount to be supplied

In hospital the pharmacist will organize this. Many hospitals have a policy to supply drugs sufficient for a predetermined period on discharge, and a prescription written for drugs for the patient to take home after a stay in hospital will generally have to take account of that. In general practice one should indicate the quantities of drugs one wants to be dispensed. This may be done by indicating, for example, the precise number of tablets required, but it is often simpler to indicate the period of treatment. There is a space on the prescription form (see Fig. 19.1) for indicating the duration of treatment.

19.1.8 Instructions for labelling

In the National Health Service a drug container will be labelled with whatever drug name the practitioner uses on the prescription, whether it be an approved name or a proprietary name (see below). The standard prescription sheet used in general practice (the FP10, see Fig. 19.1) contains the instruction 'NP' (*nomen proprium* or 'proper name'). If the prescriber does not want the name of the drug to be written on the label he or she must strike out the letters 'NP'. Generally it is best if the drug name is included on the label, although occasionally an exception may arise. Drugs given by private prescription need to be labelled 'NP' by the prescriber if he or she wants the name of the drug to be included on the label. Drugs prescribed by a hospital pharmacy will generally be labelled with the name of the drug, unless specific instructions are given otherwise, but local practices may vary.

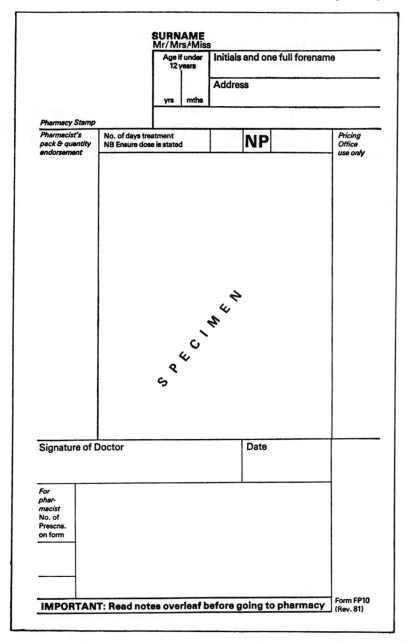

SURNAME
Mr/Mrs/Miss

Age if under 12 years	Initials and one full forename
	Address
yrs	mths

Pharmacy Stamp

| *Pharmacist's pack & quantity endorsement* | No. of days treatment NB Ensure dose is stated | **NP** | *Pricing Office use only* |

S P E C I M E N

| Signature of Doctor | Date |

| *For pharmacist No. of Prescns. on form* | |

IMPORTANT: Read notes overleaf before going to pharmacy | Form FP10 (Rev. 81)

■ **Fig. 19.1** The FP10, the prescription form used in the UK by general practitioners. (Reproduced with the permission of the Controller of her Majesty's Stationery Office. Crown Copyright.)

19.1.9 The prescriber's signature

The prescription must be signed by the prescriber, must contain some indication of the prescriber's qualifications, and should show his or her address. Then if there are any queries the pharmacist can contact the prescriber. Private prescriptions are best written on the prescriber's personal headed notepaper or on a specially printed form, in order to avoid doubts about authenticity.

19.2 Proprietary names versus approved names

A drug may be called by one of several different kinds of name.

1. Its chemical name, whose form generally follows the rules issued by the International Union of Pure and Applied Chemistry (IUPAC).
2. Its approved (official or generic) name. This is usually the International Nonproprietary Name, recommended or proposed by the World Health Organization (WHO), but may be some locally approved name (for example British Approved Name or United States Adopted Name).
3. Its proprietary name (brand-name or trade-name), given to it by a pharmaceutical manufacturer.

Take the following example:

chemical name: 6-[[amino(4-hydroxyphenyl)
acetyl]-amino]-3,3-dimethyl-7-oxo-4-thia-1-
azabicyclo[3.2.0]heptane-2-carboxylic acid;
approved name: amoxycillin;
proprietary names: Almodan®, Amoxil®.

Since the chemical name is often, as in this case, unsuitable for routine prescribing, one has to use either the approved name or the proprietary name. Which should one choose? For some drugs the question is somewhat academic, since only one proprietary formulation exists. When a pharmaceutical firm produces a unique drug their brand, which carries their proprietary registered name (trademark), is the only one available (for example enalapril currently is available only as Innovace®). However, sometimes, on the basis of a commercial agreement, a new drug might be marketed by two different firms, for example in two different countries, with two different proprietary names. Examples of this kind of marketing include Bactrim® and Septrin® (both co-trimoxazole), Norpace® and Rythmodan® (both disopyramide), and Carace® and Zestril® (both lisinopril).

Note that these are examples of drugs which were marketed under different proprietary names by different companies before the original patents on the compounds had expired. However, several proprietary formulations of the same chemical entity may become available when the patent expires on a drug with a previously unique proprietary name. For instance, diazepam (approved name) was first marketed as Valium® (proprietary name). When the patent on diazepam expired the number of proprietary brands of diazepam multiplied. Oral formulations currently available include Alupram®, Atensine®, Solis®, Tensium®, and Valium®. When this happens prescribing and dispensing problems may arise. For example, whether the prescriber writes 'enalapril BP' or 'Innovace' the patient will receive Innovace®. However, if the prescriber writes 'diazepam BP' the pharmacist may dispense any formulation of diazepam he or she chooses, provided that the formulation conforms to the description laid out in the BP (British Pharmacopoeia, see Chapter 20). Thus, he or she might dispense Valium®, or Atensine®, or any of the other formulations mentioned above. However, if the prescriber writes 'caps diazepam' the pharmacist may prescribe only Solis® or Valium®, since the other formulations are not available as capsules. Generally the dispenser will dispense the cheapest acceptable formulation available.

By writing the proprietary name the prescriber can ensure that a particular formulation of a drug is prescribed. However, in hospitals in the UK it is frequently the case that the hospital pharmacy stocks only one formulation, and even if the hospital doctor writes 'Valium' on an in-patient prescription chart the pharmacist may dispense Atensine®, or some other approved formulation of diazepam. For this reason it is generally better in hospital to prescribe drugs by their generic names.

There are certain advantages and disadvantages to the prescribing of drugs by their generic as opposed to their proprietary names.

19.2.1 Advantages of prescribing by approved name

(a) Awareness of one's prescription
Consider the list of proprietary names in the left-hand column of Table 19.1. This list of proprietary names was actually typed on the formal

∎ **Table 19.1** Proprietary and aproved names of the drugs listed on the referral letter illustrated in Fig. 19.2

Proprietary name	Approved name(s)
Maxolon®	Metoclopramide monohydrochloride
Largactil®	Chlorpromazine hydrochloride
Stemetil®	Prochlorperazine maleate
Triptafen Minor®	Perphenazine + amitriptyline hydrochloride
Merital®	Nomifensine hydrogen maleate
Valium®	Diazepam
Halcion®	Triazolam
Tegretol®	Carbamazepine
Epilim®	Sodium valproate
Stugeron®	Cinnarizine
Norgesic®	Orphenadrine citrate + paracetamol
Solpadeine®	Paracetamol + codeine phosphate + caffeine
Dolobid®	Diflunisal
Zomax®	Zomepirac
Ipral®	Trimethoprim
Co-Fram®	Trimethoprim + sulphamoxole

referral letter that a patient brought into hospital (reproduced in Fig. 19.2). It is hard to imagine that the practitioner who prepared that referral letter really knew what the drugs were that the prescribed formulations contained, since no-one who did know would have prescribed two formulations containing trimethoprim, two containing paracetamol, two containing different benzodiazepines, and three containing different phenothiazines. There is a danger that in prescribing by proprietary name the nature of the drugs being prescribed will be forgotten.

(b) Drug stocks

If one prescribes say 'Almodan' rather than 'amoxycillin', and the pharmacist who is to dispense the prescription stocks only Amoxil®, he or she cannot legally dispense the prescription without first consulting the doctor. Clearly this can cause inconvenience to all concerned and might result in delayed treatment.

(c) Expense

It will generally be cheaper to prescribe by the approved name, since the pharmacist will dispense the cheapest variant held in stock. The actual cash saving will vary widely from drug to drug. That is because firstly many drugs are still available in only one manufacturer's formulation and no saving will be made by prescribing by approved name, and secondly because competition between manufacturers often means that the difference between the cheapest and dearest brands may not be large. However, it has been estimated that prescribing the cheapest formulations of all available drugs could be about 5 per cent cheaper than prescribing the dearest. In an annual budget of, say, £3000 million that would represent a saving of £150 million.

19.2.2 Advantages of prescribing by proprietary name

(a) Remembering names

Proprietary names are chosen by pharmaceutical companies because they are catchy, usually easier to remember than the corresponding generic name, and shorter and easier to spell (compare, for example, 'Librium'® with 'chlordiazepoxide'). Furthermore, a single proprietary name will do when the formulation may in fact contain two or more drugs (compare, for example, 'Fefol' with 'ferrous sulphate and folic acid'). However, in recent years there has been a move to counteract this problem, by giving single approved names to some common combinations of drugs. For example, the combination of paracetamol with dextropropoxyphene is now known as co-proxamol. The common feature of these combination terms is that they begin with the syllable 'co-'. A list of some of these is given in Table 19.2.

(b) Quality of product

For some drugs a change in tablet excipients may have important effects on the absorption of the drug from the formulation. This has been demonstrated for drugs such as digoxin and phenytoin, and is an argument for prescribing such drugs by the same proprietary name every time for the same patient, so that variations in formulation do not lead to variations in systemically available dose. This is certainly important for formulations of lithium salts and theophylline, which should always be prescribed by brand name (see p. 73).

INDICATION OF DRUG TREATMENT FROM GENERAL PRACTITIONERS

Please take this form to your General Practitioner *before* coming into hospital so that he may fill in the relevant details below.

PLEASE BRING TO HOSPITAL WITH YOU

Doctor,

Could you please list the drugs etc., if any, that this patient is taking:

Zomax, Valium, Stemetil, Merital 50mg, Norgesic,
....

Solpadeine, Maxolon, Ipral, Dolobid, Triptafen Minor,

PLEASE PRINT ....

Epilim, Halcion, Tegretol, Stugeron, Co Fram, Largactil
....

Has patient been on *STEROIDS* during the past 2 years?

Yes ....

No   NO
....

Has this patient any known *ALLERGIES* (Drug or otherwise)?

   NO
....

If patient is taking one of the tranquillisers containing a *MONO-AMINE OXIDASE INHIBITOR* then he/she should be off these drugs for two weeks prior to surgery. If necessary, could you please notify the Waiting List Clerk so that the patient's admission may be delayed.

■ **Fig. 19.2** Part of a letter which a patient brought into hospital after being referred for acute admission. The drugs named in the letter are listed in Table 19.1 in both brand-name and generic-name forms.

(c) Continuity of treatment

Patients not infrequently become confused if the drug they are being given changes its form with every prescription. Continuity can be achieved by prescribing the same proprietary formulation every time.

19.2.3 Proprietary or approved name?

It is clear that there is no simple answer to the question 'Should I prescribe by approved name or proprietary name?' In hospital it is usually better to prescribe by approved name, since the pharmacy will dispense whatever formulation is held in stock. The proprietary name may be used when a combination product is prescribed for which no single approved name exists (for example 'Burinex-K'). In general practice we would recommend prescribing by approved name also, although we recognize that many practitioners will find it easier to prescribe by proprietary name and in some cases (for example lithium

salts and theophylline) we would recommend it. However, if a doctor makes the effort to prescribe where possible by approved name, particularly from the start of his or her career, he or she will generally find it just as easy as prescribing by proprietary name. Currently in the UK about 41 per cent of prescriptions for drugs in the community are by approved name.

19.3 Prescribing controlled drugs

Because of the problem of drug addiction and misuse of drugs, drugs likely to be abused are the subject, in the UK, of the Misuse of Drugs Act (1971), the Misuse of Drugs (Notification of and Supply to Addicts) Regulations (1973), and the Misuse of Drugs Regulations, which are updated from time to time, the latest version being that of 1985.

The Misuse of Drugs Act divides drugs into three classes.

▮ **Table 19.2** Approved names for some common drug combinations

Approved name	Combination
Co-amilofruse	Amiloride + frusemide
Co-amilozide	Amiloride + hydrochlorothiazide
Co-amoxiclav	Amoxycillin + clavulanic acid
Co-beneldopa	Benserazide + L-dopa
Co-careldopa	Carbidopa + L-dopa
Co-codamol	Codeine phosphate + paracetamol
Co-codaprin	Codeine phosphate + aspirin
Co-danthramer	Danthron + poloxamer '188'
Co-danthrusate	Danthron + docusate
Co-dergocrine	Dihydroergocornine mesylate + dihydroergocristine mesylate + α- and β-dihydroergocryptine mesylates
Co-dydramol	Dihydrocodeine tartrate + paracetamol
Co-fluampicil	Flucloxacillin + ampicillin
Co-flumactone	Hydroflumethiazide + spironolactone
Co-phenotrope	Diphenoxylate + atropine
Co-prenozide	Oxprenolol + cyclopenthiazide
Co-proxamol	Dextropropoxyphene + paracetamol
Co-simalcite	Activated dimethicone + hydrotalcite
Co-tenidone	Atenolol + chlorthalidone
Co-trimoxazole	Trimethoprim + sulphamethoxazole

1. Class A includes alfentanil, cocaine, dextromoramide, diamorphine (heroin), dipipanone, LSD, methadone, morphine, opium, pethidine, and phencyclidine. It also includes the compounds in Class B when they are formulated for intravenous injection.

2. Class B includes oral amphetamines, barbiturates, cannabis, codeine, ethylmorphine, glutethimide, pentazocine, phenmetrazine, and pholcodine.

3. Class C includes certain drugs related to the amphetamines, such as benzphetamine and chlorphentermine, most benzodiazepines, buprenorphine, diethylpropion, mazindol, meprobamate, pemoline, and pipradrol.

The Misuse of Drugs Regulations define five schedules of person who are authorized to supply and possess controlled drugs.

1. Schedule 1 includes cannabis and LSD, possession and supply of which requires the authorization of the Home Office.

2. Schedule 2 includes amphetamine, cocaine, diamorphine, glutethimide, morphine, pethidine, and quinalbarbitone. These are subject to the full restrictions on controlled drugs laid down in the Act.

3. Schedule 3 includes most barbiturates, buprenorphine, diethylpropion, mazindol, meprobamate, pentazocine, and phentermine. These are subject to the special prescription requirements of the Act, but not to the other restrictions.

4. Schedule 4 includes benzodiazepines and pemoline, over which minimal control is exerted.

5. Schedule 5 is a list of drugs which are exempted from the requirements of the Act, apart from the need to keep invoices for 2 years.

Under the Misuse of Drugs (Notification of and Supply to Addicts) Regulations (1973), practitioners in the UK have an obligation to notify drug addicts to the Home Office within seven days of the patient's attendance and annually thereafter. The Home Office maintains an Index of Addicts, which may be consulted in confidence by doctors.

The drugs which are specified in the 1973 Regulations in defining addicts include cocaine, dextromoramide, diamorphine, dipipanone, hydrocodone, hydromorphone, levorphanol, methadone, morphine, opium, oxycodone, pethidine, and phenazocine.

Only medical practitioners who hold a special licence may prescribe diamorphine, dipipanone, or cocaine for addicts. Other practitioners must refer addicts to a treatment centre. All general practitioners may prescribe diamorphine, dipipanone, and cocaine for the treatment of pain and organic disease (even in addicts).

All practitioners have a responsibility to try to curb drug dependence by careful and thoughtful prescribing, and by avoiding being duped by addicts skilled in wheedling drugs out of doctors.

Prescriptions for controlled drugs must:

(1) be completely written in the prescriber's handwriting in ink;

(2) be signed and dated;

(3) carry the prescriber's address;

(4) carry the name and address of the patient;

(5) state the form of the drug;

(6) state the total quantity of the drug or the number of dose units to be dispensed in both words and figures;

(7) state the exact size of each dose in both words and figures.

If these rules are not followed the pharmacist will not dispense the prescription. For other information see the British National Formulary.

19.4 Abbreviations

Some abbreviations are used in prescribing and one should be familiar with them. Those which are commonly used and are acceptable are listed in Table 19.3, although they are becoming less fashionable in favour of plain English. Other abbreviations, more obscure, should be avoided and instructions should be written in plain English.

∎ **Table 19.3** Abbreviations commonly used in prescribing

Abbreviation	Latin meaning	English translation
b.d. or b.i.d.	*bis in die*	twice a day
gutt.	*guttae*	drops
i.m.	–	intramuscular(ly)
i.v.	–	intravenous(ly)
NP	*nomen proprium*	the proper name
o.d.	*omni die*	(once) every day
o.m.	*omni mane**	(once) every morning
o.n.	*omni nocte**	(once) every night
p.o.	*per os*	by mouth
PR	*per rectum*	by the anal route
p.r.n.	*pro re nata*	whenever required
PV	*per vaginam*	by the vaginal route
q.d.s.	*quater die sumendum†*	four times a day
s.c.	–	subcutaneous(ly)
stat.	*statim*	immediately
t.d.s.	*ter die sumendum†*	three times a day

*Sometimes written simply as *mane* or *nocte*.
†The abbreviations t.i.d. or q.i.d. (*ter* or *quater in die*) are sometimes used instead.

20 Sources of information on drugs

There are several different types of sources of information on the different aspects of clinical pharmacology and therapeutics:

(1) textbooks;
(2) monographs;
(3) review articles in journals;
(4) manufacturers' literature (see Chapter 15);
(5) original scientific papers;
(6) computerized databases.

It is as well to become familiar with a handful of reference texts in which you will be able to find information for most problems (see the bibliography below), going only to the more detailed texts when studying a particular topic in greater depth. In addition you may be able to find out information about drugs from your local community pharmacy, from your hospital pharmacy, from your Regional Drug Information service (see the *British National Formulary* (Joint Formulary Committee) for telephone numbers), or from your University's Department of Clinical Pharmacology. The medical information departments of pharmaceutical companies may also sometimes be useful sources of information, although some pieces of information will be confidential.

20.1 Pharmaceutical information

For general pharmaceutical information the *Pharmaceutical Handbook* (edited by R.G. Todd) is useful, although it is now somewhat out of date.

The *British Pharmacopoeia* and the *Pharmaceutical Codex* contain information about the pharmaceutical requirements for formulations in the UK, and there are comparable publications in other countries (for example the *US Pharmacopoeia and National Formulary*).

The *British National Formulary* (Joint Formulary Committee) contains comprehensive lists of the different drug formulations available, as does *Martindale's Extra Pharmacopoeia* (edited by Reynolds).

20.2 Pharmacokinetics

20.2.1 General principles

There are several texts of varying degrees of inscrutability in which the principles of pharmacokinetics are outlined. The shortest introduction to the subject is *An Introduction to Pharmacokinetics* by Clark and Smith, but for those who want a more comprehensive introductory text *Clinical Pharmacokinetics. Concepts and Applications* by Rowland and Tozer may be preferred. *Pharmacokinetics* by Gibaldi and Perrier and *Fundamentals of Clinical Pharmacokinetics* by J.G. Wagner are useful for those who are conversant with the basic principles and want to explore further. *Basic Clinical Pharmacokinetics* by Winter shows how the principles of pharmacokinetics may be applied to clinical problems. Drug metabolism is discussed in detail in *Introduction to Drug Metabolism* by Gibson and Shett. *Variability in Human Drug Response* by Smith and Rawlins contains highly readable introductory accounts of the various aspects of clinical pharmacokinetics.

20.2.2 Specific pharmacokinetic information

We have given only a limited amount of pharmacokinetic information on specific drugs in the Pharmacopoeia and in the tables in Chapter 3. More detailed information on individual drugs is to be found in the *Handbook of Clinical Pharmacology* by Bochner *et al.*, in *Therapeutic Drugs* edited by Sir Colin Dollery, and in the lists published in *Drug Treatment* edited by G.S. Avery and in *Goodman and Gilman's The Pharmacological Basis of Therapeutics* edited by Gilman *et al.* The monthly journals *Clinical Pharmacokinetics* and *Drugs* publish long review articles about specific drugs. They contain much useful and readily accessible information and extensive lists of references.

20.3 Pharmacological effects of drugs

The standard texts on basic pharmacology are *Goodman and Gilman's The Pharmacological Basis of Therapeutics* edited by Gilman *et al.* and the *Textbook of Pharmacology* by Bowman and Rand. These texts also contain a large selection of primary and secondary source references. The review journal *Drugs* is also informative. A general discussion of relevant pharmacological principles is contained in *Goldstein's Principles of Drug Action for Physicians and Medical Students* by Goldstein, Aronow, and Kalman.

20.4 Therapeutics

There are few texts devoted solely to therapeutics, and large textbooks of medicine and medical monographs tend to concentrate more on other aspects of disease. The following are devoted mainly to therapeutics: *Conn's Current Therapy* edited by R.E. Rakel; *Drug Treatment* edited by G.S. Avery; *Emergencies in Clinical Medicine* edited by H.J. Kennedy.

Self-poisoning is dealt with as a separate subject in several monographs, of which the following may be found useful: *Diagnosis and Management of Acute Poisoning* by A.T. Proudfoot and *A Concise Guide to the Management of Poisoning* edited by Vale and Meredith. For immediate information on individual drugs contact your nearest poisons information service (see the *British National Formulary*). In some places computerized poisons information may be available by Viewdata (see below).

20.5 Pharmacogenetics

There are few monographs on pharmacogenetics and they are not widely available. The chapter in *Goldstein's Principles of Drug Action for Physicians and Medical Students* by Goldstein, Aronow, and Kalman is useful. *Pharmacogenetics. Principles and Paediatric Aspects* by I. Szorady and *Pharmacogenetics, Heredity and the Response to Drugs* by W. Kalow are good but out of date. *Geigy Scientific Tables* (ed. Lentner) contains a short helpful section.

20.6 Adverse effects of drugs

The most useful sources of information about adverse effects of specific drugs are the various editions of *Meyler's Side Effects of Drugs* and its companion annual update volumes (all edited by M.N.G. Dukes and others). *Martindale's Extra Pharmacopoeia* (also available on CD ROM) is also useful.

Adverse drug effects are also discussed in terms of the ways in which organ systems may be affected in the *Textbook of Adverse Drug Reactions* edited by D.M. Davies and *Iatrogenic Diseases* by D'Arcy and Griffin.

Mechanisms of adverse effects of drugs are discussed in *Goodman and Gilman's The Pharmacological Basis of Therapeutics* edited by Gilman *et al.* The weekly journal *Reactions* publishes vignettes, short reviews, and abstracts of case reports, giving up-to-date information on adverse drug reactions.

20.7 Drug interactions

Comprehensive listings of drug interactions are to be found in *Drug Interactions* by P.D. Hansten and *Drug Interactions* by I. Stockley.

20.8 Clinical trials

Clinical Trials edited by Johnson and Johnson, *Clinical Trials, A Practical Approach* by

S.J. Pocock, and *The Principles and Practice of Clinical Trials* edited by C.S. Good, deal with the subject in different ways. For statistical discussions see the texts by Bradford Hill, Armitage, and Gore and Altman (see the Bibliography).

20.9 Patient compliance

The monograph on compliance edited by Sackett and Haynes, *Compliance with Therapeutic Regimens*, is very informative. Other information must largely be gleaned from primary sources.

20.10 Prescribing information

Notes on writing prescriptions are to be found in the *British National Formulary* (Joint Formulary Committee).

Information about the different available formulations of drugs, proprietary or otherwise, is to be found in the *British National Formulary* (Joint Formulary Committee), *MIMS* (the Monthly Index of Medical Specialties), the *Data Sheet Compendium* compiled by the Association of British Pharmaceutical Industries, and the *Physician's Desk Reference* compiled by the Medical Economics Company Inc.

All of these texts are described in the Bibliography which follows, along with some additional texts to which we have not alluded.

20.11 Computerized databases

Several types of computerized databases are available. These include Viewdata Service, CD ROM, and on-line services. Specialists may also use other types of computerized databases.

20.11.1 Viewdata services

Viewdata services such as VADIS®, TOXBASE®, and TRAVAX® are available to users (for example libraries, drug information centres) on subscription. They are accessed via a telephone line to a centralized computer, and the information is displayed on the user's VDU.

VADIS® gives up-to-date information on drugs, synthesizing information from standard texts, such as the *British National Formulary* and *Martindale's Extra Pharmacopoeia*, supplemented by information from specialist texts and other sources.

TOXBASE® gives information on drug toxicity and the management of poisoning, and TRAVAX® gives information on immunizations and malaria prophylaxis for travel abroad.

20.11.2 CD ROM

Information on CD ROM is purchased on a subscription basis and is supplied on compact discs, which are read by the user on conventional equipment.

Information systems which are available in this way include Medline® (computerized *Index Medicus*), *Martindale's Extra Pharmacopoeia*, and the *American Hospital Formulary System* (available on the software known as Compact Cambridge®).

20.11.3 On-line information

On-line information is available to subscribers via telephone and modem attached to their own VDU. Available host systems include Datastar® and Maxwell On-line®. The information available includes *Index Medicus*, *Excerpta Medica*, *Chemistry Abstracts*, *Pharmline*, and many others.

20.12 Drug information services

Many Regional and District Health Authorities in the UK have set up their own drug information services, staffed by pharmacists. Drug information pharmacists are responsible for collecting, collating, and disseminating information about all aspects of drug use, often in collaboration with an academic Department of Clinical Pharmacology. They may be consulted by any doctor, nurse, or other member of the health care team about any drug-related problem.

20.13 Bibliography

In this annotated bibliography we have listed some textual sources of information which may be useful either for reference or for general reading.

Adverse Drug Reaction Bulletin. Adverse Drug Reaction Research Unit, Co. Durham. Published bimonthly. Contains review articles on various different aspects of adverse drug reactions. Clear, concise; well referenced.

Armitage, P. (1971). *Statistical methods in medical research*. Blackwell Scientific Publications, Oxford. Good introductory textbook, but does not deal specifically with clinical trials. Easy to read, but has a lot of mathematics (cf. Bradford Hill).

Association of British Pharmaceutical Industries. *Data sheet compendium*. Datapharm Publications, London. Published annually. Voluntary compilation of the data sheets of the pharmaceutical companies which are members of the Association, as issued by individual companies in compliance with legal requirements for drug marketing. Listed as individual drugs under the name of each manufacturer. Each describes the formulations available, the drug's licensed indications for use, notes on dosages and administration, adverse effects, precautions and contra-indications, treatment of overdosage, and interactions, and adds a little pharmaceutical information (for example special storage instructions). Two indexes: one of proprietary names the other of approved names with corresponding proprietary names.

Avery, G.S. (ed.) (1987). *Drug treatment* (3rd edn). Adis Press, Sydney; Churchill Livingstone, Edinburgh and London. Introductory chapters on basic clinical pharmacology followed by chapters on the therapeutics of disease discussed by system. Appendices contain numerous tables listing physicochemical and pharmacokinetic properties of drugs, adverse reactions, interactions, details of antibacterial drugs, and dosages in renal and hepatic disease.

Bland, M. (1987). *An introduction to medical statistics*. Oxford University Press, Oxford. Good introductory text on statistics with clear examples and relatively little mathematics.

Bochner, F., Carruthers, G., Kampmann, J., and Steiner, J. (1983). *Handbook of clinical pharmacology* (2nd edn). Little, Brown, Boston. Monographs on individual drugs or groups of closely related drugs (for example penicillins) containing notes on mode of action, pharmacokinetic properties, dosages, therapeutic concentrations, adverse reactions, and interactions. Well referenced. Abbreviated introductory chapters on some aspects of basic clinical pharmacology.

Bowman, W.C. and Rand, M.J. (1980). *Textbook of pharmacology* (2nd edn). Blackwell Scientific Publications, Oxford. Excellent reference text covering the basic pharmacology of drugs mostly by organ systems (for example the blood, the heart) but in some cases by indication (for example pain, anaesthesia, hypnotics, and sedatives). Six introductory chapters deal with some relevant matters of anatomy, physiology, and biochemistry. The last five chapters deal with the principles of drug action, pharmacokinetics, relevant statistics, 'social' pharmacology, and diet.

Bradford Hill, A. (1985). *Short textbook of medical statistics* (2nd edn). Hodder, London. Good introductory text, well oriented towards specific problems (for example chapters on clinical trials, problems of sampling, collection of statistics). Relatively little mathematics.

British Pharmacopoeia (1988; 2 volumes) and *Addenda* (1989, 1990, 1991). HMSO, London. Monographs on individual therapeutic agents giving (Vol. 1) structural formulae, chemical properties, preparations, notes on storage, assay techniques, and (Vol. 2) descriptions of individual formulations describing identification, strengths available, and details of requirements for dissolution rates and uniformity of content where necessary.

British Pharmacopoeia Commission (1990). *British approved names* and *Supplements* 1, 2, and 3. Department of Health via HMSO, London. Lists approved names alphabetically, giving corresponding chemical names, proprietary names, and a note on the actions and uses.

Budavari, S. (ed) (1989). *The Merck index* (11th edn). Merck B Co. Inc., Rahway, N.J. Comprehensive list of chemical substances. Includes structures, chemical information, a few references (usually on synthesis but sometimes on uses etc), and occasionally other information (for example LD_{50}, pharmaceutical incompatibilities). Useful appendices, containing miscellaneous tables and other information.

Clark, B. and Smith, D.A. (1986). *An introduction to pharmacokinetics* (2nd edn). Blackwell Scientific Publications, Oxford. A simple introduction to pharmacokinetics without excessive emphasis on mathematics; but you would still have to follow the mathematics to understand it thoroughly. Contains practical examples.

Clinical Pharmacokinetics. Adis Press, Australia. Published bimonthly. Journal containing detailed review articles on all aspects of the pharmacokinetics of drugs relevant to clinical practice. Well referenced.

Dale, J.R. and Appelbe, G.E. (1989). *Pharmacy, law and ethics* (4th edn). The Pharmaceutical Press, London. Deals with most legal aspects of drugs. Mainly intended for pharmacists but has much information of interest to doctors.

D'Arcy, P.F. and Griffin, J.P. (1986). *Iatrogenic diseases* (3rd edn). Oxford University Press, Oxford. Introductory chapters on interactions and on the monitoring and epidemiology of adverse reactions, followed by chapters in which adverse reactions in body systems (for example blood dyscrasias) are discussed in relation to the drugs which may cause them. Well referenced. Two appendices contain lists of interactions and matching of approved with proprietary names.

Davies, D.M. (ed.) (1991). *Textbook of adverse drug reactions* (4th edn). Oxford University Press, Oxford. Adverse drug reactions classified by organ systems. Introductory chapters deal with history, epidemiology, pathogenesis, detection, and investigation. The final chapter covers medicolegal aspects, and there are four useful appendices (for example 'Effect of drugs on laboratory tests').

Dollery, Sir Colin (ed.) (1991). *Therapeutic drugs*. Churchill Livingstone, Edinburgh. A comprehensive collection of monographs on most therapeutic drugs, organized in the same way as the monographs in the Pharmacopoeia of this book, with additional material on the results of clinical trials. Well referenced.

Drug and Therapeutics Bulletin. Consumers' Association, London. Published fortnightly. Contains reviews of new drugs or treatment procedures, providing advice on the value of such therapies, generally in comparison with other available therapies. Clear and concise, with primary references.

Drugs. Adis Press, Australia. Published monthly. Journal containing detailed review articles on the pharmacology and clinical pharmacology of drugs. Includes information on basic pharmacology, pharmacokinetics, therapeutic trials, adverse effects, interactions, dosages and administration, and assessments of the value of the drugs in clinical practice. Also contains other more specific reviews.

Dukes, M.N.G. (ed.) (1980, 1983, 1988). *Meyler's side effects of drugs* (Vols 9, 10, 11). Excerpta Medica, Amsterdam. Adverse reactions to drugs discussed under the headings of the individual drugs or groups of drugs, arranged in chapters according to class of drug. The earlier volumes sometimes contain information not included in later volumes, whose format is slightly different. Good indexes with separate listings for drugs and diseases. Vol 12 is due to be published in 1992.

Dukes, M.N.G. *et al.* (eds) *Meyler's side effects of drugs annuals*. Excerpta Medica, Amsterdam. Published annually since 1977. Companion volumes to *Meyler's side effects of drugs* (ed. Dukes), using the same format, but mostly covering only reports published during the relevant year. A special feature is the 'reviews', in which specific topics are reviewed carefully and distinguished from the rest of the text typographically.

Gibaldi, M. and Perrier, D. (1982). *Pharmacokinetics* (2nd edn). Marcel Dekker, New York. An excellent text on the mathematics of pharmacokinetics, although it probably contains too much mathematics to be used as an introduction to the subject, much of the text can be read for the purpose of learning principles without needing attention to the mathematics.

Gibson, G.G. and Skett, P. (1986) *Introduction to drug metabolism*. Chapman and Hall, London and New York. Very good introduction to all aspects of drug metabolism. Well referenced.

Gilman, A.G., Rall, T.W., Nies, A.S., and Taylor, P. (1990) *Goodman and Gilman's The pharmacological basis of therapeutics* (8th edn). Macmillan, New York. Comprehensive account of basic pharmacology as relevant to therapeutics, arranged by groups of drugs. Useful appendices on prescribing, pharmacokinetic data of individual drugs, and interactions. Very well referenced with both primary and secondary sources.

Goldstein, A., Aronow, L., and Kalman, S.M. (1988). *Goldstein's Principles of drug action for physicians and medical students*. John Wiley, New York. Broad-ranging text on numerous aspects of both basic and clinical pharmacology, including molecular aspects of drug action (mostly about drug–receptor interactions), descriptive pharmacokinetics, drug toxicity in its various aspects, pharmacogenetics, and drug development and evaluation.

Good, C.S. (ed.) (1976). *The principles and practice of clinical trials*. Churchill Livingstone, Edinburgh. Proceedings of a symposium covering the setting up, running, and evaluation of clinical trials. Well illustrated with examples throughout, with references.

Gore, S.M. and Altman, D.G. (1982). *Statistics in practice*. British Medical Association. A compilation of articles originally published in the *British Medical Journal*. Deals in a readable introductory way with a variety of aspects of statistics in clinical practice, particularly in relation to clinical trials. Well referenced.

Gross, F.H. and Inman, W.H.W. (eds) (1977). *Drug monitoring*. Academic Press, London. Proceedings of a symposium on methods of monitoring for adverse drug reactions. Covers virtually every aspect, with references to primary sources.

Hansten, P.D. (1989). *Drug interactions* (6th edn; annual updates.). Lea and Febiger, Philadelphia. Drug interactions listed by class of drug (for example antiarrhythmics, oral anticoagulants). Within classes subdivided according to whether the effect of the object drug is increased or decreased. The clinical significance of the interactions is both shown typographically and discussed. Management is also mentioned. Also contains detailed lists of drug effects on laboratory tests.

Hay, C.E. and Pearce, M.E. (1984). *Medicines and poisons guide* (4th edn). The Pharmaceutical Press, London. Legal classification of medicinal products and non-medicinal poisons. Includes sections on prescriptions, dispensing, and labelling. Comprehensive lists of medicines for human and veterinary use and on non-medicinal poisons for retail use or supply.

Johnson, F.N. and Johnson, S. (eds) (1977). *Clinical trials*. Blackwell Scientific Publications, Oxford. Clear, comprehensive descriptions of most aspects of clinical trials, including Phase I and Phase II trials during drug development, organization of trials, statistical analysis, interpretation, and ethics.

Joint Formulary Committee. *British National Formulary*. British Medical Association and The Pharmaceutical Society of Great Britain, London. Published about every 6 months since 1981. Excellent guide to currently available formulations, with notes on dosages, uses, adverse effects, and interactions. Appendices include lists of interactions and intravenous additives. Introductory chapters on prescribing, especially in renal failure, in liver disease, in pregnancy, and during breast-feeding.

Kalow, W. (1962). *Pharmacogenetics, heredity and the response to drugs*. W.B. Saunders, Philadelphia. Thorough, well-referenced, but out-of-date review covering pharmacokinetic and pharmacodynamic types of genetic variability, and the effects of race, in addition to drug resistance in bacteria and insects.

Kennedy, H.J. (ed.) (1985). *Emergencies in clinical medicine*. Blackwell Scientific Publications, Oxford. Well-written straightforward accounts of the management of common acute medical emergencies (for example cardiac arrest, acute respiratory failure, status epilepticus, upper gastrointestinal haemorrhage, and poisoning). Well referenced.

Lentner, C. (ed.) (1981 onward; several volumes). *Geigy scientific tables*. Ciba–Geigy Ltd, Basle. Invaluable sets of tables for most branches of medical science. Includes mathematical and statistical tables and tables of chemical and biochemical data. Also has a large section on descriptive statistics useful for reference.

MIMS (*Monthly Index of Medical Specialities*). Medical Publications, London. Published monthly. Lists proprietary formulations by the proprietary names arranged alphabetically with class headings. Gives names of manufacturers, approved name(s) of the drug(s) contained in the formulations, types of formulation available, costs, doses, indications, contra-indications, and special precautions. Each month's issue contains a list of newly issued formulations with a little extra pharmacological information. *MIMS* is sent free to all general practitioners and to a few other selected doctors in the UK.

Notari, R.E. (1986). *Biopharmaceutics and pharmacokinetics. An introduction* (4th edn). Marcel Dekker, New York. A step-by-step account of pharmacokinetics. A lot of algebra and good sample problems. Mainly aimed at pharmacists.

The Pharmaceutical Codex (1979). (11th edn). The Pharmaceutical Press, London. Monographs on specific therapeutic agents and diseases, arranged alphabetically. The drug monographs include the following information to a greater or lesser extent: chemical characteristics, means of identification, available formulations, pharmacokinetic characteristics, adverse effects, contra-indications and precautions, interactions, and uses. Has references for further reading. A new edition is expected in a year or two.

Physician's Desk Reference. Edward R Barnhart for the Medical Economics Company Inc. Oradell, NJ. Published annually. The US equivalent of the *British National Formulary* and the *Data Sheet Compendium* in one volume, but the product information sheets contain more information than their UK equivalents.

Pocock, S.J. (1983) *Clinical trials, a practical approach*. John Wiley, Chichester. A comprehensive introduction to the design, performance, and analysis of clinical trials, with a short bibliography.

Prescribers' Journal. HMSO, London. Published monthly. Short clear articles on the treatment of disease, the adverse effects of drugs, drug interactions, and other topics relevant to drug therapy. Sent free to all prescribing doctors in the UK.

Proudfoot, A.T. (1982). *Diagnosis and management of acute poisoning*. Blackwell Scientific Publications, Oxford. Clearly written text with introductory chapters on the classification, diagnosis, and general plan for management of acute poisoning, followed by monographs on individual drugs.

Rakel, R.E. (ed.) *Conn's current therapy*. W.B. Saunders, Philadelphia, Published annually. Individualistic accounts of the management of specific diseases arranged in monographs under systematic headings.

Reactions. Weekly journal which publishes vignettes, short reviews, and abstracts of case reports, giving up-to-date information on adverse drug reactions.

Reynolds, J.E.F. (ed). (1989). *Martindale: the extra pharmacopoeia* (29th edn.). The Pharmaceutical Press, London. Lists virtually every therapeutic agent, with notes on dosages, relevant chemical and pharmaceutical properties, adverse effects, precautions, absorption and fate, uses, and formulations (both proprietary and non-proprietary). Extensively illustrated by quotations from published reports, with references.

Riggs, D.S. (1963). *The mathematical approach to physiological problems*. A critical primer. The MIT Press, Cambridge, Mass. Essential reading for anyone who intends making any kind of scientific calculations.

Rowland, M. and Tozer, T.N. (1989). *Clinical pharmacokinetics. Concepts and applications* (2nd edn). Lea and Febiger, Philadelphia, London. An excellent introductory text which needs to be worked through systematically. Covers basic concepts, principles of kinetics as applied to drugs, therapeutic regimens, and individualization of therapy. Well illustrated with practical problems throughout. Light on maths, but appendices deal with some of the practicalities of the mathematical treatment of kinetic data.

Sackett, D.L. and Haynes, R.B. (eds) (1976). *Compliance with therapeutic regimens*. Johns Hopkins University Press, Baltimore. A lively collection of papers on a variety of aspects of patient compliance.

Smith, S.E. and Rawlins, M.D. (1973). *Variability in human drug response*. Butterworth, London. Excellent, easy-to-read introduction to basic clinical pharmacology including descriptive and mathematical pharmacokinetics, pharmacogenetics, tissue sensitivity, and monitoring drug therapy.

Stockley, I. (1991). *Drug interactions* (2nd edn). Blackwell Scientific Publications, Oxford. Monographs on individual drug interactions arranged in chapters by object drug. Each well-referenced monograph contains a description of the interaction and its mechanism, and an assessment of its importance, with guidance on management. The introductory chapter contains an abbreviated account of basic mechanisms.

Szorady, I. (1973). *Pharmacogenetics. Principles and paediatric aspects*. Akademiai Kiado, Budapest. Comprehensive, well-referenced text, but difficult to read and out of date.

Todd, R.G. (ed.) (1980). *Pharmaceutical handbook* (19th edn). The Pharmaceutical Press, London. Contains a wide variety of information on numerous pharmaceutical matters, including the preparation of medicines, posology, microbiology, immunology, nomenclature, mensuration. Contains several comprehensive glossaries (for example 'Terms used in pharmacology', 'Approved names and their synonyms').

Vale, J.A. and Meredith, T.J. (1985). *A concise guide to the management of poisoning* (3rd edn). Churchill Livingstone, Edinburgh. Notes on the general and specific management of self-poisoning.

Wagner, J.G. (1971) *Biopharmaceutics and relevant pharmacokinetics* (1st edn). Drug Intelligence Publications, Hamilton, Ill. Technical account, mostly of pharmaceutical matters, for example disintegration and dissolution of dosage forms, special formulations (sustained-release, enteric-coated), systemic availability, and quality control. Useful chapters on mechanisms of drug transport in the body.

Wagner, J.G. (1975) *Fundamentals of clinical pharmacokinetics*. Drug Intelligence Publications, Hamilton, Ill. Eclectic text on various aspects of pharmacokinetics. Contains many useful equations, but is difficult to use without a good basic understanding of the subject. Deals extensively with compartment models (linear and non-linear), dosage regimen calculations, the effects of disease on pharmacokinetics, and concentration–response relationships.

Winter, M.E. (1988). *Basic clinical pharmacokinetics* (2nd edn). Applied Therapeutics Inc., Vancouver, Washington. The basic principles of clinical pharmacokinetics outlined, with only essential mathematics. Followed by sections on practical applications for all important drugs, including case studies.

Section III

The drug therapy of disease

21 Introduction to drug therapy

In Section I we discussed the basic principles of clinical pharmacology, breaking down drug therapy into its component processes (pharmaceutical, pharmacokinetic, pharmacodynamic, and therapeutic). In Section II we discussed some principles relating to the prescribing of drugs. Section IV (the Pharmacopoeia) contains details of the properties of individual drugs or groups of drugs.

In this section it is our aim to marry the properties of the drugs with the basic principles, and to link both with the pathology of the disease and its manifestations, in order to illustrate the ways in which drugs are used in the treatment of disease.

It is not always easy to state precisely the molecular mechanisms responsible for causing disease (for example hypertension, depression, cancer), nor in fact the precise mechanisms through which drugs exert their therapeutic effects (for example β-adrenoceptor antagonists in hypertension, ergotamine in migraine, phenytoin in epilepsy), and in such cases attempts at a purely rational approach to drug therapy are to some extent thwarted. None the less, an interpretation at some level of understanding (see

	PATHOPHYSIOLOGY	SYMPTOMS	THERAPEUTIC POINTS
CAUSE	Coronary atheroma and obstruction (thrombosis). Risk factors: diet smoking hypertension genetic thrombotic potential		?Reduce chlosterol intake Stop smoking Treat hypertension early Treat hyperlipidaemia Aspirin, ?warfarin
PRIMARY PATHOLOGY	Myocardial ischaemia (± previous episodes of myocardial infarction) ↓ Ventricular dysfunction (poor pump) ↓ Altered haemodynamics reduced cardiac output increased left ventricular end-diastolic pressure pulmonary oedema ⟶ hypoxia increased venous pressure ⟶ hepatomegaly	Angina, acute chest pain	Nitrates, nifedipine, β-adrenoceptor antagonists
			Rest, positive inotropic drugs (digoxin, β-adrenoceptor agonists), vasodilators
		Breathlessness} Liver pain	Acutely diamorphine/ morphine, vasodilators, oxygen; chronically diuretics, vasodilators
SECONDARY PATHOLOGY	Poor renal perfusion (+congestion) ⟶ oedema Poor tissue perfusion (including brain)	Legs swell Exhaustion	Diuretics

■ **Fig. 21.1** Pathophysiological changes in acute myocardial infarction with corresponding therapeutic points.

Chapter 4) is usually possible. For example, although we do not understand precisely how corticosteroids act at the molecular level, many of their actions at the cellular and organ levels are known and can be related to their therapeutic effects.

Take the treatment of cardiac failure as an example. In Fig. 21.1 are shown the underlying pathophysiological changes and the drugs or other manoeuvres which one might use in therapy. Of course, there are various different possible presentations of cardiac failure, each demanding some fine tuning of drug therapy and other approaches, but the broad essentials are shown in Fig. 21.1. Now compare the treatment of acute left ventricular failure associated with a myocardial infarction with the treatment of chronic congestive cardiac failure associated with chronic severe myocardial ischaemia.

Acute left ventricular failure will require:

(1) oxygen;

(2) diamorphine or morphine i.v.;

(3) frusemide i.v.;

(4) then perhaps a vasodilator i.v. (for example isosorbide dinitrate).

Chronic congestive cardiac failure will require:

(1) oral diuretics (for example thiazides, frusemide or bumetanide, potassium-sparing diuretics);

(2) then perhaps digitalis (for example digoxin orally);

(3) or an oral vasodilator (for example enalapril).

In each case we are guided by our knowledge of the pathophysiology of the disease and of the properties of the drugs used, and by our cumulative corporate experience of the results of using those drugs in those circumstances.

Where appropriate in the chapters which follow in this section, we shall describe drug therapy starting with the relevant pathophysiology, stating the nature of the problem, and continuing with the details of specific drug use, referring to the Pharmacopoeia as necessary.

22 The drug therapy of infectious diseases

Co-authors: N. J. White and C. P. Conlon

For practical reasons our aim in this chapter is to deal with the general principles governing the ways in which drugs are used in the treatment of diseases caused by infective agents. These can be classified according to the type of infective agent against which the drug is directed:

(1) antibacterial drugs;

(2) antiviral drugs;

(3) antiprotozoal drugs;

(4) antihelminthic drugs;

(5) antitrematodal drugs;

(6) antifungal drugs.

We shall deal with each class separately. Many specific infections are dealt with in other chapters (for example infective endocarditis in Chapter 23, pneumonias in Chapter 24, and so on). Because sexually transmitted disorders are generally dealt with by specialists in the branch of infectious diseases known as genitourinary medicine, they will be dealt with in a separate section at the end of this chapter.

22.1 Antibacterial drugs: the treatment of bacterial infections

The list of antibacterial drugs which one has at one's disposal is a formidable, and is given in Table 22.1. However, it is possible to pare back this list to a much shorter list of drugs, covering about 85 per cent of all the antibiotics prescribed in the UK. The list is as follows:

Penicillins
  benzylpenicillin
  penicillin V
  amoxycillin
  flucloxacillin
  piperacillin
Cephalosporins
  cefaclor
  cefuroxime
  cephalexin
Tetracyclines
  doxycycline
  tetracycline
Aminoglycosides
  gentamicin
Macrolides
  erythromycin
Sulphonamides
  sulphamethoxazole (in co-trimoxazole)
Trimethoprim
Quinolones
  ciprofloxacin
Metronidazole
Vancomycin

Adding the antituberculous and antileprotic drugs which are commonly used world-wide extends the list as follows:

Antituberculous drugs
  rifampicin
  ethambutol
  isoniazid
  thiacetazone
  pyrazinamide
  streptomycin
Antileprotic drugs
  dapsone

■ **Table 22.1** A list of antibiotics (drugs in bold print are first-choice antibiotics within their group)

Penicillins (p. 658)
 β-Lactamase-sensitive penicillins
  Benzylpenicillin (penicillin G)
  Procaine penicillin (a salt of benzylpenicillin)
  Benethamine penicillin (a salt of
   benzylpenicillin)
  Phenoxymethylpenicillin (penicillin V)
 Broad-spectrum penicillins
  Ampicillin
  Amoxycillin (+ clavulanic acid = co-
   amoxiclav)
  Azlocillin
  Mezlocillin
  Piperacillin
 β-Lactamase-resistant penicillins
  Flucloxacillin
  Methicillin
 Antipseudomonal penicillins
  Piperacillin
  Ticarcillin
Cephalosporins and cephamycins (p. 575)
 ([1,2,3]first-, second-, and third-generation drugs)
 Orally-active cephalosporins (*can also be given
 by injection)
  Cefaclor[2]
  Cefadroxil[3]
  Cefixime[3]
  *Cefuroxime[2]
  Cephalexin[2]
  *Cephradine[1]
  Cefetamet[3]
 Injectable cephalosporins
  Cefamandole[2]
  Cefotaxime[3]
  Cefoxitin[2]
  Cefsulodin[3]
  Ceftazidime[3]
  Ceftizoxime[3]
  Ceftriaxone[3]
  Cefuroxime[2]
  Cephamandole[2]
  Cephazolin[2]
  Latamoxef[3]
Other β-Lactam related antibiotics
 Aztreonam
 Imipenem (+cilastin)
 Mecillinam
 Pivmecillinam
Tetracyclines (p. 692)
 Tetracycline
 Doxycycline
 Minocycline

Aminoglycosides (p. 552)
 Amikacin
 Gentamicin
 Kanamycin
 Neomycin
 Netilmicin
 Tobramycin
Macrolides
 Azithromycin
 Erythromycin (p. 602)
 Oleandomycin
 Roxithromycin
 Spiramycin
Lincomycin and clindamycin (p. 628)
Sulphonamides (p. 689)
 Sulphadiazine
 Sulphamethizole
 Sulphamethoxazole (in co-trimoxazole)
Trimethoprim (p. 589)
*Co-trimoxazole (sulphamethoxazole+
 trimethoprim)* (p. 589)
Quinolones (p. 673)
 Cinoxacin
 Ciprofloxacin
 Enoxacin
 Nalidixic acid
 Norfloxacin
 Ofloxacin
Chloramphenicol (p. 578)
Nitroimidazoles (p. 558)
 Metronidazole
 Tinidazole
Sodium fusidate (p. 609)
Spectinomycin
Teicoplanin
Vancomycin (p. 701)
Antituberculous drugs
 Ethambutol (p. 603)
 Isoniazid (p. 621)
 Pyrazinamide
 Rifampicin (p. 676)
 Streptomycin (p. 552)
 Thiacetazone
Antileprotic drugs
 Clofazimine
 Dapsone (p. 593)
 Rifampicin
Urinary antimicrobials
 Nitrofurantoin (p. 652)

22.1.1 Mechanisms of action of antibiotics

Antibacterial therapy depends on the action of a drug either to kill or to prevent the growth of bacteria without harming the host. Antibacterial drugs do this by three main mechanisms (Fig. 22.1).

(a) Impairment of bacterial cell wall synthesis

Drugs which do this, usually by interfering with structurally important peptidoglycans, include the penicillins, cephalosporins, vancomycin, and bacitracin.

(b) Impairment of bacterial protein synthesis

Several antibiotics do this, but by different mechanisms: the tetracyclines interfere with tRNA function and the aminoglycosides with mRNA function; chloramphenicol inhibits peptidyl transferase; erythromycin, lincomycin, and clindamycin interfere with translocation.

(c) Impairment of bacterial nucleic acid synthesis

Several antibiotics do this, but by different mechanisms: metronidazole and nitrofurantoin damage DNA; the quinolones inhibit DNA gyrase; rifampicin inhibits RNA polymerase; the sulphonamides and trimethoprim inhibit folic acid synthesis.

Antibacterial agents, when tested *in vitro*, are either bacteriocidal (they kill bacteria) or bacteriostatic (they arrest their growth) (see Table 22.2). Some drugs are bacteriocidal against

■ **Table 22.2** Some bacteriocidal and bacteriostatic antibiotics

Bacteriocidal	Bacteriostatic
Penicillins	Sulphonamides
Cephalosporins	Tetracyclines
Aminoglycosides	Chloramphenicol
	Erythromycin
	Trimethoprim

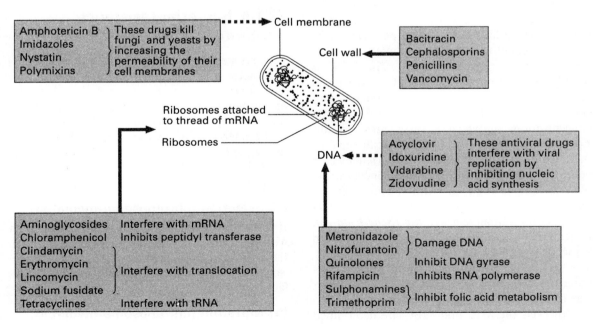

■ **Fig. 22.1** A stylized representation of a bacterium showing the sites of action of some antibiotics. Also shown are the actions of some antifungal and antiviral drugs.

some organisms but bacteriostatic against others; for example, erythromycin is bacteriocidal against *Strep. pneumoniae* but bacteriostatic against *Strep. faecalis*.

To some extent bacteriostatic agents rely upon the host's immune and cellular defence mechanisms to clear the bacteria, and this is a factor to consider in patients whose defence mechanisms are compromised (for example in patients with AIDS or patients taking immunosuppressive drugs). In such patients a bacteriocidal drug would be preferred. Bacteriocidal drugs would also be preferred when the site of infection is avascular, as in infective endocarditis, and in severe infections. However, outside of these important considerations the distinction between bacteriocidal and bacteriostatic action is not of great clinical importance.

22.1.2 Concentration/effect relationships in antibiotic therapy

Crucial factors in antibacterial chemotherapy are the minimal inhibitory concentration (MIC) and the minimal bacteriocidal concentration (MBC) of the drug against a specified organism. The MIC for a given culture system is the lowest concentration of the drug which inhibits bacterial growth. The MBC is the lowest concentration of the drug which kills at least 99.9 per cent of the organisms in culture. The lower these concentrations the more potent the drug. The MBC is usually two to four times the MIC. The clinical value of the drug then depends upon the relationship between the MIC and MBC and the plasma concentrations at which adverse effects occur. For instance, the MIC for benzylpenicillin against the pneumococcus (*Streptococcus pneumoniae*) is generally greatly below the plasma concentration of penicillin associated with adverse effects (excluding penicillin hypersensitivity), whereas the MIC for gentamicin against *Escherichia coli* is generally close to the plasma concentration associated with renal toxicity and ototoxicity. The MIC and MBC are the factors which determine the denominator in the therapeutic index (see p. 54) for an antibiotic.

However, the MIC and MBC are determined in homogeneous culture *in vitro*. *In vivo* the drug must pass from the plasma and cross tissue barriers into the infected tissue to destroy bacteria. Thus, while it may be possible to obtain a plasma concentration close to the MIC, if the concentration in the tissue is lower than that in the plasma, treatment failure may nevertheless occur. For instance, the passage of antibiotics into abscess cavities may be poor, and surgical drainage is often necessary. Antibiotics may enter cells poorly, and intracellular pathogens may therefore be difficult to eradicate; examples of intracellular pathogens include *Brucella*, *Legionella*, *Mycobacteria*, *Salmonella*, and *Toxoplasma*.

22.1.3 The post-antibiotic effect

Many antibiotics continue to exert an antibacterial effect after the plasma concentration of the antibiotic has fallen below the MIC. This is known as the post-antibiotic effect. Nearly all antibiotics have a post-antibiotic effect against Gram-positive organisms. The aminoglycosides have a post-antibiotic effect against Gram-negative organisms, while the β-lactam antibiotics do not; this means that for Gram-negative infections the aminoglycosides are effective when given once or twice a day, whereas β-lactam antibiotics need to be given every 4–6 h.

22.1.4 Bacterial resistance to antibiotics

True resistance of bacteria to antibacterial agents is a factor affecting the whole approach to the chemotherapy of infectious disease. Profligate use of antibiotics without careful consideration of their appropriate indications leads more readily to the emergence of resistant strains. The sensible use of antibiotics, as described below, reduces the risk of this. The known mechanisms of bacterial resistance to antibiotics are detailed below.

(a) Selection (chromosome-mediated)

If within a bacterial population there are bacteria with a natural resistance to an antibiotic, then the antibiotic will eliminate the sensitive organisms and the resistant forms will proliferate. This factor operates particularly in hospitals.

(b) Mutation (chromosome-mediated)

Within a population of bacteria, mutants which are resistant to an antibiotic may arise spontaneously. These bacteria are then selected for proliferation as described above.

(c) Transferred resistance

Resistance may be transferred from one organism to another by the exchange of genes which confer antibiotic resistance. Such genes may either be contained within bacteriophages (viruses which infect bacteria) or within plasmids. Plasmids which confer resistance are transferred into other bacteria by conjugation and the actual passage of DNA from one bacterial cell to another. Either way, new DNA enters the bacterium and codes for a mechanism which confers resistance. Such mechanisms involve:

(i) Enzymatic inactivation of the antibiotic

For example, β-lactamases confer resistance to some penicillins and cephalosporins, chloramphenicol acetyltransferase confers resistance to chloramphenicol, and various transferases confer resistance to aminoglycosides.

(ii) Substitution of a metabolic pathway resistant to the antibacterial agent

This type of resistance has been described for sulphonamides and trimethoprim.

(iii) Altered site of action

This type of resistance has been described for chloramphenicol, erythromycin, rifampicin, and streptomycin. Alterations in penicillin binding proteins may confer resistance in this way.

(iv) Altered transport of the antibiotic to its site of action

This type of resistance has been described for tetracyclines, aminoglycosides, and β-lactams.

Emergence of bacterial resistance can be minimized by prescribing antibiotics only when really necessary, by ensuring adequate dosages, by carefully reserving certain drugs for certain infections, and by using narrow-spectrum antibiotics. In some infections resistance develops very rapidly when certain antibiotics are used on their own (for example rifampicin and fusidic acid used to treat infection with *Staphylococcus aureus*), but resistance develops very slowly when two or more antibiotics are used in combination; the risk of bacterial resistance in these cases can be reduced by using drug combinations (for example in tuberculosis).

22.1.5 Principles of antibacterial chemotherapy

There is a great deal of unnecessary prescribing of antibiotics. The hazards of this are several.

Firstly, resistant organisms may arise. This is a particular hazard in hospitals and can lead to disastrous wound infections on surgical wards and cross-infections in urology wards, oncology wards, and intensive care units.

Secondly, the presence of a resistant organism other than that for which therapy was originally intended brings the risk of superinfection with that organism. For example, superinfection with *Candida albicans* is very common, particularly in old or very ill patients; pseudomembranous colitis is due to superinfection in the bowel with *Clostridium difficile*, which is resistant to the antibiotics used for the primary infection.

Thirdly, the unnecessary use of antibiotics carries the risk of adverse effects, for example hypersensitivity.

If antibiotics are prescribed for a bacterial infection before a diagnosis is made and if treatment does not eradicate the infection, subsequent diagnosis can be very difficult, because of confusion caused by alteration of the clinical signs, alteration in bacterial flora, and the problems of culturing bacteria and determining bacterial sensitivities, even of resistant organisms, in the presence of an antibiotic.

If the following principles are followed many of these problems will be avoided.

(a) Make a diagnosis

It would be perfect if before starting antibiotic therapy the precise bacteriological diagnosis was known in every case. However, this ideal is not possible. For instance, in life-threatening infections 'best-guess' antibiotic therapy must be started quickly on the basis of the clinical features of the illness, although in all such cases specimens (blood, urine, sputum, etc.) must be taken before treatment, so that rational antibiotic therapy can be applied later if an organism is identified.

Sheer numbers of patients and economic realities in various parts of the world pose the problem of whether it is really necessary to establish the precise laboratory diagnosis in some common infections when the infecting organism is predictable with a high degree of certainty. Examples of such infections would be uncomplicated urinary tract infection in women (mostly due to *E. coli*, *S. saprophyticus*, or *Pr. mirabilis*), acute follicular tonsillitis (*Strep. pyogenes*), and acute bronchitis complicating chronic bronchitis (*H. influenzae* and *Strep. pneumoniae*). Of course, if circumstances permit one should certainly take relevant specimens in such cases, but if this is impracticable then one would be warranted in starting therapy with an antibiotic which would be expected to be effective, without formal identification of the organism.

Whether or not bacteriological investigation in such cases should be undertaken depends upon the prevailing clinical practice in the particular socio-economic circumstances. The infections mentioned above do have a reasonable chance of being due to the named organisms, and a fair guess can be made in a particular environment as to their likely sensitivities to antibiotics. However, there are many conditions in which there is a low likelihood of making a correct clinical guess about the infecting organism and/or its antibiotic sensitivities, and indeed in which the correct answer may be essential for a favourable outcome. Meningitis is a case in point. A Gram stain of the cerebrospinal fluid (CSF) may show many polymorphonuclear leucocytes and Gram-negative kidney-shaped diplococci. Bacteriological culture may later reveal *Neisseria meningitidis* (the meningococcus) in the CSF or blood, but treatment with benzylpenicillin may be started on the basis of the Gram stain of the CSF alone, although a cloudy CSF in a patient with meningism and a rash is also highly suggestive. Gram-positive diplococci in the CSF are likely to be pneumococci, which should also be responsive to penicillin. Small Gram-negative bacilli in the CSF are likely to be *H. influenzae*, for which a third-generation cephalosporin (for example cefotaxime) or chloramphenicol would be the treatment of choice. However, in no case would one start therapy without some indication of the identity of the infecting organism, and the simple procedure of making a Gram stain of the

CSF can be very useful in this life-threatening infection.

In some cases it may be possible to make a diagnosis by using one of an increasing number of rapid antigen detection methods instead of bacterial culture. The organisms which can be detected in this way include streptococci (*Strep. pyogenes* Groups A and B, *Strep. pneumoniae*), *Neisseria meningitidis*, *Haemophilus influenzae*, *Mycobacterium tuberculosis*, and *Chlamydia trachomatis*.

In summary, therefore, the counsel of perfection is to make an exact bacteriological or antigenic diagnosis before treatment. If this is not possible, because of practical difficulties or the urgency of the problem, one should take appropriate specimens for bacteriological examination, make a clinical guess at the responsible organism, and start treatment with the 'best guess' antibiotic. If there are problems about the bacterial diagnosis consult a bacteriologist at the earliest opportunity.

(b) Decide whether antibiotic therapy is really necessary

Not all bacterial infections need to be treated with antibiotics. For example, not all boils need antibiotic therapy, although this needs careful clinical judgement as to the likelihood of complications and spread, and the need for surgical drainage. Generally speaking, bacillary dysentery and food poisoning with *Salmonella* organisms do not need antibiotic therapy.

(c) Choose the appropriate antibiotic

Several different factors influence one's choice of antibiotic:

(1) the spectrum of antibacterial activity;

(2) bacterial resistance;

(3) pharmacokinetics (for example the distribution to the infected tissues);

(4) adverse effects and drug interactions;

(5) clinical trial evidence of efficacy in the clinical problem;

(6) synergy with other antibiotics (combination therapy);

(7) cost.

(i) The spectrum of antibacterial activity

It is helpful to make yourself acquainted with the patterns of antibiotic sensitivities of organisms which are commonly cultured in your hospital or area, and many hospitals have lists of common sensitivities. It is also increasingly common for hospitals to have local formularies or antibiotics policies in which indications, dosages, and costs of antibiotics are detailed.

Ideally the antibacterial activity for a given organism should be tested *in vitro* by determining the ability of antibiotics to inhibit the growth of the causative organism. However, in cases in which the organism has not, or not yet, been isolated it has to be assumed that the suspected organism is sensitive to a particular antibiotic because of the known characteristics of such organisms in general. In Table 22.3 are listed the infections for which particular antibiotics are usually the first choice, and in Table 22.4 are shown the usual sensitivities of organisms to the commonly used antibiotics. Whenever possible a narrow-spectrum antibiotic should be chosen, in order to minimize the risk of the emergence of resistant organisms. For example, one would use flucloxacillin for an infection with penicillin-resistant *S. aureus* and penicillin V for a streptococcal sore throat.

(ii) Bacterial resistance

This is also ideally tested by direct examination of the causative organism, but it may have to be assumed. For example, the staphylococci found in hospitals are generally resistant to certain penicillins because they produce a β-lactamase (penicillinase). In such circumstances one would choose a β-lactamase-resistant penicillin, such as flucloxacillin, or add clavulanic acid, a β-lactamase inhibitor, to the penicillin regimen.

(iii) Pharmacokinetics

Various aspects of the pharmacokinetics of an antibiotic may govern its use in different circumstances, but particularly important is its distribution to specific tissues for the treatment of infections in those tissues.

For example, in meningitis one must be sure that the antibiotic will enter the CSF well enough to achieve a concentration sufficient to kill the organism. Some antibiotics penetrate the CSF well across normal meninges, others penetrate well only when the meninges are inflamed, and others still do not penetrate well under either circumstance (see Table 22.5).

The ability of lincomycin, clindamycin, fusidic acid, and penicillinase-resistant penicillins to penetrate bone is of importance in the treatment of staphylococcal osteomyelitis.

Ampicillin, amoxycillin, and tetracyclines are concentrated in the functioning gall-bladder and may therefore be useful in the treatment of biliary tract infections.

Abscesses should be drained whenever possible, since they are poorly penetrated by antibiotics, and their low pH inhibits the antibacterial activity of many antibiotics.

In infective endocarditis relatively high dosages of antibiotics, particularly penicillins, are usually recommended, for two reasons: the penetration of antibiotics into vegetations and valve tissue (which is relatively avascular) may be poor, and tissue defence mechanisms in the infected area are often inadequate.

In the treatment of urinary tract infections, where there is tissue inflammation, with many pus cells and bacteria in the urine, it is logical to use antibiotics which not only reach the bacteria in the tissues but which also reach sufficiently high concentrations in the urine to act on the bacteria there. Amoxycillin, the quinolones (for example ciprofloxacin), trimethoprim, the sulphonamides, gentamicin, and nitrofurantoin do that.

(iv) Adverse effects and drug interactions

These are discussed below (p. 237).

(v) Clinical trial evidence of efficacy

The use of chloramphenicol in the treatment of typhoid fever rests on the clinical observation that it works and that other antibiotics to which the organism is sensitive *in vitro* (for example gentamicin) may not always be as effective. Sometimes it is clinical experience of this kind which determines the choice of antibiotic.

(vi) Synergy

In the treatment of bacterial endocarditis penicillin and gentamicin are used together, because they have been shown to be synergistic in killing

■ **Table 22.3** Infections for which the listed antibiotics are usually first choice

Benzylpenicillin
Streptococcus pyogenes	Acute follicular tonsillitis
	Cellulitis/erysipelas
	Acute otitis media (over 5 years; see also co-amoxiclav)
'Viridans' streptococci	Endocarditis (+ gentamicin)
Streptococcus pneumoniae	Pneumococcal pneumonia
Enterococcus faecalis	Endocarditis (+gentamicin)
Neisseria gonorrhoeae	Gonorrhoea
Neisseria meningitidis	Meningococcal meningitis
Treponema pallidum	Syphilis

Amoxycillin
Streptococcus pneumoniae	Exacerbations of chronic bronchitis, acute bronchitis/pneumonia
Streptococcus pyogenes	Acute otitis media (under 5 years)
Streptococcus pneumoniae	Sinusitis
Streptococcus pyogenes	Sinusitis
Escherichia coli	Urinary tract infection (+clavulanic acid if resistant)
Enterococcus faecalis	Urinary tract infection (+clavulanic acid if resistant)
Listeria monocytogenes	Listeria septicaemia and meningitis

Co-amoxiclav
Haemophilus influenzae	Exacerbations of chronic bronchitis, acute bronchitis/pneumonia, sinusitis, acute otitis media (under 5 years)

Flucloxacillin
Staphylococcus aureus (penicillin-resistant)	Wounds, boils (if necessary), and abscesses
	Septic arthritis
	Osteomyelitis
	Pneumonia
	Endocarditis
	Impetigo

Piperacillin
Pseudomonas aeruginosa	Septicaemia (+gentamicin)
	Urinary tract infection
	Pneumonia (+ gentamicin)

Tetracyclines
Rickettsiae	Typhus, Q fever
Chlamydiae	Trachoma
	Psittacosis
	Lymphogranuloma venereum
	Non-specific urethritis

Gentamicin
'Viridans' streptococci	Endocarditis (+ benzylpenicillin)
Enterococcus faecalis	Endocarditis (+ benzylpenicillin)
Escherichia coli ⎤	
Klebsiella ⎥	In severe infections, for example septicaemia, acute pyelonephritis, pneumonia, biliary tract infection
Enterobacter ⎥	
Proteus ⎦	
Pseudomonas aeruginosa	(+azlocillin) urinary tract infection, pneumonia

Erythromycin
Mycoplasma pneumoniae	Mycoplasma ('atypical') pneumonia
Legionella pneumophila	Legionnaires' pneumonia

Trimethoprim
    Escherichia coli   Pyelonephritis
                                          Urinary tract infection
    Haemophilus influenzae   Exacerbations of chronic bronchitis
    Streptococcus pneumoniae Exacerbations of chronic bronchitis
Chloramphenicol
    Salmonella typhi   Typhoid fever
    Haemophilus influenzae   Meningitis
Metronidazole
    Anaerobic organisms   Intra-abdominal infections, for example:
    (for example *Bacteroides* spp.)   liver abscess
                                          pelvic inflammatory disease
                                        cholangitis
                                        peritonitis
                                        female genital tract infections
                        Lung infections: abscess
                        Brain abscess
                        Endocarditis
    Clostridium difficile   Antibiotic-associated diarrhoea
Vancomycin
    Staphylococcus aureus   Infections resistant to methicillin
    Coagulase-negative   All infections
       staphylococci
    Clostridium difficile   Antibiotic-associated diarrhoea resistant to metronidazole

---

bacteria *in vitro*. The synergy of trimethoprim with sulphamethoxazole (co-trimoxazole) is discussed in the Pharmacopoeia (p. 589).

(d) Consider patient (host) factors

(i) Severity of infection

If the infection is very severe, the general condition of the patient may be poor and absorption unpredictable (for example because of nausea, vomiting, gastric stasis). It is wiser in such cases to give intramuscular or intravenous antibiotics. In hospital the intravenous route is preferred.

After the infection is brought under control and the patient's general condition has improved, it may be possible to achieve adequate antibiotic concentrations in the infected tissues by oral administration. An exception in some circumstances is infective endocarditis (see p. 293).

(ii) Host defence mechanisms

The patient's ability to mount a complete defence response against a bacterial infection is of great importance in determining the overall outcome of treatment. If defence mechanisms are impaired (for example in old age, malignant disease, treatment with immunosuppressive drugs, malnutrition, or AIDS), then bacteriocidal drugs are preferable to bacteriostatic drugs.

(iii) Individual pharmacokinetic factors

Age: The newborn (because of poor renal and hepatic function) and old people (mainly because of poor renal function) may have altered rates of elimination of antibiotics, and dosage adjustments may have to be made accordingly (see Chapter 11).

Renal failure: Severe infections may be associated with impaired renal function, particularly in old people. Infections of the urinary tract, both acute and chronic, particularly when associated with urinary obstruction, can produce renal failure. In addition, some antibiotics are themselves nephrotoxic (see Table 26.6). For example, gentamicin (particularly when used with frusemide) can produce tubular damage; the penicillins may produce acute interstitial nephritis. In all grades of renal failure the dosages of cephalosporins, ethambutol, and vancomycin should be reduced; the plasma concentrations of gentamicin and other aminoglycosides must be monitored if ototoxicity and renal damage are to be avoided and

Table 22.4 The sensitivities of some organisms to commonly used antibiotics

	Staphylococcus aureus (penicillin-sensitive)	Staphylococcus aureus (penicillin-resistant)	Streptococcus pyogenes	Streptococcus pneumoniae	Enterococcus faecalis	'Viridans' streptococci	Neisseria meningitidis	Neisseria gonorrhoeae	Haemophilus influenzae	Escherichia coli	Klebsiella	Proteus mirabilis	Pseudomonas aeruginosa	Brucella	Legionella pneumophila	Salmonella typhi	Bacteroides spp. and other anaerobes	Mycoplasma pneumoniae	Chlamydiae	Listeria monocytogenes	Rickettsiae
Penicillin G/penicillin V	++		++	++	++	++	++									+					
Ampicillin/amoxycillin	+	+	+	++	+	+	++	++	+	++							++				
Flucloxacillin	+	++																			
Piperacillin					+								++								
Cefoxitin																	+				
Ceftazidime													++								
Cefuroxime/cefotaxime/cefamandole		+					+	+	++	+	+	+									
Chloramphenicol			+			+			+										+	+	
Co-trimoxazole	+	+						+	+	++	++	++				+					
Erythromycin	+	+	+			+									++			++	+		
Gentamicin	+	+								+	+	+	++								
Metronidazole																	++				
Quinolones		+						+	+	+	+		++			+					
Tetracyclines	+		+					+	+					++	+			+	++		++

++ Drugs of first choice. + Drugs of second choice.

■ **Table 22.5** Penetration of antibiotics into CSF

Meninges normal: good penetration	Meninges inflamed: good penetration	Meninges inflamed: poor penetration
Sulphonamides	Benzylpenicillin	Streptomycin
Trimethoprim	Ampicillin	Gentamicin
Metronidazole	Tetracycline	Most cephalosporins
Rifampicin	Macrolides	Ethambutol
Isoniazid		
Chloramphenicol		
Third-generation cephalosporins		

efficacy maintained (see Chapter 7). In more severe grades of renal failure the dosages of metronidazole, co-trimoxazole, and the β-lactams need modification. Tetracyclines (except doxycycline), nitrofurantoin, and nalidixic acid should be avoided in renal failure.

Hepatic disease: If an antibiotic is excreted by the liver its dosages may have to be reduced in liver disease, for example erythromycin, clindamycin, lincomycin, and chloramphenicol. In the case of erythromycin it is now thought that the risk of liver damage is independent of the ester used (for example estolate, stearate, or ethylsuccinate). In cirrhosis of the liver the half-times of rifampicin and isoniazid are prolonged, and this poses problems in the treatment of tuberculosis in patients with alcoholic cirrhosis, a not uncommon combination. Dosages of these drugs may need to be reduced, particularly as both rifampicin and isoniazid may themselves cause liver damage.

(iv) Pharmacogenetic factors (see Chapter 8)

Sulphonamides, nitrofurantoin, and chloramphenicol can produce acute haemolysis in patients with glucose-6-phosphate dehydrogenase (G6PD) deficiency. Sulphonamides and griseofulvin should be avoided in patients with porphyria.

(e) Consider the chances of adverse effects

(i) Allergic reactions

Never give a patient an antibiotic without having taken, as best you can, a history of allergy to antibiotics (see Chapter 17). This applies particularly to the penicillins, with which anaphylactic shock and other serious reactions occur not uncommonly. It is estimated that 1 in 2000 patients treated with a penicillin will have a type I hypersensitivity reaction. Although this seems a small frequency, very large numbers of patients are treated with penicillins, and thus the actual numbers of patients affected may be quite large. Some but by no means all patients allergic to penicillin will also be allergic to cephalosporins (see p. 575). Unfortunately it is not possible to tell whether an individual is allergic to both.

Ampicillin and amoxycillin both produce a measles-like rash in almost all patients with infectious mononucleosis, and in some patients with cytomegalovirus infections and chronic lymphocytic leukaemia, but this reaction is not a type I hypersensitivity reaction, nor apparently any sort of hypersensitivity reaction, although it may be difficult to distinguish it from true hypersensitivity (see p. 110).

(ii) Superinfection

There is always a risk of superinfection in patients taking antibiotics. This is particularly so in frail and immunosuppressed patients. Severely ill patients requiring mechanical ventilation will frequently develop superinfection of the lower airways with organisms resistant to the antibiotics being used. Careful oral and general hygiene and attention to nutritional factors, particularly in old people, are essential in any severe infection during treatment with antibiotics. The organism which most commonly causes superinfection is

Candida albicans, which can usually be treated effectively with nystatin.

(iii) General comments

If patients are not allergic to penicillins they are fairly safe drugs with a high toxic/therapeutic ratio (a high therapeutic index). Sulphonamides quite frequently produce hypersensitivity reactions. Do not forget, therefore, that co-trimoxazole contains sulphamethoxazole. Trimethoprim does not seem to produce hypersensitivity reactions frequently, but it can cause bone-marrow suppression with neutropenia and thrombocytopenia.

Erythromycin can cause liver damage, but rarely. Otherwise it is a safe antibiotic.

Tetracyclines (apart from doxycycline) may worsen renal failure and they should not be used in patients with pre-existing renal impairment. They stain teeth in children up to 7 years of age. They can produce antibiotic-associated diarrhoea (in up to 50 per cent of patients) and rarely pseudomembranous colitis. Overgrowth of *Candida albicans* is common. Photosensitive skin rashes often occur.

The aminoglycosides are ototoxic and nephrotoxic and dosages need careful control.

The adverse effects of the cephalosporins, if one excludes allergy, are not frequent. Occasionally neutropenia and thrombocytopenia occur. Some cephalosporins may also cause bleeding, because of interference with clotting mechanisms; this has been a particular problem with latamoxef, with which concurrent vitamin K therapy (10 mg weekly orally) is recommended. Nephrotoxicity was a problem with cephaloridine and cephalothin, but these have been superseded by safer cephalosporins.

The quinolones may cause skin rashes, gastrointestinal adverse effects, and changes in liver function tests. Since they increase the threshold for seizures they should be used with care in patients with a history of epilepsy.

Clindamycin and lincomycin may cause pseudomembranous colitis, a serious and potentially fatal adverse reaction. Their use should be reserved for the treatment of severe anaerobic infections and for infections in bones and joints.

Chloramphenicol commonly causes mild anaemia and may rarely cause aplastic anaemia.

It is therefore reserved for the treatment of typhoid fever, cerebral abscesses, meningitis due to sensitive *H. influenzae*, and Rickettsial infections.

Serious adverse effects with metronidazole are uncommon, although peripheral neuropathy can occur with prolonged use. It should be avoided in patients with porphyria.

(iv) Drug interactions

Drug interactions may produce toxicity or inefficacy. Some of the more common interactions with antibiotics are shown in Table 22.6.

(f) Consider the route of administration, the dose, and the frequency and duration of therapy

The dosage of an antibiotic must be designed to produce adequate bacteriocidal or bacteriostatic concentrations at the site of infection. The frequency of dosage must be sufficient to maintain appropriate concentrations at the site of infection for an appropriate length of time. The duration of treatment should be sufficient to eradicate the infection completely.

Each of these factors needs careful consideration in each individual patient. The guidelines on dosages in the Pharmacopoeia indicate the usual dosage ranges, but adjustments must be made according to age, weight, renal and hepatic function, and the severity of the infection. In severe infections in hospital dosage schedules may be guided by the MIC of the antibiotic against the offending organism.

Take, for example, the use of amoxycillin in different circumstances. An uncomplicated *E. coli* urinary tract infection in a young woman may be treated effectively with two 3 g doses of amoxycillin spaced 10–12 h apart. On the other hand, an episode of acute bronchitis associated with *H. influenzae* or *Strep. pneumoniae* may require amoxycillin in a dose of 250–500 mg t.d.s. for a week or more.

Or take the treatment of infective endocarditis due to 'viridans' streptococci. Assuming the organism is sensitive to benzylpenicillin in a concentration of 0.2 mg/mL, a usual initial regimen would be benzylpenicillin 7.2 g (12 million i.u.) daily i.v. (in four divided doses), together with gentamicin 5 mg/kg body weight daily,

∎ **Table 22.6** Drug interactions with antibiotics

Antibiotic	Interacting drug	Mechanism	Effect
Gentamicin	Frusemide	Additive	Ototoxicity
Gentamicin	Ethacrynic acid	Additive	Ototoxicity
Chloramphenicol	Warfarin	Inhibition of metabolism	Potentiation of anticoagulation
Quinolones	Theophylline	Inhibition of metabolism	Reduced clearance of theophylline
Isoniazid (slow acetylators)	Phenytoin	Inhibition of metabolism	Phenytoin toxicity
Metronidazole	Warfarin	Inhibition of metabolism	Potentiation of anticoagulation
Metronidazole	Alcohol	Inhibition of aldehyde dehydrogenase	'Disulfiram reaction'
Rifampicin	Warfarin	Induction of metabolism	Diminished effect of warfarin
Rifampicin	Oestrogens (oral contraceptives)	Induction of metabolism	Decreased contraceptive effect
Tetracycline	Antacids	Chelation	Decreased effect of tetracycline
Tetracycline	Warfarin	Altered clotting factor activity	Potentiation of anticoagulation

divided into two doses given at 12-hourly intervals i.v. if renal function is normal. However, there are various opinions as to how this treatment should be continued thereafter. If the organism is very sensitive to penicillin and the patient is not very ill, some physicians would discontinue the gentamicin after a week and continue the benzylpenicillin for four weeks. Others would discontinue the gentamicin after a week and change from i.v. benzylpenicillin to oral amoxycillin plus probenecid. Others more conservative would continue with both drugs for a full four weeks. Whichever regimen is adopted, treatment should be based upon the MICs of the organism, adequate plasma or serum concentrations of the antibiotic (i.e. serum bacteriocidal activity), avoidance of gentamicin toxicity, and the patient's clinical condition, which must be carefully monitored, in order to anticipate the need for cardiac valve replacement.

(g) Consider the use of adjunctive drugs

In some cases it may be possible to increase the efficacy of an antibiotic by adding other types of drugs.

(i) Probenecid

Probenecid is an organic acid which competes with penicillins for tubular secretion in the kidney (see p. 131). It thus inhibits the excretion of penicillins and can be used to prolong their action. This has been particularly helpful in the treatment of gonorrhoea with a single dose of penicillin (in order to circumvent the problem of poor compliance) and in maintaining adequate plasma penicillin concentrations in the treatment of infective endocarditis.

(ii) Clavulanic acid

Clavulanic acid is an inhibitor of penicillinase, and if it is given in combination with a penicillinase-sensitive penicillin it will make it penicil-linase-resistant, thus broadening its antibacterial spectrum to include *S. aureus*, and a wider range of Gram-negative and anaerobic organisms. Clavulanic acid has been marketed in combination with amoxycillin as co-amoxiclav (Augmentin®) and with ticarcillin (Timentin®).

(iii) Imipenem + cilastin

Imipenem is a carbapenem antibiotic related to the penicillins; it is used in combination with cilastin, a dipeptidase inhibitor. Imipenem is a broad-spectrum antibiotic with activity against a large range of organisms, including staphylococci, *Ps. aeruginosa*, *Listeria monocytogenes*, and enterococci; it is resistant to β-lactamases. However, it is inactivated by a renal dipeptidase, dihydropeptidase I, which is in turn inhibited by cilastin. Thus, cilastin reduces the rate of renal clearance of imipenem and increases the concentrations of imipenem in the urine to above the MIC for most infective organisms. The half-time of imipenem is not prolonged by cilastin, because the systemic clearance is reduced.

(iv) Centoxin

In patients with severe Gram-negative septicaemias, in which there is a circulating lipopolysaccharide endotoxin derived from the infective organism, the antilipopolysaccharide monoclonal immunoglobulin, centoxin, given as a single intravenous dose, has been found to be effective in reducing mortality. It is currently available on a limited basis and is very expensive, but it may be life-saving in selected cases.

22.2 Chemotherapy of viral infections

Until recently the only therapeutic approach to viral illnesses was to attempt to prevent them. Immunization has been very effective for smallpox, measles, rubella, poliomyelitis, and yellow fever. Although immunization against influenza viruses is effective, the influenza virus changes its antigenic properties so frequently and unpredict-

■ **Table 22.7**   Antiviral drugs

Acyclovir
Amantadine
Ganciclovir
Idoxuridine (p. 616)
Inosine pranobex
Interferons
Tribavirin
Vidarabine
Zidovudine (p. 717)

---

ably that it is difficult to provide effective vaccines to order.

During the past few years important chemotherapeutic agents have been produced which are effective, albeit of limited usefulness, and which pave the way for further advances. These drugs are listed in Table 22.7.

22.2.1 Mechanisms of action of antiviral drugs

Most of the commonly used antiviral drugs are analogues of nucleosides and are converted by intracellular kinases to active phosphorylated derivatives, mono-, bis-, and triphosphates (nucleotides). These nucleotides have a variety of effects on DNA and RNA synthesis and replication.

(a) Acyclovir

Acyclovir is a nucleoside which enters all cells and is phosphorylated by intracellular kinases to active phosphorylated derivatives (nucleotides) which inhibit DNA polymerase, thus blocking viral replication. The triphosphate is also incorporated into viral DNA, thus blocking DNA chain prolongation. Acyclovir has a much greater affinity for viral kinases than for human kinases, and because of the selectivity of its activation it has a high therapeutic index compared with idoxuridine and vidarabine.

Acyclovir is active when applied topically, and is used as an ointment in the treatment of *Herpes simplex* eye infections. It also has some activity when used topically as a cream in herpetic labial and genital lesions if started early. In the prevention of recurrent genital *Herpes simplex* infection acyclovir can be given orally, as tablets or a suspension. If started within 72 h of the onset of infection high-dose oral acyclovir is also effective in the treatment of shingles, particularly in patients with severe pain. Acyclovir is also available for i.v. administration in the treatment of systemic infections caused by *H. simplex* and *H. zoster*.

(b) Ganciclovir

Ganciclovir is a nucleoside, a guanine derivative, which is phosphorylated by intracellular kinases to nucleotides which inhibit DNA polymerase and block DNA prolongation. It is used to treat severe cytomegalovirus (CMV) infections in immunocompromized patients (for example patients with AIDS or who are taking immuno-suppressive drugs), and is particularly used for CMV retinitis and pneumonia. It is given in a dose of 5 mg/kg by i.v. infusion over 1 h repeated every 12 h for 14–21 days. This initial therapy may be followed by maintenance therapy (for example in patients at risk of relapse of CMV retinitis) in a dose of 6 mg/kg daily for 5 days of the week or 5 mg/kg daily.

Ganciclovir is cytotoxic and may cause neutro-penia, thrombocytopenia, anaemia, and impaired fertility. Its other adverse effects include rash, nausea, vomiting, and diarrhoea, fever, phlebitis at the infusion site, confusion, seizures, and abnormal liver function tests. It should not be given in pregnancy.

(c) Idoxuridine

Idoxuridine is a nucleoside structurally similar to thymidine and it is phosphorylated by intracellular kinases to active nucleotides, which inhibit DNA polymerase. However, in contrast to acy-clovir and ganciclovir (see above) it does not block DNA synthesis and its main action is by its incorporation into viral DNA, making it more susceptible to breakage and faulty transcription. Nor is idoxuridine specific for viral DNA, and it can therefore cause bone-marrow suppression with neutropenia when used systemically. It is therefore be used locally for *Herpes simplex* infections of the eye, skin, and external genitalia, and also for the skin lesions of *Herpes zoster*.

(d) Tribavirin

Tribavirin (ribavirin) is a nucleoside structurally related to guanosine. It is activated by intracellular kinases, and interferes with mRNA function and inhibits viral RNA polymerase. It is used by inhalation in the treatment of infants and children with bronchiolitis due to the respiratory syncytial virus and has also been used intravenously for Lassa fever.

Inhaled tribavirin is given via a small-particle aerosol generator for 12–18 h daily for at least 3 and not more than 7 d. Given in this way it has few adverse effects, but may cause impaired res-piration and pneumothorax and may increase the risk of bacterial pneumonia; it should not be used in pregnancy.

(e) Vidarabine

Vidarabine is a nucleoside (adenosine arabino-side) which is phosphorylated by intracellular kinases to a triphosphate which inhibits DNA polymerase and therefore DNA synthesis. It inhibits DNA synthesis in all cells, producing bone-marrow suppression, but is more specific for viral DNA than for host cell DNA.

Vidarabine is used systemically for the treat-ment of chicken-pox and *H. zoster* infections in immunosuppressed patients, in whom such infec-tions are life-threatening, and as topical therapy in the treatment of *H. simplex* infections of the eye. It has also been used to treat *H. simplex* encephalitis.

(f) Zidovudine

Zidovudine (azidothymidine, AZT) is discussed in the section on sexually transmitted diseases (p. 254).

(g) Amantadine

Amantadine is active against RNA viruses, of which influenza A virus is the most important. It is thought that it inhibits viral uncoating within the cell. To be effective amantadine has to be taken prophylactically against influenza A infec-tion, and it must therefore be given during the whole course of an epidemic, for perhaps 8 weeks or so. It accumulates in renal failure, and dosages should be reduced. Adverse effects, such as confu-sion, depression, insomnia, and agitation are not uncommon, and although usually mild they can be a nuisance in old people. Amantadine has therefore never become popular. It was during trials of its prophylactic effect against influenza

A that its anti-Parkinsonian effect (see p. 430) was discovered.

22.2.2 The uses of antiviral drugs

The uses of the antiviral drugs are mentioned under the several headings in the previous section and their modes of administration and current uses are summarized in Table 22.8.

22.3 Chemotherapy of protozoal infections

Because of increased international travel it is not uncommon in the UK to encounter patients with malaria, amoebiasis, and giardiasis, and an acquaintance with the therapy of these diseases is important, although facility in its application requires experience. For this reason, when an imported protozoal infection which is uncommon in local medical practice occurs, expert advice should be sought.

The drugs used in the treatment of protozoal infections are listed in Table 22.9.

22.3.1 Mechanisms of action of antimalarial drugs

In Fig. 22.2 is shown the life-cycle of the malaria parasite (*Plasmodium*) and the sites of action of the various antimalarial drugs. The molecular mechanisms of the actions of these drugs are still obscure. Their selective toxicity probably depends either on their concentration by the parasite, or on their binding to high-affinity binding sites in the parasite. Proguanil, pyrimethamine, the sulphonamides, and the sulphones interfere with folic acid production and therefore inhibit parasitic nucleic acid synthesis.

22.3.2 Drug treatment of malaria

The aims of therapy in malaria are the preservation of life in severe acute infections, the elimination of parasitaemia in the acute attack, and the prevention of infection in areas of risk.

(a) Malarial attacks in adults infected by *Plasmodium vivax*, *Plasmodium ovale*, or *Plasmodium malariae*

Oral treatment with chloroquine is usually sufficient, unless the patient cannot take it.

■ **Table 22.8** Routes of administration of antiviral drugs and their indications

Drug	Route of administration	Indication
Acyclovir	3% eye ointment	*H. simplex* keratitis
	5% cream	*H. simplex* labialis or genitalis
	Oral (early treatment)	*H. simplex* labialis or genitalis and *H. zoster* infections (primary infections and prevention of recurrence)
	i.v.	Systemic *H. simplex* and *H. zoster* infections; acute *H. simplex* and *H. zoster* infections in immunocompromized patients
Amantadine	Oral	Prophylaxis of influenza
Ganciclovir	i.v. infusion	CMV infections in immunocompromized patients
Idoxuridine	1% eye-drops	*H. simplex* keratitis
	0.1% paint	Oral herpes
	5% in dimethyl sulphoxide	*H. simplex* and *H. zoster* of skin (must be started early)
Inosine pranobex	Oral	Mucocutaneous *H. simplex* infections; genital warts
Tribavirin	Aerosol	Severe respiratory syncytial virus bronchiolitis
Vidarabine	3% eye ointment	*H. simplex* keratitis
	i.v.	Chicken pox and *H. zoster* infections in immunosuppressed patients
Zidovudine	Oral	HIV infection

■ **Table 22.9** Drugs used in the treatment of protozoal infections

1. *Drug therapy of malaria*
Treatment	*Prophylaxis*
Chloroquine (p. 580)	Chloroquine
Quinine (p. 672)	Proguanil
Primaquine	Pyrimethamine + dapsone (Maloprim®) (p. 593)
Pyrimethamine + sulphonamide	Mefloquine
Tetracycline	

2. *Drug therapy of amoebiasis*
   Metronidazole (p. 635)
   Tinidazole
   Diloxanide furoate

3. *Drug therapy of giardiasis*
   Metronidazole
   Tinidazole
   Mepacrine (rarely needed)

4. *Drug therapy of trichomonal infections*
   Metronidazole

5. *Drug therapy of leishmaniasis*
   Sodium stilbogluconate
   Meglumine antimoniate
   Pentamidine

First day: chloroquine base 10 mg/kg followed in 6–8 h by chloroquine base 5 mg/kg.
Second day: chloroquine base 5 mg/kg.
Third day: chloroquine base 5 mg/kg.
Days 4–18: primaquine 7.5 mg b.d. to prevent relapse.

Relapse may occur in infection with *P. vivax* or *P. ovale*, because of persistent hepatic forms known as hypnozoites. In such cases follow a short-term course of antimalarials with a course of primaquine. Primaquine should not be used in pregnant women or in patients with G6PD deficiency. However, in areas in which mild variants of G6PD deficiency are common primaquine is given in a single dose of 45 mg weekly for 6 weeks.

(b) Uncomplicated *P. falciparum* malaria

Treatment depends on whether the local parasite is sensitive or resistant to chloroquine.

(i) Chloroquine-sensitive areas

Oral therapy is usually adequate in the doses given above and primaquine is not needed.

(ii) Chloroquine-resistant areas

Chloroquine resistance requires one to tailor the treatment to the known sensitivities in particular geographical areas. The continual emergence of resistant strains provides a perpetual problem in the effective treatment of malaria.

Oral therapy is usually adequate. Quinine salt 10 mg/kg is given every 8 h for 7 d. In areas of quinine resistance add tetracycline 250 mg q.d.s.; doxycycline may be used instead. However, remember that tetracyclines should not be given to pregnant women or children under 12 years of age; instead mefloquine may be used in a single dose of 15–25 mg/kg.

(c) Complicated attacks of *P. falciparum* malaria

Here one should start with parenteral treatment and switch to oral therapy when the patient can swallow.

(i) Chloroquine-sensitive areas

Give chloroquine 10 mg/kg by constant i.v. infusion over 8 h then 15 mg/kg over the next 24 h. Rapid i.v. administration is dangerous and if

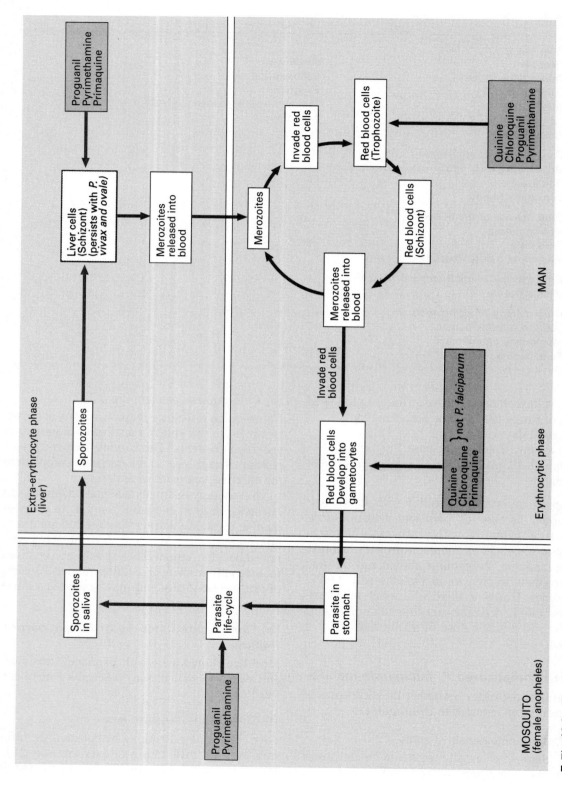

▪ **Fig. 22.2**   The life-cycle of the malaria parasite and the sites of action of antimalarial drugs.

slow infusion is not possible give 3.5 mg/kg by i.m. injection every 6 h until oral therapy can be taken.

(ii) Chloroquine-resistant areas

Give i.v. quinine salt 20 mg/kg by i.v. infusion over 4 h and then 10 mg/kg 8 hourly thereafter. When the patient can swallow, give oral quinine 10 mg/kg t.d.s. for a total of 7 d.

(iii) Treatment of complications in *P. falciparum* malaria

The principles complications in *P. falciparum* malaria are:

> cerebral malaria + convulsions
> blackwater fever (acute haemolysis + acute renal failure)
> acute pulmonary oedema
> hypoglycaemia
> lactic acidosis
> in pregnancy fetal death

The complications of *P. falciparum* malaria require prompt chemotherapy and full supportive treatment (maintenance of fluid and electrolyte balance, careful monitoring of blood glucose concentrations, anticonvulsants, renal dialysis, blood transfusion). Dexamethasone is not effective in the treatment of cerebral malaria and may in fact be deleterious.

22.3.3 Prevention of malaria

Because drug resistance varies with the geographical area, advice should be sought from the appropriate advisory body on which drug to use for which area. In the UK advice on special problems can be obtained by telephoning specialist centres (see the *British National Formulary* for details). Treatment should be started with the prophylactic drug before entering the area, and should be continued for 4 weeks after leaving it. The following drugs are recommended at the time of writing (1991) for the relevant areas:

(a) Areas in which chloroquine-resistant *P. falciparum* is absent

This currently includes parts of Asia (Afghanistan, Iran, Iraq, Maldives, Mauritius, Oman, Saudi Arabia, Syria, Yemen), North Africa (Algeria, Egypt, Libya, Morocco), and the Americas (Argentina, Belize, Costa Rica, El Salvador, Guatemala, Haiti, Honduras, Mexico, Nicaragua, and Paraguay).

> Chloroquine 300 mg once a week (short-term treatment)
> or proguanil 200 mg daily (long-term treatment).

(b) Areas in which chloroquine-resistant *P. falciparum* occurs, but is not widespread and is of low resistance to chloroquine

This currently includes some of China, parts of South Asia (Bangladesh, India, Nepal, Pakistan, Sri Lanka), most of Africa (south of the Sahara), and the jungle areas of South America (Brazil, Colombia, Ecuador, Peru). However, chloroquine resistance is spreading rapidly and it is not possible to generalize about which areas are affected at any time; up-to-date local advice will be needed.

> Chloroquine 300 mg once a week
> + proguanil 200 mg once a day.

(c) Areas in which highly chloroquine-resistant *P. falciparum* occurs

This currently includes parts of South-east Asia (Burma, Cambodia, Indonesia, Laos, Malaysia, Papua New Guinea, Philippines, Solomon Islands, Thailand, Vietnam).

> Chloroquine 300 mg once a week to prevent infection due to *P. vivax*.

During prophylactic treatment with chloroquine, febrile illnesses should be treated immediately with mefloquine on the presumption that they are due to *P. falciparum* malaria; in definite high-risk areas in which medical treatment might be delayed mefloquine should be added prophylactically in a dose of 250 mg/week.

Note that most major cities in East Asia are free of malaria and many seasoned travellers prefer to omit prophylaxis if their visits are to be confined to those cities.

22.3.4 Adverse effects of antimalarials

Serious adverse effects during the short-term treatment of malaria are uncommon and usually mild (see the Pharmacopoeia). However, hypersensitivity reactions may occur, and in individuals with G6PD deficiency acute haemolysis may result from treatment with primaquine or sulphonamides (see Chapter 8). Chloroquine commonly causes itching in dark-skinned patients, and this may be severe.

The most serious adverse effect of long-term chloroquine therapy is a retinopathy which is dose- and time-related (see p. 114), the risk being particularly high in those who have taken a cumulative total of 100 g or more. Patients should either have yearly ophthalmological assessment after they have been taking chloroquine for more than 5 years or they should switch to proguanil.

In the treatment of acute severe malaria quinine may cause hypoglycaemia, perhaps by stimulating the release of insulin from pancreatic beta cells via an effect on potassium channels.

22.3.5. Drug therapy of amoebiasis

(a) Mechanisms of action of amoebicides

Entamoeba histolytica exists in two forms:

(1) trophozoites, which are found in the stools of patients with active and acute amoebic dysentery;

(2) cysts, which are characteristically found in the stools of patients with chronic intestinal amoebiasis, whether or not they have symptoms.

Metronidazole and tinidazole are most active against trophozoites. Diloxanide furoate is active against cysts. Metronidazole is thought to act via a reduced derivative, which interferes with protozoal DNA function. The mechanism of action of diloxanide is unknown.

(b) Treatment of amoebiasis

(i) Acute amoebic dysentery

Metronidazole 800 mg t.d.s. for 5 d or tinidazole 2 g daily for 3 d, followed by diloxanide furoate 500 mg t.d.s. for 10 d (to eradicate cysts).

(ii) Cysts in stools with minimal or no symptoms

Diloxanide furoate 500 mg t.d.s. for 10 d.

(iii) Hepatic amoebiasis

Metronidazole 400 mg t.d.s. for 5 d or tinidazole 2 g daily for 3 d, followed by diloxanide furoate 500 mg t.d.s. for 10 d (to eradicate cysts in the intestine). Hepatic abscesses may require aspiration.

22.3.6 Drug therapy of giardiasis

Giardiasis is an infection of the duodenum and jejunum with the protozoan *Giardia lamblia*. The protozoan exists in two forms:

(1) trophozoites, which attach themselves to the small intestinal mucosa and somehow cause diarrhoea;

(2) cysts, which spread in the faeces and transmit the infection.

Chronic infection with *Giardia* may cause chronic diarrhoea, which may be associated with intestinal malabsorption.

Treatment is with metronidazole, 2 g daily orally for 3 d, or a single dose of tinidazole (2 g). This treatment may have to be repeated. The adverse effects of metronidazole include a metallic taste, nausea, vomiting, headache, discoloured urine, and dizziness. Patients should be warned not to drink alcohol and not to drive or handle complex and dangerous machinery. Tinidazole has similar adverse effects to metronidazole. Rarely, if these drugs fail, mepacrine (100 mg t.d.s. for 7 d) would be required. However, it has more severe adverse effects, including nausea, vomiting, yellow staining of the skin and sclera, skin rashes, psychosis, and blood dyscrasias.

22.3.7 Drug therapy of trichomonal infections

This is dealt with in the section on sexually transmitted diseases (p. 254).

22.3.8 Drug therapy of toxoplasmosis

Toxoplasmosis is caused by a protozoon, *Toxoplasma gondii*. It may be acquired or congenital. The acquired form is usually mild and asymptomatic. Occasionally, however, there is lymph gland enlargement, sometimes with spleen and liver enlargement, headache, fever, and a rash.

Treatment of acquired toxoplasmosis is necessary only in severe cases, which should be treated with oral pyrimethamine 25–50 mg t.d.s. for 3–5 d, followed by pyrimethamine 25–50 mg daily plus sulphadiazine 4–6 g daily for 3–4 weeks. Pyrimethamine may cause leucopenia and thrombocytopenia, in which case treatment should be withdrawn and folinic acid (15 mg daily) given. Spiramycin (500 mg q.d.s. for 3 weeks) is an alternative to pyrimethamine, particularly in pregnancy, since pyrimethamine in high dosages is theoretically teratogenic during the first trimester. However, spiramycin is not suitable for patients with ocular involvement. Sulphadiazine should not be used in late pregnancy (see p. 155).

22.3.9 Drug therapy of leishmaniasis

Leishmaniasis is caused by protozoa of the genus *Leishmania*. They all respond to treatment with a pentavalent antimony salt (either sodium stilbogluconate or meglumine antimoniate) or pentamidine. The antimonials are given in a dose of 10–20 mg/kg i.v. or i.m. once or twice daily and pentamidine in a dose of 4 mg/kg i.m. weekly. Most types of infection will respond to treatment for 3–6 weeks, although in some cases longer periods may be required. There is evidence that the combination of a pentavalent antimonial with γ-interferon is more effective than an antimonial alone, but this is not yet a licensed indication for interferon.

In low doses the pentavalent antimonials have few adverse effects. In high doses they may cause anorexia, nausea, vomiting, malaise, muscle pains, liver damage, anaemia, and cardiac arrhythmias. Intravenous injections may cause venous thrombosis and intramuscular injections are painful.

Pentamidine may cause severe hypotension after injection, particularly i.v., and it should be given by deep intramuscular injection, with the patient recumbent, and with careful blood pressure monitoring. Intramuscular injection is painful and may cause muscle necrosis and abscess formation. Other adverse effects include nausea and vomiting, hypocalcaemia, blood dyscrasias (leucopenia, thrombocytopenia, and anaemia),

renal failure, cardiac arrhythmias, hyper- and hypoglycaemia, and pancreatitis.

22.4 Chemotherapy of helminthic infections

The drugs used in the treatment of helminthic infections are listed in Table 22.10. These drugs are not discussed in the Pharmacopoeia. For information consult the *British National Formulary* or the manufacturers' literature. Other drugs are available for the infections listed, but the drugs listed are usually the first choices in the UK.

22.5 Chemotherapy of trematode infections

Many trematode infections respond to treatment with praziquantel, including schistomiasis, liver fluke infections (for example opisthorchiasis, clonorchiasis, and fascioliasis), intestinal infections (for example fasciolopsiasis and echinostomiasis), and lung fluke infections (paragonimiasis).

In schistosomiasis praziquantel is given in a single dose of 40 mg/kg (*S. mansoni* and *S. haematobium*) or in three doses of 20 mg/kg (*S. japonicum*). For liver fluke infections it is given in a dosage of 25 mg/kg t.d.s. for one or two days. For intestinal infections it is given in a single dose of 15 mg/kg last thing at night. For lung fluke infections it is given in a dosage of 25 mg/kg t.d.s. for two or three days.

Adverse effects of praziquantel include nausea and abdominal discomfort, fever, sweating, and sedation.

22.6 Chemotherapy of fungal infections

The drugs used in the treatment of fungal infections are listed in Table 22.11 and their pharmacological properties are discussed in the Pharmacopoeia.

In Tables 22.12 and 22.13 are shown the indications and routes of administration. Adverse

■ **Table 22.10** Drug therapy of infestations

Worm	Drug	Comments
Ascariasis (roundworm)	Pyrantel	Useful in multiple infections; use with caution in liver disease; occasional nausea
	Mebendazole	Teratogenic in animals: avoid in pregnancy
	Levamisole	Occasional blood dyscrasias
	Piperazine	Very cheap and effective; nausea, vomiting, diarrhoea
	Pyrantel	As above
Trichuriasis (whipworm)	Mebendazole	As above
	Albendazole	Avoid in pregnancy
Ankylostomiasis (hookworm)	Mebendazole	As above
	Albendazole	As above
	Bephenium	Cheap; nausea and vomiting
Strongyloidiasis	Thiabendazole	As above
Enterobiasis (threadworm or pinworm)	Piperazine	As above
	Mebendazole	As above
	Pyrantel	As above
Taenia saginata (tapeworm)	Praziquantel	Occasional nausea and abdominal pain
	Niclosamide	Gastrointestinal discomfort
Taenia solium	Praziquantel	As above
	Niclosamide	As above
Cysticercosis	Praziquantel	As above
	Albendazole	As above

■ **Table 22.11** Drugs used in the treatment of fungal infections

Amphotericin (p. 555)
Flucytosine
Griseofulvin (p. 611)
Imidazoles (p. 558)
   Clotrimazole
   Econazole
   Fluconazole
   Itraconazole
   Ketoconazole
   Miconazole
   Tioconazole
Nystatin (p. 654)

effects and dosages are listed in the Pharmacopoeia.

The following points should be noted in using these drugs.

1. Drug interactions due to enzyme induction may occur with griseofulvin.

2. Amphotericin has a low toxic:therapeutic ratio and dosages must be carefully adjusted, with frequent monitoring of renal function and plasma potassium concentrations. Amphotericin penetrates the CSF poorly.

3. The most important adverse effect of flucytosine is bone-marrow suppression, which is dose-related.

4. Imidazoles (particularly ketoconazole) (see Table 22.11) can cause hepatic dysfunction and liver damage and can cause drug interactions by enzyme inhibition.

22.7 Prevention of infections using vaccines and immunoglobulins

22.7.1 Vaccines

The term 'vaccine' was originally used to describe the extract of cowpox (Latin *vacca* = cow) used

■ **Table 22.12** Preferred antifungal therapy for superficial my

	Topical amphotericin	Topical clotrimazole	Topical miconazole	Topical econazole	Topical nystatin	Oral griseofulvin	Oral ketoconazole	
Candidiasis								
Skin	+ +	+ +	+ +	+ +	+ +	−	+[1]	[1]Chronic mucocutaneous candidiasis.
Mouth	+ +	−	+	−	+	−	+[2]	[2]Not responding to local therapy or chronic and recurrent.
Vagina	+	+ +	+ +	+ +	+ +	−	+[2]	[2]Not responding to local therapy or chronic and recurrent.
Dermatophytes								
Tinea cruris, Tinea pedis, Tinea corporis, Tinea capitis	−	+ +	+ +	+ +	−	+ +	+ +	Don't forget Whitfield's ointment for local lesions. If at all severe use griseofulvin. Ketoconazole is also active, but is not useful for nail infections.
Tinea versicolor (pityriasis)	−	+	+	+	−	−	+ +	2% selenium sulphide or 20% sodium hyposulphate also used.

■ **Table 22.13** Drug therapy of some systemic mycoses

	Amphotericin B, i.v.	Flucytosine, oral or i.v.	Miconazole, i.v. or oral	Ketoconazole, oral	Fluconazole, oral or i.v.	Itraconazole, oral
Systemic candidiasis	+*	+	+	+	+	
Histoplasmosis	+*			+		
Coccidioidomycosis	+*		+	+		
Blastomycosis	+*			?		
Cryptococcosis (meningitis)	+*	+*			+	+
Systemic aspergillosis**	+*					?

*First choice.
Cryptococcal meningitis: combine amphotericin with flucytosine.
?=under investigation.
**Not aspergilloma or allergic bronchopulmonary aspergillosis.

to inoculate against smallpox in the eighteenth century. However, it is now used to describe any formulation used for active immunization against any infectious disease.

Vaccines are available for immunization against both bacterial and viral infections and are of three types.

1. Live organisms given in attenuated form.

2. Inactivated organisms.

3. Extracts of organisms or exotoxins produced by organisms (toxoids).

Live organisms usually require to be given in only a single dose. They produce immunity lasting almost as long as that of a natural infection. This group includes vaccines against tuberculosis (BCG), influenza, measles, poliomyelitis (oral formulation), rubella, smallpox, and yellow fever.

Inactivated organisms usually require an initial series of injections to stimulate antibody production, and booster doses may be required at later times. This group includes cholera, pertussis, hepatitis B, poliomyelitis (subcutaneous and intramuscular formulations), rabies, and typhoid.

Toxoids require schedules similar to those for inactivated organisms. This group includes diphtheria and tetanus.

(a) Schedules of immunization

A list of commonly used vaccines is given in Table 22.14, showing their sources and usual times of initial administration. In the UK the Department of Health has laid down a recommended schedule of administration for many of these vaccines, and an outline is given in Table 22.15.

Recommendations on vaccination before travel abroad are issued by government agencies. A set of recommendations is summarized in Table 22.16, but requirements change from time to time and it is always best to obtain up-to-date information locally (for the UK see the *British National Formulary*).

(b) Adverse effects of vaccines

Reactions at the site of injection of a vaccine are very common, and often provide evidence of a good antibody response. When this occurs, there will in most cases be some local swelling and inflammation; in some cases there may also be local lymph node enlargement, and occasionally this may be accompanied by fever, headache, and general malaise, lasting for up to a few days.

Hypersensitivity reactions may occur with vaccines made from viruses grown in chick or duck embryos (for example influenza and measles vaccines), and it is important to ask about hypersensitivity to eggs before giving these vaccines. However, measles vaccine may be used, even in those with a history of hypersensitivity reactions to eggs, except in cases of previous anaphylactoid reactions; hypersensitivity to chickens' feathers does not constitute a contra-indication.

For vaccines which contain antibiotics or animal serum (for example neomycin in rubella and poliomyelitis vaccines), hypersensitivity reactions are a theoretical risk. However, these vaccines need only be withheld from those who give a history of severe allergic reactions.

Care should be taken when vaccinating patients who have allergic disorders, such as eczema or asthma. Smallpox vaccine (which may still be indicated for laboratory workers handling pox viruses) should never be given to individuals with eczema, because of the risk of vaccinatum gangrenosum.

Vaccines containing live organisms may cause severe local reactions, or even systemic infections in patients with infections and other acute febrile illnesses, and in patients whose immune responsiveness is impaired for any reason (for example due to disease, radiotherapy, or drugs, see below). Live vaccines should therefore not generally be used in such patients. However, in patients with HIV infection all vaccines except BCG and yellow fever may be used.

Pertussis vaccine has been reported to have caused on rare occasions neurological complications resulting in convulsions and permanent brain damage. Despite past controversy it is generally felt that the benefit of immunization outweighs the risk of complications in most cases. However, if a child has had a severe local or general reaction on one occasion pertussis vaccine should not be given again. Furthermore, the vaccine should not be given to a child with a history of a disorder of the central nervous system or who has an acute infection at the time.

■ **Table 22.14** Immunization schedules

Vaccine	Source	Usual times of administration
BCG	Live attenuated bovine *M. tuberculosis*	Age 10–14 years (if tuberculin-negative)
Cholera	Killed *Vibrio cholerae*	Before entering an endemic zone; 6-monthly in endemic zones
Diphtheria	Toxoid, prepared from toxin of *C. diphtheriae*	First dose at 3 months, second dose 6–8 weeks later, third dose 4–6 months later
Tetanus	Toxoid, prepared from toxin of *C. tetani*	First dose at 3 months, second dose 6–8 weeks later, third dose 4–6 months later
Pertussis	Killed *Bordetella pertussis*	First dose at 3 months, second dose 6–8 weeks later, third dose 4–6 months later
Hepatitis A	Normal immunoglobulin	Before entering an endemic zone
Hepatitis B	Hepatitis B surface antigen (biosynthetic)	When risk of infection is high; at birth in endemic areas
Influenza	Live attenuated influenza viruses (grown in chick embryos)	In high-risk patients when infection is anticipated
Japanese B encephalitis	Inactivated virus	Before entering an endemic zone
Measles	Live attenuated measles virus (grown in chick embryos)	Age 2 years
Meningococcus	Polysaccharide from *Neisseria meningitidis*	Before entering an endemic zone
Mumps	Live attenuated mumps virus (grown in chick embryos)	Age 2 years
Poliomyelitis	(a) Live attenuated polio virus (oral)	As for diphtheria, tetanus, and pertussis
	(b) Inactivated polio virus	If live vaccine contra-indicated (for example pregnancy and immune suppression)
Rabies	Inactivated rabies virus	After an infection (combined with antirabies immunoglobulin) and when the risk of infection is high
Rubella	Live attenuated rubella virus	Girls aged 10–13 years and women of child-bearing age (if seronegative for rubella)
Smallpox	Live attenuated smallpox	Research workers studying pox virus
Typhoid	Killed *Salmonella typhi*	Before entering an endemic zone; every 2–3 years in endemic zones
Yellow fever	Live attenuated yellow fever virus	Before entering an endemic zone

Live vaccines should not in general be used in pregnancy. However, if a woman finds herself to be pregnant shortly after having been immunized, she should be reassured, since no cases of fetal abnormality have been attributed to vaccines in current use.

(c) Interactions with vaccines

Vaccines prepared from live organisms should not be given to patients taking cytotoxic chemo-therapy, because of the risks of severe local reactions, and even overwhelming systemic infection. Patients taking long-term corticosteroid therapy may be similarly at risk.

22.7.2 Immunoglobulins

Immunoglobulins are used to provide immediate protection against infection, but they confer passive immunity and their effects last for only 1–6 months.

■ **Table 22.15** Recommended immunization schedules in the UK

Time	Vaccine(s)	Comments
First year	Diphtheria/tetanus/pertussis	Pertussis may be omitted if
	Poliomyelitis	contra-indicated or refused
2 years old	Measles/mumps/rubella	
On first going to school	Diphtheria/tetanus	At least 3 years after first course
	Poliomyelitis	At least 3 years after first course
	Measles/mumps/rubella	Unless previously immunized or contra-indicated
10–14 years old	BCG	If tuberculin negative
	Rubella	Girls only
On leaving school	Poliomyelitis	
	Tetanus	
Adults	Poliomyelitis	If not previously immunized and travelling to an endemic area or own child being immunized
	Rubella	Women, if seronegative; exclude pregnancy first and avoid pregnancy for 3 months
	Tetanus	If unvaccinated for 5 years

■ **Table 22.16** Recommended immunization for travellers

Region[1]	Immunization[2]
S. Europe	Poliomyelitis
Central and S. America	Yellow fever, typhoid, polio, hepatitis[3], rabies[4]
Middle East and N. Africa	Typhoid, polio, cholera, rabies, hepatitis
Central Africa, E. Africa, and W. Africa	Yellow fever, typhoid, polio, hepatitis[3], rabies[4]
S. Africa	Typhoid, polio, hepatitis[3]
Indian subcontinent, China, and S. E. Asia	Typhoid, polio, rabies, hepatitis[3], Japanese B encephalitis in some areas

[1]Precautions are not necessary for travel in N. Europe, N. America, Japan, Australia, and New Zealand.

[2]Malaria prophylaxis should also be considered for all the areas listed in the table, except for S. Europe and S. Africa to the south of Johannesburg.

[3]Gamma globulin is sometimes given to short-term visitors as passive immunization against hepatitis A.

[4]Antirabies immunization is not always necessary, but should be offered to travellers to primitive areas or if medical facilities will not be available.

(a) Normal immunoglobulin

Normal immunoglobulin is gamma globulin prepared from normal human plasma. It is used in short-term prophylaxis against and in the modification of infective hepatitis (A and B) and measles, and in the prevention of rubella in women exposed to infection. It is also used in the treatment of hypogammaglobulinaemia. Its effects last for 4–6 months.

The recommended dosages of the 16 per cent solution are as follows:

Infective hepatitis: 0.02–0.04 mL/kg i.m. as routine prophylaxis; 0.06–0.12 mL/kg i.m. in circumstances in which the risk of infection is high.

Measles: 0.02 mL/kg i.m. within 5 d of exposure.

Rubella: (in pregnant women) 20 mL i.m. as soon as possible after exposure.

(b) Specific immunoglobulins

Immunoglobulins for specific disorders are prepared from the plasma of patients who have had the disorders. They include immunoglobulins for the prevention of rhesus incompatibility, for short-term prophylaxis of hepatitis B, measles, pertussis, rabies, tetanus, and vaccinia infections, and in an attempt to prevent these infections after exposure.

Recently it has been shown that a single injection of a monoclonal antibody directed against the lipopolysaccharide that constitutes the endotoxin of Gram-negative bacteria can reduce the mortality from Gram-negative septicaemia (see p. 240).

(c) Important adverse effects of immunoglobulins

Hypersensitivity reactions may occur and occasionally result in anaphylaxis. Pain and tenderness at the site of immunization are common.

Anti-D (rhesus negative) immunoglobulin should not be given to rhesus-positive or rhesus-immunized patients, since it may cause haemolysis.

Immunoglobulin may impair the efficacy of live vaccines (excluding yellow fever). Vaccines for measles, mumps, rubella, and poliomyelitis (oral) should not be given within 3 months of immunoglobulin.

22.8 The drug treatment of sexually transmitted diseases

The drugs used in the treatment of sexually transmitted diseases are listed in Table 22.17.

22.8.1 Syphilis

The drug of choice in all forms of syphilis is a penicillin, and procaine penicillin (600 mg i.m. daily) or oral benzathine penicillin (10 mL q.d.s.) are the formulations of choice. The duration of treatment should be 10 days in primary and secondary syphilis, 14 d in early and late latent syphilis, and 21 d in cardiovascular or neurosyphilis. The alternatives, in patients with penicillin allergy, are erythromycin (1 g orally b.d. for 2 weeks) or tetracycline (500 mg orally q.d.s. for 2 weeks).

In addition to the usual risk of penicillin hypersensitivity there is an additional risk in early syphilis of the Jarisch–Herxheimer reaction. This is a systemic reaction which is thought to be due to the release of endotoxin from killed spirochaetes. It comes on within a few hours of the first injection of penicillin and lasts for up to a day. It consists of fever, flushing, tachycardia, myalgia, and hypotension. It is rare in late syphilis, but when it occurs it can cause progression of neurosyphilis or exacerbation of the local effects of gummata. Pretreatment with prednisolone, 40 mg, on the day before treatment and in subsequently decreasing doses can mitigate the effects. Aspirin may give symptomatic relief.

Asymptomatic sexual contacts of syphilitic patients should be traced and treated. Patients should be warned to avoid sexual intercourse for 2 weeks.

22.8.2 Gonococcal infections

(a) Gonorrhoea

A single dose of a penicillin is the treatment of choice in most cases of uncomplicated gonorrhoea, for example ampicillin (2 g orally) plus probenecid (1 g orally). In penicillin allergy or for penicillin-resistant organisms the alternatives are:

co-trimoxazole, 4 tablets b.d. for 2 d, or 5 tablets repeated after 8 h, or 8 tablets as a single dose;
spectinomycin, 2 g i.m. in men, 4 g i.m. in women as a single dose;
cefotaxime, 1.0 g i.m. as a single dose;
ciprofloxacin, 0.5 g orally as a single dose.

When gonorrhoea is complicated by pelvic inflammation or is affecting other organs, 2-week courses of a penicillin or one of its alternatives will be required.

■ **Table 22.17**   Drugs used in the treatment of sexually transmitted diseases

Disease	Anti-infective drug	Alternative
Syphilis	Procaine or benzathine penicillin	Erythromycin or tetracycline
Gonorrhoea	Ampicillin + probenecid	Co-trimoxazole, spectinomycin, ciprofloxacin
Non-gonococcal urethritis	Tetracycline	Erythromycin
HIV infection	Zidovudine	Didanosine

(b) Gonococcal conjunctivitis

Gonococcal conjunctivitis may be prevented in the new-born child of an infected mother by the use of silver nitrate eye-drops (1 per cent) immediately after delivery. However, this treatment may cause a chemical conjunctivitis, and many doctors prefer to treat only those in whom infection has occurred.

In an established infection penicillin eye-drops should be given 4-hourly plus procaine penicillin 300 000 i.u./day i.m. for 5 d.

Chloramphenicol ointment, 1 per cent applied 4-hourly, is an alternative to penicillin eye-drops.

22.8.3 Non-gonococcal urethritis

Non-gonococcal (or 'non-specific') urethritis is most commonly caused by *Chlamydia trachomatis* or *Ureaplasma urealyticum* organisms. Both are sensitive to tetracyclines and erythromycin. The dosages are oxytetracycline 250 mg orally q.d.s. or chlortetracycline 300 mg b.d. for 2 weeks, and erythromycin 500 mg orally b.d. for 2 weeks. In pregnancy use erythromycin.

22.8.4 *Trichomonas vaginalis* infection

Trichomonas vaginalis most commonly causes vaginitis and sometimes urethritis. Treatment is with metronidazole, and various dosage regimens are recommended, good compliance being most likely with the first of the following.

1. Metronidazole in a single dose of 2 g. Sexual partners should be treated also.

2. Metronidazole 800 g in the morning and 1.2 g at night for 2 d.

3 Metronidazole 200 mg t.d.s. for 7 d.

22.8.5 The acquired immune deficiency syndrome (AIDS), AIDS-related complex (ARC), and asymptomatic HIV infections

Infection with the human immunodeficiency virus (HIV) eventually leads to disease through increasing immunosuppression, and usually results in the clinical condition of AIDS. Early problems include thrombocytopenia, *Herpes zoster*, and oropharyngeal candidiasis. As immunosuppression advances, the individual is at increasing risk of a variety of opportunistic infections and tumours. Many of the infections, such as *Pneumocystis carinii* pneumonia and *Toxoplasma* encephalitis, are treatable with standard drugs (for example see p. 246), but after acute treatment long-term antimicrobial therapy is required to prevent relapse.

Currently, zidovudine is the only licensed drug that has been shown to reduce the incidence of opportunistic infections and to prolong survival in patients with AIDS. It also delays the progression to AIDS in patients with symptomatic HIV disease (the so-called AIDS-related complex or ARC). It is not known whether it is of benefit to patients with asymptomatic HIV infection, and this is currently under study.

Zidovudine is a nucleoside analogue which is taken up by cells and phosphorylated by intracellular kinases to mono-, bis-, and triphosphates, which inhibit reverse transcriptase and block nucleic acid chain elongation. Its is more potent at doing this in viral cells than in human cells, but some of its adverse effects (for example on the bone-marrow) come from this action.

Zidovudine is usually given initially in a dosage of 500–1000 mg per day in 2–4 divided doses. Minor adverse effects, such as myalgia, headache, and insomnia, are common but usually subside within a few weeks. The most important problem is bone-marrow toxicity, and a macrocytic anaemia occurs in up to 25 per cent of patients taking the higher dosages. Reducing the dosage or withdrawing the drug usually reverses the anaemia, but if dosage reduction is not possible patients may require blood transfusions. Selected patients may benefit from erythropoietin.

Although zidovudine interacts with several other drugs, the clinical relevance of these is not clear. The important interactions are detailed in the Pharmacopoeia.

In patients taking long-term zidovudine, HIV cultured from the blood may show *in vitro* resistance to zidovudine. The clinical relevance of this is not yet clear, but it is widely recognized that the benefits of zidovudine wear off after a year or two, and the disease then progresses despite treatment. In these circumstances other drugs currently undergoing clinical trial, such as the reverse transcriptase inhibitor dideoxyinosine (didanosine), may have a role.

22.8.6 *Herpes* genitalis

Genital infections with *Herpes simplex* virus type 2 (and sometimes type 1) usually present with painful vesicles or ulcers. Occasionally women may have asymptomatic cervical herpes infection. Primary attacks are usually worse than recurrent ones and may be associated with systemic symptoms.

Treatment is usually with oral acyclovir, 200 mg 5 times a day for 5 d, but mild attacks will subside without specific therapy. For individuals with frequent recurrences prophylactic therapy (200–400 mg daily) may be justified. Alternatively, these patients may be given a course of tablets to be used to abort attacks as soon as the first symptoms occur.

22.8.7 Anaerobic vaginosis

Anaerobic vaginosis usually presents as a vaginal discharge, occasionally with pelvic discomfort. Although *Gardnerella vaginalis*, a coccobacillus, is often isolated, the condition is thought to be primarily due to anaerobic organisms. The usual treatment is with an imidazole, either metronidazole 200 mg 8-hourly for a week or tinidazole in a single dose of 2 g.

23 The drug therapy of cardiovascular disorders

Co-author: T.R. Cripps

23.1 Hypertension

Hypertension may either be of unknown cause (so-called 'essential') or secondary to some definite abnormality, for example renal parenchymal disease, renovascular disease, a variety of endocrine diseases, coarctation of the aorta, and drugs. In the majority of cases there is no underlying cause, but an underlying cause should always be sought and should be particularly actively pursued in young patients with severe hypertension resistant to therapy.

Where the primary abnormality can be reversed (for example renal artery stenosis, phaeochromocytoma) there may be no need to use drugs for long-term treatment of the hypertension. However, in many cases treatment of the underlying cause is not possible, and treatment of secondary hypertension generally follows the same principles as the treatment of essential hypertension. In the following discussion we shall deal principally with essential hypertension and note some special points about secondary forms of hypertension. A list of drugs which may commonly cause or exacerbate hypertension, or which may oppose the effects of antihypertensive drugs is given in Table 23.1.

Hypertension is usually asymptomatic. However, chronic hypertension has certain complications (cardiac failure, renal failure, stroke, and myocardial ischaemia). In addition, severe hypertension may be associated with necrotizing vascular changes, so-called 'malignant' or 'accelerated' hypertension. The sizes of the risks of these complications are known. For example, there is a 50 per cent increase in mortality from ischaemic heart disease in middle-aged men with a blood pressure of 140/95 mmHg, and the risks increase with increasing blood pressure (b.p.).

Although it is difficult to give precise definitions of degrees of severity of hypertension, a rough working guide is as follows (the diastolic pressures are phase V pressures):

> mild hypertension, b.p. 130/90−140/100 mmHg;
>
> moderate hypertension, b.p. 140/100−160/120 mmHg;
>
> severe hypertension, b.p. above 160/120 mmHg (although if there is severe retinopathy or nephropathy, hypertension should be considered to be severe, whatever the b.p.);
>
> hypertensive emergency, diastolic b.p. above 130 mmHg or if there is encephalopathy, whatever the b.p.

These values apply to adults in the age range 20–65 years (roughly). In young children increases in blood pressure to 160/110 mmHg (for example in acute glomerulonephritis) can result in accelerated hypertension. Conversely, people in their seventies may have no arteriolar damage with a blood pressure of 220/120 mmHg. In pregnancy the blood pressure normally tends to fall, and a value of 130/90 mmHg may constitute serious hypertension. Hard and fast rules are therefore difficult to apply. None the less, the individual doctor has to decide when to treat, and some guidance is necessary.

There is no doubt that the effective treatment of accelerated or malignant hypertension is lifesaving. The natural history of malignant hypertension is that 90 per cent of untreated patients die within a year. On the other hand, treated

■ **Table 23.1** Drugs which may commonly cause or exacerbate hypertension or oppose the effects of antihypertensives

1. By sodium and water retention
Sodium salts of drugs (for example sodium penicillin, sodium-containing antacids)
Steroids
   glucocorticoids
   mineralocorticoids
   oestrogens and progestogens (for example oral contraceptives)
Non-steroidal anti-inflammatory drugs (for example indomethacin)
Carbenoxolone

2. By vasoconstriction
Sympathomimetics (for example adrenaline, noradrenaline)
Monoamine oxidase (MAO) inhibitors (in interaction with vasoactive amines, such as dietary tyramine: the 'cheese reaction')

3. After withdrawal of antihypertensive drugs (rebound hypertension)
Clonidine (potentially dangerous)
α-Methyldopa
β-Adrenoceptor antagonists

patients have a similar prognosis to patients with chronic hypertension.

Lowering the blood pressure in patients with moderate or severe chronic hypertension considerably reduces the risk of stroke, renal failure, and cardiac failure, and may also reduce the risk of myocardial ischaemia. In such cases the benefit of treatment undoubtedly outweighs the risk of adverse drug effects. However, in people over 80 years of age little benefit has been shown and the adverse effects of treatment may be troublesome; in them the risks may outweigh the benefits.

However, in mild hypertension the case for antihypertensive drug therapy is still not absolutely proven. There is certainly evidence from large-scale clinical trials that the risks of the complications of mild hypertension are reduced by treatment. However, the morbidity and mortality among patients with mild hypertension without tissue damage is only slightly greater than those in the non-hypertensive population, and it is not clear that the benefit:risk ratio in the population is in favour of treatment, particularly because one can never tell whether or to what extent one is reducing the risks of complications in an individual patient, and whether the change in risk outweighs the risk of adverse

effects in that individual. Despite these uncertainties many doctors are now prescribing antihypertensive drugs for patients with mild hypertension without evidence of tissue damage. Although the value of doing this is debatable, one would certainly offer treatment to patients who have definite evidence of tissue damage, for example in the form of signs, such as left ventricular hypertrophy or failure, renal failure, or retinopathy, or of symptoms, such as a history of angina pectoris or symptoms of cerebral ischaemia, or to patients with certain high risk factors for arterial damage, such as diabetes, hyperlipidaemia, or a strong family history of vascular disease.

Antihypertensive therapy generally implies a lifelong commitment to drug therapy, and one should therefore be careful to ensure that the diagnosis is correct. This involves measurement of the blood pressure on at least three separate occasions after the patient has been resting for a few minutes. Repeated measurement is important, since the b.p. tends to fall on successive visits to the doctor.

If treatment is instituted, the aim in young and middle-aged patients should be to reduce the blood pressure to about 130/90 mmHg if possible.

23.1.1 Mechanisms of action of drugs used in hypertension

In Fig. 23.1 are shown the mechanisms involved in the actions of antihypertensive drugs, and in Table 23.2 are listed the various drugs used, arranged according to their mechanisms of action.

(a) Diuretics

The mechanism of action of the thiazide diuretics in hypertension is not yet understood and cannot be solely related to their effects on salt and water balance. More potent diuretics, such as frusemide, are not more potent antihypertensive drugs, and diazoxide, a chemically related compound causing sodium retention, is a powerful antihypertensive drug which acts by peripheral vasodilatation by opening potassium channels.

Although intravascular fluid volume and total body sodium fall during the first few weeks of diuretic therapy, there follows an increase in circulating renin, and within a few weeks the intravascular volume and sodium content return to normal, but the antihypertensive effect persists. It may be that diuretics act by a direct effect on vascular smooth muscle, causing vasodilatation. Such an effect could be mediated through a decrease in vessel wall sodium content or through an action on potassium channels.

(b) β-adrenoceptor antagonists (β-blockers)

The mechanism of action of the β-adrenoceptor antagonists is not fully understood. Currently favoured is the idea that they produce a fall in cardiac output, that the baroreflex mechanisms do not fully compensate for this, that the baroreflex receptors are reset, and so peripheral resistance falls. However, all the details of this suggested mechanism of action have not been worked out. Other hypotheses are that the β-adrenoceptor antagonists have a central effect, altering sympathetic tone (unlikely, since β-adrenoceptor antagonists which enter the brain relatively poorly, such as atenolol, are equally good antihypertensives), or that they inhibit renin release from the kidney.

(c) Vasodilators

Several drugs act as direct vasodilators of arterioles. The angiotensin converting enzyme (ACE) inhibitors, such as captopril and enalapril, act by reducing circulating concentrations of the vasoconstrictor angiotensin II, and to a lesser extent by increasing the concentrations of vasodilator kinins. They also reduce aldosterone production and thus decrease sodium retention. The calcium antagonists act by reducing calcium entry into cells via potential-operated calcium channels. Sodium nitroprusside probably acts by mimicking the action of the endogenous endothelium-derived relaxing factor (nitric oxide) on vascular smooth muscle. The mechanisms of action of other vasodilators, such as hydralazine, minoxidil, and diazoxide, which act directly on the arterioles, are not known, but some of them may act by stimulating potassium efflux from cells via potassium channels.

Since most of these drugs cause salt and water retention they are generally used in combination with a diuretic, although the ACE inhibitors can be used alone. Furthermore, since hydralazine causes a reflex tachycardia, its effects are enhanced by the concurrent administration of a β-adrenoceptor antagonist.

(d) α-adrenoceptor antagonists (α-blockers)

Certain drugs have direct vasodilatory actions on vascular smooth muscle by virtue of their inhibitory effects on α-adrenoceptors, and particularly postsynaptic (α_1)-adrenoceptors. Examples include prazosin and indoramin. Labetalol combines non-specific α-adrenoceptor and non-specific β-adrenoceptor antagonist actions.

(e) Drugs affecting the nervous control of blood pressure

These drugs act in diverse ways. Drugs which are α-adrenoceptor agonists act by stimulating α-adrenoceptors in the brain stem, and this causes a reduction in peripheral sympathetic nervous system function. It is thought that α-methyldopa acts in this way, by being converted in noradrenergic neurones to α-methylnoradrenaline, a potent α-adrenoceptor agonist. Clonidine has a similar action, in that it is a direct α-adrenoceptor agonist.

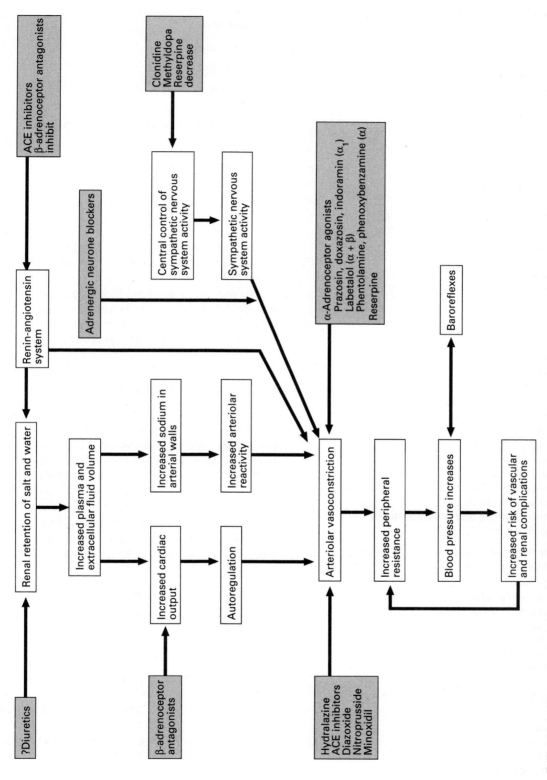

◼ **Fig. 23.1** The pathophysiology of hypertension and the sites and mechanisms of action of antihypertensive drugs.

■ **Table 23.2** Drugs used in the treatment of hypertension

1. *Diuretics*
   Thiazides (p. 695)
   Other thiazide-like diuretics
   Chlorthalidone
   Clopamide
   Clorexolone
   Indapamide
   Mefruside
   Metolazone
   Quinethazone
   Xipamide

2. *β-Adrenoceptor antagonists* (p. 544)
   Acebutolol
   Atenolol
   Betaxolol
   Bisoprolol
   Metoprolol
   Nadolol
   Oxprenolol
   Penbutolol
   Pindolol
   Propranolol
   Sotalol
   Timolol

3. *α-Adrenoceptor antagonists*
   Selective (α_1) (p. 543)
   Doxazosin
   Prazosin
   Terazosin
   Indoramin
   Non-selective (α_1 and α_2) (generally only used in phaeochromocytoma)
   Phentolamine and phenoxybenzamine (p. 542)

4. *Mixed α- and β-adrenoceptor antagonist*
   Labetalol (p. 622)

5. *Angiotensin converting enzyme (ACE) inhibitors* (p. 556)
   Captopril
   Enalapril
   Lisinopril
   Perindropril
   Quinapril

6. *Calcium antagonists* (p. 569)
   Dihydropyridines
   Amlodipine
   Isradipine
   Nicardipine
   Nifedipine
   Nimodipine

   Others
   Verapamil

7. *Vasodilators*
   Diazoxide
   Hydralazine (p. 614)
   Minoxidil (p. 636)
   Sodium nitroprusside (p. 686)

8. *Drugs affecting nervous control of blood pressure*
   Methyldopa (p. 633)
   Clonidine
   Reserpine

Reserpine acts by causing depletion of neuronal stores of catecholamines both centrally and peripherally.

The adrenergic neurone-blocking drugs, which include bethanidine, debrisoquine, and guanethidine, inhibit the release of noradrenaline from peripheral sympathetic nerve-endings.

23.1.2 The practical use of antihypertensive drugs

Exercise, reduction in weight, reduced alcohol and cigarette consumption, and reduced dietary salt intake may all contribute to a lowering of the blood pressure. We shall not deal further here with these and other non-pharmacological methods of treatment, although in mild cases they may obviate the need for drugs.

The different choices of drug regimens in essential hypertension are summarized in Table 23.3 in the order in which they are generally used.

(a) Moderate hypertension

In the initial treatment of mild or moderate hypertension the choice of drug is from among a diuretic, a β-adrenoceptor antagonist, a calcium antagonist, or an ACE inhibitor. The decision which to use may depend upon the doctor's personal preferences and habits of medical practice. However, in some cases a knowledge of the actions of the drugs and the attributes of the patient may dictate a logical choice. For example, in a hypertensive patient with cardiac failure a diuretic and/or an ACE inhibitor would be the

■ **Table 23.3** Summary of the drug therapy of hypertension

---

1. *Moderate hypertension*
   (a) *β*-blocker not contra-indicated
      (i) Diuretic or *β*-blocker or calcium antagonist or ACE inhibitor
      (ii) Diuretic + *β*-blocker or diuretic + ACE inhibitor or *β*-blocker + calcium antagonist
      (iii) Diuretic + *β*-blocker + calcium antagonist or diuretic + *β*-blocker + ACE inhibitor
   (b) *β*-blocker contra-indicated
      (i) Diuretic or ACE inhibitor
      (ii) Diuretic + calcium antagonist or diuretic + ACE inhibitor
      (iii) Diuretic + calcium antagonist + ACE inhibitor

2. *Severe hypertension*
   (a) *β*-blocker not contra-indicated
      (i) *β*-blocker + diuretic or ACE inhibitor + diuretic
      (ii) *β*-blocker + calcium antagonist + diuretic or *β*-blocker + ACE inhibitor + diuretic
      (iii) *β*-blocker + calcium antagonist + ACE inhibitor + diuretic
   (b) *β*-blocker contra-indicated
      (i) Diuretic + ACE inhibitor
      (ii) Diuretic + ACE inhibitor + calcium antagonist or diuretic + ACE inhibitor + prazosin
   (c) Patients not responding to these regimens
      Add methyldopa or minoxidil or an adrenergic neurone-blocking drug

---

logical choices, while a *β*-adrenoceptor antagonist or a calcium antagonist would be preferred in a hypertensive patient who also had angina pectoris.

(i) Diuretics

The choice of a diuretic is restricted to a thiazide or thiazide-like diuretic (see Table 23.2), other diuretics (for example loop diuretics) conferring no special advantages.

Commonly one would choose a thiazide, such as bendrofluazide 2.5–5 mg o.d. orally or cyclopenthiazide 0.5–1.0 mg o.d. orally. Potassium depletion is not usually a problem when diuretics are used to treat hypertension, but in some cases potassium conservation or replacement may be required. The use of potassium supplements, potassium-sparing diuretics, and ACE inhibitors in maintaining potassium balance in patients taking diuretics is discussed in detail in Chapter 26.

Besides potassium depletion the major adverse effects of the thiazides are excessive salt and water loss, hyperuricaemia, and impairment of glucose tolerance. There is also an increased prevalence of erectile impotence in men with hypertension taking thiazide diuretics. Patients do not often complain of this, since they generally do not link it with the drug and in any case do not like to mention it spontaneously.

(ii) *β*-adrenoceptor antagonists

Of the wide variety of *β*-adrenoceptor antagonists atenolol is usually chosen: it penetrates the brain relatively poorly and consequently may have fewer central adverse effects, it can be given once a day in the hope of improving compliance, and it is relatively β_1-cardioselective. The usual dose is 50–100 mg o.d. orally. Metoprolol is similar, but needs to be given twice daily and is less cardioselective. The usual dosage is 50–100 mg b.d. orally. Despite their relative cardioselectivity, these drugs may nevertheless cause bronchospasm in patients with a history of reversible airways obstruction, in whom they are better avoided. Their other adverse effects include bradycardia and impairment of cardiac output, which may result in heart failure, an increased susceptibility of the hands and feet to the cold, especially in patients with peripheral vascular disease and Raynaud's phenomenon, and a general feeling of fatigue, particularly muscular weakness and fatigue on severe muscular effort. In men erectile impotence is not uncommon.

(iii) Calcium antagonists

The most commonly used calcium antagonist of those licensed for use in hypertension is nifedipine, although there are no important differences among the calcium antagonists available (Table 23.2). The usual dosage is 20–40 mg b.d. orally. The most common adverse effects of these drugs are headache, flushing, and dizziness, all due to dilatation of cranial blood vessels. They may also cause fluid retention with ankle swelling.

(iv) Angiotensin converting enzyme (ACE) inhibitors

The most commonly used ACE inhibitors are captopril and enalapril, although there is little to choose from among any of the alternatives. The most important adverse effect of these drugs is their tendency to cause severe hypotension after the first dose, especially in patients already taking a diuretic. It is therefore advisable to withdraw the diuretic for a few (say three) days before starting treatment with the ACE inhibitor and to start with a low dose (captopril 12.5 mg or 6.25 mg in a patient with renal impairment; enalapril 5 mg); the dose of the ACE inhibitor can then be increased gradually and the diuretic can be restarted after another few days, when ACE inhibitory therapy is established. Ideally, ACE inhibitor therapy in patients who have been taking diuretics should be started in hospital, where the patient can be kept in bed for careful monitoring of the blood pressure after the administration of the first few doses. However, the risk of severe hypotension is not so great in patients with hypertension as it is in those with cardiac failure and it is also less in those not already taking a diuretic or in patients in whom a diuretic and an ACE inhibitor are started at the same time.

Other important adverse effects of the ACE inhibitors are skin rashes, neutropenia, and renal damage, which usually first manifests as proteinuria. Cough and transient taste disturbances are troublesome, if not serious, adverse effects in some patients.

(v) Alternatives to monotherapy

The use of a single agent, whether a diuretic, a β-adrenoceptor antagonist, a calcium antagonist, or an ACE inhibitor, will lower the blood pressure satisfactorily in up to 80 per cent of patients with moderate hypertension. This figure can be increased to about 90 per cent by combining two types of treatment.

If the patient is already taking a diuretic or an ACE inhibitor, such as captopril or enalapril, then it is logical to combine them, for two reasons. Firstly, the action of the ACE inhibitors is increased by the reduction in fluid volume caused by diuretics; and secondly, the ACE inhibitors cause potassium retention via decreased aldosterone secretion, and this may counteract any potassium depletion due to the diuretic. The ACE inhibitors are also valuable in the patient with heart failure, because of their vasodilator action.

If the patient is already taking a β-adrenoceptor antagonist or a calcium antagonist as monotherapy then it is logical to combine them, since the calcium antagonist may counteract any peripheral vasoconstriction due to the β-adrenoceptor antagonist, while the β-adrenoceptor antagonist will inhibit any reflex tachycardia due to the calcium antagonist.

Other alternatives for combination therapy include the α_1-adrenoceptor antagonists prazosin and doxazosin. These drugs can be combined with a β-adrenoceptor antagonist and are also useful alternatives in the treatment of patients already taking a diuretic, in patients in whom a β-adrenoceptor antagonist is contra-indicated, and in patients with heart failure, for which their vasodilator properties are also helpful.

Like the ACE inhibitors, prazosin can cause severe hypotension after the first dose. The first dose should therefore be low and it should be given when the patient is lying in bed. The usual dose is 0.5 mg t.d.s initially, increasing gradually as required to a maximum of 5 mg q.d.s.

Labetalol is an alternative to the combination of a peripheral vasodilator and a β-adrenoceptor antagonist, since it combines α- and β-adrenoceptor antagonist properties, albeit non-selective ones. The usual dose is 100–800 mg t.d.s. and it is often combined with a diuretic.

Hydralazine has also been used in combination with a β-adrenoceptor antagonist. Hydralazine alone is an effective vasodilator, but its blood pressure lowering effect is counteracted by reflex tachycardia. High doses of hydralazine are therefore required if it is to be an effective antihypertensive when used alone, and high doses cause a lupus-like syndrome. However, in combination with a β-adrenoceptor antagonist, which blocks the reflex tachycardia, it is effective in lower doses (less than 200 mg daily in all). The usual dose is 25–50 mg t.d.s. or q.d.s. However, even in these low doses it can cause a lupus-like syndrome, particularly in women, and its long-term use is not therefore recommended. Its other important adverse effects are postural hypotension, nausea, vomiting, and diarrhoea.

(b) Severe hypertension

In severe hypertension various combinations of drugs can be used. One method is to start with a β-adrenoceptor antagonist, such as atenolol 100 mg o.d., increasing to 200 mg o.d. if the desired response is not achieved within a week or two weeks, and then adding nifedipine, an ACE inhibitor, or prazosin. In patients in whom a β-adrenoceptor antagonist is contra-indicated a diuretic with an ACE inhibitor or prazosin can be used.

(c) Last-line alternatives

Well over 95 per cent of patients will respond to one of the regimens mentioned above. In the few patients who do not respond well, one should consider poor compliance and an undiagnosed underlying cause. In some cases the blood pressure is only raised during the visit to the hospital clinic and communication between the hospital and the general practitioner may reveal the discrepancy; in such cases a non-invasive 24-h ambulatory recording will help determine how serious the hypertension is. If these factors have been ruled out, other drugs must be added. The main alternatives are α-methyldopa, minoxidil, and the adrenergic neurone-blocking drugs.

(i) α-methyldopa

α-methyldopa is an effective antihypertensive drug which, with diuretics, was first-line treatment for moderate and severe hypertension before the advent of β-adrenoceptor antagonists. However, it often makes patients feel depressed and generally lacking in physical and mental energy, and is now a reserve drug for that reason. It is given in an initial dose of 250 mg t.d.s. orally, and this may be increased to a maximum of 3 g daily. Dosages should be reduced in renal failure (see Table 3.5).

(ii) Minoxidil

Minoxidil is a potent vasodilator which causes marked fluid retention, hirsutism, and reflex tachycardia. It is therefore reserved for the treatment of hypertension which has failed to respond to the above measures, and it must be used in combination with both a diuretic and a β-adrenoceptor antagonist. Fluid retention may be severe enough to require the use of a loop diuretic.

(iii) Adrenergic neurone-blocking drugs

These drugs (bethanidine, debrisoquine, and guanethidine) are now little used because of their adverse effects, which include severe postural hypotension, diarrhoea, and erectile impotence.

23.1.3 Some aspects of the treatment of secondary hypertension

(a) Renal disease

The treatment of hypertension secondary to renal disease is similar to that of essential hypertension. However, fluid retention can be a particular problem when vasodilators are used and a loop diuretic may then be preferable to a thiazide diuretic. Some antihypertensive drugs are excreted unchanged by the kidneys and have to be used in lower dosages in renal impairment. The important examples are α-methyldopa and the β-adrenoceptor antagonists sotalol and nadolol. The ACE inhibitors are particularly effective in patients with renal parenchymal disease and hypertension, but they may impair renal function and make hypertension worse in patients with renovascular disease. Their effects in patients with renal impairment need careful monitoring.

(b) Types of hypertension for which non-selective α-adrenoceptor antagonists are indicated

There are some circumstances in which the non-selective α-adrenoceptor antagonists phenoxybenzamine and phentolamine should be used in treating hypertension.

(i) Phaeochromocytoma (see also p. 370)

For long-term treatment of hypertension due to phaeochromocytoma before surgery or when surgery is not possible, oral phenoxybenzamine should be used (10 mg o.d. to start with, increasing to a maximum of 60 mg t.d.s. if required).

At operation an i.v. infusion of phentolamine should be used to prevent sudden severe hypertension due to release of noradrenaline during handling of the tumour. The mixed α- and β-adrenoceptor antagonist labetalol is an alternative to α-antagonists both before and during surgery.

(ii) Certain causes of acute hypertensive crisis

There are certain circumstances in which an acute hypertensive crisis should be treated with i.v. phentolamine. They are:

acute hypertension after abrupt clonidine withdrawal;

a hypertensive crisis in a patient taking a monoamine oxidase inhibitor (for example the 'cheese reaction');

hypertension after an overdose with an α-adrenoceptor agonist.

(c) Endocrine disorders

In hypertension due to Conn's syndrome (primary hyperaldosteronism) if surgical treatment is not possible the aldosterone antagonist spironolactone may be used. In Cushing's syndrome β-adrenoceptor antagonists may provide nonspecific hypotensive effects, although more specific medical or surgical treatment may be indicated. In both of these conditions hypokalaemia is a particular risk and care must be taken with thiazides and loop diuretics.

(d) Hypertension in pregnancy (see also Chapter 12)

Hypertension in pregnancy may be due either to pre-existing hypertension (for example essential or renal hypertension) or to the specific entity called pre-eclampsia or toxaemia of pregnancy, which occurs in the third trimester, and in which there is hypertension with persistent proteinuria and peripheral oedema. Pre-eclampsia carries the risks of slowed intrauterine fetal growth, an increased incidence of stillbirth, and the occurrence of eclampsia (fits), with danger to the life of the mother and fetus. Other complications include disseminated intravascular coagulation, renal failure, acute left ventricular failure, and stroke.

Since the blood pressure normally falls during pregnancy, the criteria for the diagnosis of hypertension are difficult to establish, but one would usually define hypertension in pre-eclampsia as a persistently increased blood pressure at least 30/15 mmHg higher than the pressure first recorded before 20 weeks of gestation. In some women with chronic hypertension it is possible to withhold treatment during pregnancy, but if drug treatment is necessary, either for chronic hypertension or pre-eclampsia, then the drug of choice is a calcium antagonist, such as nifedipine, α-methyldopa, or a β-adrenoceptor antagonist, such as atenolol. Diuretics should be avoided because intravascular volume is already reduced in pregnancy. The aim of treatment should be to reduce the diastolic pressure to around 90 mmHg.

If pre-eclampsia occurs rapidly late in pregnancy the best treatment is immediate termination (i.e. delivery of the child), but if the blood pressure needs to be lowered rapidly nifedipine can be given orally, or hydralazine parenterally. If fits occur they should be treated with chlormethiazole; in the US magnesium sulphate is used for this purpose (4 g i.v. over 15 min followed by 2 g/h).

23.1.4 Hypertensive emergencies

The definition of a hypertensive emergency is a diastolic blood pressure greater than 130 mmHg.

Although it is desirable to reduce the diastolic pressure below 120 mmHg within 24 h in accelerated or malignant hypertension, it is usually unnecessary to reduce it more rapidly, and indeed it may be dangerous to do so. That is because the mechanisms which maintain cerebral blood flow at a constant level independent of peripheral blood pressure are impaired in hypertension. If the blood pressure is lowered too rapidly in such cases cerebral blood flow may fall and brain damage and death can occur from cerebral anoxia, oedema, and even infarction.

When lowering of the blood pressure is not urgent the treatment of choice is an oral β-adrenoceptor antagonist, such as atenolol, or oral nifedipine in patients in whom a β-adrenoceptor antagonist is contra-indicated.

However, there are some circumstances in which a raised blood pressure is life-threatening.

In these cases the blood pressure must be lowered quickly and the need to do so outweighs the risk of reducing cerebral blood flow. They include:

accelerated or malignant hypertension with hypertensive encephalopathy;

acute dissecting aneurysm of the aorta;

severe hypertensive left ventricular failure;

pre-eclampsia (see above).

If the blood pressure has to be lowered rapidly the choice of drugs includes hydralazine, sodium nitroprusside, labetalol, and diazoxide. Hydralazine is given by slow i.v. or i.m injection of 5–20 mg. This dose can be repeated after 30 min if required. If hydralazine causes a reflex tachycardia this can be blunted by concomitant administration of a β-adrenoceptor antagonist.

Sodium nitroprusside has the advantage of having a rapid 'on-off' effect. Its half-time is very short and its effects come on and wear off in a few minutes. It is thus possible to control the blood pressure by varying the infusion rate (usual dosage 0.5–1.5 micrograms/kg/min, increasing if necessary to 8 micrograms/kg/min). It is therefore an ideal drug for precise control of blood pressure. However, because of the rapidity of its action its use requires constant medical supervision with frequently repeated, or preferably continuous, blood pressure measurement. It should not be given to patients with renal failure because of the danger of cyanide poisoning, nor in pregnancy.

Labetalol can be given either as a continuous i.v. infusion at a rate of 1–4 mg/min or as bolus doses of 50 mg i.v. repeated at 15 min intervals up to a maximum total of 200 mg. Patients should always be kept supine because of the risk of severe postural hypotension. The effects of labetalol after bolus injection occur within a few minutes and last for up to 6 h, and in some cases as long as 24 h.

Diazoxide is given as a rapid i.v. bolus of 150 or 300 mg, but it should be used with great care, since the blood pressure may fall markedly within a few minutes of administration. It has a long half-time (25 h) and is excreted unchanged in the urine. Dosages should not therefore be repeated too often in renal failure. It is not now used in the long-term management of hypertension because of its adverse effects, which include impairment of glucose tolerance, salt and water retention, hyperuricaemia, hirsutism, and hypersensitivity reactions (skin rashes, thrombocytopenia, and leucopenia). Its adverse effects after acute i.v. administration include tachycardia and cardiac pain, and it may occasionally cause acute pancreatitis with severe epigastric pain.

23.1.5 Contra-indications to treatment of hypertension

There are two circumstances in which one must be cautious about treating hypertension: in patients with stroke or with acute myocardial infarction. Only if there is severe hypertension (diastolic pressure greater than 120 mmHg) should antihypertensive drugs be used acutely. In stroke thiazide diuretics and/or β-adrenoceptor antagonists are safe, and in acute myocardial infarction treatment of pain with opiates and of heart failure with diuretics may result in satisfactory lowering of the blood pressure without the need for other specific measures.

Treatment of hypertension in old people is still controversial, despite the encouraging results of recent large trials, since the benefits may be small and the benefit:risk ratio is not clearly in favour of therapy. Diuretics and β-adrenoceptor antagonists are the drugs of choice if it is decided to give treatment. Nifedipine and the ACE inhibitors may also be used.

23.1.6 Monitoring therapy in hypertension

When measuring the blood pressure it is always desirable to do so with the patient first supine and then standing, in order to detect postural falls. It may also be useful to measure the blood pressure after the patient has exercised (for example by stepping up and down on a step half-a-dozen times). This is particularly helpful in patients taking a β-adrenoceptor antagonist, in whom the pressure may fall on exercise. If more information about the blood pressure is required it is relatively simple for patients to measure their own blood pressure at home, and it should be remembered that the blood pressure taken in the clinic or surgery is often higher than at other times. Self-monitoring in this way can give information about the day-to-day variability of the blood pressure and its response to treatment. More accurate information about the blood pressure can be obtained by 24 h monitoring. This can be done either by continuous measurement with an intra-arterial catheter (not a technique which is suitable for routine use), or by other devices, such as a cuff which is left in position on the arm and which automatically inflates, measures, and records the blood pressure at predetermined intervals.

23.1.7 Compliance in hypertension

There is a special case for discussing compliance in the treatment of hypertension, since patients are usually asymptomatic and may not understand the potential advantages of taking long-term drug treatment. It is therefore important to take the time to explain carefully to every hypertensive patient why treatment is advantageous. Careful education has been shown to improve compliance. Once-daily therapy may also help but is not always possible.

There are ways of monitoring for the specific actions of some antihypertensive drugs. One can usually tell if a patient is taking a β-adrenoceptor antagonist by taking the pulse and blood pressure at rest and after exercise; the pulse and blood pressure should be little affected by exercise, or the blood pressure may even fall. In the patient who is taking a diuretic, plasma urea and uric acid concentrations should increase. There may be changes in plasma potassium concentrations in patients taking ACE inhibitors, but this is not a reliable method of determining compliance, particularly in patients who are also taking diuretics.

If compliance is a suspected problem in severe resistant hypertension, supervized therapy in hospital may help to clarify the problem, although there is also a blood pressure-lowering effect of hospitalization.

23.2 Angina pectoris

The syndrome of angina pectoris occurs when there is an acute imbalance between the oxygen requirements of the myocardium and the oxygen available to it. This occurs either when there is a sudden increase in demand for oxygen in a chronically ischaemic heart or when there is spasm of a coronary artery (so-called 'variant', 'atypical', or 'Prinzmetal' angina). There is also the condition of so-called 'unstable angina', which is usually due to the rupture of an atheromatous plaque in a coronary artery. The treatment of unstable angina is dealt with under myocardial infarction.

An increase in oxygen demand may result from any stimulus which causes an increase in systolic ventricular pressure or size, an increase in heart rate, or an increase in the rate or force of contractility of the myocardium. The commonest precipitating factor of an acute attack of angina is exercise, but angina pectoris can also occur in response to other forms of stress, such as emotion, cold, or a heavy meal. Other factors which may be associated with attacks of angina pectoris in patients with chronic myocardial ischaemia include anaemia (poor oxygen-carrying capacity of the blood), aortic stenosis (inadequate supply of blood to the coronary arteries during diastole), paroxysmal arrhythmias (impaired blood supply), and thyrotoxicosis (increased metabolic requirements).

23.2.1 Mechanisms of action of the drugs used to relieve or prevent angina pectoris

The drugs used in the treatment of an acute attack of angina pectoris or in the prevention of attacks are listed in Table 23.4, and their mechanisms of action are illustrated in Fig. 23.2.

Nitrates, such as glyceryl trinitrate, isosorbide dinitrate, and isosorbide mononitrate, relieve angina pectoris by several mechanisms.

1. By causing arteriolar dilatation, lowering peripheral resistance, and reducing myocardial work and oxygen demand.
2. By causing peripheral vasodilatation, decreasing venous return, and thereby reducing left ventricular end-diastolic pressure and volume, and again reducing myocardial work and oxygen demand.
3. By relieving coronary arterial spasm in variant angina, and any spasm occurring as part of common angina.
4. By redistribution of myocardial blood flow to improve the perfusion of ischaemic areas.

∎ **Table 23.4**   Drugs used in angina pectoris

---

1. *Treatment of an acute attack in chronic stable angina*
   Glyceryl trinitrate (p. 651)
   Isosorbide mononitrate or dinitrate (p. 651)

2. *Prevention of acute attacks and treatment of unstable angina*
   Glyceryl trinitrate (topical application)
   Isosorbide mononitrate or dinitrate
   β-adrenoceptor antagonists (p. 544)
   Calcium antagonists (p. 569)
   Aspirin (p. 677)
   Heparin (p. 612)

β-adrenoceptor antagonists act by blocking the action of noradrenaline released from cardiac sympathetic nerve-endings, thereby decreasing the effects of endogenous sympathomimetic amines on cardiac β-adrenoceptors. This has two effects: firstly the increase in heart rate in response to physical or emotional stress is reduced, and secondly the force of contractility of the myocardium is reduced. Both of these effects result in prevention of increased oxygen requirements at times of stress.

The antagonists of calcium ion flux, such as nifedipine and diltiazem, cause peripheral arterial and venous vasodilatation. In this respect they act like the nitrates. They also dilate normal coronary arteries.

23.2.2 The use of antianginal drugs

(a) The treatment of acute attacks of angina pectoris in chronic stable angina

If a patient has acute attacks of angina pectoris, whether on a background of chronic ischaemic myocardial disease or because of coronary artery spasm, the treatment of choice for the acute attack is a nitrate, and glyceryl trinitrate is the nitrate usually chosen. It is taken as a tablet which is allowed to dissolve under the tongue, because the rapid absorption of glyceryl trinitrate through the oral mucosa provides rapid relief of anginal pain, and because this route of administration also avoids the extensive first-pass metabolism of glyceryl trinitrate in the liver after oral administration. In other words the sublingual route improves both the rate and extent of the systemic availability of glyceryl trinitrate.

The antianginal action of glyceryl trinitrate begins within a minute or two and lasts for up to half an hour. The chief adverse effects when it is taken in this way are secondary to vasodilatation and include palpitation, headache, flushing, dizziness, and postural hypotension.

Usually one tablet (0.5 mg) is enough to relieve the pain of an attack, but two tablets may sometimes be necessary. Patients should be told that if pain relief does not occur within a few minutes they should not continue to use glyceryl trinitrate but should consult a doctor. They should also be advised of the use of a tablet of glyceryl trinitrate taken sublingually in order to prevent a single attack of angina pectoris which may be anticipated (for example just before unusual exertion, in anticipation of an emotional stress, or before going out on a very cold morning). There is no limit on the number of tablets a patient may use for the treatment of repeated attacks.

Glyceryl trinitrate in tablets is unstable and deterioration can lead to loss of efficacy within a month or two. Patients should be told to keep their tablets in a dark container, only taking out enough tablets for a day's supply at a time, if it is their habit to carry tablets loose. The bottle in which the tablets are stored should have an aluminium-foil lined cap. Neither cotton wool nor other drugs should be kept in the same bottle. For patients who cannot manage all this, or for those in whom attacks are infrequent, there is an alternative, more expensive, formulation of glyceryl trinitrate in a stable aerosol spray for sublingual administration.

(b) The prevention of acute attacks in chronic stable angina

The choices of therapy in the prevention of acute anginal attacks in chronic stable angina are shown in Table 23.4.

(i) Nitrates

Glyceryl trinitrate, isosorbide dinitrate, and isosorbide mononitrate are equally effective alternatives.

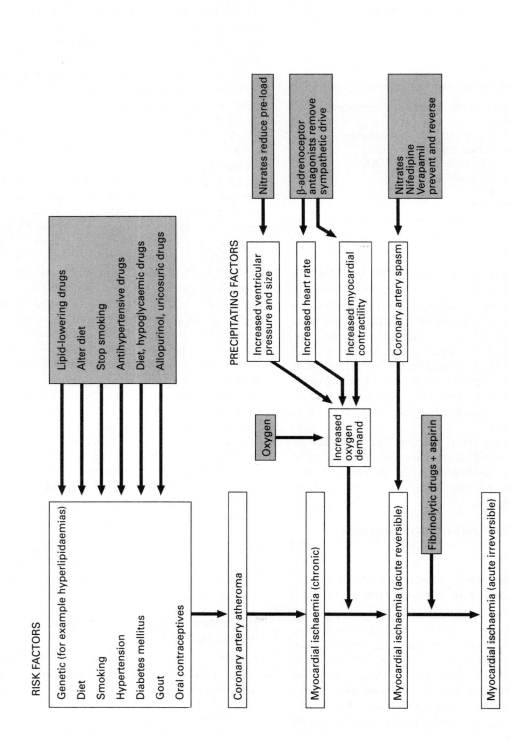

■ **Fig. 23.2** The pathophysiology of ischaemic heart disease and the sites and mechanisms of action of drugs used in its treatment.

Glyceryl trinitrate is available in several different formulations for long-term use. As an ointment it can be rubbed into the skin (usually of the anterior chest) whence it is slowly absorbed, maintaining therapeutic plasma concentrations for up to 8 h. The ointment is also available in adhesive patches, which are applied to the skin and from which slow release occurs into the blood. In order to prevent the development of long-term tolerance (see p. 60) and a consequent reduction in therapeutic efficacy, patients should be advised to remove glyceryl trinitrate patches for a few hours each day. If patients are free from attacks overnight it is usual to remove the patch before going to bed. Glyceryl trinitrate can also be given in buccal tablets, from which it is slowly absorbed into the systemic circulation via the buccal mucosa.

Isosorbide dinitrate and isosorbide mononitrate are the most commonly used nitrates and are given in a dosage of 5–30 mg q.d.s. Both of these drugs are also available in slow-release formulations for once daily dosage (mononitrate, 40–120 mg) or twice-daily dosage (dinitrate, 20–60 mg b.d.). Their adverse effects are the same as those of sublingual glyceryl trinitrate. Isosorbide mononitrate is generally preferred to the dinitrate, since it is not subject to first-pass metabolism and the therapeutic response is therefore more predictable.

(ii) β-adrenoceptor antagonists

All β-adrenoceptor antagonists are probably equally effective in preventing acute anginal attacks. Atenolol is a good choice, for the reasons outlined under the treatment of hypertension. It is given in a dose of 50–200 mg o.d. orally. Alternatives include propranolol, metoprolol, and oxprenolol (see the Pharmacopoeia, p. 544). Cardiac failure is usually a contra-indication to the use of β-adrenoceptor antagonists. If there is concern about left ventricular function in a patient with angina on β-adrenoceptor antagonists, it is wise to prescribe a diuretic or a cardiac glycoside and further consider the possible treatment of cardiac failure (see p. 287). Other contra-indications are the same as for the use of β-adrenoceptor antagonists in hypertension.

(iii) Calcium antagonists

The calcium antagonist nifedipine is commonly used in the prevention of attacks of angina. It is given in a dosage of 10–20 mg t.d.s. Its main adverse effects are headache, hypotension, and tachycardia. It is therefore better used in combination with a β-adrenoceptor antagonist, which will oppose the tachycardia. The same considerations apply to other dihydropyridines, such as nicardipine (20–30 mg t.d.s.) and amlodipine (5–10 mg o.d.)

Diltiazem is a useful alternative to the dihydropyridine calcium antagonists, since it tends to cause a sinus bradycardia, although for that reason it should not be used with a β-adrenoceptor antagonist.

Verapamil (40–80 mg t.d.s.) has been used, but is better avoided, since it has a negative inotropic effect on the heart and may cause heart failure; it also causes atrioventricular (AV) block and should be avoided if the QRS complex is widened on the electrocardiogram (ECG). Verapamil should generally not be used in combination with a β-adrenoceptor antagonist, because of the increased risk of heart failure and cardiac arrhythmias with this combination.

In variant angina one would generally start with a nitrate, such as isosorbide dinitrate or mononitrate and add a calcium antagonist if necessary; β-adrenoceptor antagonists are usually avoided, since there is concern that they may cause coronary vasospasm in patients with variant angina. In patients with coronary atheroma one would start with a nitrate and then add a β-adrenoceptor antagonist, which may be helpful in preventing reflex tachycardia due to the vasodilator types of drugs (the long-acting nitrates and the calcium antagonists). However, if there are contra-indications to a β-adrenoceptor antagonist one would add a calcium antagonist instead. Sometimes it may be necessary to use a combination of all three types of drug.

Treatment with one or a combination of these drugs will either prevent or markedly reduce the frequency of attacks of angina pectoris in over 90 per cent of patients, but it is not known whether effective treatment leads to a reduction in the death rate from coronary artery disease. However, there is some evidence that long-term therapy with β-adrenoceptor antagonists may reduce the incidence of myocardial infarction.

Ideally one would refer all patients with angina to a cardiologist for exercise testing and, where indicated, coronary angiography. However, if every patient were referred in this way the cardiological services would be overburdened by those patients alone. Patients who have angina pectoris after a myocardial infarction or who have left ventricular impairment should be referred, at least for an exercise test. Patients who do not respond satisfactorily to drugs should also be referred with a view to considering angiography followed by coronary angioplasty or by-pass graft surgery. There may also be some patients who are asymptomatic because they restrict their activities; if they can be identified, they too should be referred for exercise testing, since they may be more severely restricted by their disease than they or the doctor appreciates.

(c) Unstable angina

Unstable angina is a state in which there is acute cardiac pain at rest or during minimal exercise; it may lead on to myocardial infarction (i.e. irreversible ischaemic damage) and/or sudden death. Angina of recent onset (within the previous month) should also be considered to be an emergency.

The patient should be admitted to hospital and asked to remain in bed. Intravenous infusions of heparin (1500 i.u./h) and isosorbide dinitrate or glyceryl trinitrate (2–10 mg/h) should be started. If an infusion is not possible glyceryl trinitrate ointment (1–2 inches rubbed into the chest) or oral isosorbide (10 mg t.d.s. increasing to 20 mg t.d.s. if necessary) are alternatives. If there is ST elevation on the electrocardiogram or if the pain is not relieved within 20 min, the patient should be treated as if for a myocardial infarction (see below). If the pain does resolve, a β-adrenoceptor antagonist (for example metoprolol 50 mg b.d. initially, increasing if required to 100 mg q.d.s.) should be given. If the patient then remains pain-free, exercise testing after 2–3 d will give guidance to the need for further intervention, but if the pain recurs the patient should be referred immediately for coronary angiography with a view to angioplasty or by-pass graft surgery.

Aspirin approximately halves the risk of death or progression to complete infarction in unstable angina. It should be given orally in a dose of 150 mg daily.

During the acute phase careful review of the patient should be undertaken twice a day and dosages of drugs increased if the pain is not controlled.

23.3 Acute myocardial infarction

Acute myocardial infarction occurs when there is occlusion of a coronary artery, because of thrombosis, spasm, or rarely embolism, with subsequent irreversible tissue damage. Treatment can be considered in terms of prevention and treatment of the acute attack.

23.3.1 Prevention of myocardial infarction

The risk factors for coronary atheroma are illustrated in Fig. 23.2. Drugs may be needed for the treatment of hyperlipidaemias, diabetes mellitus, and hypertension. So far there have been no studies showing convincing overall benefit from any drug therapy in the primary prevention of myocardial infarction, outside of the treatment of risk factors; although there is some evidence that aspirin may be effective it is too early to recommend it as a routine. The secondary prevention of myocardial infarction is discussed below.

23.3.2 Mechanisms of action of drugs used in the treatment of acute myocardial infarction

The drugs used in the treatment of acute myocardial infarction and its complications are listed in Table 23.5.

(a) Oxygen

The rationale for the use of oxygen in acute myocardial infarction is that the partial pressure of oxygen in the arterial blood (P_AO_2) is often reduced and an increase in inhaled oxygen will correct that, thereby increasing tissue oxygena-

■ **Table 23.5** Drugs used in the treatment of acute myocardial infarction and its major complications

1. *Hypoxia*
   Oxygen

2. *Relief of pain and distress*
   Opiate analgesics (p. 641)

3. *Limiting infarct size*
   Thrombolytics + aspirin + heparin
   β-adrenoceptor antagonists (p. 544)

4. *Nausea and vomiting*
   Antiemetics (for example phenothiazines,
   p. 645)

5. *Cardiac failure*
   Oxygen
   Loop diuretics (pp. 566 and 608)
   Opiates
   Vasodilators (Table 23.9)
   Dopamine (p. 597)
   β-adrenoceptor agonists (for example
   dobutamine) (p. 541)

6. *Arrhythmias*
   Antiarrhythmics (Table 23.6)

7. *Prevention of secondary venous thrombosis*
   Heparin (p. 612)

8. *Pericarditis and Dressler's syndrome*
   Aspirin (p. 677)
   Indomethacin (p. 653)
   Corticosteroids (p. 584)

tion. Oxygen should therefore be used if there is evidence of arterial hypoxia, for example in patients with acute left ventricular failure or cardiogenic shock. Oxygen must be used with caution in patients with chronic obstructive airways disease (see p. 301).

(b) Opiate analgesics

Opiate analgesics have several different valuable properties for use in myocardial infarction. They relieve pain and mental distress, and presumably reduce sympathetic nervous system activity. They are dilators of peripheral blood vessels, both arterioles and venules, thereby reducing cardiac preload and afterload, and relieving cardiac failure.

However, they may cause hypotension, nausea, and vomiting. They should be used with caution in patients with chronic lung disease because they depress the respiratory centre.

(c) Antiemetics

Patients with acute myocardial infarction frequently feel sick and vomit. Opiate analgesics make this worse and antiemetics are therefore given. However, great care must be taken with some commonly used antiemetics, such as the phenothiazines and related antihistamines, since they can cause hypotension, because of α-adrenoceptor blockade, particularly in patients with hypovolaemia.

(d) Diuretics

Many patients have some degree of left ventricular failure after an acute myocardial infarction. Intravenous frusemide relieves this by causing both peripheral venous vasodilatation and a diuresis.

(e) Antiarrhythmic drugs

The treatment of cardiac arrhythmias after acute myocardial infarction is described later in this Chapter (see pp. 276–87).

(f) Heparin

Patients who have had an acute myocardial infarction have an increased risk of deep venous thrombosis and therefore of pulmonary embolism. Normally low-dose heparin subcutaneously is given to prevent this (see p. 612) if full-dose heparin is not used after thrombolytic therapy (see below).

(g) Drugs used to limit infarct size

Acute coronary occlusion produces an area of irreversibly damaged (i.e. dead) myocardium surrounded by normal myocardium. Between these two regions there is an intermediate zone of tissue which is ischaemic but which theoretically might recover, saving useful myocardium from permanent damage. In recent years, therefore, efforts have been made to prevent irreversible damage in this intermediate ischaemic zone. Since prognosis is related to infarct size this approach is of considerable importance.

The most commonly used type of treatment is the i.v. administration of a thrombolytic agent, such as streptokinase or its analogues, which act by dissolving the thrombus in the affected coronary arteries. The mechanism of this action at the molecular level is via changes in fibrinolysis (see Fig. P3, p. 558). The beneficial outcome with thrombolytic drugs is enhanced by the addition of oral aspirin.

β-adrenoceptor antagonists have also been used in acute myocardial infarction to limit infarct size. The rationale is that the reduction in myocardial contractility and heart rate produced by β-adrenoceptor antagonists results in reduced myocardial oxygen requirements and thus a greater likelihood that the compromised tissue will survive the ischaemic insult. The earlier the β-adrenoceptor antagonist is given after the onset of pain the greater the beneficial effect will be. β-adrenoceptor antagonists also reduce the risk of cardiac rupture, which may be important after thrombolytic therapy, which tends to produce a soft haemorrhagic infarct.

23.3.3 Drug therapy in acute myocardial infarction

About 50 per cent of those who die after an acute myocardial infarction die immediately or within the first few hours, mostly because of arrhythmias, such as ventricular fibrillation. This observation has led to the introduction in some centres of schemes to improve the availability of facilities for cardiopulmonary resuscitation. Such schemes include the provision of rapidly mobilized coronary-care ambulances, whose staff are specially trained in the appropriate techniques.

(a) General measures

(i) Oxygen

Oxygen should be given if there is suspicion of hypoxia, for example in patients with cardiac failure or cardiogenic shock. It should be given either via a face-mask capable of delivering high concentrations in the inspired air (see p. 301) or via nasal tubing. If the patient has obstructive airways disease only 24 or 28 per cent oxygen should be used, because of the danger of CO_2 narcosis with higher concentrations (see p. 301).

(ii) Pain relief

The treatment of choice for pain relief is either morphine or diamorphine (heroin). Diamorphine is widely used in the UK, but it is rapidly metabolized to morphine ($t_{1/2}$ 10 min) and there are no major important differences between the two besides dosage: morphine 10–20 mg i.m. or i.v.; diamorphine 5–10 mg i.m. or i.v. A single dose is usually enough to relieve the pain of myocardial infarction, but the dose may be repeated if it has not taken effect within 15 min of an i.v. injection or within 30 min of an i.m. injection.

The opiate analgesics cause peripheral venous and arteriolar vasodilatation, and while this may be beneficial in patients with left ventricular failure, too much opiate may cause severe hypotension, and excessive doses must be avoided. Because they depress the respiratory centre, opiates must be used with caution in patients with chronic lung disease.

(iii) Antiemetics

The opiate analgesics commonly cause nausea and vomiting and are often given with an antiemetic. There is no clear-cut guidance as to the best choice of antiemetic in these circumstances, but phenothiazines or related antihistamines are commonly used (for example cyclizine 50 mg i.v.). However, these drugs are liable to cause hypotension, via α-adrenoceptor blockade, and so metoclopramide (10 mg i.v.) is a better choice.

(iv) Sedatives

The opiates and phenothiazines or antihistamines together have the added benefit of causing sedation, and this is generally welcome. However, if it is felt necessary to continue to relieve mental distress after the initial acute stage, when opiates are no longer required, then a benzodiazepine, such as diazepam 5–10 mg t.d.s., may have this effect, and may also help patients to sleep, especially if they are being treated in the unfamiliar and perhaps worrying environment of the coronary care unit. The use of a benzodiazepine in such circumstances should be a temporary measure.

(v) Thrombolysis

In patients in whom thrombolysis is not contraindicated streptokinase should be given as soon as possible, in order to limit the size of the infarct. Streptokinase is currently the thrombolytic drug of choice, since it is of proven efficacy, may carry a lower risk of bleeding than other thrombolytic agents, and is cheaper. If streptokinase has been used in the previous 6 months there is a theoretical risk of an allergic response to a further dose and in such a case another thrombolytic drug would be used, for example anistreplase (APSAC, anisoylated plasminogen–streptokinase activator complex) or alteplase (tPA, tissue-type plasminogen activator). Other thrombolytic drugs which are currently under trial include urokinase, and pro-urokinase.

Aspirin (150 mg orally) should be given at once, followed by streptokinase by i.v. infusion of 1.5 million units over 60 min. Oral aspirin should then be continued (150 mg for at least 4 weeks), since this combination has a greater effect on subsequent mortality that either treatment alone.

Anistreplase has the advantage in general practice that if the diagnosis of myocardial infarction has been made it can be given as a single dose of 30 units i.v. over 4–5 min, whereas streptokinase must be given by i.v. infusion over 60 min. Theoretically, the sooner thrombolytic therapy is given, the better the result will be and anistreplase might therefore be have an advantage in such cases. However, this has yet to be definitively established. Another alternative to streptokinase in hospital, alteplase, is given by i.v infusion of 10 mg over 1–2 min, 50 mg over 1 h, and finally 40 mg over the next 2 h.

The adverse effects of, and the contra-indications to, thrombolytic agents are discussed under the treatment of thromboembolic disorders (see Table 23.16). However, it is important to note that one of the contra-indications is an acute dissecting aneurysm of the aorta, which may be confused with acute myocardial infarction. If there is any doubt one should look for mediastinal widening on a chest X-ray, in the absence of which thrombolysis may be given. Hypotension may occur during thrombolysis, and if it is severe treatment may have to be withdrawn.

(vi) Anticoagulation

There is some evidence that high-dose subcutaneous heparin (12 500 i.u. b.d.) may reduce mortality after acute myocardial infarction, albeit with a small increase in the risk of stroke. Some physicians therefore use this form of anticoagulation, or even full i.v. heparin (1500 i.u./h), for 2–3 d after acute myocardial infarction, instead of low-dose subcutaneous heparin.

There is an increased risk of deep venous thrombosis, and therefore of pulmonary embolism, after acute myocardial infarction. The risk can be reduced by the use of heparin given subcutaneously in the low dose of 5000 i.u. b.d. or t.d.s. Patients should also be encouraged to move their leg muscles in order to reduce the risk of venous thrombosis. If deep venous thrombosis or pulmonary embolism occurs, or if the patient develops a ventricular aneurysm, which carries a risk of ventricular clot and systemic emboli, full anticoagulation may be required, starting with i.v. heparin and continuing with warfarin (see the treatment of thromboembolism, p. 296). Patients with pericarditis should not be given full anticoagulation because of a theoretical risk of pericardial haemorrhage and tamponade.

(vii) β-adrenoceptor antagonists

If a β-adrenoceptor antagonist is used in an attempt to limit infarct size and prevent cardiac rupture, it should be given as soon as possible after the onset of pain, but only in those for whom such treatment is not contra-indicated. This excludes patients with asthma, chronic bronchitis with bronchoconstriction, moderate or severe left ventricular failure, heart block of any degree, bradycardia, or a systolic blood pressure below 100 mmHg. Treatment, if used, should start with i.v. administration (for example atenolol 5–10 mg by slow i.v. injection, followed by 50 mg after 15 min, 50 mg after 12 h) and then continuing with the usual oral dosages. Generally, such treatment should be undertaken only in coronary care units, with continuous electrocardiogram monitoring and facilities for resuscitation. If excessive bradycardia or hypotension occurs, treatment should be withheld immediately. The use of a β-adrenoceptor antagonist may have the additional advantage of relieving ischaemic pain. Note that this use of β-adrenoceptor antagonists in acute myocardial infarction is quite different from their use in the secondary prevention of myocardial infarction.

(b) Treatment of immediate complications

(i) Acute left ventricular failure with pulmonary oedema

This is diagnosed on the basis of the signs and symptoms of pulmonary oedema when present (orthopnoea, crackles at the lung bases), evidence of pulmonary congestion on the chest X-ray, and haemodynamic measurements (if available) showing a raised pulmonary capillary wedge pressure. It is an adverse prognostic feature, even if it resolves quickly with treatment.

In myocardial infarction left ventricular failure may be transient, and often responds to oxygen and the opiate given to relieve pain. However, not infrequently it is also necessary to give a diuretic, such as frusemide (either 40–80 mg orally or if more severe 20–40 mg i.v.) or bumetanide (1–2 mg orally or i.v.). The dosage and frequency of administration of diuretics may have to be increased in more severe cases, for instance to doses of 160 mg i.v. of frusemide or 5 mg i.v. of bumetanide. However, great care should be taken not to overuse diuretics, since that may cause a reduction in cardiac output due to a reduced intravascular volume.

Severe left ventricular failure may be fatal, and requires vigorous treatment. If there is evidence of low cardiac output (cool peripheries and a poor urinary output) dobutamine and low-dose dopamine should be given (see below) and evidence of mechanical problems (for example rupture of the mitral valve or interventricular septum) should be sought. On the other hand, if there is evidence of a good cardiac output start treatment with vasodilators to reduce afterload. This should preferably be carried out in a coronary care unit under haemodynamic control, with measurement of right atrial (i.e. central venous) pressure, pulmonary capillary wedge pressure (left ventricular filling pressure), and cardiac output. The choice of vasodilator is from glyceryl trinitrate i.v., isosorbide dinitrate i.v., or sodium nitroprusside i.v. The administration of these drugs requires meticulous attention to cardiac haemodynamic state. For the use of vasodilators see below under cardiogenic shock.

(ii) Cardiogenic shock

In cardiogenic shock the patient is hypotensive (systolic pressure below 90 mmHg), cold, clammy, cyanosed, hyperventilating, and oliguric. The peripheral veins are constricted and the pulse rapid and thready. The prognosis is very poor, with a 90 per cent mortality, even with modern methods of management. Ideally, all drug therapy in cardiogenic shock should be accompanied by haemodynamic monitoring of central venous pressure and pulmonary capillary wedge pressure, but of course that may not be possible. The aims should be to improve cardiac output and renal function with positive inotropic drugs and dopamine, and to reduce afterload with a vasodilator; if these measures are successful the left ventricular filling pressure (preload) will in turn fall.

When there is low cardiac output the combination of dopamine and dobutamine is generally used. Dopamine is given in low doses (1–3 micrograms/kg/min) for its agonist effect on dopamine receptors in the kidney, which causes renal vasodilatation. It can also be used in higher dosages (up to 20 micrograms/kg/min) for its positive inotropic action on cardiac β_1-adrenoceptors. However, its use in this way carries a risk of cardiac arrhythmias and peripheral vasoconstriction, since at high doses it also has α-adrenoceptor agonist properties. Dobutamine also has a positive inotropic action, is equally arrhythmogenic, and may cause peripheral vasoconstriction, but it does not have the dopaminergic effect necessary to dilate renal arteries. It is therefore usually given (5–20 micrograms/kg/min) in combination with low-dose dopamine. If cardiac arrhythmias occur i.v. amiodarone may be used.

If hypotension is not too severe and peripheral perfusion adequate, one can give an i.v. infusion of a vasodilator, such as glyceryl trinitrate (100–200 micrograms/min), isosorbide dinitrate (2–7 mg/h), or sodium nitroprusside (initially in a dosage of 0.5–1.5 micrograms/kg/min, increasing if required to 8 micrograms/kg/min) with careful continuous monitoring. These can be combined with low-dose dopamine (3–5 micrograms/kg/min).

In general, cardiac glycosides should be avoided as positive inotropic drugs in myocardial infarction. For the patient in mild heart failure they tend to increase myocardial oxygen consumption and enhance the risk of arrhythmias.

Their inotropic effect is in any case relatively small and in severe heart failure dobutamine at least is a more potent inotropic drug. However i.v. ouabain or oral digoxin should be used in patients with atrial fibrillation with a fast ventricular rate (for the treatment of arrhythmias see p. 281). Digoxin may also be of help later on when i.v. inotropic drugs have been withdrawn.

If drug therapy fails, balloon counter-pulsation may be used, although this is generally reserved for cases in which a mechanical problem has been identified (for example mitral valve rupture) or where cardiac transplant is being considered.

Whatever method of treatment is used the prognosis in acute cardiogenic shock is uniformly poor.

(ii) Cardiac arrhythmias

The common arrhythmias in acute myocardial infarction are: ventricular extra beats, ventricular tachycardia, and ventricular fibrillation; sinus tachycardia; atrial fibrillation and flutter; supraventricular tachycardia; and heart block (which we include for convenience under this heading). Their treatment is dealt with in the section on arrhythmias. Cardiac arrest (also dealt with below) may occur as a result of ventricular arrhythmias, asystole, bradycardia, or electromechanical dissociation.

(iii) Pericarditis

Acute pericarditis occurs in about 10 per cent of patients with an acute myocardial infarction, and causes severe, sharp, stabbing chest pain, made worse by coughing, by inspiration, and by sitting forward. It may be associated with breathlessness. The treatment of choice for mild or moderate pain due to acute pericarditis is indomethacin 50 mg t.d.s.

(c) Treatment of late complications

(i) Dressler's syndrome

This consists of fever with pericarditis and sometimes pleurisy. It occurs in about 4 per cent of patients. In some cases aspirin or other non-steroidal anti-inflammatory drugs may be sufficient. In patients who do not respond to aspirin, or if there is severe pain, a short course of corticosteroids should be given (for example prednisolone 60 mg o.d., reducing the dose to complete withdrawal in 4–6 days, or hydrocortisone 100 mg i.v. six-hourly). Occasionally attacks may be recurrent, requiring repeated courses of corticosteroid therapy.

(ii) Ventricular aneurysm

The formation of a left ventricular aneurysm may be suggested by persistent ST segment elevation on the electrocardiogram and it can be confirmed by echocardiography. Some cardiologists recommend the use of full dosages of oral anticoagulants in order to minimize the risk of mural thrombus and consequent cerebral embolism. These patients may also require treatment for heart failure and recurrent ventricular tachycardia.

Surgical resection is usually only considered when heart failure or arrhythmias do not respond to drugs.

(iii) Recurrent ischaemic pain

If ischaemic chest pain recurs without evidence of re-infarction or extension of infarction it should be treated in the same way as unstable angina (see section 23.2.2c, p. 270).

23.3.4 Treatment in the postinfarction period

Rehabilitation after myocardial infarction includes attention to physical and psychological well-being. Patients should be told to stop smoking, they should be instructed on how much exercise to take, on how to modify their diet, on when to return to work, when to drive again, and when and how sexual activity can be resumed. We shall not discuss these matters in detail.

Drug therapy after myocardial infarction generally consists of treatment for heart failure and arrhythmias (which are dealt with elsewhere, see pp. 287 and 276). There is also the question of the secondary prevention of myocardial infarction, which we shall consider here.

23.3.5 Secondary prevention of myocardial infarction

Various types of therapy have been investigated in the hope that it may be possible to prevent a recurrence of myocardial infarction after a first episode.

(a) Drugs which reduce platelet aggregation

Drugs such as aspirin, sulphinpyrazone, and dipyridamole have been used for this purpose. The evidence that dipyridamole and sulphinpyrazone are effective in secondary prevention is limited. However, there is considerable evidence that aspirin may reduce re-infarction rate by about 10 per cent, and when long-term aspirin therapy is given after a dose of streptokinase in the acute phase of myocardial infarction there is a 25 per cent reduction in subsequent mortality.

(b) β-adrenoceptor antagonists

There is now convincing evidence that β-adrenoceptor antagonists given after myocardial infarction reduce the subsequent incidence of both re-infarction and sudden death. The precise mechanism of this effect is unknown and could involve prevention of arrhythmias, reduction of myocardial oxygen requirements, and prevention of increased blood pressure.

Propranolol, sotalol, timolol, and metoprolol have individually been shown to be effective in the secondary prevention of myocardial infarction. However, the exact place of such therapy remains to be worked out: it is not clear, for example, which patients are most likely to benefit from this therapy, which (if any) of the numerous β-adrenoceptor antagonists is the drug of choice, what the optimum dose should be, for how long therapy should be continued, and whether or not the effects of β-adrenoceptor antagonists and aspirin are additive. Despite these uncertainties, most authorities would recommend β-blockade in the secondary prevention of myocardial infarction, unless the first event has been completely uncomplicated.

(c) Anticoagulants

There was a vogue some years ago for the use of long-term anticoagulant therapy with coumarin anticoagulants after myocardial infarction. The early studies which were said to show efficacy in preventing re-infarction were later heavily criticized and the practice was dropped. Recently there has been a revival of interest in this mode of treatment, but the current consensus is that the benefits do not outweigh the risks, except in a patient with a large anterior infarct, especially if there is an aneurysm, or if there have been arrhythmias or transient ischaemic attacks.

23.4 Cardiac arrhythmias

Cardiac arrhythmias are most commonly associated with ischaemic heart disease, but may also be due to congenital abnormalities of conduction pathways, to arrhythmogenic drugs, such as cardiac glycosides and antiarrhythmic drugs themselves, and to metabolic disturbances, such as hypokalaemia.

23.4.1 Classification of anti-arrhythmic drugs

The antiarrhythmic drugs have been classified pharmacologically into four main classes (classes I–IV), depending on their electrophysiological effects on the action potential (see Table 23.6 and lignocaine in the Pharmacopoeia, p. 624). This classification allows one to refer to large groups of drugs under a single banner (for example 'Class I antiarrhythmic drugs'), but it is not clear how those general classes of actions relate to the therapeutic effects of the antiarrhythmic drugs. In practice therefore the uses of these drugs are determined by empirical observations in studies of their efficacy, rather than on any strictly rational application of pharmacological understanding. An alternative method of classification, which may allow the student to remember better the uses of the antiarrhythmic drugs is based on their sites of action in the heart, and one such classification is shown in Table 23.6.

23.4.2 Principles underlying anti-arrhythmic drug therapy

There are certain practical principles at the root of antiarrhythmic drug therapy which must be considered in each case before prescribing an antiarrhythmic drug.

∎ **Table 23.6** Classifications of antiarrhythmic drugs

1. *Electrophysiological classification (based on that of Vaughan Williams)*

Class I	Ia	Ib	Ic
	Quinidine	Lignocaine	Lorcainide
	Procainamide	Phenytoin	
	Flecainide	Disopyramide	
	Mexiletine	Encainide	
	Tocainide	Propafenone	
		(also has Class II	
		activity)	

Class II

β-Adrenoceptor antagonists

Class III

Amiodarone
Sotalol (also has Class II activity)

Class IV

Verapamil

2. *Classification by site of action (the Classes refer to the drugs listed in part 1 of the Table)*

Atria	Sinoatrial node	Accessory pathways
Class Ia drugs	Class II drugs	Class Ia drugs
Class Ic drugs	Class IV drugs	Class III drugs
Class II drugs		
Class III drugs	*Atrioventricular node*	
	Class Ic drugs	
Ventricles	Class II drugs	
Class I drugs	Class IV drugs	
Class III drugs		

(a) Does the arrhythmia require treatment?

This question must be considered carefully with respect to two different aspects:

(i) Are there any treatable precipitating factors?

Not infrequently it may be possible to treat an arrhythmia by treating an underlying precipitating abnormality. Important precipitating factors in the ischaemic heart yielding to this approach are:

hypokalaemia;

acidosis and hypoxia;

drugs, for example cardiac glycosides;

heart failure;

pulmonary embolism;

pericarditis and myocarditis.

It is important to identify and treat hypokalaemia, not only because treatment may cause resolution of an arrhythmia, but because hypokalaemia may increase the arrhythmogenic effects of amiodarone and the class I antiarrhythmic drugs, such as lignocaine, quinidine, procainamide, and disopyramide. Because hypokalaemia is so common in acute myocardial infarction, perhaps because of increased influx of potassium into cells under the influence of catecholamines, patients are generally given oral potassium chloride immediately after an acute infarction, with the intention of preventing hypo-kalaemia.

(ii) Does the benefit of treatment outweigh the risk?

Compare, for example, recurrent ventricular tachycardia, which carries a high risk of ventricular fibrillation and which must be treated, with, at the other end of the spectrum, multiple supraventricular extra beats, which are harmless and which generally need no treatment. Atrial fibrillation with a fast ventricular response rate will eventually impair myocardial contractility, and the ventricular rate should be slowed.

However, atrial fibrillation with a normal ventricular rate does not need specific treatment, although in some cases anticoagulation will be necessary because of the risk of systemic emboli.

(b) Is there a non-drug treatment?

In some circumstances drug therapy can be avoided by the use of some other procedure. Examples include:

carotid sinus massage in acute supraventricular tachycardia;

d.c. cardioversion in acute supraventricular tachycardia, atrial fibrillation, ventricular tachycardia, and ventricular fibrillation;

surgical treatment in arrhythmias due to anomalous conduction pathways (for example Wolff–Parkinson–White syndrome);

overdrive pacing in *torsade de pointes*;

a permanent pacemaker in complete heart block;

specialized pacemakers for certain paroxysmal arrhythmias;

ablation of the atrioventricular (AV) node or an anomalous conduction pathway using radiofrequency discharges.

(c) Choice of drug

The drugs used in treating specific cardiac arrhythmias are listed in Table 23.7. In choosing a particular drug, consideration should be given to the following:

(i) Class of drug

Generally, treatment with antiarrhythmic drugs should be limited to one drug from any class or sub-class, because the adverse effects on the heart of two drugs from the same class will be additive. It may also be dangerous to combine amiodarone with those drugs of class I which prolong the QT interval of the electrocardiogram (for example the class Ia drugs, quinidine, procainamide, and disopyramide)

Non-cardiac adverse effects of antiarrhythmic drugs may constitute contra-indications to their use, and these are listed in Table 23.8. For example, atropine, quinidine, and disopyramide have anticholinergic effects and would be contra-indicated in patients with glaucoma or prostatic enlargement.

(ii) Drug interactions

Drug interactions involving antiarrhythmic drugs are listed in Table 23.9. These combinations should either be avoided altogether, or if they are used the dose of the object drug should be reduced.

(iii) The presence of heart failure or heart block

Those antiarrhythmic drugs which have pronounced negative inotropic effects and those which delay conduction through the AV node should be avoided or used with care in patients with heart failure or with heart block. Antiarrhythmic drugs which are particularly likely to exacerbate heart failure are quinidine, procainamide, disopyramide, β-adrenoceptor antagonists, and verapamil. Drugs likely to delay conduction through the AV node include quinidine, procainamide, disopyramide, β-adrenoceptor antagonists, and cardiac glycosides. Lignocaine does not decrease conduction velocity in normal conducting tissue but does if the tissue is ischaemic.

(d) Dose of drug

The pharmacokinetics of certain antiarrhythmic drugs are altered by cardiac failure and dosages may need to be altered accordingly (see p. 108). For example, the apparent volumes of distribution of lignocaine, quinidine, and procainamide are reduced in heart failure and loading doses should be reduced. In hepatic congestion the hepatic metabolism of these drugs will be affected and maintenance doses will also have to be reduced.

▮ **Table 23.7**   Drugs used in treating cardiac arrhythmias

Sinus node arrhythmias	
Sinus tachycardia	Treat cause
Sinus bradycardia	Atropine

Supraventricular arrhythmias

Atrial fibrillation	(D.c. cardioversion)
	Cardiac glycosides (p. 573)
	Calcium antagonists (p. 569)
	Amiodarone (p. 554)
	β-adrenoceptor antagonists (p. 544)
	Disopyramide (p. 596)
Atrial flutter	(D.c. cardioversion)
	(Atrial pacing)
	Amiodarone
	Cardiac glycosides
	Quinidine (p. 671)
Supraventricular tachycardia	(Carotid sinus massage, etc.)
	(D.c. cardioversion)
	β-adrenoceptor antagonists
	Diltiazem (p. 569)
	Verapamil (p. 569)
	Amiodarone
	Cardiac glycosides
	Disopyramide

Ventricular tachyarrhythmias	(D.c. cardioversion)
	(Overdrive pacing)
	Lignocaine (p. 624)
	Quinidine
	Procainamide (p. 667)
	Propafenone
	Disopyramide
	Mexiletine
	Tocainide
	Acecainide
	Flecainide
	Amiodarone

Digitalis-induced arrhythmias	(Withdraw digitalis)
	Antidigoxin antibody fragments
	Potassium chloride (p. 665)
	Phenytoin (p. 663)
	Lignocaine
	β-adrenoceptor antagonists
	Atropine

■ **Table 23.8** Important non-cardiac adverse effects of antiarrhythmic drugs

Drug	Class	Important non-cardiac adverse effects
Atropine	–	Anticholinergic effects
Quinidine	Ia	Cinchonism
		Anticholinergic effects
		Hypersensitivity reactions (including thrombocytopenia)
Procainamide	Ia	Lupus-like syndrome
		Hypersensitivity reactions
		Neutropenia (especially slow-release formulations)
Disopyramide	Ia	Anticholinergic effects
Lignocaine	Ib	Central nervous toxicity
Mexiletine	Ib	Central nervous toxicity
Acecainide	Ib	Central nervous toxicity
Phenytoin	Ib	Central nervous toxicity
		Long-term effects (see Pharmacopoeia)
Tocainide	Ib	Central nervous toxicity
		Neutropenia
Flecainide	Ic	Central nervous toxicity
Propafenone	Ic/II	Central nervous toxicity
β-blockers	II	Bronchoconstriction
		Peripheral vasoconstriction
Amiodarone	III	Corneal opacities
		Skin pigmentation and photosensitivity
		Thyroid dysfunction
		Fibrosing alveolitis
		Peripheral neuropathy
		Liver damage
Verapamil	IV	Headache (uncommon)

■ **Table 23.9** Drug interactions with antiarrhythmic drugs

Object drug	Precipitant drug	Result of interaction
Class I drugs	Class I drugs	Potentiation
Quinidine, procainamide, disopyramide, acecainide, amiodarone	The same drugs	Prolongation of the QT interval
Class I drugs	Drugs causing hypokalaemia	Increased risk of arrhythmias
Digoxin	Quinidine, amiodarone, verapamil	Digoxin toxicity
Warfarin	Amiodarone	Warfarin toxicity
Anticholinergic drugs	Quinidine, disopyramide	Potentiation
Class I drugs	β-adrenoceptor antagonists	Negative inotropy
Verapamil	β-adrenoceptor antagonists	Negative inotropy/ arrhythmias/asystole
Antihypertensive drugs	Bretylium	Severe hypotension

23.4.3 The practical treatment of cardiac arrhythmias

(a) Sinus node arrhythmias

(i) Sinus tachycardia

There is no specific treatment for sinus tachycardia and attention should be paid to the underlying cause. In hyperthyroidism the administration of a β-adrenoceptor antagonist will, among other things, slow a sinus tachycardia.

(ii) Sinus bradycardia

Chronic sinus bradycardia (ventricular rate below 60 per min) may be due to a number of different causes, including hypothyroidism and drugs such as β-adrenoceptor antagonists, the phenothiazines, cardiac glycosides, and acetylcholinesterase inhibitors. In these cases treatment of the underlying cause is all that is required, and in many cases when drugs are to blame no treatment at all is required, provided cardiac function otherwise remains normal. Sinus bradycardia is a normal feature in highly trained athletes and requires no treatment.

Sinus bradycardia is common after an acute myocardial infarction and need be treated only if there is clinically important lowering of the cardiac output. In that case atropine 0.5 mg i.v. should be given every 5 min until the heart rate rises above 60 per min or until a total maximum dose of 2 mg has been given.

Sinus bradycardia occurring as part of the sick sinus syndrome may require treatment with a pacemaker.

(b) Supraventricular arrhythmias

(i) Atrial fibrillation

The most common causes of atrial fibrillation are acute or chronic myocardial ischaemia, mitral stenosis, and hyperthyroidism. Less commonly it may be due to pericarditis, myocarditis, other acute infections, cardiomyopathies, sick sinus syndrome, Wolff–Parkinson–White syndrome, or an unknown cause (so-called 'lone fibrillation').

In atrial fibrillation of recent origin (for example after an acute myocardial infarction) the aim would be to convert the rhythm to sinus rhythm using d.c. shock. However, in some circumstances there is a high chance of recurrence after cardioversion (for example in mitral stenosis, severe left ventricular failure, sick sinus syndrome, and untreated hyperthyroidism), and in those cases drug therapy would be indicated. Cardioversion is unlikely to be successful if the diameter of the left atrium is over 5 cm, and ideally this should be determined by echocardiography before cardioversion is attempted. If atrial fibrillation persists in hyperthyroidism, despite the restoration of normal thyroid function, direct current (d.c.) cardioversion should be tried in the first place, followed by drugs if cardioversion fails.

Patients in whom cardioversion is to be attempted are at risk of embolism from atrial thrombus when the atria start to contract normally. It is customary, therefore, unless contraindicated, to anticoagulate patients with warfarin for 1 month before elective cardioversion, although it has not been satisfactorily proven that this prevents embolism.

If fast atrial fibrillation is of prolonged duration drugs are indicated, since reversion to sinus rhythm is unlikely. The aim of treatment will be to slow the ventricular rate to within normal limits (60–90 beats per min at rest). A cardiac glycoside is usually the treatment of choice and long-term therapy will generally be required. There is no hard-and-fast rule about the choice of cardiac glycoside, and it is best to become thoroughly acquainted with the use of one and stick to it. We prefer digoxin, and a suitable dosage regimen is outlined in the Pharmacopoeia.

Although cardiac glycosides are effective in slowing the ventricular rate at rest in patients with atrial fibrillation, they do not control it well during exercise. If the ventricular rate is not well controlled by digitalis or if there are symptoms of a fast ventricular rate during exercise (for example palpitation) a calcium antagonist with antiarrhythmic action can be added. Although many use verapamil for this purpose, we believe diltiazem (60 mg t.d.s. to 120 mg q.d.s.) to be preferable, since verapamil has a larger negative inotropic effect on the heart. Alternatively, one can use a β-adrenoceptor antagonist, such as sotalol (120–240 mg o.d.), which has the advantage over other β-blockers of having additional class III antiarrhythmic activity. Amiodarone is also very effective and useful in short-term treatment, but its adverse effects tend to limit its usefulness as a long-term antiarrhythmic drug.

In patients with hyperthyroidism one would start with a β-adrenoceptor antagonist, such as propranolol (see p. 544), and add digitalis or a calcium antagonist if there was a poor response, or in the presence of heart failure, or if a β-adrenoceptor antagonist were contra-indicated. In sick sinus syndrome digitalis is not helpful and may even worsen arrhythmias. Amiodarone may be used instead. In some cases it may be necessary to ablate the AV node by surgery or a discharge of radiofrequency energy and insert a pacemaker.

Atrial fibrillation in Wolff–Parkinson–White syndrome, and other syndromes associated with accessory conduction pathways, is particularly difficult to treat. Digitalis should not be used, since it blocks the conduction of impulses via the AV node but does not affect the accessory pathways. A single episode may be treated by d.c. cardioversion, but if drug therapy is required to prevent recurrent atrial fibrillation diltiazem or amiodarone may be used. In some cases surgery to ablate the accessory pathway may be required.

In patients with chronic atrial fibrillation secondary to mitral stenosis there is an increased risk of embolism from atrial mural thrombus, and lifelong anticoagulation with warfarin is required. It is not clear whether anticoagulation is beneficial in patients with atrial fibrillation due to other causes, although it is often used.

Attacks of paroxysmal atrial fibrillation are very difficult to prevent. Digitalis should not be used, since it is ineffective and may exacerbate arrhythmias. Currently a β-adrenoceptor antagonist is probably the treatment of choice, and we would use sotalol. Quinidine, amiodarone, and flecainide have also been used with variable success. Flecainide is perhaps the best of these, but its adverse effects in patients with ventricular arrhythmias after acute myocardial infarction have led to its being abandoned for all but the most resistant arrhythmias.

(ii) Atrial flutter with a fast ventricular rate

The causes of atrial flutter with a fast ventricular rate (for example over 150 per min) are the same as those of atrial fibrillation. Digitalis should be

tried first, although it is less likely to be effective than in atrial fibrillation. If it is ineffective, or if it converts the atrial flutter to atrial fibrillation, as sometimes happens, then d.c. cardioversion may be used. There is an increased risk of digitalis-induced arrhythmias after d.c. shock, and it is therefore important to start with very low energies (10 J) in patients who have had digoxin within the previous 2 or 3 d or digitoxin within the previous 1 or 2 weeks, increasing the energy gradually until cardioversion occurs. Ideally digoxin should be withdrawn for 24–48 h before cardioversion.

The main alternatives to digitalis or cardioversion are oral quinidine and i.v. amiodarone. Quinidine is given in a dose of 200 mg four-hourly to a total of 1.2 g in an attempt to convert the rhythm to atrial fibrillation, followed, if successful, by digitalis. If digoxin is used in combination with quinidine the dose of digoxin should be halved (see p. 131). A suitable i.v. dosage regimen for amiodarone is given in the Pharmacopoeia.

(iii) Supraventricular tachycardia

Acute supraventricular tachycardia can occur in acute myocardial infarction, in digitalis intoxication (often in combination with heart block), in myocarditis, and after cardiac surgery. Paroxysmal atrial tachycardia may be due to chronic ischaemia, sinoatrial disease, the pre-excitation syndromes (for example Wolff–Parkinson–White syndrome), other congenital conduction defects, and digitalis toxicity. Digitalis toxicity should be strongly suspected if a patient taking digitalis develops paroxysmal atrial tachycardia with heart block ('PAT with block').

Acute supraventricular tachycardia may not need treatment if the patient is otherwise well with a good cardiac output, and in such cases spontaneous reversion to sinus rhythm may occur. However, if it persists or if cardiac function is being impaired treatment is indicated. The first recourse is to try non-pharmacological manoeuvres aimed at stimulating the vagal innervation of the heart. Carotid sinus massage is the most commonly used of these, but it should not be carried out if there is a history or evidence of carotid disease (for example a carotid bruit or a history of transient cerebral ischaemic attacks) and it should always be performed with continuous electrocardiographic monitoring, since some individuals have a sensitive carotid sinus and may go into asystole with even light pressure on the carotid sinus. Firm pressure with circular massage using the thumb over the right carotid artery for 10–20 seconds is recommended.

If carotid sinus massage has no effect and there is severe embarrassment of cardiac function then d.c. cardioversion is the treatment of choice. It will successfully restore sinus rhythm in over 90 per cent of cases.

If there is no urgency, or if d.c. cardioversion fails or is not available, then drugs should be used. The main choices are from verapamil or a β-adrenoceptor antagonist. Verapamil is given as a slow i.v. injection of up to 10 mg at a rate of 1 mg/min, stopping if the ventricular rate falls below 100 per min. Verapamil should not be used in digitalis toxicity and sick sinus syndrome or if there is severe cardiac failure, because of its negative inotropic effect. It should not be given i.v. within 24 h of a β-adrenoceptor antagonist (see p. 132).

The alternative to verapamil is a β-adrenoceptor antagonist, especially in myocardial infarction, because of the other benefits of using β-adrenoceptor antagonists in such circumstances. Practolol should be used i.v. in an initial test dose of 1 mg, followed 5 min later by up to 20 mg at a rate of 1 mg/min. During its infusion the blood pressure must be continually monitored. Practolol should not be used in severe heart failure.

For those in whom these drugs are contraindicated, i.v. amiodarone is a suitable alternative, but it should not be used in digitalis toxicity.

For the treatment of digitalis-induced cardiac arrhythmias see below (p. 285).

Attacks of paroxysmal atrial tachycardia are very difficult to prevent. Digitalis should not be used, since it is ineffective and may exacerbate arrhythmias. Currently a β-adrenoceptor antagonist, such as sotalol, is probably the treatment of choice. Quinidine, amiodarone, and flecainide have also been used with variable success (see the treatment of paroxysmal atrial fibrillation, p. 282).

(c) Ventricular arrhythmias

Ventricular extra beats, ventricular tachycardia, and ventricular fibrillation occur most commonly after acute myocardial infarction, but can also occur in otherwise healthy individuals, or because of chronic ischaemia, digitalis toxicity, and the effects of other antiarrhythmic drugs and of tricyclic antidepressants (especially in overdose). When they are due to antiarrhythmic drugs they are more likely in patients with potassium depletion and those with poor left ventricular function.

(i) Treatment of ventricular arrhythmias immediately after acute myocardial infarction

The treatment of ventricular extra beats in acute myocardial infarction is somewhat controversial. The difficulty is that there is a high risk of ventricular tachycardia or fibrillation, arrhythmias which are potentially fatal, and which it has been presumed can be prevented by suppressing the extra beats, any one of which might initiate tachycardia or fibrillation. However, there is no clear guidance as to when to use antiarrhythmic drugs in these circumstances and poor understanding of the exact benefit:risk ratios. The difficulty is increased by the fact that the drugs used in the suppression of ventricular extra beats are all cardiotoxic and may cause cardiac failure or arrhythmias, especially in patients with myocardial infarction.

The traditional guidelines for the use of antiarrhythmic drugs are as follows:

more than five ventricular extra beats in a minute; or

multifocal extra beats; or

salvos of extra beats (i.e. runs of more than two beats at a time); or

recurrent bouts of ventricular tachycardia; or premature extra beats (also called 'R on T' phenomenon).

However, there are some problems with these guidelines. For example, the premise for treating extra beats which fall very shortly after the T wave of the preceding sinus beat is based on the experimental observation that introducing an extra beat during ventricular repolarization (i.e. at the same time as the T wave) virtually always results in a fatal ventricular arrhythmia. However, there is no clear evidence that the nearer an extra beat is to the preceding T wave the more likely it is that the next extra beat will occur during ventricular repolarization. Furthermore, not all patients who develop ventricular tachyarrhythmias have 'warning' extra beats, nor do all those with extra beats go on to develop serious tachyarrhythmias.

Different authorities therefore adopt different attitudes to the use of antiarrhythmic drugs after myocardial infarction. Some recommend using drugs in all patients, on the assumption that this will reduce the incidence of ventricular tachyarrhythmias. At the other extreme, some prefer simply to observe patients with extra beats, using drugs only if ventricular tachycardia or fibrillation occur. If the latter policy is adopted then it should be in circumstances in which facilities for resuscitation are immediately available (see cardiac arrest below).

We feel that the following set of guidelines is a reasonable one:

1. Potassium depletion should be corrected or prevented by the oral administration of potassium chloride.

2. Since there is no evidence that the use of antiarrhythmic drugs prevents serious arrhythmias in patients without arrhythmias to start with, the risk of such treatment outweighs the benefit and should be avoided.

3. Ventricular extra beats should be treated (especially if facilities for resuscitation are not readily available) if they occur repeatedly in salvos.

4. If suppression of ventricular extra beats does not occur with a single drug then it is best to observe, since the use of more antiarrhythmic drugs increases the risk of adverse effects, particularly of arrhythmias.

Not only is there no general agreement as to when to treat ventricular extra beats, but there is also no general agreement as to the best drug to use when treatment is indicated. However, i.v. lignocaine is still widely regarded as the treatment of choice. The usual loading dose is 100 mg, followed by a maintenance infusion at decreasing rates (see Chapter 6, p. 68). In this way therapeutic concentrations may be rapidly achieved and then maintained. Because it has active and potentially toxic metabolites which may accumulate, lignocaine cannot be used for longer than 24–48 h, but in most cases suppression of ventricular extra beats after myocardial infarction does not need to be continued for longer than 48 h.

If lignocaine does not suppress ventricular extra beats, other possibilities are another class I antiarrhythmic drug or amiodarone. Amiodarone is given initially in a dose of 5 mg/kg i.v. over 20 min, followed by another 12 mg/kg over the next 24 h. Oral maintenance therapy can then be started in a dosage of 200 mg daily. For patients who have already had lignocaine it carries the advantage of having a different effect on the action potential from the class I drugs.

The major alternative to lignocaine from among the class I drugs is disopyramide. It can be given i.v., but because it has a potent negative inotropic effect it must be given by slow infusion at a rate of 2 mg/kg over 15 min, 2 mg/kg over the next 45 min, and then 0.4 mg/kg/h as a maintenance infusion. The dose in the first hour should not exceed 300 mg and the total daily dose should not exceed 800 mg.

There are no other good alternatives to lignocaine and disopyramide from among the class I drugs. Although flecainide is a very effective antiarrhythmic drug, it has recently been shown to increase the risk of sudden death after myocardial infarction in certain patients, and as a result its use is now restricted in all patients to life-threatening sustained resistant arrhythmias. It is then given in a dose of 2 mg/kg (maximum 150 mg) by i.v. infusion over 30 min, followed by a maintenance infusion at a rate of 1.5 mg/kg/h for 1 h then 100–250 micrograms/kg/h. Dosages of flecainide should be reduced in severe renal impairment.

Procainamide may be used, and is given at a rate of 25 mg/min until either the extra beats are abolished or 1000 mg have been given. An i.v. infusion can then be continued at a rate of 0.25–2 mg/min. However, procainamide has a marked negative inotropic effect and may cause hypersensitivity reactions.

Other alternatives which are less suitable are quinidine, mexiletine, and tocainide. Mexiletine has a high rate of dose-related adverse effects, particularly on the CNS, and since it resembles lignocaine in action it is better avoided after lignocaine has already been used. Quinidine is not available in i.v. form in some countries and is pharmaceutically quite difficult to prepare. Tocainide has actions similar to those of lignocaine, but its use is restricted to the treatment of life-threatening and otherwise resistant arrhythmias because of the risk of bone-marrow toxicity.

Other anti-arrhythmic drugs which have been used in these circumstances include the class I drugs lorcainide and propafenone (which also has some β-blocking action), and the class III drug acecainide (*N*-acetylprocainamide). However, experience with these drugs is too limited for them to be freely recommended.

(ii) Treatment of chronic ventricular arrhythmias

Chronic ventricular extra beats do not generally require therapy. However, symptomatic ventricular extra beats in a patient asking for therapy pose a problem, since it is not clear that the benefit of treatment outweighs the risks. After careful explanation of this to the patient, one may use either amiodarone or a class I antiarrhythmic drug, as described below for sustained ventricular tachycardia.

Episodes of sustained ventricular tachycardia more than 48 h after a myocardial infarct have grave prognostic significance and should be investigated thoroughly. Any drugs which may be causing arrhythmias (for example digitalis) should be withdrawn, and cardiac failure and potassium depletion should be treated appropriately (see pp. 287 and 347). Left ventricular aneurysm and thrombus should be sought by echocardiography, and left ventricular function should be assessed, since it will affect the choice of antiarrhythmic drug. Angiography should also be considered, since in some cases arrhythmias are due to ischaemia in a critical area and this may be treatable by angioplasty or by-pass graft surgery.

If there is severe impairment of left ventricular function (ejection fraction less than 30 per cent) amiodarone is the drug of choice, since the risk of causing arrhythmias with class I drugs is relatively high in such cases. Amiodarone is given in an initial oral dose of 200 mg t.d.s. for 1–4 weeks, depending on the response, thereafter reducing gradually to a suitable maintenance dose, often 200 mg o.d.

If left ventricular function is moderately good a class I drug should be used, since the risk of drug-induced arrhythmias is less than when left ventricular function is poor and preferable to the risk of the long-term adverse effects of amiodarone. The choice of a class I drug is disopyramide, given in a dosage of 100–200 mg q.d.s. However, it should not be used in patients with severe cardiac failure or if its anticholinergic actions are likely to prove a problem (for example in patients with prostatic enlargement or glaucoma).

However, in such cases there is no good alternative drug: quinidine is anticholinergic and often causes ventricular arrhythmias (so-called 'quinidine syncope'); procainamide and tocainide cause neutropenias; flecainide and encainide are associated with an increased death rate in patients who have had a myocardial infarction. Newer drugs, such as propafenone, moricizine, and acecainide, may become useful, but it is too soon to be sure.

If it is available, programmed electrical stimulation will help choose the appropriate drug in these circumstances, since there is a good correlation between the short-term effects of class I antiarrhythmic drugs in treating electrically induced ventricular tachycardia and their long-term efficacy. The technique involves the introduction of a ventricular pacing wire, which is used to deliver timed extrasystoles; if ventricular tachycardia can be induced the effects of different drugs of class I may be tested and the most effective drug can be chosen for long-term therapy. Alternatively, specialist surgical management may be considered.

The approach to the treatment of episodes of sustained ventricular tachycardia in patients who have not had a myocardial infarct is similar to that outlined above.

(d) Digitalis-induced arrhythmias

Digitalis toxicity commonly causes ectopic ventricular and supraventricular arrhythmias, or heart block, or a combination of the two. In all cases one should withhold digitalis and measure the plasma potassium concentration, giving oral or i.v. potassium chloride if necessary (see p. 347). In severe cases the treatment of choice is Fab fragments of antidigoxin antibody, which are effective in toxicity due to digoxin and other cardiac glycosides, such as digitoxin and lanatoside C. Antidigoxin antibody doses can be calculated as shown in Table 34.5. If antidigoxin antibody is not available then activated charcoal may be given by mouth, since it enhances the rate of excretion of digoxin and digitoxin. Alternatively, in the case of digitoxin, a steroid binding resin may do the same (for example cholestyramine 12–24 g daily in divided doses). If antiarrhythmic drugs are required the following are the choices.

(i) Ventricular tachyarrhythmias

Phenytoin is the treatment of choice. Of all the class I drugs it is the only one to increase conduction velocity in the AV node. However, very careful electrocardiographic monitoring is required, since serious arrhythmias may occur during its use. It should not be used if there is second- or third-degree heart block, since it decreases ventricular automaticity. The dose is 4 mg/kg given i.v. at a rate not exceeding 50 mg/min. This dose may be repeated after 10 min if necessary, and oral therapy can then be given in dosages similar to those used in epilepsy. If phenytoin is ineffective the alternatives are i.v. lignocaine or an i.v. β-adrenoceptor antagonist. If there is concurrent heart block then these drugs should be used only if there is a pacemaker in position. Direct current cardioversion is not contra-indicated in the face of a life-threatening arrhythmia.

(ii) Paroxysmal atrial tachycardia with block

Phenytoin, lignocaine, or an i.v. β-adrenoceptor antagonist should be used with a pacemaker in position, in case these drugs worsen heart block.

(iii) Sinus bradycardia

This should be treated only if it causes hypotension. It will often respond to atropine (see above), but sometimes a pacemaker may be necessary.

(e) Cardiac arrest after myocardial infarction

Cardiac arrest is usually due to acute ventricular tachycardia or fibrillation, or to cardiac asystole, the last having the worst prognosis. Cardiac arrest is an acute medical emergency, since cerebral hypoxia lasting more than 2–4 min results in irreversible brain damage. The aims of treatment are therefore to provide oxygen to the tissues and to restore normal cardiac rhythm. The following procedures should be carried out, if possible more or less simultaneously by several assistants.

1. Give a sharp blow over the sternum with a clenched fist. This wastes little time and occasionally restores normal rhythm.

2. Make sure the patient is on a hard surface (for example in a bed with a hard base or on the floor), otherwise effective cardiac massage will be difficult.

3. Make sure the airways are patent. Remove dentures, suck out vomit, and if possible insert an endotracheal tube and give oxygen. Otherwise give respiration by the mouth-to-mouth method or with an Ambu bag and check that the chest moves with each inspiration.

4. Start cardiac massage.

5. Correct acidosis by giving sodium bicarbonate 50 mmol i.v. (50 mL of an 8.4 per cent solution). This should be done only in patients in whom effective ventilation is being carried out, otherwise the carbon dioxide formed from the bicarbonate will diffuse into cells, causing further intracellular acidosis. The bicarbonate, and all other drugs, should be given via a cannula inserted into a jugular or subclavian vein rather than a more peripheral vein.

6. Direct current cardioversion should be carried out as soon as possible. Ideally one should first identify the cardiac rhythm, since d.c. cardioversion is of no use in asystole. However, if an electrocardiogram cannot be obtained, blind cardioversion should be carried out at 200 J. If ventricular fibrillation or ventricular tachycardia are not terminated, cardioversion should not be tried again for another 2 min or so. In the meantime cardiac massage and oxygenation should be continued. If then second and third cardioversions (200 J and 360 J respectively) fail, adrenaline (1.0 mL of a 1:1000 solution, i.e. 1.0 mg) should be given i.v. and a further defibrillation (360 J) tried. If that is unsuccessful i.v. lignocaine should be given (100 mg), followed by repeated attempts at cardioversion (360 J). If this does not work bretylium tosylate (5 mg/kg) should be given i.v. followed by

further attempts at cardioversion. Sometimes changing the positions of the defibrillating paddles may help. Do not mix adrenaline with bicarbonate, which inactivates it. Wait two minutes after each drug administration before trying another cardioversion and meanwhile continue cardiac massage and ventilation.

7. If there is cardiac asystole give adrenaline (1 mL of a 1:1000 solution, i.e. 1.0 mg) i.v. followed by atropine (2 mg i.v.). Calcium chloride (10 mL of a 10 per cent solution) is no longer recommended in these circumstances, except in the case of overdose with a calcium antagonist. It is important not to infuse calcium salts at the same time as sodium bicarbonate, since this will result in precipitation of the insoluble salt calcium carbonate.

There are two main indications for the use of other drugs in cardiac arrest: to treat arrhythmias and cardiac failure.

Not infrequently the result of cardioversion of a ventricular tachyarrhythmia is not sinus rhythm, but some other rhythm, such as sinus or nodal bradycardia, or idioventricular rhythm. If cardioversion results in some supraventricular arrhythmia, whether sinus or not, lignocaine should be given to try to prevent recurrence of the ventricular arrhythmia. If there is a bradycardia, atropine 0.5 mg i.v. should be given and heart block should be treated by transvenous pacing. Idioventricular rhythm may also respond to atropine, which increases the rate of sinus depolarization, or to overdrive pacing (i.e. pacing the right atrium at a faster rate than the ventricular rate). It is important at this stage to continue to assess cardiac output, by feeling the volume of the carotid pulse, and to continue cardiac massage until the heart rate increases.

Occasionally cardiographic sinus rhythm may be restored but without a palpable pulse (electro-mechanical dissociation). In that case give adrenaline (1 mg i.v.) and look for possible treatable causes, such as hypovolaemic shock, pneumothorax, or cardiac tamponade.

Cardiac failure should be treated as discussed in the section on myocardial infarction.

If resuscitation is successful check the arterial blood gases, the plasma electrolytes, and the chest X-ray, and treat any complications (for example aspiration pneumonia).

23.5 Cardiac failure

23.5.1. Mechanisms of action of drugs used to treat cardiac failure

The ways in which drugs affect the major pathophysiological abnormalities of cardiac failure are shown in Fig. 23.3, and a list of the drugs used is given in Table 23.10.

There are two principles in the treatment of cardiac failure.

(a) Removal of the underlying cause

In Table 23.11 are listed the major causes of cardiac failure. In some cases treating the cause will remove the problem of cardiac failure. Cardiac failure due to valvular disease, hypertension, anaemia, and hyperthyroidism, if treated early enough, may be amenable to this approach without the need for further specific therapy.

(b) Control of the signs and symptoms of cardiac failure

This can be done using three types of drug:

diuretics to remove excess sodium and water;

positive inotropic drugs to increase cardiac contractility;

vasodilators to reduce the workload of the heart.

Before discussing these facets of drug therapy of cardiac failure, we must first consider the relationship between cardiac output and ventricular end-diastolic pressure. This is called the Frank–Starling curve, after the physiologists who first described the relationship between cardiac output and venous pressure in an isolated heart–lung preparation. The relationship is illustrated in Fig. 23.4(a). The normal curve shows that cardiac output increases with an increase in ventricular end-diastolic pressure, but only up to a certain point, past which cardiac output starts to fall. In established cardiac failure the curve is set lower down; that is, at any given value of ventricular end-diastolic pressure cardiac output is lower than normal. Cardiac output may be able to be increased (for example by increased endogenous sympathetic drive), but that can only happen at the expense of an increased ventricular end-diastolic pressure, and eventually signs and

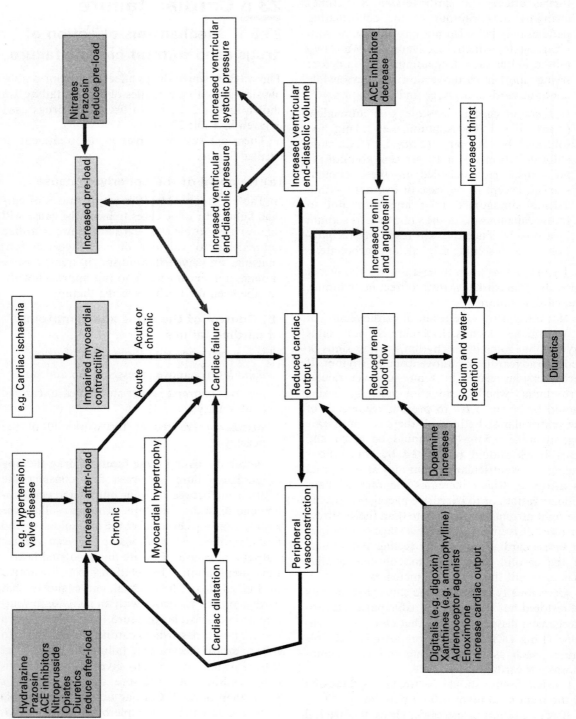

∎ **Fig. 23.3** The pathophysiology of cardiac failure and the sites and mechanisms of action of drugs used in its treatment.

▮ **Table 23.10** Drugs used in the treatment of cardiac failure

1. Diuretics
   Thiazide diuretics (p. 695)
   Thiazide-like diuretics (see Table 23.2)
   Loop diuretics
      Frusemide (p. 608)
      Bumetanide (p. 566)
   Potassium-sparing diuretics
      Amiloride (p. 551)
      Triamterene (p. 697)
      Spironolactone (p. 687)

2. Positive inotropic drugs
   Cardiac glycosides (p. 573)
   Phosphodiesterase inhibitors
      Non-specific
         Xanthines (for example aminophylline;
         p. 715)
      Specific (phosphodiesterase III)
         Enoximone
         Milrinone
   Adrenoceptor agonists (p. 541)

3. Vasodilators
   Opiates (morphine and diamorphine) (p. 641)
   Nitrates (p. 651)
   ACE inhibitors (p. 556)
   Sodium nitroprusside (p. 686)
   Hydralazine (p. 614)
   Prazosin (p. 543)

▮ **Table 23.11** Causes of cardiac failure

1. Decreased contractility
   Chronic ischaemia
   Acute myocardial infarction
   Cardiomyopathies
   Drugs
      Negative inotropic drugs
         β-adrenoceptor antagonists
         verapamil
         some class I antiarrhythmics
   Drug-induced cardiomyopathy
      doxorubicin

2. Increased afterload
   Hypertension
   Aortic valve disease
   Hypertrophic obstructive cardiomyopathy

3. Increased output
   Mitral incompetence
   Cardiac arrhythmias
   Anaemia
   Hyperthyroidism
   Peripheral shunts (for example arteriovenous
      shunts, Paget's disease)

4. Pulmonary heart disease (cor pulmonale)
   Chronic airways obstruction
   Recurrent pulmonary embolism

symptoms of congestion occur. If cardiac output cannot be increased then the signs are of low output (for example in cardiogenic shock).

(i) Diuretics

Sodium and water retention occur in cardiac failure through a combination of a variety of mechanisms, including reduced renal blood flow, increased antidiuretic hormone (ADH) secretion, and increased renin secretion, leading to increased secretion of angiotensin and aldosterone. Diuretics act to reduce the body sodium and water content. However, in the treatment of acute left ventricular failure the effects of frusemide and bumetanide occur more quickly than would be expected from the rate of onset of their diuretic actions, and vasodilator effects may be involved in their acute actions. Spironolactone is an aldo-

sterone antagonist which counteracts the hyperaldosteronism which can occur from cardiac failure itself and as a secondary response to the natriuresis produced by other diuretics. The effect of diuretics on the Frank–Starling curve is to lower the ventricular end-diastolic pressure (for example from point P towards point O in Fig. 23.4(a)).

(ii) Positive inotropic drugs

The end effect of positive inotropic drugs is to increase the cardiac output at any given value of ventricular end-diastolic pressure. Thus, the Frank–Starling curve is shifted upwards (see Fig. 23.4(a)). Consider, for example, a man whose normal state is at point N in Fig. 23.4(a). In heart failure with the same ventricular end-diastolic pressure his cardiac output would fall to point O, and if he were able to increase his cardiac output by increased sympathetic drive he

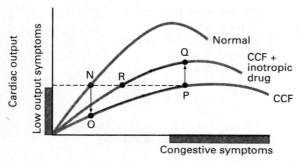

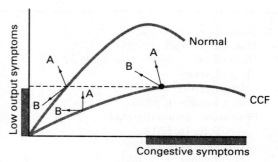

Ventricular end-diastolic pressure

■ **Fig. 23.4** The Frank–Starling curve illustrated here for the relationship between ventricular end-diastolic pressure and cardiac output. (a) The effect of positive inotropic drugs: inotropic drugs increase the cardiac output for any given value of end-diastolic pressure. (b) The effect of vasodilators: the effects of vasodilators depend on whether they are predominantly arterial vasodilators (A: for example hydralazine) or mixed vasodilators (B: for example prazosin). ((a) Adapted from Mason (1973). *Am. J. Cardiol.* **32**, 437–48 and (b) Adapted from Braunwald (1980). *Heart Disease* p. 548, W. B. Saunders, Philadelphia, with permission.)

would do so at the expense of an increased ventricular end-diastolic pressure (point P) and would develop the signs and symptoms of congestive cardiac failure. A positive inotropic drug would increase the cardiac output (point Q) and that would allow the ventricular end-diastolic pressure to fall without cardiac output falling below normal (point R). Thus, a normal cardiac output can be maintained, albeit with an increased ventricular end-diastolic pressure, and the signs and symptoms of congestive cardiac failure will be relieved if the ventricular end-diastolic pressure is low enough.

The most commonly used inotropic drugs are the cardiac glycosides. They probably act by inhibition of sodium transport out of cells through inhibition of the Na^+K^+ pump enzyme $Na^+K^+ATPase$. The resultant increase in intracellular sodium concentration leads to altered calcium flux via the Na^+/Ca^{2+} exchange mechanism, and thus to an increased intracellular calcium concentration. This leads to increased contractility through excitation–contraction coupling.

The β-adrenoceptor agonists (for example dopamine and dobutamine) cause an increase in myocardial cellular cyclic AMP concentrations, and this increases the availability of calcium to contractile sites.

Phosphodiesterase inhibitors cause an increase in tissue cyclic AMP. Xanthines, such as aminophylline, are non-specific inhibitors of phosphodiesterase, while enoximone, milrinone, and related compounds are specific for myocardial phosphodiesterase type III.

(iii) Vasodilators

Vasodilators reduce the workload of the heart by dilating either arterioles, or venules, or both. Dilatation of arterioles results in a reduction in cardiac afterload and dilatation of venules results in a reduction in cardiac preload. A pure reduction in afterload will increase the cardiac output at a given ventricular end-diastolic pressure, while a pure reduction in preload will reduce the ventricular end-diastolic pressure and hence the cardiac output along the Frank–Starling curve (Fig. 23.4(b)). In practice vasodilators cause both of these effects. That is because a reduction in arterial resistance (reduction in afterload) increases ventricular emptying, which in turn reduces preload, and venous dilatation (reduction in preload) decreases ventricular volume, which in turn reduces afterload. In both cases cardiac output increases and ventricular end-diastolic pressure falls. However, the extent to which these two effects occur depends on whether the vasodilator acts predominantly on arterioles or venules. For example, in a patient with congestive cardiac failure hydralazine, which is a pure arteriolar dilator, has a larger effect on cardiac output than on ventricular end-diastolic pressure. In contrast, prazosin, which is both an arteriolar and a venular vasodilator, alters both cardiac output and ventricular end-diastolic pressure equally (see Fig. 23.4(b)). Furthermore, the extent and direction of the effects of these vasodilators also depend on the severity of the disease, as shown in Fig. 23.4(b): compare the effects in normal individuals with those in patients with cardiac failure with normal ventricular end-diastolic pressure and those in patients with congestive cardiac failure.

23.5.2 Practical treatment of cardiac failure

(a) Left ventricular failure

Acute left ventricular failure producing pulmonary oedema is a medical emergency, requiring treatment with oxygen, morphine or diamorphine, a loop diuretic, and vasodilators if required, as described above under the treatment of acute left ventricular failure in myocardial infarction. Oxygen should be given in a high concentration by face mask or nasal cannulae. Frusemide is given i.v. in a dose of 40 mg; bumetanide can be given instead (1 mg i.v.). This is followed by i.v. morphine, 10 mg via the same needle.

If there is a poor response to this regimen then the dose of morphine may be repeated and higher doses of diuretic given. However, in severe left ventricular failure i.v. vasodilators, such as glyceryl trinitrate or isosorbide dinitrate, should be used, as described under the treatment of left ventricular failure and cardiogenic shock in the section on myocardial infarction.

Cardiac glycosides may also be used in acute left ventricular failure, particularly when it is associated with fast atrial fibrillation. The use of digoxin is described in the Pharmacopoeia (p. 573) In acute left ventricular failure due to acute severe hypertension the blood pressure should be lowered using hydralazine, nitroprusside, or diazoxide (see under hypertension).

Acute left ventricular failure due to iatrogenic fluid overload can be prevented by the use of a loop diuretic. For example, during blood transfusion in a patient with chronic anaemia, and therefore a normal intravascular volume, frusemide 20 mg i.v. should be given immediately before each unit of blood.

(b) Congestive cardiac failure

The initial treatment of cardiac failure is generally with diuretics. If the response to diuretics is felt to be inadequate a vasodilator may be added and nowadays most would choose an ACE inhibitor. An alternative in patients with cardiac failure due to ischaemic heart disease, mitral valve disease, or hypertensive heart disease is a cardiac glycoside. In severe cardiac failure one may use a combination of a diuretic with either a vasodilator or a cardiac glycoside from the start, proceeding to a combination of all three if necessary.

(i) Diuretics

The choice of diuretic depends on the severity of cardiac failure. In mild cardiac failure a thiazide or thiazide-like diuretic is sufficient (see Table 26.1). The most commonly used of these diuretics in the UK are bendrofluazide (5–10 mg o.d. orally) and cyclopenthiazide (0.5–1.0 mg o.d. orally), but there is no particular advantage in using any one of these diuretics rather than another.

In more severe cardiac failure oral loop diuretics are used, for example frusemide 40–160 mg o.d. or bumetanide 1–5 mg o.d. If there is a poor response to thiazides or loop diuretics the two types may be combined.

In using these diuretics care must be taken to avoid hypokalaemia, especially in old people and in patients taking cardiac glycosides, and potassium chloride supplements or a potassium-sparing diuretic will generally be required. Thus, it is common to prescribe a thiazide diuretic or a loop diuretic in combination with a potassium-sparing diuretic (amiloride, triamterene, or spironolactone). The use of potassium chloride supplements and of potassium-sparing diuretics is discussed in Chapter 26. In some cases it may be necessary to use a combination of all three types of diuretic.

(ii) Vasodilators

It has recently become common practice to introduce vasodilators early on in the treatment of cardiac failure. The choice is from among those with predominantly arteriolar actions and those with mixed arteriolar and venular actions (Table 23.12). The outcome of the physiology discussed above is that the arteriolar dilators are primarily useful for those who have symptoms of low cardiac output while the mixed dilators will be more useful for those with congestive signs and symptoms (see Fig. 23.4(b)).

In most patients a mixed vasodilator is indicated, and the first choice is an ACE inhibitor, such as captopril or enalapril. These drugs have the advantage over other vasodilators that they have additional actions besides vasodilatation, including inhibition of aldosterone release. They thus reduce sodium and water retention and promote potassium retention, which is helpful in patients also taking diuretics. In contrast, other vasodilators may promote sodium and water retention. The ACE inhibitors also reduce myocardial oxygen demand, which other vasodilators do not do. Hydralazine would be the arteriolar dilator of choice if a pure arteriolar dilator were required. However, it has important adverse effects (see p. 262) and nifedipine, which has some venular effects, is generally preferred in most cases. The dosages of all these drugs are as discussed under hypertension (see p. 260).

■ **Table 23.12** Effects of different vasodilators on arterioles and venules

Drug	Arterial dilatation	Venous dilatation
Hydralazine	+ +	−
Calcium antagonists	+ +	+
ACE inhibitors	+ +	+ +
Prazosin	+ +	+ +
Salbutamol	+ +	+ +
Nitroprusside	+ +	+ +
Nitrates	+	+ +
Opiates	+	+ +

(iii) Cardiac glycosides

A cardiac glycoside may be added to diuretic therapy if diuretics have not been completely effective. Cardiac glycosides are likely to be effective in patients with cardiac failure due to chronic ischaemia, mitral valve disease, and hypertension. They should not be used, or are ineffective, in the following conditions:

left ventricular outflow obstruction (for example aortic stenosis, hypertrophic obstructive cardiomyopathy), since they increase the force of contraction against a fixed obstruction;

constrictive pericarditis, for an analogous reason;

chronic cor pulmonale, because of decreased efficacy and an increased risk of toxicity, perhaps secondary to hypoxia and acidosis;

hyperthyroidism, because of decreased efficacy and an increased risk of toxicity, although they may be useful in addition to a β-adrenoceptor antagonist in patients with atrial fibrillation (see p. 282).

The question of the long-term efficacy of cardiac glycosides in cardiac failure in sinus rhythm has been the subject of much study. There is no doubt that digitalis is effective in the short-term treatment of some forms of cardiac failure (see above), but it has been thought that in some patients its efficacy is not maintained in the long term. This is partly due to the fact that when cardiac failure has resolved it may remain in remission for some time before further treatment is required. However, it is now common practice to give continuous treatment for cardiac failure in order to prevent relapse. On the other hand, there is a high risk of toxicity in using digitalis and some prefer not to use it in long-term therapy. The following are practical guidelines:

1. If the patient's condition is stable and there has been some identifiable precipitant of cardiac failure which has since been treated (for example anaemia, hyperthyroidism), then one may withdraw the cardiac glycoside.

2. If the patient's condition is stable and the plasma glycoside concentration is below the lower end of the accepted therapeutic range

(0.8 ng/mL for digoxin, see Chapter 7), then one may withdraw the cardiac glycoside.

3. If digitalis is withheld from other patients whose condition is stable, then in about a third of cases there will be subsequent clinical deterioration. The risk is particularly high in patients with evidence of poor left ventricular function (for example a third heart sound). In general it is therefore better to continue treatment, unless there is an increased risk of digitalis toxicity (for example in a patient with severe impairment of renal function or at high risk of potassium depletion). If withdrawal is undertaken in such patients then careful observations should be made over the next few weeks in anticipation of possible worsening of cardiac function.

(iv) Anticoagulants

In immobile patients with severe cardiac failure with swollen legs due to oedema there is an increased risk of venous thrombosis. Prophylactic anticoagulation is therefore advisable in such patients, using either an oral anticoagulant (for example warfarin) or low-dose subcutaneous heparin.

23.6 Infective endocarditis

The principles of the treatment of infection are outlined in Chapter 22. In infective endocarditis the aims are:

(1) to prevent the infection from occurring;

(2) to identify the infective organism when infection occurs;

(3) to eradicate the organism, by using the appropriate antibiotics in sufficient doses for sufficient a period of time;

(4) to make continual careful observations of the patient's condition and to consider the indications for surgical intervention.

23.6.1 Prevention of infective endocarditis

There are two factors which combine to cause infective endocarditis. They are as follows:

(a) The presence of a cardiac abnormality

A cardiac abnormality, such as a valvular or septal defect or an artificial valve, provides a site for infection. Some abnormalities are associated with a high risk of endocarditis and some with a lower risk (Table 23.13).

(b) The occurrence of bacteraemia

Infective endocarditis occurs when an abnormal heart is infected by bacteria released into the circulation from an infected site, for example bad teeth or a skin abscess, or after some surgical procedure. The most commonly incriminated procedure is dental surgery, but other procedures also carry a risk, including gastrointestinal, biliary, and genitourinary surgery, upper respiratory surgery, and cardiac surgery with extracorporeal circulation. Drug addicts (main-liners) have an increased risk of endocarditis, particularly in the right side of the heart.

■ **Table 23.13** Cardiac abnormalities associated with a risk of infective endocarditis

1. *High risk*
   Aortic valve disease (acquired or congenital)
   Aortic coarctation
   Mitral regurgitation
   Prosthetic valves
   Ventricular septal defect
   Atrial septal defect (ostium primum)
   Tetralogy of Fallot
   Transposition of the great vessels
   A previous episode of infective endocarditis

2. *Intermediate risk*
   Mitral valve prolapse if accompanied
      by mitral regurgitation
      (no risk otherwise)
   Hypertrophic obstructive cardiomyopathy
   Pulmonary stenosis
   Marfan's syndrome

3. *Low risk*
   Mitral stenosis
   Tricuspid valve disease
      (but high risk in drug addicts)
   Atrial septal defect
      (other than ostium primum)

For each of these types of procedure different prophylactic regimens are recommended, since the organisms likely to cause infection vary. In Table 23.13 are listed the various therapeutic regimens appropriate to the different surgical procedures. A few points about these regimens should be stressed.

1. All involve a penicillin. If the patient gives a history of penicillin hypersensitivity then an alternative should be used, either vancomycin or erythromycin, as shown in Table 23.14.

2. Intramuscular or intravenous antibiotics should be given 30 min before any procedure. Oral antibiotics should usually be given 60 min before any procedure (with some exceptions, see Table 23.14). If preoperative treatment is more prolonged there is a risk that resistant organisms will emerge and cause an infection that will be difficult to treat. The main aim of prophylaxis is to cover the transient bacteraemia which occurs during surgical procedures.

3. In some cases it is also necessary to give another dose of antibiotic after the procedure (see Table 23.14).

4. Vancomycin is ototoxic and nephrotoxic and should not be used in patients with pre-existing hearing impairment or renal damage. In a patient who is hypersensitive to penicillin and in whom vancomycin is contra-indicated a cephalosporin should be used, for example cefotaxime 1 g i.v. or i.m.

23.6.2 Identification of the organism

If you suspect infective endocarditis do not give antibiotics before taking at least three separate sets of blood samples for culture and one sample for serological examination (for *Chlamydia* and *Coxiella*). In a clear-cut case of infective endocarditis it is best to proceed with treatment as soon as blood samples have been taken. Treatment should initially be with benzylpenicillin and gentamicin, since streptococcal and penicillin-sensitive staphylococcal infections account for 80 per cent of all cases. However, in drug addicts and patients with artificial valves one would add flucloxacillin, because of the risk of penicillin-

resistant staphylococcal infection. When the organism has been identified therapy may be changed if required. Culture-negative and serology-negative endocarditis should be treated as for enterococcal endocarditis, with ampicillin and gentamicin.

23.6.3 Antibiotics

(a) Choice of antibiotic

The choice of antibiotic depends, as always, on the type and sensitivities of the infecting organism. The usual treatments for a variety of organisms in infective endocarditis are listed in Table 23.15.

(b) Routes of administration and dosages of antibiotics

For most of the antibiotics used in infective endocarditis the dosages are as given in the Pharmacopoeia. However, the following points should be noted.

1. The route of administration should be i.v. and bolus doses are said to be more effective than continuous infusion. After the first two or three weeks oral antibiotics may be substituted.

2. Recommended penicillin dosages vary widely. The dosage in an individual should be tailored to the sensitivity of the organism, and as a rule the antibiotic should be present in the plasma in a peak plasma concentration which is in at least in eightfold excess of the minimum inhibitory concentration (MIC) or bactericidal concentration (MBC) for the organism (see Chapter 22, p. 230). This is so that enough penicillin can get into the cardiac vegetations and valves to kill the organism. A typical dose of benzylpenicillin (penicillin G) would be 7.2 g (12 megaunits) four-hourly.

3. When oral penicillin is substituted for i.v. penicillin it may be given in combination with probenecid to decrease the tubular secretion of penicillin and thus to maintain plasma penicillin concentrations for a longer period of time.

23.6.4 Duration of treatment

In most cases treatment should be continued for 4 weeks, but infections with *Enterococcus faecalis*

∎ **Table 23.14** Surgical procedures associated with a risk of infective endocarditis and the prophylactic regimens appropriate to each

Procedure	Likely organisms	Initial prophylactic drug (dose; time before procedure) [Follow-up drug (dose; frequency)]	Alternative(s) in penicillin hypersensitivity
1. Dental surgery	Streptococci/Enterococci/Staphylococci (a) Local or no anaesthesia (excluding fillings)	Amoxycillin p.o. (3 g; 1 h) [erythromycin p.o. (500 mg; 6 h)]	Erythromycin p.o. (1.5 g; 1–2 h) or Clindamycin p.o. (600 mg; 1 h)
	(b) General anaesthesia (no special risk)	Amoxycillin i.m. (1 g; just before procedure) [amoxycillin p.o. (500 mg; 6 h)] or amoxycillin p.o. (3 g; 4 h) [amoxycillin p.o. (3 g; as soon as possible)] or amoxycillin/probenecid (3 g/1 g; 4 h)	Vancomycin i.v. (1 g over 60 min) + gentamicin i.v. (120 mg; just before induction or 15 min before procedure)
	(c) Artificial valves or patients who have had endocarditis	Amoxycillin/gentamicin i.m. (1 g/120 mg; just before procedure) (amoxycillin p.o. (500 mg; 6 h))	Vancomycin i.v. (1 g over 60 min) + gentamicin i.v. (120 mg; just before induction or 15 min before procedure)
2. Tonsillectomy, adenoidectomy,	Streptococci/Enterococci/Staphylococci	As for dental procedures with anaesthesia and no special risk and other ENT surgery	
3. Genitourinary surgery	Streptococci/Gram-negative bacteria/ *Bacteroides* spp.	As for dental procedures in patients with prosthetic valves	
4. Obstetric, gynaecological	Streptococci/Gram-negative bacteria/ *Bacteroides* spp.	As for dental procedures in patients with prosthetic valves, gastrointestinal, and biliary surgery (prosthetic valves only)	
5. Cardiac surgery	*Staphylococcus aureus*	Gentamicin/cloxacillin i.v. (120 mg/2 g; 30 min)	Gentamicin/vancomycin i.v. (120 mg/1 g; 30 min)

∎ **Table 23.15**   Choice of antibiotic in infective endocarditis

Organism	First choice	Alternatives
Viridans streptococci	Penicillin G + gentamicin	Vancomycin
Enterococci		
(for example *Enterococcus faecalis*)	Ampicillin + gentamicin	Vancomycin
Streptococcus bovis	Penicillin G	Cephalosporin/vancomycin
Streptococcus pneumoniae	Penicillin G	Cephalosporin/vancomycin
Staphylococcus aureus		
Penicillin-sensitive	Penicillin G + gentamicin	Cephalosporin/vancomycin
Penicillin-resistant	Flucloxacillin + gentamicin	Vancomycin
Staphylococcus epidermidis	Flucloxacillin + gentamicin	Vancomycin
Haemophilus	Ampicillin	Cephalosporin/vancomycin
Escherichia coli	Cephalosporin	Ampicillin
Proteus	Ampicillin	Cephalosporin/vancomycin
Klebsiella	Cephalosporin	Gentamicin
Pseudomonas	Tobramycin + antipseudomonal penicillin (for example piperacillin)	Gentamicin or amikacin + cephalosporin
Yeasts and fungi	Amphotericin B + flucytosine	
Chlamydia and *Coxiella*	Tetracycline + clindamycin	Chloramphenicol
Culture and serology negative	Ampicillin + gentamicin	Vancomycin

and *Staphylococcus* spp. need 6–8 weeks of treatment. If the organism has been shown to have good sensitivity to penicillin, gentamicin may be withdrawn after 2 weeks and oral penicillin substituted for i.v. penicillin. However, if the organism has relatively poor sensitivity to penicillin, as judged by a high MBC, i.v. penicillin and gentamicin should be continued for 4 weeks.

23.6.5 Monitoring therapy

Body temperature and the erythrocyte sedimentation rate or C-reactive protein should be measured regularly. Fever should resolve within a week of successful therapy. If it does not one should suspect persisting infection, abscess formation, embolic infection, or a drug reaction. Regular echocardiography will help in the diagnosis of persisting infection with valvular vegetations and of abscess formation.

The toxic effects of gentamicin are common and great care should be taken to minimize the risks by careful plasma concentration measurement (see Chapter 7).

23.7 Venous thromboembolic disease

There are three aspects to the treatment of venous thromboembolic disease:

(1) prevention;

(2) treatment of established venous thrombosis;

(3) treatment of pulmonary embolism.

23.7.1 Prevention of venous thrombosis

The circumstances in which there is an increased risk of venous thrombosis are listed in Table 23.16. In some cases short-term prophylaxis is sufficient, but occasionally long-term prophylaxis is appropriate.

For short-term prophylaxis heparin is the usual choice. It reduces the incidence of venous thrombosis in patients with acute myocardial infarction and in patients undergoing general

■ **Table 23.16** Circumstances in which there is an increased risk of venous thrombosis

1. *Conditions associated with an increased risk*
   *Myocardial infarction
   †*Severe congestive cardiac failure
   *Surgical operations:
      General surgery
      ‡Fractured hip
      ‡Elective hip surgery
      ‡Pelvic operations
      *Trauma
   Malignant disease
   Pregnancy
   Severe varicose veins
   Polycythaemia
   Oral contraceptive therapy

2. *Factors which increase the risk*
   A previous episode of venous thrombosis
   Advanced age
   Immobility

*Short-term prevention may be appropriate.
†Long-term prevention may be appropriate.
‡Higher risk than general surgery.

surgical operations. It is given in a dose of 5000 i.u. b.d. or t.d.s. subcutaneously into the anterior abdominal wall, varying the site of injection each time. For patients undergoing general surgery an extra dose should be given 2 h before the operation. Treatment should be continued for as long as the patient is immobile. The major worry concerning its use after surgery is that of bleeding, and some surgeons are not keen on taking this risk as a routine, reserving treatment for those whom they consider to be at high risk.

The effect of heparin in patients undergoing orthopaedic surgery on the leg (for example hip replacement) or pelvic surgery (for example prostatectomy or gynaecological operations) is not so marked as in other forms of surgery, and the alternative is dextran. Dextran has been shown to reduce the incidence of postoperative thrombosis in hip surgery, but is no more effective than heparin in urological and gynaecological surgery. It acts by reducing blood viscosity, reducing platelet aggregation, and promoting fibrinolysis. Dextran 40 or dextran 70 (molecular weights

40 000 and 70 000 daltons respectively) are used. They are given as an initial 500 mL infusion over 30 min, followed by 1000–2000 mL/day for 2 d and 500–1000 mL/d for 3 d by continuous i.v. infusion. The main adverse effects are bleeding, which is usually not excessive, and allergic reactions, which are rare and which occur less commonly with dextran 40. Fluid overload can occur if care is not taken.

Because of the high risk of venous thrombosis in patients undergoing hip surgery, and the relative ineffectiveness of heparin and dextran, some recommend full oral anticoagulation with warfarin in selected patients (for dosages see below and in the Pharmacopoeia, p. 709). Warfarin is effective in patients with fractured hips, but in elective hip surgery it is not recommended because of the increased risk of bleeding.

Because of the adverse effects of heparin and dextran, many surgeons prefer to use mechanical methods for preventing venous thrombosis. These methods include electrical calf stimulation during the operation and intermittent calf compression both during the operation and for one or more days after. Intermittent compression, using an inflatable pulsatile stocking or other methods, reduces the incidence of venous thrombosis after most forms of surgery and is free from adverse effects. It is of no value in hip surgery for fractures. Some orthopaedic surgeons prefer to use warfarin in patients with a low risk of postoperative bleeding.

Long-term prophylaxis can be carried out using either subcutaneous heparin (5000 i.u. b.d. or t.d.s.) or oral anticoagulants (for example warfarin). This may be required in high-risk patients who are rendered immobile for long periods of time (for example patients with severe congestive cardiac failure).

If shunt thrombosis is a problem in patients undergoing regular haemodialysis, it may be prevented by the use of epoprostenol (prostacyclin) given by i.v. infusion (5 nanograms/kg/min) just before and during a dialysis.

For women who need prophylaxis during pregnancy give subcutaneous heparin 10 000 i.u. b.d. or t.d.s up to 16 weeks and after 36 weeks. Warfarin should be used between 16 and 36 weeks. Heparin is not used throughout pregnancy, because its continued use carries a risk of osteoporosis.

23.7.2 Treatment of venous thrombosis

(a) Deep vein thrombosis in the calf

Definite thrombosis in the calf should be treated with full anticoagulation in the absence of contra-indications (see Table 23.17). However, some would treat thrombosis in the soleal veins with an elastic stocking only, provided the patient is mobile. The aims of treatment are to prevent extension of the existing clot, to prevent contralateral thrombosis, and to prevent pulmonary embolism.

Treatment should begin with heparin given by continuous i.v. infusion. It is usual to give an intravenous loading dose of 5000 i.u. followed by an infusion of 1000–1500 i.u./h. It is important to control the rate of infusion carefully, and so one should if possible use an infusion pump, rather than the usual, less easily controlled, i.v. infusion methods.

Therapy may be monitored by measuring the partial thromboplastin time, and adjustments in dose may be made as required to prolong the time about twofold (see the Pharmacopoeia, p. 612).

Bleeding is the only important short-term adverse effect of heparin. If minor bleeding occurs stop the infusion and measure the partial thromboplastin time. Generally no specific treatment will be needed, since heparin has a rapid half-time at these dosages (about 1 h). However, if there is major bleeding protamine sulphate should be given to reverse the effects of heparin. The dose of protamine can be calculated on the basis of the calculated amount of heparin in the body, since 1 mg of protamine neutralizes 100 i.u. of heparin. If bleeding occurs within 15 min of a single dose of heparin the dose of protamine can be calculated directly on this basis; if bleeding occurs later the dose of protamine can be calculated on the basis of the predicted amount left in the body, given that the half-time is 1 h (for example 50 per cent left after 1 h, 25 per cent left after 2 h, etc; see Table 3.3). During steady-state administration the amount of heparin in

■ **Table 23.17** Contra-indications to the use of anti-coagulants and thrombolytic drugs

1. *Contra-indications to the use of heparin and warfarin*
   - (a) Absolute
     - Current gastrointestinal bleeding
     - Recurrent intracranial or intraocular bleeding
     - Pericarditis
     - Pregnancy (warfarin before 16 weeks and after 36 weeks)
   - (b) Relative (altered dosages may be required)
     - Haemostatic disorders (congenital or acquired, for example liver disease)
     - Past history of gastrointestinal bleeding
     - Thrombocytopenia
     - Drug interactions (see Pharmacopoeia)

2. *Contra-indications to the use of thrombolytic drugs*
   - (a) Absolute
     - Active bleeding (including menstruation)
     - Recent intracranial or intraocular bleeding
     - Children (urokinase)
   - (b) Relative
     - Recent surgery (within 10 days)
     - Recent obstetric delivery
     - Recent puncture of a non-compressible blood vessel
     - Recent gastrointestinal bleeding
     - Recent trauma
     - Severe hypertension (systolic pressure over 200 mmHg or diastolic pressure over 110 mmHg)
     - Haemostatic disorders (congenital or acquired, for example liver disease)
     - Pregnancy
     - Infective endocarditis
     - Age over 75 years
     - Diabetic haemorrhagic retinopathy
     - Streptococcal infection
     - Recent cavitating pulmonary tuberculosis

the body can be calculated from the following relationship (see eqn (3.38), p. 37):

$$\text{amount in body} = (\text{rate of infusion} \times t_{1/2})/0.7$$

Thus, if the rate of infusion is 1500 i.u./h and the $t_{1/2}$ is 1 h, the amount in the body at steady state is $1500 \times 1/0.7$, i.e. about 2100 i.u. Protamine is given by slow i.v. injection of no more than 50 mg (see heparin in the Pharmacopoeia). Rebound hypercoagulability may occur after reversal of heparin, but if the bleeding is serious this risk may have to be taken.

Once heparin therapy has been started there is no rush to start oral anticoagulation, and warfarin can be started the next day, after the prothrombin time has been measured, in order to be sure that it is not already reduced because of parenchymal liver disease or hepatic congestion secondary to cardiac failure. When the prothrombin time is known warfarin can be given using the sort of regimen described in detail in the Pharmacopoeia, i.e. daily loading doses of 10 mg until the prothrombin time is from 1.5 to 2 times normal (using the International Normalized Ratio), followed by a maintenance dose depending on the loading dose. Remember that lower dosages than normal will be required in patients with liver disease, congestive cardiac failure, or hypothyroidism, and in those who are taking some drugs, the most important of which are amiodarone, chloramphenicol, cimetidine, isoniazid, metronidazole and ketoconazole, and phenylbutazone (all of which inhibit warfarin metabolism), and anabolic steroids, clofibrate, and tetracyclines (all of which increase the effect of warfarin on clotting factor synthesis); avoid tetracyclines and phenylbutazone altogether in patients taking warfarin.

Higher dosages of warfarin may be required in patients on enzyme inducing drugs, such as carbamazepine, griseofulvin, phenobarbitone, phenytoin, primidone, and rifampicin. Remember also that when these drugs are withdrawn warfarin requirements will fall.

Care should be taken in patients on aspirin, dipyridamole, and sulphinpyrazone, because if bleeding occurs haemostasis may be impaired by their actions on platelets. Aspirin should be avoided completely in patients taking warfarin, because it can also cause gastric erosions.

As with heparin, the most important adverse effect of warfarin is bleeding. In most cases withdrawal of warfarin is all that will be required, but if bleeding is serious give fresh frozen plasma as a source of clotting factors. If plasma is not available give vitamin K_1 (phytomenadione) 10 mg i.v. over at least 10 min (not i.m. because of the risk of haematoma). Because of the risk of anaphylactoid reactions to phytomenadione have parenteral adrenaline, hydrocortisone, and an antihistamine to hand (see p. 524).

Heparin treatment should be continued until the prothrombin time has been stable for at least 3 d on a regular maintenance dose of warfarin. Warfarin should then be continued for at least 3 months before it is withdrawn.

It should be noted that there is no guarantee that one will necessarily prevent pulmonary embolism from an existing clot simply by prolonging the clotting time as long as it can be prolonged without bleeding. That is because neither heparin nor warfarin is thrombolytic in action. Their use is aimed at preventing extension of the existing clot, and preventing clot formation elsewhere (for example in the other leg). thereby allowing the body a chance to disperse the existing clot by natural thrombolysis and to recanalize the affected vessel.

In venous thrombosis in pregnancy use only heparin up to 16 weeks and after 36 weeks. Heparin and warfarin may be used between 16 and 36 weeks. If heparin alone is used it should be given by continuous i.v. infusion, in dosages according to the partial thromboplastin time, for 1 week, followed by 10 000 i.u. s.c. b.d. Heparin should be continued in a dosage of 8000 i.u. b.d. for 10 d postpartum, when warfarin can be started. Anticoagulation should be continued for at least 6 weeks postpartum, whatever the duration of preceding therapy.

23.7.3 Iliofemoral and other large vein thrombosis

Thrombosis in large veins is a more serious condition than thrombosis in the veins of the calf, carrying a high risk of pulmonary embolism. The risk of pulmonary embolism is higher in thigh and pelvic vein thrombosis than in thrombosis of the axillary vein of the arm.

Here there is a choice of treatment between heparin plus warfarin on the one hand and the thrombolytic agents streptokinase and urokinase on the other. The newer thrombolytic agents alteplase and anistreplase are not yet licensed for this use.

The main advantage of the thrombolytic agents is that they cause lysis of clot. This results in a reduced risk of embolism, more rapid relief of local signs and symptoms, and a reduction in the risk of damage to the venous valves and therefore of subsequent symptoms due to venous stasis. The combination of heparin and warfarin does none of this. The main disadvantage of the thrombolytic agents is that the risk of bleeding is higher than with heparin/warfarin. However, if patients are chosen carefully according to the contra-indications listed in Table 23.17, the risk of bleeding is outweighed by the therapeutic benefit. In addition, thrombolytic agents should not be used unless the diagnosis has been established by venography or some other detection technique (for example [^{125}I]-fibrinogen uptake) and should not be used unless the thrombosis is of recent origin (within 7 d).

Before treatment starts the thrombin time, activated partial thromboplastin time, prothrombin time, platelet count, and packed cell volume should all be measured, to check that there are no important coagulation abnormalities and to provide a baseline for monitoring therapy. Treatment should be given as described in the Pharmacopoeia (see p. 605) with monitoring by thrombin time or thromboplastin time measurement. Heparin and warfarin should be discontinued before thrombolytic drugs are given, and the thrombin time and prothrombin time should not be prolonged more than twofold.

Bleeding from puncture sites is almost inevitable and does not usually necessitate withdrawal. The number of such sites should be kept to a minimum (for example one venous line and, if blood gas measurements are required, one arterial line). If major bleeding occurs, stop therapy and give whole fresh blood, packed cells, or fresh frozen plasma. It may also be necessary to give tranexamic acid (see p. 557).

Streptokinase is the thrombolytic drug of choice, and urokinase should be used only in patients with a history of streptokinase hypersensitivity. Streptokinase is given for 7 d, after which heparin and warfarin should be started, the heparin being continued until the prothrombin time is stable for at least 3 d on the same dose of warfarin. Warfarin should then be continued for at least 6 months.

If a thrombolytic drug is contra-indicated then heparin and warfarin should be used, in the absence of contra-indications (Table 23.17).

23.7.4 Treatment of pulmonary embolism

Here the choice of drug treatment lies between heparin plus warfarin on the one hand and the thrombolytic drugs on the other.

Heparin and warfarin are used in patients with a small pulmonary embolism in whom there is little or no haemodynamic disturbance, and in patients in whom thrombolytic drugs are contra-indicated (Table 23.17).

In large pulmonary embolism when there is haemodynamic disturbance heparin should be used in the first instance, followed as soon as possible, once the diagnosis has been definitely established (preferably by angiography), by thrombolytic agents, provided that there are no contra-indications. Heart failure and cardiac arrest should also be treated as required.

The main advantage of the thrombolytic agents is that they cause lysis of clot. This results in more rapid relief of haemodynamic and pulmonary disturbance and minimal damage to the pulmonary vascular bed. The combination of heparin and warfarin does none of this.

The dosages of drugs in pulmonary embolism are the same as in venous thrombosis. The warfarin therapy given after heparin or streptokinase should be continued for at least 6 months. Recurrent multiple emboli may require lifelong therapy.

24 The drug therapy of respiratory disorders

Co-author: J Efthimiou

24.1 The use of oxygen in respiratory disorders

When there is hypoxia (as in the conditions listed in Table 24.1) it is therapeutically useful to increase the concentration of oxygen in the inspired air, whose normal oxygen concentration is about 20 per cent.

Oxygen may be added to the inspired air to produce concentrations ranging from 24 to 60 per cent. The dose one chooses depends not simply on the degree of hypoxia, but also on the presence or absence of hypercapnia. If the partial pressure of carbon dioxide in arterial blood (P_ACO_2) is normal (up to 6.0 kPa or 45 mmHg) then high concentrations of oxygen may usually be given safely. However, if there is hypercapnia (P_ACO_2 over 6.6 kPa or 50 mmHg) then high concentrations of oxygen may be dangerous. This is because the respiratory centre responds mainly to the P_ACO_2 and arterial pH, and to a lesser extent to the P_AO_2. However, in chronic hypercapnia the respiratory centre responds poorly to carbon dioxide and relies on hypoxia as a stimulus. If arterial hypoxia is removed, by giving a high concentration of inspired oxygen, the hypoxic drive to respiration is lost and hypercapnia worsens. It is therefore important when giving oxygen to monitor the arterial blood gases regularly. The problem of avoiding hypercapnia most often occurs in patients with chronic obstructive lung disease.

High concentrations of oxygen (up to 60 per cent) can be given via either nasal catheters or facial mask. Nasal catheters may be preferred by some patients, but they tend to produce uncomfortable drying of the nasal mucosa, and if oxygen is given in this way it should ideally be humidified first.

Lower concentrations of oxygen (24–35 per cent) can be given via masks which are designed to deliver different concentrations of oxygen in the inspired air, depending on the design of the mask and on the flow rate of oxygen. Examples are the Edinburgh mask and Venturi masks. The Edinburgh mask can be tuned to give any desired concentration of oxygen within a particular range, depending on the flow rate. Venturi masks, on the other hand, come in different varieties, which give different concentrations of oxygen depending on the sizes of the holes admitting air to the mixture. Three types of mask are available, giving 24, 28, or 35 per cent oxygen, at flow rates of 4–8 L/min.

When low concentrations of oxygen are required it is best to start with a concentration of 24 per cent and to increase the concentration only if the blood gases show continuing hypoxia (P_AO_2 below 8 kPa) without worsening hypercapnia, compared with pretreatment values.

■ **Table 24.1** Common conditions in which oxygen therapy may be useful

Chronic bronchitis and emphysema
Asthma
Pneumonia
Pulmonary oedema
Pulmonary embolism
Pneumothorax
Fibrosing alveolitis

Oxygen is not without adverse effects. The risk of worsening hypercapnia is mentioned above. Prolonged inhalation of high concentrations of inspired oxygen may have adverse effects in both neonates and adults. In neonates it can cause retrolental fibroplasia and consequent blindness. In adults it may cause irritation of the respiratory tract, with coughing, sore throat, tracheobronchitis, pulmonary oedema, and atelectasis.

24.2 Cough

If a cough is irritating and unproductive of sputum it may be suppressed. If it is associated with production of sputum, but difficulty in expectoration, then some would use expectorant drugs. These measures are used only for the symptomatic treatment of cough, and where possible the underlying condition should also be treated.

24.2.1 Cough suppressants

Opiates act as cough suppressants by a direct effect on the medullary mechanisms subserving cough. Codeine phosphate and pholcodine can be used when a dry cough is disturbing sleep, but rarely otherwise. They may cause sputum retention, and should therefore be used with caution in chronic bronchitis or bronchiectasis. The potent opiates, such as morphine and diamorphine, may sometimes be useful in the treatment of intractable dry cough in patients with terminal illness, particularly bronchogenic carcinoma.

In addition to drugs which suppress cough directly, symptomatic relief may sometimes be obtained from a simple linctus, which feels soothing to the throat.

24.2.2 Expectorants

Various compounds have been purported to act as expectorants, but there is little evidence that any of them is of any practical value. The inhalation of steam, with or without a volatile inhalant, such as menthol or benzoin, is soothing in bronchitis and bronchiectasis, and is harmless. It may be used as an adjunct to physiotherapy to aid expectoration of viscid sputum.

Mucolytic expectorants supposedly act by decreasing sputum viscosity. Although they can certainly be shown to have that effect *in vitro*, their clinical efficacy is unproven, and they are probably no better than inhalations of steam or menthol. There is a wide variety of other expectorants available, containing drugs which supposedly increase watery bronchial secretions, but which probably act as expectorants only if they cause vomiting (for example squill, ipecacuanha, ammonium chloride). There is no evidence that any of these is of any value and they are certainly toxic.

Recently, nebulized hypertonic saline (3 mL of a 6 per cent solution) and nebulized amiloride (3 mL of a 10^{-3} molar solution) have been used as expectorants in patients with bronchiectasis and cystic fibrosis, but although they may increase the volume and water content (i.e. reduce the viscosity) of the sputum, their clinical benefit is not clear.

24.3 Pneumonias

A list of infective causes of pneumonia is given in Table 24.2, along with the first-line and alternative antibiotics indicated in such cases.

The principles of treatment of infections are outlined in Chapter 22, but the following points are worth emphasizing in regard to pneumonia.

24.3.1 Drug therapy besides antibiotics

Oxygen should be given for hypoxia. If there is severe hypoxia (P_AO_2 less than 6.5 kPa) or worsening hypercapnia, ventilation may be required. Fluids should be given if there is dehydration. Mild pleuritic pain can be relieved by analgesics such as aspirin and paracetamol, or by non-steroidal anti-inflammatory drugs such as naproxen and indomethacin. More severe pain may be treated with more potent analgesics, such as buprenorphine, morphine, or pethidine, but care must be taken in patients with hypercapnia,

∎ **Table 24.2**   Common causes of pneumonia and their treatment

Organism	Antibiotic(s) of choice	Alternative(s)
1. Bacterial		
Streptococcus pneumoniae	Benzylpenicillin or amoxycillin	Erythromycin or cefuroxime
Staphylococcus aureus (penicillin-sensitive)	Benzylpenicillin	Erythromycin
Staphylococcus aureus (penicillinase-producing)	Flucloxacillin	According to local sensitivities
Klebsiella pneumoniae	Gentamicin + cephalosporin	Chloramphenicol or co-trimoxazole
Haemophilus influenzae	Amoxycillin or ampicillin	Cephalosporin or chloramphenicol
Legionella pneumophila	Erythromycin	Rifampicin
Mycobacterium tuberculosis	See text	
2. Viral	Treat secondary bacterial infection	
3. Others		
Chlamydia psittaci	Tetracyclines	Erythromycin
Coxiella burneti	Tetracyclines	Erythromycin
Mycoplasma pneumoniae	Erythromycin	Tetracyclines
*4. Severe pneumonia of unknown origin**	Amoxycillin + flucloxacillin + erythromycin	Cefuroxime + erythromycin

*Microbiological proof of pneumonia is not found in about 30 per cent of patients.

since narcotic analgesics can cause respiratory depression.

22.3.2 Route of administration of antibiotics

In severe cases (for example if the patient is ill enough to be admitted to hospital) parenteral antibiotics should be used. A change to oral treatment should be possible when there is clinical improvement. In mild or moderate cases the oral route will usually be satisfactory.

24.3.3 Duration of treatment

Treatment for 7–10 d is usually sufficient, but antibiotics should be continued for at least 3 d after the temperature has returned to normal. However, there are exceptions. Infections with *Staph. aureus* and *Kl. pneumoniae* can be very difficult to eradicate, and relapse readily. In those cases parenteral treatment should be continued until the temperature is consistently normal and the sputum has cleared. Thereafter, oral therapy should be given for at least 2 weeks.

Infections with *Mycoplasma pneumoniae* tend to relapse readily, and treatment should be continued for a total of 2–3 weeks.

24.3.4 Alternatives to first-line antibiotics

The alternative antibiotics to those of first choice are listed in Table 24.2. They should be used if the first choice is contra-indicated (for example penicillin in a patient with penicillin hypersensitivity, or tetracycline in a young child or a patient with renal failure), or if the organism proves to be resistant to the first choice (for example a β-lactamase-producing *Staph. aureus*), or if the patient is failing to respond.

24.3.5 Failure to respond to initial treatment

Failure to improve in response to initial therapy may occur for several reasons.

1. Because the diagnosis is wrong. Pulmonary infarction or oedema should be ruled out.
2. Because the organism is resistant. An alternative antibiotic may help. Ask the microbiologist for advice.
3. Because of other pulmonary disease, for example pre-existing obstruction or bronchiectasis or complications of pneumonia, such as abscess and empyema.

If the patient's fever does not resolve despite other evidence of resolving infection, consider the possibility of an allergic drug reaction.

24.3.6 Pneumonia acquired in hospital

Because pneumonia acquired in hospital is likely to be due to a resistant organism, intravenous treatment should be started with a broad-spectrum drug, such as a cephalosporin, for example cefuroxime, plus gentamicin.

24.3.7 Inhalation pneumonia

The organisms which complicate aspiration pneumonia are unusual. Outside of hospital they may be fusiform bacteria from the gingivae, anaerobes, and unusual cocci. In cases acquired in hospital the organisms are more likely to be Gram-negative bacilli and penicillin-resistant staphylococci, in addition to anaerobes. For infections acquired outside hospital treatment should be with parenteral penicillin G (4–10 megaunits per day) plus metronidazole (for anaerobic organisms). Clindamycin (150–300 mg 6-hourly) is the recommended alternative in patients with penicillin hypersensitivity. For aspiration pneumonia acquired in hospital a cephalosporin, such as cefuroxime, plus gentamicin plus metronidazole should be used. Treatment should be continued for 3–6 weeks. Some would also give corticosteroids (for example hydrocortisone 200 mg q.d.s.), although their value is not proven.

24.3.8 Pneumonia in the immunocompromised patient

With the increasing incidence of AIDS and the use of drugs with immunosuppressive effects in the treatment of cancer and organ transplants, the treatment of pneumonia in the immunocompromised patient is becoming a common problem. Unusual organisms are to be expected in such cases, including viruses (especially cytomegalovirus), fungi (especially cryptococcus), and protozoa (especially *Pneumocystis carinii*).

Pneumonia in these patients is serious, and it should always be treated in hospital if possible. If there is a fever and pulmonary infiltrates, treatment should be started immediately with a cephalosporin and gentamicin. If the infiltrates are diffuse and bilateral, high-dose co-trimoxazole (see below) should also be given. Aggressive efforts should be made to reach a specific diagnosis (for example by bronchoscopy and lavage) and appropriate therapy given. Specialist guidance should be sought.

Treatment of *Pneumocystis* pneumonia is with high dosages of co-trimoxazole, 30 mg/kg q.d.s. orally or i.v. Since one tablet and one i.v. ampoule of co-trimoxazole contains 480 mg (80 mg of trimethoprim and 400 mg of sulphamethoxazole), this dosage is equivalent to about 3 or 4 tablets or ampoules of co-trimoxazole q.d.s. Alternatively (for example in patients with sulphonamide hypersensitivity) one can use pentamidine by nebulizer, 600 mg in 6 mL daily. Pentamidine can also be given i.v. in a dosage of 4 mg/kg/d, but it has many serious adverse effects, including hypotension, cardiac arrhythmias, pancreatitis, neutropenia, thrombocytopenia, hypoglycaemia, hypocalcaemia, and acute renal failure.

Long-term administration of co-trimoxazole, 2 tablets once or twice a day, effectively prevents infection with *Pneumocystis carinii*.

24.4 Chronic obstructive lung disease

In chronic obstructive lung disease the main aims of treatment are to prevent infections, to relieve reversible airways obstruction (due to broncho-spasm and secretions), and to treat acute exacer-bations and heart failure. In addition, patients should be advised to stop smoking.

24.4.1 Infection in chronic obstructive lung disease

Antibiotics are not used prophylactically as con-tinuous therapy, since their use in this way leads to the emergence of resistant organisms. Instead, patients may be given a supply of an antibiotic (amoxycillin, co-trimoxazole, or a tetracycline) to take when they get an upper respiratory tract infection (for example a winter cold) or at the first signs of acute infective bronchitis, so that the risks of infection can be reduced. Influenza vaccine should be given in the winter, since serious bacterial infection often occurs in these patients secondary to viral infections.

24.4.2 Bronchospasm in chronic obstructive lung disease

Chronic obstructive lung disease may be revers-ible or irreversible. Reversible obstruction is due to mucus secretion and bronchospasm. Broncho-spasm can be treated as in bronchial asthma, with aerosol inhalations of bronchodilators and corticosteroids (see below). There is little evidence that drugs used as expectorants are of value in relieving obstruction due to viscid mucus, but steam inhalations soothe and may be used in combination with physiotherapy.

24.4.3 Acute exacerbations of chronic obstructive lung disease

Acute exacerbations are generally caused by infections, and prompt treatment of infection is important. In an acute exacerbation hypoxia should be treated with oxygen, starting with a low concentration (for example 24 per cent) and increasing slowly according to response (see above under oxygen). Dehydration should be treated as necessary. Infection is usually due to *H. influenzae* or *Strep. pneumoniae*, and treatment with amoxycillin, co-trimoxazole, or a tetra-cycline is indicated. Bronchospasm should be treated as in acute asthma with inhaled or i.v.

bronchodilators, such as salbutamol and amino-phylline.

24.4.4 Cardiac failure in chronic obstructive lung disease

Congestive cardiac failure should be treated with diuretics, as described in Chapter 23 (p. 291). In the acute stage, loop diuretics should be used, and later it may be possible to switch to a thiazide. However, in some cases long-term treat-ment with a loop diuretic or with a combination of diuretics may be necessary. Potassium chloride supplements or a potassium-sparing diuretic are usually necessary in these patients (see Chap-ter 26, p. 346).

Cardiac glycosides should not be used in chronic cor pulmonale in the absence of atrial fibrillation, since they are poorly effective and the risk of digitalis toxicity is high.

24.4.5 Oxygen therapy in chronic obstructive lung disease

Some patients may benefit from having oxygen available at home. In some cases short-term oxygen may be useful for acute exacerbations of symptoms of chronic obstructive lung disease, and may, in combination with early antibiotic therapy, obviate the need for hospital admission. In selected patients long-term oxygen may be of therapeutic benefit, in which case it has to be given for at least 15 h a day at a rate of 1–3 L/min, and this is best achieved using an oxygen concentrator. The recommended criteria for this treatment are as follows:

P_AO_2 less than 7.3 kPa;
P_ACO_2 more than 6.0 kPa;
FEV_1 less than 1.5 L;
FVC less than 2.0 L.

24.4.6 Respiratory stimulants in chronic obstructive lung disease

Patients with respiratory failure and hypercapnia in whom respiratory drive is thought to be low may benefit from respiratory stimulation with analeptic drugs, such as doxapram and nitheram-ide. Nikethamide is little used now because of its common and severe adverse effects. The primary sites of action of doxapram are the peripheral chemoreceptors, and central nervous system stimulation only occurs with high dosages. The normal dosage by i.v. infusion is 1–4 mg/min, depending on the patient's condition and level of hypercapnia. Respiratory stimulants should be avoided in patients already maximally stimulated by hypoxia or hypercapnia, as respiratory muscle fatigue may be precipitated and harm done.

24.5 Bronchial asthma

24.5.1 Pharmacological factors in the production of asthma and the mechanisms of action of the drugs used in its treatment

Impairment of airflow in asthma is caused by three bronchial abnormalities.

1. Excessive contraction of bronchial smooth muscle (bronchoconstriction). The extent to which bronchoconstriction occurs in response to a stimulus at any time varies with bronchial reactivity, which is generally increased in asthma.
2. Swelling of bronchial mucosa (bronchial oedema)
3. Excessive bronchial mucus secretion.

These abnormalities are caused by the release of chemical inflammatory and bronchoconstricting mediators within the bronchial wall, mainly from mast cells, but also from leucocytes, macrophages, platelets, and epithelial cells. The mediators involved include histamine, peptides (kinins), and arachidonic acid derivatives (prostaglandins, leukotrienes, and platelet activating factor). The release of these substances from cells, and their actions on bronchial tissues involve intracellular mediators, such as cyclic AMP and cyclic GMP. In addition to their direct bronchoconstrictive and inflammatory effects these substances may also enhance axon reflexes in the lung, causing further release of inflammatory neuropeptides, such as substance P. There is also an alteration in the balance of nervous innervation of the airways in asthma, with increased cholinergic drive and decreased β-adrenergic drive.

Occasionally, asthma may be drug-induced. It may be precipitated by pseudoallergy to aspirin, which is discussed elsewhere (see p. 111), and by the direct action of β-adrenoceptor antagonists, particularly non-cardioselective antagonists, such as propranolol and oxprenolol. The pathogenetic mechanisms in asthma are summarized in Fig. 24.1, in which are also shown the effects of drugs used to treat it. The drugs are also listed in Table 24.3.

(a) β_2-adrenoceptor agonists

These drugs (salbutamol, terbutaline, rimiterol, fenoterol, reproterol, and salmeterol) are direct β-adrenoceptor agonists with some selectivity for β_2-adrenoceptors. They therefore act mainly on adrenoceptors in bronchial tissue, and when used in the recommended doses have much less effect on cardiac (β_1) adrenoceptors than non-selective β-agonists. Their actions on mast cells and bronchial smooth muscle cells result in increases in adenylate cyclase activity and cellular cyclic AMP concentrations. This leads to bronchodilatation, and to decreased cellular release of inflammatory mediators.

Salmeterol is the first long-acting β_2-adrenoceptor agonist, whose bronchodilatory effect lasts for up to 12 h (compare with salbutamol, 4 h). Salmeterol not only prevents early bronchoconstriction after allergen challenge, as do all the β-adrenoceptor agonists, but may also prevent the late phase reaction, which suggests that it also has an anti-inflammatory action.

(b) Xanthine derivatives

Theophylline and its congeners (for example aminophylline) reduce the breakdown of cyclic AMP by inhibition of phosphodiesterase. The result is an increase in cellular cyclic AMP concentrations, with similar effects to those of the β_2-adrenoceptor agonists. Since the two types of drug produce the same effect by different routes one would expect their therapeutic effects to be at least additive, and there is experimental evidence that that is so.

(c) Anticholinergic drugs

Ipratropium, an atropine analogue, inhibits the action of acetylcholine at tissue cholinoceptors, and thereby inhibits the bronchoconstrictive

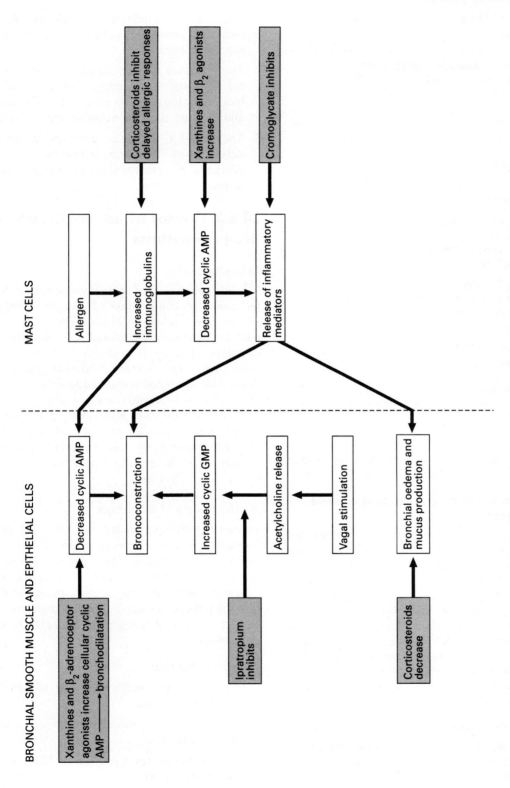

■ **Fig. 24.1** The pathophysiology of bronchial asthma and the sites and mechanisms of action of drugs used in its treatment.

■ **Table 24.3**   Drugs used in the treatment of bronchial asthma

---

1. *β₂-Adrenoceptor agonists* (p. 541)
   Salbutamol (albuterol)
   Terbutaline
   Fenoterol
   Pirbuterol
   Reproterol
   Rimiterol
   Salmeterol

2. *Anticholinergic drugs* (p. 538)
   Ipratropium

3. *Xanthine derivatives* (p. 715)
   Aminophylline
   Choline theophyllinate
   Theophylline

4. *Mast cell stabilizers*
   Sodium cromoglycate (p. 590)
   Nedocromil sodium
   Ketotifen

5. *Corticosteroids* (p. 584)
   Beclomethasone
   Betamethasone
   Budesonide

---

effects of vagus nerve activity. It also reduces bronchial mucus secretion.

(d) Sodium cromoglycate and related compounds

Sodium cromoglycate (cromolyn sodium) and related compounds (ketotifen and nedocromil sodium) are supposed to act by inhibiting the release of inflammatory mediators from cells. However, it has also been suggested that sodium cromoglycate may act by inhibiting local axon reflexes in the bronchioles. Ketotifen is also an antihistamine and may have some additional action through that mechanism. Whatever their mechanism of action these drugs are used in the prevention of attacks rather than in the treatment of an acute attack.

(e) Corticosteroids

The mechanisms of action of corticosteroids in asthma are not fully understood, but they probably act in several different ways.

1. They have anti-inflammatory effects, thereby reducing bronchial oedema and bronchial mucus production.

2. They enhance the actions of the β-adrenoceptor agonists, both endogenous (catecholamines) and exogenous (for example salbutamol), and increase their bronchodilating properties.

3. They inhibit the IgE- and IgG-dependent delayed (type III) allergic responses to extrinsic allergens, but not the immediate (type I) IgE-mediated response.

24.5.2 Routes of administration of drugs in asthma

(a) Inhalation

The administration of some anti-asthmatic drugs by inhalation confers two advantages. Firstly, it allows rapid relief of bronchospasm with β₂-adrenoceptor agonists; secondly, it allows the use of smaller dosages of drugs, with the result that there are fewer systemic adverse effects. In Table 24.4 are listed some of the different kinds of inhalational formulations available.

It is important when prescribing these formulations to ensure that the patient understands how to use them properly. There are two important points to be made about the mechanics and regularity of their use.

(i) Mechanics of inhalation

Incorrect technique in the use of inhalational formulations is a common cause of failure to respond to treatment. The patient should be taught the correct method of inhalation by demonstration, and the doctor should confirm that the patient can use the inhaler correctly. The correct method of using a traditional inhaler is as follows:

breathe out fully;

put the inhaler just inside the mouth and depress the canister;

at the same time breathe in slowly and as deeply as possible;

hold the breath for a few (up to 10) seconds; breathe out slowly.

■ **Table 24.4** Some types of inhalational formulations used in the treatment of bronchial asthma

Formulation	Drug	Dose (mg) in one puff	Dose (mg) in one oral formulation
Aerosol*	β_2-adrenoceptor agonists		
	Fenoterol	0.2	–
	Pirbuterol	0.2	10
	Reproterol	0.5	20
	Rimiterol	0.2	–
	Salbutamol	0.1	2/4
	Terbutaline	0.25	5
	Salmeterol	0.025	–
	Corticosteroids		
	Beclomethasone	0.05/0.1/0.25	–
	Betamethasone	0.1	0.5
	Budesonide	0.05/0.2	–
	Anticholinergic drugs		
	Ipratropium	0.02/0.04	–
	Mast cell stabilizers		
	Sodium cromoglycate	5.0	100
	Nedocromil sodium	2.0	–
Aerosol (breath-activated)	β_2-adrenoceptor agonists		
	Rimiterol	0.2	–
	Salbutamol	0.1	2/4
Micro-fine powder (breath-activated)	β_2-adrenoceptor agonists		
	Salbutamol	0.2/0.4	2/4
	Terbutaline	0.5	5
	Beclomethasone	0.1/0.2/0.4	–
	Sodium cromoglycate	20.0	100
Solutions for nebulizing	β_2-adrenoceptor agonists		
	Fenoterol		
	Reproterol		
	Salbutamol		
	Terbutaline		
	Beclomethasone		
	Ipratropium		

*Aerosol combinations of β-adrenoceptor agonists with corticosteroids are not recommended.

Some patients have difficulty in co-ordinating this procedure (for example old people, very young people, and people with arthritis), and for them alternative types of inhaler are available. Conventional inhalers can have a 'spacer' fitted to the mouthpiece; this allows a little extra time after depression of the canister before inhalation is required (for example Bricanyl Nebuhaler Spacer®, Ventolin Volumatic Spacer®). Alternatively, there are inhalers which merely require the patient to breathe in, without separately activat-ing a drug release mechanism (for example Ventolin Rotacaps®).

(ii) Frequency of administration

The β_2-adrenoceptor agonists act very rapidly in relieving bronchospasm, and are therefore often used to treat acute attacks. Because of this inter-mittent use of β_2-adrenoceptor agonists, patients often believe that other drugs can be taken intermittently. However, that is not the case, and corticosteroids, cromoglycate, and ipratropium should be taken at regular intervals during the day, usually four times. Some patients with chronic asthma may benefit from regular use of the β_2-adrenoceptor agonists, three or four times a day, although doubt has recently been cast on this method of treatment because of a suspicion that the β_2-adrenoceptor agonists may increase the risk of death from asthma. This issue remains to be resolved.

24.5.3 The practical treatment of bronchial asthma

The practical treatment of bronchial asthma has several aspects:

(a) The avoidance of precipitating factors.

(b) The treatment of reversible airways obstruction.

   (i) acute severe asthma (status asthmaticus);

   (ii) acute mild or moderate asthma;

   (iii) chronic asthma.

(c) Prevention of acute attacks.

(a) Avoidance of precipitating factors

If allergenic precipitating factors can be identified, attacks may be avoidable by avoidance of the allergen. The role of desensitization is controversial, but there is little evidence to support its use.

Drugs which can cause asthma should be avoided. Non-selective (i.e. β_1 and β_2) adrenoceptor antagonists should never be used in patients with asthma, and the relatively selective β_1-adrenoceptor antagonists (for example bisoprolol, practolol, atenolol, and metoprolol) should be used with great caution, if at all. Aspirin and other salicylates should not be used in patients with known aspirin pseudoallergy (see p. 111), and such patients should be warned of the vast number of over-the-counter medicines which contain aspirin. These patients may also be sensitive to other non-steroidal anti-inflammatory drugs and to some food colouring agents, including tartrazine (E102).

Infection is an important complication to avoid, and patients whose asthma is clearly associated with chest infections should be given a supply of an antibiotic, such as amoxycillin, to take at the first sign of an upper or lower respiratory tract infection. In all asthmatics lower respiratory tract infections should be treated vigorously, and in patients with influenza prophylactic antibiotics should be given to prevent secondary bacterial infection. Influenza vaccine should be given in the winter.

(b) Treatment of reversible airways obstruction

(i) Acute severe asthma (status asthmaticus)

Acute severe asthma is an acute medical emergency characterized by severe wheeze, incapacitating breathlessness (to the extent that the patient can hardly speak), tachycardia, central cyanosis, and pulsus paradoxus.

An acute severe attack of asthma should be treated with oxygen, nebulized or i.v. bronchodilators, i.v. fluids, i.v. corticosteroids, antibiotics, and ventilation if required. Although these patients are excessively anxious, it is important not to sedate them, unless they are to be ventilated, since sedation will reduce their respiratory drive.

Oxygen may be given in a high concentration (up to 60 per cent), but only if there is hypoxia and a low $P_A CO_2$. A high normal or raised $P_A CO_2$ accompanied by hypoxia is a sign of very severe asthma, in which case the initial concentration of oxygen in the inspired air should be 24 per cent, increasing, if necessary, according to the arterial blood gases (see above under oxygen).

Bronchodilators A β_2-adrenoceptor agonist should be given by nebulizer. The doses of salbutamol or terbutaline given in this way are 2.5–10.0 mg by continuous inhalation every 2–6 h. It is important to remember that when nebulized drugs are given in oxygen rather than in air as a vehicle the concentration of inspired oxygen should be chosen carefully according to the arterial blood gases (see above). The therapeutic effect of the β_2-adrenoceptor agonists when given by nebulizer is so good that this method has almost completely replaced i.v. administration. If nebulized salbutamol does not produce a therapeutic effect ipratropium may be added to the nebulizer in a dose of 250–500 micrograms. However, some patients (for example those with very severe bronchoconstriction, which limits the access of the drug to the site of action) will not respond to nebulized drugs, and in them i.v. salbutamol may be tried. Start with a continuous infusion at a rate of 5 microgram/min and increase it to 20 microgram/min according to the clinical response. When clinical improvement occurs the i.v. infusion can be replaced by a nebulizer.

Aminophylline may also be given by i.v. infusion, although some prefer not to use it, because of the risk of cardiac arrhythmias, particularly in patients also receiving a β_2-adrenoceptor agonist. Aminophylline is given in a loading dose of 6 mg/kg i.v. over 15 min, followed by a continuous infusion at a rate of 0.5–0.9 mg/kg/h. Lower maintenance doses should be used if the patient has chronic obstructive lung disease, congestive cardiac failure, or impaired liver function, and in patients over 50 years of age (for dosages see Table P11, p. 716). Some would not use aminophylline in patients who have previously been taking oral theophylline formulations, on the grounds that it is unlikely to be effective and may even be dangerous if the plasma theophylline concentration is already in the therapeutic range. (Note that in addition to prescribable formulations there are other formulations, available over the counter as 'cold cures', which contain theophylline (for example Dodo® tablets).) If aminophylline is to be used in such cases the loading dose should be omitted and the plasma theophylline concentration should be measured as a guide to the maintenance dose. Plasma theophylline concentrations should be monitored during treatment (see Chapter 7).

Corticosteroids should be given i.v., for example hydrocortisone 200 mg 8-hourly, until oral prednisolone can be given, starting with a dosage of 30–40 mg o.d.

Antibiotics Chest infections should be treated with an appropriate antibiotic. Ampicillin should be given i.v. and a cephalosporin can be used as an alternative in patients with penicillin hypersensitivity. If oral therapy is possible cotrimoxazole and tetracyclines are alternatives.

Fluid and electrolyte replacement These patients are generally dehydrated, and adequate fluid replacement is essential. Hypokalaemia can occur as a result of the disease (through hyperventilation) or its treatment (β_2-adrenoceptor agonists and corticosteroids), and it should be corrected with i.v. potassium chloride (see p. 349).

Intermittent positive pressure ventilation (IPPV) In patients who do not respond to the above treatment IPPV will be necessary. IPPV should be considered if the $P_A O_2$ remains low (less than 6.6 kPa), if the $P_A CO_2$ rises above 6.6 kPa, if acidosis persists (arterial pH less than 7.3), or if there is severe drowsiness, confusion, or exhaustion leading to worsening hypoxia and hypercapnia.

If the patient improves in response to these measures, then oral and inhaled therapy should be continued, using oxygen, nebulized salbutamol or terbutaline with or without ipratropium, oral corticosteroids gradually reducing in dosage to eventual withdrawal, and an oral antibiotic. Physiotherapy should be started. Later, bronchodilators by nebulizer may be replaced by regular aerosols, with or without oral bronchodilators as required (see below). In addition, regular inhaled corticosteroids (for example beclomethasone 2 puffs b.d., see p. 586) should probably be started before discharge from hospital and continued for at least several months in most patients who have had a severe attack of asthma.

(ii) Acute mild or moderate attacks of asthma

Acute intermittent asthmatic attacks are best treated with a β_2-adrenoceptor agonist by inhalation (see Table 24.4). These drugs relieve bronchospasm within a few minutes, reach a peak at 15–30 min, and last for 3–4 h. Ipratropium by inhaler is an alternative, but its effects take longer to come on, and it is probably better reserved for the regular treatment of chronic asthma.

An inhalation of a β_2-adrenoceptor agonist before exposure to a known precipitant (for example in patients with cold-induced or exercise-induced asthma) may help to prevent the anticipated acute attack. Those who wake at night with an acute attack may also benefit from a dose of a β_2-adrenoceptor agonist immediately before going to sleep.

(iii) Chronic asthma

In maintenance therapy of chronic asthma a β_2-adrenoceptor agonist (for example salbutamol) by aerosol four times a day was until recently the treatment of choice. However, evidence is emerging that the risk of death from asthma may be increased in patients who take β_2-adrenoceptor agonists as long-term therapy, for reasons which are not clear. Partly because of this and partly because asthma is increasingly being regarded as an inflammatory disease, attention has turned to the use of regular inhaled corticosteroids, such as beclomethasone 2 puffs b.d., see p. 586, in all patients who require inhaled β_2-adrenoceptor agonists more than once a day.

In patients who do not respond to inhaled corticosteroids (with or without a β_2-adrenoceptor agonist), ipratropium or cromoglycate (each 2 puffs q.d.s., see pp. 539, 590) may be added. In addition, salbutamol and ipratropium may be taken regularly via a portable nebulizer if the response to simple aerosol inhalers is not good. Alternatively, regular inhaled salmeterol (2 puffs b.d., see p. 541) may be tried.

If the response is still poor, one can try an oral xanthine, for example theophylline or aminophylline. Because the toxic:therapeutic ratio of the xanthines is low, initial dosages should be low, and ideally therapy should be monitored by plasma theophylline concentration measurements (see Chapter 7). Slow-release aminophylline is particularly useful for patients who have nocturnal or early-morning symptoms, as is not uncommon and may be difficult to treat. Slow-release salbutamol is an alternative available for this purpose.

(c) Prevention of acute attacks

Prevention of asthmatic attacks may be achieved by regular maintenance therapy with inhaled corticosteroids or sodium cromoglycate. These are given up to four times a day, even if the patient is not chronically wheezy. Cromoglycate may also be a useful alternative to a β_2-adrenoceptor agonist in preventing exercise-induced asthma.

In patients with severe asthma, in whom other drug therapy has been ineffective, oral corticosteroids may be required. They may also be used in short courses in the case of a severe attack when the patient's usual treatment becomes ineffective in controlling symptoms.

24.5.4 Adverse effects of drugs in asthma

Adverse effects are very uncommon with the use of inhaled drugs, because the dosages used are much lower than the equivalent oral dosages (see Table 24.4).

Occasionally with high dosages of β_2-adrenoceptor agonists sinus tachycardia and cardiac arrhythmias may occur; this is particularly important in patients being treated with a β_2-adrenoceptor agonist by inhalation via a nebulizer. The increased risk of death from asthma in patients taking β_2-adrenoceptor agonists has been mentioned above.

Inhalation of corticosteroids may occasionally cause oropharyngeal infection with *Candida albicans*, the risk of which can be minimized by regular rinsing of the mouth after inhalation and by using an inhaler with a spacer. A reversible dysphonia may occur, due to myopathic weakening of the adductor muscles of the vocal cords. Some suppression of the hypothalamic–pituitary axis may occasionally occur with high dosages (over 15×100 microgram puffs, i.e. 1.5 mg, per day).

Intravenous β_2-adrenoceptor agonists can cause tachycardia and cardiac arrhythmias. They may worsen glucose tolerance in patients with diabetes, particularly when given i.v. with hydrocortisone in acute severe asthma, and increased dosages of insulin may be required.

Xanthines can cause cardiac arrhythmias, and ideally electrocardiographic monitoring should be available when xanthines and β_2-adrenoceptor agonists are given together i.v. in acute severe attacks. During chronic therapy the adverse effects of the xanthines can be minimized by monitoring plasma theophylline concentrations.

The numerous adverse effects of oral corticosteroids are detailed in the Pharmacopoeia (p. 584).

24.5.5 Monitoring therapy in asthma

During the treatment of asthma it is important to monitor progress by measuring either the forced expiratory volume in one second (FEV_1), or more simply the peak expiratory flow rate (PEFR). This has been discussed in Chapter 7, but it is worth stressing that there is a large diurnal variation in these measurements. There is often a dip early in the morning, and the fact that lung function is apparently normal later in the day may not reflect the true severity of the disease. Patients should be encouraged to measure their own PEFR at home, in order to monitor their own progress. Monitoring of plasma theophylline concentrations is discussed in Chapter 7.

24.6 Pulmonary tuberculosis

The general principles of treating infection (see Chapter 22) apply to the treatment of pulmonary tuberculosis. However, in all cases at least two, and usually three or four, drugs are used concurrently, because the causative organisms are often resistant to at least one antituberculous drug, and further resistance will develop if only one drug is used.

Drug regimens vary throughout the world, depending on socio-economic conditions. The drugs used are listed in Table 24.5, with details of adult dosages, important adverse effects, drug interactions, comments about monitoring various aspects of therapy, and comments about circumstances in which the drugs should be avoided.

24.6.1 Prevention

BCG immunization should be given to contacts of tuberculosis cases who have a weak tuberculin response, except in those who have previously been immunized and in people with HIV infection. Other high-risk individuals for whom BCG immunization is recommended include health workers and immigrants from countries in which tuberculosis is common.

In a few cases drug prevention of tuberculosis may be required. Primary prevention is chiefly used in breast-feeding children whose mothers are sputum positive. Secondary prevention (i.e. the prevention of full infection in someone who has already acquired the organism) is used in children under 5 years of age who are tuberculin positive (since they have a high risk of tuberculous meningitis and miliary tuberculosis), in people under 20 years of age who are close contacts of infected individuals, in those who have recently become tuberculin positive, and in those who are taking long-term immunosuppressive drugs. Its value in HIV-infected individuals has yet to be demonstrated.

Preventive treatment in these cases should be with isoniazid, 5 mg/kg/d for 6 months. Pyridoxine need not be given if the dose of isoniazid is not above 5 mg/kg/d. If compliance is a problem with a 6-month regimen or if there is isoniazid resistance, rifampicin plus isoniazid can be used for 3 months.

24.6.2 The treatment of tuberculosis in developed countries

The most usual regimen used in the initial therapy of tuberculosis in developed countries is the combination of rifampicin, isoniazid (with pyridoxine), ethambutol, and pyrazinamide. The addition of pyrazinamide to the previously standard three-drug regimen has shortened the duration of treatment from 9 months to 6 months. In the initial phase these drugs should be given once daily as single oral doses (see Table 24.5) 30–60 min before food. Initial treatment should be continued for 2 months. When the results of drug sensitivity tests are known, treatment in the continuation phase can be with two drugs only, one of which should be isoniazid. The usual combination is isoniazid with rifampicin, and treatment should be continued for a further 4 months (i.e. 6 months in all).

The nine-month regimen is the same as the six-month regimen, but pyrazinamide is omitted. Ethambutol is stopped after 2 months and isoniazid and rifampicin are continued for a further 7 months.

Sometimes alternative drugs are used, for the following reasons.

(a) Resistant organisms

If a patient fails to improve on the standard regimen of rifampicin, isoniazid, ethambutol, and pyrazinamide, and if sensitivity tests suggest that bacterial resistance is the cause, alternative drugs may be used, as suggested by the sensitivity tests (see Table 24.5).

(b) Poor compliance

If compliance is a problem, supervised therapy with the following thrice-weekly regimen is recommended:

■ **Table 24.5** Drugs used in the treatment of tuberculosis

Drug	Daily adult dosages		Important adverse effects and interactions	Comments
	Daily therapy	Intermittent therapy		
1. *Routine therapy (developed countries)*				
Isoniazid (p. 621)	5 mg/kg (max. 300 mg)	15 mg/kg (max. 1 g)	Peripheral neuropathy (must be given with pyridoxine) Hepatitis	Monitor liver function Pharmacogenetic variability in metabolism (see Chapter 8)
Rifampicin (p. 676)	8–12 mg/kg	600–900 mg	Hepatotoxicity Induces metabolism of warfarin and oral contraceptive	Monitor liver function Avoid in pregnancy
Pyrazinamide	30 mg/kg (max. 3 g)	40 mg/kg (max. 3 g)	Liver damage Hyperuricaemia	Monitor liver function
Ethambutol (p. 603)	15 mg/kg	30–45 mg/kg	Optic neuritis	Monitor visual fields/colour vision Reduce dosage in renal failure
Thiacetazone	2 mg/kg	–	Jaundice Anorexia, nausea, vomiting Vestibular toxicity	Initial dose 0.5 mg/kg
2. *Second-line drugs (developing countries and for resistant organisms)*				
Streptomycin (p. 552)	7.5–15 mg/kg	1 g i.m.	Hypersensitivity Nephrotoxicity (enhanced by frusemide and ethacrynic acid) Ototoxicity Enhances effects of neuromuscular blockers	Wear gloves when administering i.m. Avoid in pregnancy Monitor plasma concentrations (if possible)
p-Amino-salicylic acid (PAS)	150 mg/kg in divided doses	12 g in divided doses	Anorexia, nausea, vomiting Liver damage Hypersensitivity	Avoid in renal failure
3. *Other drugs for resistant organisms*				
Ethionamide	0.75–1.0 g in 3 doses	–	Anorexia, nausea, vomiting Mental disturbances Peripheral neuropathy	Avoid in liver disease and pregnancy
Capreomycin	1 g i.m. (maximum 20 mg/kg)	–	Ototoxicity Potassium depletion Nephrotoxicity Hepatotoxicity	Avoid in pregnancy Monitor auditory, renal, and hepatic function
Cycloserine	250 mg b.d. or t.d.s	–	CNS toxicity Psychosis Convulsions	Reduce dosages in renal failure Avoid in epilepsy or psychosis

isoniazid (15 mg/kg orally, to a maximum of 1 g, with pyridoxine 10 mg orally);

rifampicin (15 mg/kg orally, to a maximum of 900 mg);

pyrazinamide (2 g orally for patients weighing less than 50 kg, otherwise 2.5 g);

streptomycin (1 g i.m.) or ethambutol (25 mg/kg orally).

This regimen is continued for 2 months and is followed by thrice-weekly rifampicin and isoniazid for 4 months.

(c) Contra-indications

The main contra-indications to antituberculous drugs are shown in Table 24.5. For example, in pregnancy rifampicin, streptomycin, ethionamide, and capreomycin should not be used. Isoniazid and ethambutol would be the drugs of choice.

(d) Adverse reactions

Transient increases in liver enzymes are common soon after starting treatment with regimens which include rifampicin, isoniazid, and pyrazinamide, but they require no action, unless the patient develops jaundice or symptoms of hepatitis.

If a serious adverse reaction occurs and can be attributed to a single drug (for example visual disturbance due to ethambutol) the drug should be withdrawn and therapy continued with the other three drugs. Other drugs can be added later if the response is poor. Infrequently, serious blood dyscrasias or hypersensitivity reactions occur, in which case all antituberculous drugs should be withdrawn for at least two weeks. Alternative drugs should then be used.

Ethambutol can cause optic neuropathy, and ideally visual acuity and colour vision should be tested formally before starting treatment, particularly with daily dosages above 15 mg/kg.

Streptomycin and ethambutol are eliminated by the kidneys. Renal function should therefore be checked before starting treatment and dosages altered accordingly.

24.6.3 Treatment in developing countries

The regimens detailed above are relatively expensive. At the prices current in the UK at the time of writing the 6-month regimen would cost about £250 and the 9-month regimen about £300. In countries in which the cost of expensive regimens cannot be met, cheaper regimens are used for longer periods of time. Three typical regimens are:

1. Daily streptomycin and isoniazid (with pyridoxine) for 3 months followed by twice-weekly streptomycin and isoniazid for a further 9 months. In this regimen the dosages of the drugs are different when they are given daily during the first 3 months from when they are given twice weekly (see Table 24.5).

2. Streptomycin, isoniazid, and pyrazinamide thrice weekly for 9 months. This regimen is less effective than the foregoing, although shorter in duration. It is best used when compliance is a problem.

3. Daily streptomycin, isoniazid, rifampicin, and pyrazinamide for 2 months followed by daily thiacetazone and isoniazid for 6 months. This regimen is as effective as the first regimen above. Because it is of shorter duration it is also less expensive.

At UK prices at the time of writing the first two regimens would cost about £200 in all, the third about £160. PAS may be used instead of thiacetazone if adverse effects are a problem (for example in the Chinese, who tolerate thiacetazone poorly).

24.6.4 Relapse

If a first-line regimen (for example rifampicin, isoniazid, ethambutol, and pyrazinamide) is complied with strictly there should be eradication of the tubercle bacillus in 100 per cent of cases. In patients treated with a twice-weekly regimen 5–10 per cent will need to be retreated at a later time. Relapse rates are not higher after the cheaper regimens detailed above, but they increase in frequency with shorter courses of therapy. For example, the relapse rate after 18 months of therapy with streptomycin, PAS, and isoniazid is about 3 per cent, but it is up to 15 per cent after a 12-month course.

Initial treatment in relapse should be with isoniazid plus two drugs which the patient has not previously taken. Subsequently changes may be made in the light of *in vitro* sensitivities.

■ **Table 24.6** Drug-induced respiratory disorders

Type of disorder	Drugs commonly involved
Acute pulmonary oedema/adult respiratory distress syndrome	Hydrochlorothiazide Naloxone Salicylates
Acute infiltration and eosinophilia	Nitrofurantoin
Chronic eosinophilic infiltration	Aspirin Carbamazepine Chlorpromazine Chlorpropamide Gold salts Imipramine Methotrexate Naproxen Penicillamine Penicillins Phenytoin Procarbazine Sulphasalazine Sulphonamides Tetracyclines

Interstitial pneumonia and fibrosis	Amiodarone
	Cytotoxic/immunosuppressive drugs
	  Azathioprine
	  Bleomycin
	  Busulphan
	  Carmustine
	  Chlorambucil
	  Cyclophosphamide
	  Cytosine arabinoside
	  Lomustine
	  Melphalan
	  Mercaptopurine
	  Methotrexate
	  Mitomycin C
	Nitrofurantoin

Pleural effusions and fibrosis	Bromocriptine Dantrolene Methotrexate Methysergide
Lupus-like syndrome	Hydralazine Phenytoin Procainamide
Asthma	β-adrenoceptor antagonists Cholinergic drugs (for example carbachol, pilocarpine, pyridostigmine) Prostaglandin $F_{2\alpha}$ Salicylates Tartrazine (E102) Anaphylaxis (any drug)

Type of disorder	Drugs commonly involved
Pulmonary embolism	Oral contraceptives
Respiratory depression	Alcohol
	Antidepressants
	Antihistamines
	Benzodiazepines
	Chloral derivatives
	Opioid analgesics

24.6.5 Monitoring therapy

It is important to monitor therapy when treating tuberculosis, particularly in patients in whom compliance may be poor. Some antituberculous drugs, such as isoniazid, PAS, and ethambutol, can be detected in the urine using simple chemical tests. Rifampicin colours the urine reddish-brown and is readily detected by eye.

The desirability of measuring colour vision and visual acuity to establish a baseline before starting treatment with ethambutol has been mentioned above. These tests are not used in routine monitoring, but should be used if the patient complains of visual symptoms during treatment.

If streptomycin is used then, ideally, plasma concentrations should be monitored, so that dosages can be tailored to individual requirements in order to minimize the risk of damage to the eighth cranial nerve. This is particularly important in patients with renal impairment. Unfortunately, in developing countries, in which streptomycin is most commonly used, monitoring is too expensive. The steady-state plasma concentration, measured 24 h after a daily dose, should be no higher than 20 µg/mL.

24.7 Inflammatory lung disorders

24.7.1 Cryptogenic fibrosing alveolitis

Cryptogenic fibrosing alveolitis is a disorder of unknown cause associated with alveolar inflammation and fibrosis. Most patients present with progressive dyspnoea and the mortality is high, half the patients dying within 5 years of diagnosis.

Corticosteroids in high dosages (for example prednisolone 40–80 mg/d) is the standard therapy. It produces subjective improvement in about 50 per cent of patients and objective improvement in lung function in about 15 per cent. Immunosuppressive drugs, such as azathioprine, cyclophosphamide, chlorambucil, and cyclosporin, may be effective in some patients who fail to respond to corticosteroids, and the combination of corticosteroids and azathioprine (150–200 mg/d) or cyclophosphamide (100–200 mg/d) may be superior to prednisolone alone.

Fibrosing alveolitis may be associated with various collagen diseases, such as rheumatoid arthritis, scleroderma, systemic lupus erythematosus, dermatomyositis, and mixed connective tissue disease. When it is associated with rheumatoid arthritis and scleroderma it is generally resistant to treatment. However, when it is associated with the other diseases mentioned it may respond dramatically to prednisolone and/ or azathioprine or cyclophosphamide.

24.7.2 Pulmonary vasculitis

Pulmonary vasculitis is an inflammatory disorder which results in various degrees of destruction and occlusion of pulmonary blood vessels, leading to infarction, haemorrhage, and aneurysm formation. It is often part of a systemic process in which vasculitis occurs in a variety of organs. Different types of vasculitis have different propensities for involving different organs. Those which may have a predominant effect on the lungs include Wegener's granulomatosis, polyarteritis nodosa, and the Churg–Strauss syndrome.

Corticosteroids are often beneficial, at least in the short term, but the most effective treatment is a combination of cyclophosphamide and corticosteroids (usually prednisolone). Azathioprine is useful in patients who cannot tolerate cyclophosphamide because of adverse effects.

24.8 Drug-induced respiratory disorders

A variety of drugs can cause respiratory disorders. Some important examples are given in Table 24.6.

25 The drug therapy of gastrointestinal, hepatic, and biliary disorders

Co-author: H. R. Dalton

25.1 Antacids

Antacids are used for the symptomatic relief of dyspepsia, whether it be 'functional' or associated with identifiable pathology, for example heartburn due to oesophageal reflux, pain, and discomfort associated with peptic ulceration, or gastritis.

25.1.1 Mechanisms of action of antacids

Antacids are bases which raise the pH of the gastric contents. Examples of commonly used antacids are listed in Table 25.1 along with the additives which are often incorporated in proprietary formulations.

The normal pH of gastric contents is 1–2, although food may increase the pH to as much as 5. The administration of 5–10 mL of a liquid antacid formulation may raise the pH to 3–4 on average, but the alkalinizing effects of proprietary formulations of antacids vary widely. The relative neutralizing capacities of some antacid formulations are listed in Table 25.2.

Other effects of antacids include decreased pepsin activity secondary to the increase in gastric pH, and increased oesophageal sphincter pressure. Some antacids also adsorb bile acids.

The duration of action of antacids depends on the rate of gastric emptying. If they are taken on an empty stomach the buffering effect lasts for about 30 min; if after a meal it lasts for up to 2 h or more. Calcium-containing antacids may cause rebound hyperacidity and are better avoided.

Alginates are often added to antacid formulations as foaming agents. They act by forming a layer of foam on top of gastric contents and are thereby supposed to reduce oesophageal reflux. In contrast the anti-foaming agent dimethicone decreases the surface tension of gastric fluid, thereby reducing bubble formation – it too is supposed to reduce oesophageal reflux.

Oxethazaine is sometimes also added, particularly for the treatment of symptoms associated

■ **Table 25.1** Examples of commonly used antacids and antacid formulations

---

1. *Antacids*
   (a) Aluminium salts, for example aluminium hydroxide
   (b) Magnesium salts, for example magnesium trisilicate
   (c) Sodium salts, for example sodium bicarbonate

2. *Common additives*
   (a) Foaming agents, for example alginates
   (b) Anti-foaming agents, for example dimethicone (simethicone)
   (c) Surface (local) anaesthetics, for example oxethazaine

3. *Examples of common combinations*
   Aluminium + magnesium salts
   Aluminium + magnesium salts + dimethicone
   Sodium bicarbonate + alginic acid
   Sodium + aluminium + magnesium salts
     + alginic acid

■ **Table 25.2**   Relative neutralizing capacities and sodium contents of some antacid formulations

Antacid formulation	Relative neutralizing capacity (aluminium hydroxide=1)	Sodium content
Aluminium hydroxide gel BPC	1.00	
Magnesium hydroxide BP	1.00	
Magnesium trisilicate BPC	0.62 (liquid)	High
Magnesium carbonate BPC	0.57	High
Magnesium trisilicate BPC	0.25 (tablets)	

with oesophageal reflux. It is supposed to act as a surface anaesthetic, but is of doubtful efficacy.

25.1.2 Uses of antacids

(a) Symptomatic relief of dyspeptic symptoms

Antacids are commonly used for symptomatic relief of dyspeptic symptoms, whether or not a cause, such as oesophageal reflux, has been found. The usual dosages are 5–10 mL of a liquid formulation or one to two tablets whenever required, but higher dosages can be used if necessary to relieve symptoms.

(b) Peptic ulceration

In small doses antacids relieve pain but do not heal the ulcer. On the other hand, large dosages of antacids (for example 30 mL seven times a day) have been shown to be effective in healing duodenal ulcers. However, the large volumes of antacid required for such therapy, the need for obsessive compliance, and the high incidence of adverse effects make this approach to the treatment of duodenal ulcer unacceptable, compared with the use of drugs such as the histamine (H_2) antagonists.

(c) During labour

Antacids may be given at regular intervals to women in labour, who may have to have an emergency operation. The rationale is that if buffered gastric acid is inhaled during the operation it is less likely to damage the lungs than unbuffered acid. The histamine (H_2) antagonists are often used as an alternative to antacids in these circumstances.

25.1.3 Choice of an antacid

The following considerations may influence the choice of an antacid.

1. Liquid antacids act faster than tablets, but have a shorter duration of action.
2. Aluminium salts may cause constipation and magnesium salts diarrhoea. The choice may therefore be dictated by the patient's bowel habit. Many proprietary formulations contain both types of antacid salts, in the hope of minimizing bowel disturbances of these kinds.
3. In patients with congestive cardiac failure or hypertension, in whom a high intake of salt is thought to be undesirable, one would choose an antacid with a low sodium content. Some examples of antacids with a high sodium content are shown in Table 25.2.

25.1.4 Adverse effects of antacids

Antacids are generally safe, but certain adverse effects peculiar to individual antacids should be noted.

(a) Sodium bicarbonate

Sodium bicarbonate is water soluble and is readily absorbed from the gastrointestinal tract. It therefore acts as a systemic alkali as well as having a local effect in the stomach. In patients who take large volumes of sodium bicarbonate systemic alkalosis may occur and result in hypercalcaemia with nephrocalcinosis and renal failure. This has been called the 'milk-alkali syndrome'.

(b) Magnesium and aluminium salts

These antacids are water insoluble and are less well absorbed than sodium bicarbonate. Their most common adverse effects are therefore on the bowel. Aluminium salts tend to cause constipation, while magnesium salts are laxative. These salts (particularly aluminium hydroxide) also form insoluble phosphate salts in the gut and thus reduce phosphate absorption.

Normally, little aluminium is absorbed. However, if patients with renal failure are treated with high doses of aluminium hydroxide for hyperphosphataemia and are exposed to aluminium in dialysis fluids, large amounts of aluminium may be absorbed and accumulate in the body, leading to aluminium toxicity and causing the encephalopathy known as 'aluminium dementia'.

Although it has been suggested that excess intake of aluminium may be associated with Alzheimer's disease the link has not been proven and chronic dementia is not currently regarded as a potential long-term adverse effect of antacids.

25.1.5 Interactions with antacids

Antacids inhibit the action of colloidal bismuth (tripotassium dicitratobismuthate) and the two should not be given within 30 min of each other.

Antacids may bind other drugs and prevent their absorption. Drugs which may be affected include tetracyclines (but not doxycycline), digoxin, iron, and prednisone.

The absorption of L-dopa is increased by antacids, with enhancement of its effects in Parkinson's disease.

If urinary pH is increased by large doses of sodium bicarbonate the passive reabsorption of some drugs may be altered. This may lead to an increased rate of clearance of salicylates and decreased rates of clearance of quinine and quinidine.

It is not clear to what extent these interactions are of clinical importance. For example, only very large doses of antacids reduce digoxin absorption significantly. However, it is wise to advise patients to take drugs at a different time of day from antacids (at least 30 min apart).

25.2 Antiemetics

The primary aim in the treatment of vomiting is to remove the underlying cause, but antiemetics may be given for symptomatic relief.

25.2.1 Mechanisms of action of drugs used to treat vomiting

The drugs used in the treatment of vomiting are listed in Table 25.3, and some current views on their mechanisms of action are illustrated in Fig. 25.1. Stimuli from peripheral tissues, such as the stomach and lungs, pass via afferent nerves to the group of nuclei known collectively as the vomiting centre in the medulla oblongata in the brain stem. The vomiting centre also receives impulses from the labyrinth via the vestibular nucleus and reticular formation, from higher centres following stimuli such as sight and emotion, and from the chemoreceptor trigger zone in the area postrema in the floor of the fourth ventricle, which itself receives input from various stimuli, such as drugs with emetic effects. It is known that nerve impulses in these areas are subserved by different neurotransmitters: acetylcholine (muscarinic) and histamine (H_1) in the vestibular system and vomiting centre; dopamine (D_2) in the chemoreceptor trigger zone; and 5-hydroxytryptamine in the area postrema and NTS. It is likely that antiemetics acting at these sites do so by effects on these neurotransmitters, but the detailed mechanisms whereby these antiemetic effects occur are not fully understood. Some antiemetics also have peripheral actions. For example, 5-HT_3 antagonists block the actions of 5-HT on afferent vagal nerve terminals in the gut.

Hyoscine (scopolamine) seems to act primarily on the vomiting centre in the medulla, where it has an anticholinergic (antimuscarinic) action. It also has an effect on the vestibular apparatus, which explains its efficacy in motion sickness.

▍ **Table 25.3** Drugs used in the treatment of nausea and vomiting

Antihistamines (p. 559)
Hyoscine hydrobromide (p. 538)
Metoclopramide (p. 633)
Phenothiazines (p. 645)
Domperidone (p. 597)
Ondansetron
Granisetron

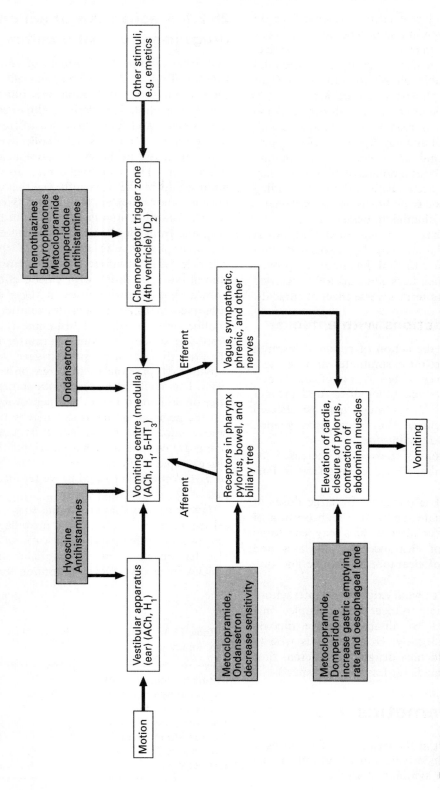

■ **Fig. 25.1** The pathophysiology of vomiting and the sites and mechanisms of actions of antiemetic drugs. ACh, acetylcholine (muscarinic) receptors; H_1, histamine (H_1) receptors; D_2, dopamine (D_2) receptors; 5-HT_3, 5-hydroxytryptamine (5-HT_3) receptors.

The phenothiazines, butyrophenones, domperidone, and metoclopramide are all dopamine receptor antagonists acting on the chemoreceptor trigger zone.

Antihistamines act on the vestibular apparatus, vomiting centre, and chemoreceptor trigger zone. However, their effects in these areas vary, since they have varying potencies as anticholinergic, antihistaminic, and antidopaminergic drugs.

Ondansetron and granisetron are selective antagonists at 5-HT$_3$ receptors in the area postrema and NTS and at the afferent vagal nerve terminals in the gut.

Some other antiemetics also have peripheral effects. For example, hyoscine reduces gastrointestinal motility. Metoclopramide reduces the sensitivity of the afferent impulses to the brain and alters gastric function by increasing oesophageal tone, stimulating pyloric contraction, and increasing the rate of gastric emptying, effects which it shares with domperidone.

25.2.2 Uses of antiemetic drugs

The drugs of choice in the treatment of vomiting due to different disorders are summarized in Table 25.3. For dosages, adverse effects, and interactions of these drugs see the Pharmacopoeia.

(a) Motion sickness

Hyoscine is the most effective drug available. It is usually given orally, but recently a transdermal formulation has become available: a patch impregnated with the drug is stuck on to the skin, usually behind the ear, and there is slow absorption into the bloodstream, providing a prolonged effect. Hyoscine should not be used in people with glaucoma or prostatic enlargement. The alternatives are the antihistamines, but they may cause more drowsiness than hyoscine. Travellers should therefore be cautious about driving when they take hyoscine or an antihistamine for travel sickness.

(b) Drug-induced nausea and vomiting

Withdrawal of the drug is best, but if it has to be continued then treatment depends on the mechanism of the drug-induced emesis. Local gastric irritation may be minimized by spreading the doses out during the day (for example L-dopa, spironolactone) and by taking the drug with food (for example proguanil). Central effects, such as opiate-induced vomiting after myocardial infarction, may be treated or prevented with a phenothiazine, such as prochlorperazine, or an antihistamine, such as cyclizine. Vomiting during cytotoxic drug therapy is dealt with separately below.

(c) Postoperative vomiting

Postoperative vomiting may be due to several causes, including surgically remediable abnormalities (for example intestinal obstruction), intestinal stasis (for example gastric stasis, ileus), and drugs (for example opiate analgesics). However, postoperative vomiting occurs in up to 50 per cent of cases and is usually not associated with any of these causes.

Metoclopramide or a phenothiazine are the treatments of choice. However, metoclopramide should not be used after intestinal surgery or if there is intestinal obstruction. If there is intestinal stasis gastric suction may be required. Hyoscine is also effective for postoperative vomiting, but there may be tolerance to a second dose, particularly when the slow-release patch formulation is used.

(d) Migraine

The nausea and vomiting of migraine is accompanied by gastric stasis, and there may therefore be delayed absorption of analgesics such as aspirin and paracetamol. To speed gastric emptying and increase the rate of analgesic absorption metoclopramide may be given parenterally or orally (see Fig. 10.1). There are proprietary formulations in which metoclopramide is combined with either aspirin or paracetamol for the treatment of migraine.

(e) Pregnancy

Because of the fear of teratogenicity, drug therapy of vomiting in pregnancy should be undertaken only when it is very troublesome. Then the general opinion is that promethazine or thiethylperazine are not harmful to the fetus and can be effective.

(f) Vomiting due to cytotoxic drug therapy and radiotherapy

Nausea and vomiting occur frequently during the treatment of cancer with cytotoxic drugs or irradiation (see Chapter 37). No treatment is entirely satisfactory, but phenothiazines and butyrophenones are used regularly with some effect. Cannabinoids also have some efficacy, and a synthetic cannabinoid, nabilone, is available for this purpose. The recent advent of the 5-HT$_3$ antagonists, such as ondansetron, has provided another means of treatment, particularly for nausea and vomiting due to radiotherapy or drug regimens which include cisplatin. If a single agent is not effective a combination of drugs with different actions may be tried, for example prochlorperazine plus diphenhydramine. The 5-HT$_3$ antagonists may be more effective when combined with dexamethasone.

(g) Symptomatic relief

If the underlying cause is either self-limiting or cannot be removed in circumstances other than those discussed above, then metoclopramide is usually the drug of choice, in the absence of gastrointestinal obstruction. However, if a sedative effect is also required a phenothiazine or an antihistamine would be preferred.

25.3 Peptic ulceration

25.3.1 The mechanisms of action of drugs used in treating peptic ulceration

The main identifiable factors involved in the pathogenesis of peptic (gastric and duodenal) ulceration are acid and pepsin secretion and reduced mucosal resistance to acid and pepsin. The bacterium *Helicobacter pylori* (previously called *Campylobacter pylori*) has also been implicated. However, the precise pathogenetic mechanisms are not yet known. Certain drugs which cause peptic ulceration (for example aspirin, other non-steroidal anti-inflammatory drugs, and corticosteroids) are thought to do so by impairing mucosal resistance to acid and pepsin.

The drugs which are used in the treatment of peptic ulceration are listed in Table 25.4.

■ **Table 25.4** Drugs used in the treatment of peptic ulceration

Antacids (p. 319)
Histamine (H$_2$) antagonists (p. 613)
Omeprazole (p. 656)
Tripotassium dicitratobismuthate
Misoprostol
Sucralfate
Pirenzepine
Antibiotics

(a) Antacids

Antacids give symptomatic relief, as described in section 25.1. Their use in high doses in treating duodenal ulcer is also discussed in section 25.1.

(b) Histamine (H$_2$) antagonists

The H$_2$ antagonists cimetidine, ranitidine, famotidine, and nizatidine reduce gastric acid secretion in response to histamine, gastrin, and food. They have a relatively short duration of action (up to 12 h) compared with omeprazole (see below).

(c) Omeprazole

Omeprazole is a specific inhibitor of the H$^+$K$^+$ATPase (the proton pump), which is present only in the oxyntic cells of the gastric mucosa and which is responsible for the secretion of hydrochloric acid into the stomach. It has a long duration of action: a single dose will inhibit gastric acid secretion for about 24 h.

(d) Misoprostol

Misoprostol is an analogue of the naturally-occurring prostaglandin E$_1$, whose actions on the stomach it mimics. It thus inhibits the secretion of gastric acid and of the proteolytic enzymes normally found in the gastric juices. It also increases the secretion of bicarbonate and mucus. However, the exact mechanisms whereby prostaglandins protect the gastric mucosa are poorly understood.

(e) Pirenzepine

Pirenzepine is an antagonist at acetylcholine receptors, with specific affinity for muscarinic

(M_2) receptors. By their effects on the vagal innervation of the stomach anticholinergic drugs reduce the secretion of gastric acid and pepsin. Previous anticholinergic drugs used in the treatment of peptic ulceration (for example propantheline) were non-specific cholinoceptor antagonists, whose adverse effects, mediated via anticholinergic actions elsewhere in the body, limited their usefulness. However, pirenzepine has a relatively specific effect on gastric (M_2) muscarinic cholinoceptors and it penetrates the brain poorly. This means that it has similar therapeutic effects to the traditional anticholinergic drugs but fewer adverse effects.

(f) Colloidal bismuth

Colloidal bismuth (bismuth chelate, tripotassium dicitratobismuthate) must have a local action in the stomach, since it is poorly absorbed and is effective after oral administration. It is thought that its effects may be mediated through an inhibitory action on *Helicobacter pylori* and perhaps through stimulation of prostaglandin secretion. It may also adhere to the ulcer and prevent the access of acid and pepsin.

(g) Sucralfate

Sucralfate is a complex of aluminium hydroxide and sulphated sucrose. Despite its aluminium content it is not an antacid and its mode of action is not known. Like bismuth it is poorly absorbed and so must have a local action. Since it forms highly polar polyanions when in solution, it has been suggested that it may act by an electrostatic interaction with the ulcer, coating it, and thus preventing the access of acid, pepsin, and bile acids. It may also bind pepsin and bile acids in the gut lumen.

25.3.2 Treatment of gastro-oesophageal reflux

In mild cases symptomatic relief with an antacid and an alginate may be sufficient. Patients should also be advised to stop smoking, to lose weight, to avoid large meals before going to bed, and to raise the head of the bed. Ulcer-causing drugs should be withdrawn if possible.

If these measures do not produce relief H_2 antagonists should be used, for example ranitidine 300 mg b.d. for 8 weeks. In resistant cases omeprazole usually causes a dramatic improvement, as it virtually abolishes gastric acid secretion. Dosages of up to 40 mg a day may be required.

In some patients stimulants of gastric motility may help, by increasing the rate of gastric emptying. Metoclopramide and domperidone have been used for this purpose, and recently a novel drug, cisapride, has also become available. Cisapride probably acts by releasing acetylcholine in the gut wall and is not a dopamine receptor antagonist. It is given in a dosage of 10 mg 3–4 times a day. Cisapride is also used to stimulate gastric emptying in patients with diabetes, systemic sclerosis, and autonomic neuropathy.

25.3.3 Treatment of peptic ulceration

The aims of treatment in peptic ulceration are to relieve symptoms, to heal the ulcer, and to prevent recurrence. Ulcer-causing drugs should be withdrawn if possible and symptomatic and specific therapy should be given. Smokers should be advised to stop smoking.

(a) Antacids

The use of antacids in providing symptomatic relief is discussed in section 25.1.

(b) Histamine (H_2) antagonists

The H_2 antagonists increase the rate of healing of gastric and duodenal ulcers, of stomal ulcers, of ulceration due to oesophageal reflux, and of the multiple ulcers due to the hypergastrinaemia of the Zollinger–Ellison syndrome. They are the initial choice of treatment in all these conditions. Of the H_2 antagonists currently available, ranitidine is to be preferred. Compared with cimetidine it is as effective in healing ulcers and has fewer adverse effects and drug interactions (see the Pharmacopoeia), although cimetidine is somewhat cheaper. The other H_2 antagonists are too new for their place in clinical practice to have been properly evaluated.

Ranitidine should be given in a dosage of 150 mg b.d. or 300 mg at bedtime for 6–8 weeks.

The corresponding dosages for cimetidine are 400 mg b.d. or 800 mg at bedtime. This results in healing rates of approximately 70 per cent for gastric ulcers and 80–90 per cent for duodenal ulcers. Ranitidine has few adverse effects. It may occasionally cause gynaecomastia or breast swelling.

Antacids should also be prescribed to be taken as required, although in practice the H_2 antagonists will often cause sufficient symptomatic relief to make their use unnecessary. For ulcers that do not heal on this therapy, the dose of ranitidine can be increased to 300 mg b.d. It is important to take further endoscopic biopsies of gastric ulcers which have not healed after a standard course of an H_2 antagonist, as a few of these will prove to be carcinomatous.

(c) Omeprazole

Omeprazole is very effective in the treatment of peptic ulcer. However, the prolonged inhibition of gastric acid secretion caused by omeprazole gives cause for concern about its possible carcinogenicity, a concern which does not now apply to the H_2 antagonists. This is because reduced gastric acidity is known to be associated with an increased risk of gastric cancer (for example in patients with pernicious anaemia), perhaps because of loss of the normal action of gastric acid in inhibiting the formation of carcinogenic nitrosamines from dietary nitrates. There has also been concern about evidence in animals that long-term therapy may cause gastric carcinoid tumours, although this has not been reported in humans. Omeprazole is therefore reserved for short-term use in patients whose ulcers have not responded to maximal doses of H_2 antagonists, especially in the Zollinger–Ellison syndrome. For resistant peptic ulceration it is given in a dose of 20 mg a day for 8 weeks. The dose may be increased to 40 mg a day if there is still failure to respond. Omeprazole may cause nausea and vomiting, bowel disturbances, headache, and rashes. It should not be used in pregnancy and breast-feeding mothers. It may increase the effects of warfarin and phenytoin by inhibiting their metabolism.

Omeprazole has also recently been licensed for use in preventing gastric ulceration due to non-steroidal anti-inflammatory drugs. However, in the few cases in which such treatment would be indicated misoprostol or ranitidine would usually be preferred (see below).

(d) Misoprostol

The main use of misoprostol is in the prevention of gastric ulceration in patients taking non-steroidal anti-inflammatory drugs. However, it should not be used routinely in all such patients, but only in those in whom gastric ulceration is a known complication and in whom non-steroidal anti-inflammatory drugs cannot be withdrawn. It is given in a dosage of 200 micrograms 2–4 times a day. In patients who have duodenal ulceration in relation to non-steroidal anti-inflammatory drug therapy either misoprostol or an H_2 antagonist may be used.

Misoprostol may cause severe diarrhoea, which may limit its use. It may also cause nausea and vomiting, abdominal pain, and vaginal bleeding. It should not be used in pregnancy or if a pregnancy is planned, since it increases uterine contraction.

(e) Drugs used to eradicate *Helicobacter pylori*

Helicobacter pylori has been implicated in the pathogenesis of peptic and particularly duodenal ulceration. Although its exact role remains to be determined, it is becoming clear that eradication of *Helicobacter pylori* from patients with peptic ulceration significantly lowers the relapse rate.

Colloidal bismuth is as effective as the H_2 antagonists in treating peptic ulceration and the subsequent relapse rate is probably lower. The lower relapse rate presumably reflects the effect of bismuth on *Helicobacter pylori*, although its ulcer-healing action may also relate to physical coating of the ulcer.

A 6–8 week course of bismuth only eradicates *Helicobacter pylori* in a proportion of patients, and patients in whom ulceration is associated with *Helicobacter pylori* are therefore treated with a combination of drugs with activity against the organism. A typical regimen for such patients would be tripotassium dicitratobismuthate 240 mg b.d. for 8 weeks, plus ampicillin 500 mg q.d.s. (or tetracycline 500 mg q.d.s.), for 2 weeks, plus metronidazole 500 mg t.d.s. for 2 weeks. This regimen clears *Helicobacter pylori* completely and causes healing of the ulcer in the majority of patients; it also has a very low relapse rate.

Colloidal bismuth causes darkening of the faeces and stains the tongue and teeth black (especially the liquid formulation). it should not be used in severe renal failure, since it may cause an encephalopathy.

(f) Other drugs

Although the other drugs listed in Table 25.4 are effective in treating peptic ulceration, they are not so commonly used, either because of adverse effects or simply because of fashion.

Sucralfate is as effective as the H_2 antagonists, both in primary treatment and in maintaining remission. However, it has not been widely studied, and there are concerns about the possible long-term effects of the aluminium which it contains. Sucralfate may reduce the absorption of phenytoin.

Pirenzepine is also as effective as the H_2 antagonists and has sometimes been used in combination with them in resistant cases. Its main adverse effects are anticholinergic, namely dry mouth and blurred vision, and it is now rarely used.

Carbenoxolone, once the treatment of choice for peptic ulceration, is no longer used because of its serious adverse effects, including fluid retention and potassium depletion.

All of the drugs discussed above are effective in healing ulcers, with similar endoscopic healing rates after 6–8 weeks. The H_2 antagonists and omeprazole probably give the most rapid symptomatic relief, and the H_2 antagonists should be the first line of therapy, because of their proven safety and relatively low cost. Whether eradication of *H. pylori* should be the first line of treatment is currently under debate, but with increasing resistance to antibiotics this strategy should probably be reserved for patients with resistant ulcers.

Once an ulcer is healed maintenance therapy with H_2 antagonists will reduce the chance of relapse. However, although clinical practice varies, maintenance therapy is probably best reserved for patients who have frequent recurrences when treatment is withdrawn.

25.3.4 Zollinger–Ellison syndrome

The Zollinger–Ellison syndrome is caused by a gastrin-secreting tumour, usually of the islets of Langerhans in the pancreas. Acid output from the stomach is vastly increased and there is severe and/or resistant peptic ulceration. Most patients will have been taking H_2 antagonists before the diagnosis is made. If their symptoms have been thus controlled, treatment should be continued until the ulcers have healed endoscopically. Many patients will require large dosages to relieve symptoms and heal the ulcers (for example up to 6 g of ranitidine daily). In some cases the ulcers will be resistant, and these patients should be given omeprazole (up to 60 mg b.d.). Once the ulcers have healed, maintenance therapy should be continued with H_2 antagonists or, in severe cases, omeprazole.

25.3.5 Bleeding from peptic ulcer

Chronic bleeding from a peptic ulcer may cause iron deficiency anaemia requiring iron replacement therapy (see Chapter 28). Acute and obvious bleeding (for example haematemesis or melaena) is a medical emergency and may require haemodynamic monitoring and blood transfusion. Its management is complex, and involves endoscopic investigation and joint medical and surgical care. Reference should be made to standard medical texts (see Chapter 20). There is no evidence that any of the ulcer-healing drugs is of value in arresting acute bleeding from gastric or duodenal ulcer.

25.3.6 Surgery for peptic ulcer

It is beyond the scope of this book to discuss the surgery of peptic ulcer in detail. However, a surgical opinion should be sought in patients with malignant ulcers, in patients who fail to respond to maximum doses of H_2 antagonists and omeprazole, or if gastrointestinal bleeding becomes a problem, despite misoprostol, in a patient who needs non-steroidal anti-inflammatory drugs. Remember that malignant ulcers may appear to heal with modern drugs and that multiple biopsies must be taken in order to rule out malignancy. The indications for emergency surgery, such as perforation, acute uncontrollable bleeding, and stenosis, need no further discussion here.

25.4 Laxatives

The commonly used laxatives are listed in Table 25.5, in which they have been divided into broad categories according to their mechanisms of action. There are numerous proprietary formulations of laxatives available and dosages are to be found in standard references such as the *British National Formulary* and the *Physicians' Desk Reference*. The important principle in using laxatives is to vary the dosage until, by trial and error, the most suitable dosage for the patient is found, i.e. the dosage which regularly produces a comfortable formed stool.

All patients with simple constipation should also be advised about diet and regularity of bowel habit, so that eventually a regular pattern can be established without the use of purgatives. Patients should be encouraged to take food with a high content of 'fibre', for example fruit and vegetables, whole wheat and bran cereals, and wholemeal bread.

25.4.1 Bulk-forming agents

These are hydrophilic compounds, which act by absorbing water, swelling, and increasing stool bulk. The increased bulk stimulates rectal reflexes and promotes defaecation.

The bulk laxatives are given orally and take a few days to have their full effect. They are used to establish a normal bowel habit in patients with chronic constipation, and are particularly useful in patients with simple constipation (i.e. constipation without associated colonic disease) and with constipation associated with diverticular disease, irritable bowel syndrome, and pregnancy.

Flatulence is a common adverse effect of the bulk laxatives. They can cause intestinal obstruction in patients with intestinal diseases (for example intestinal adhesions, stenosis, or ulceration, scleroderma, or autonomic neuropathy), and they should be avoided in those circumstances.

25.4.2 Faecal softeners and lubricants

Vegetable and mineral oils act by lubricating and softening the stool. Arachis (peanut) oil is usually given as an enema and glycerol by suppository. These compounds do not cause adverse effects but they are not always effective.

Dioctyl sodium sulphosuccinate is an anionic surface-active detergent, which increases the volume of the stool by unknown mechanisms. It also acts as a gastrointestinal stimulant. Because it inhibits the secretion of bile and may damage gastric mucosa it is better reserved for rectal administration only.

The faecal softeners and lubricants are used in cases in which bulk laxatives would be indicated, but cannot be used because of intestinal pathology (see above). They are also indicated in patients with anal fissure or haemorrhoids, in whom constipation may be caused by fear of pain during defaecation. They are also of value when a rapid purgative effect is required.

■ **Table 25.5** Commonly used laxatives

1. *Bulk-forming agents*
   Bran
   Ispaghula husk
   Methylcellulose
   Sterculia

2. *Faecal softeners and lubricants*
   Arachis oil
   *Dioctyl sodium sulphosuccinate
   *Glycerol

3. *Gastrointestinal stimulants*
   Frangula
   Senna
   Anthraquinones
   Danthron
   Sodium picosulphate
   Bisacodyl
   Castor oil

4. *Osmotic laxatives*
   Lactulose
   Magnesium slats
   Sodium salts

*Also act as stimulants.

Paraffin oil ('liquid paraffin'), widely used in the past, is no longer recommended, because of a wide range of adverse effects, including malabsorption of fat-soluble vitamins, foreign body reactions in the small bowel ('paraffinoma'), and faecal leakage at the anus, causing pruritus ani.

25.4.3 Gastrointestinal stimulants

These drugs act on the bowel, stimulating peristalsis and reducing net reabsorption of water and electrolytes by unknown mechanisms. Frangula, senna, and danthron (the anthraquinones), bisacodyl (a phenylmethane), and sodium picosulphate act on the colon, and take about 6–8 h to act after oral administration. Bisacodyl can be given rectally for a faster action. Castor oil has its effects on the small bowel and acts within 1–3 h.

The gastrointestinal stimulants are used when rapid evacuation of the bowel is required, for example in preparation for radiological examination of the bowel or for colonic surgery. They are also used immediately after the treatment of faecal impaction following severe chronic constipation.

The main adverse effects of these drugs occur with repeated abuse. This leads to loss of fluid and electrolytes (particularly potassium) and colonic atony (which causes constipation, leading to further abuse). In such cases fluid and electrolyte losses should be replaced and a saline purgative, such as magnesium sulphate, given instead. Later on gradual withdrawal of the saline purgative should be attempted, and it is important to educate the patient on the dangers of continued purgation and the need for regular bowel habits. Abuse of anthraquinones can be diagnosed by observation of the typical appearances of melanosis coli at colonoscopy.

Certain phenylmethane derivatives, used in the past, are no longer recommended, because of adverse effects. They include oxyphenisatin, which is hepatotoxic, and phenolphthalein, which often causes hypersensitivity reactions.

25.4.4 Osmotic laxatives

Osmotic laxatives act by reducing water reabsorption in the bowel. Magnesium and sodium salts, such as magnesium sulphate or hydroxide (the so-called 'saline purgatives') cause large amounts of water to be retained in both small and large bowel and thus cause increased peristalsis throughout the bowel. Because of their rapid and severe effects they are usually reserved for rectal administration only, although oral magnesium sulphate is being increasingly used.

Lactulose is a disaccharide of galactose and fructose. It is hydrolysed by colonic bacteria to its component sugars, which are then fermented to acetic and lactic acids, which act as osmotic laxatives. In contrast to the saline purgatives, lactulose takes 48 h to act and is taken orally. It is also used in the treatment of hepatic encephalopathy. It may cause abdominal discomfort and flatulence.

25.4.5 Treatment of faecal impaction

In cases of faecal impaction a simple laxative, such as oral magnesium sulphate, or a suppository of glycerol or bisacodyl should be tried first. If there is no response a colonic stimulant, such as sodium picosulphate, should be tried. If that is ineffective rectal washout will be necessary. Start with a retention enema of arachis oil or another vegetable oil (100–150 mL) or of dioctyl sodium sulphosuccinate (40 mL in 80 mL of warm water). Run the enema into the rectum with the patient supine and the foot of the bed raised. The enema should be retained for 15–30 min to allow time for it to soften the stool. This should be done twice daily for one to two days, followed by rectal wash-outs with warm saline (500 mL). If treatment is urgent digital evacuation of the rectum may be required: use a well-lubricated glove and sedate the patient well, for example with pethidine 50–100 mg i.m. or diazepam 5–10 mg i.m. After disimpaction start treatment with a colonic stimulant and re-educate the patient.

25.5 Antidiarrhoeal drugs

The commonly used antidiarrhoeal drugs are listed in Table 25.6 and dosages will be found in standard references, such as the *British National Formulary* and the *Physicians' Desk Reference*.

■ **Table 25.6** Drugs used in the symptomatic treatment of diarrhoea

---

1. *Drugs which alter gastrointestinal motility*
   Codeine (p. 641)
   Diphenoxylate (combined with atropine in
      Lomotil®) (p. 641)
   Loperamide (p. 630)
   Morphine (p. 641)

2. *Fluid adsorbents*
   Kaolin

3. *Fluid absorbents*
   Bulk-forming agents (see Table 25.5)

4. *Drugs used in specific circumstances*
   Indomethacin (post-irradiation enteritis)
   Cholestyramine (diarrhoea due to excess bile
      acids)
   Pancreatic enzymes (pancreatic malabsorption)

When treating diarrhoea the underlying cause should be treated if possible, and fluid and electrolyte losses replaced if necessary. The antidiarrhoeal drugs are used for symptomatic relief and do not constitute specific therapy.

25.5.1 Drugs which alter gastrointestinal motility

This group of drugs includes the opiate analgesics, such as codeine phosphate and morphine, and opiate analogues, such as loperamide and diphenoxylate. They reduce bowel motility, giving more time for fluid reabsorption to occur. They also increase the tone of the anal sphincter and reduce central awareness of the sensory reflex arc for defaecation. These effects are caused by stimulation of opioid receptors in the bowel, and these drugs are most useful in cases of chronic diarrhoea in which there is increased motility of the small or large bowel.

Dosage requirements vary from patient to patient. Initial dosages should be at the lower end of the dosage range, increasing gradually until the diarrhoea is controlled. Note, however, that there are maximum dosages for these drugs: codeine phosphate 180 mg/d, loperamide 16 mg/d, and diphenoxylate (in combination with atrop-

ine as Lomotil®) 20 mg/d. In addition, dosages must be carefully titrated so as to avoid constipation.

The opiates should not be used in patients with acute inflammatory disease of the large bowel (for example ulcerative colitis, Crohn's disease, or pseudomembranous colitis) since they may precipitate the serious condition of acute 'toxic' dilatation of the colon. Care should also be taken in old people, because of the risk of faecal impaction.

Morphine and codeine should not be used in patients with chronic liver disease (see p. 339). In chronic diarrhoea codeine is to be preferred to morphine, since it is less likely to cause dependence. Morphine is used in short-term symptomatic treatment, usually in combination with kaolin.

25.5.2 Fluid adsorbents

About 1.0–1.5 L of water enter the colon every day, of which most is reabsorbed, about 100–200 mL being excreted in the faeces. Relatively small changes in faecal fluid volume (10–20 mL) can make the difference between a hard stool and a soft stool, or between a soft stool and a watery stool. This accounts for the efficacy of fluid adsorbents, such as kaolin, in treating diarrhoea. Kaolin is used primarily in the short-term symptomatic treatment of diarrhoea and is often combined with a small dose of morphine. Its main adverse effect is constipation.

25.5.3 Fluid absorbents

The bulk-forming agents (discussed above under laxatives) are also of use in diarrhoea, in which they act by absorbing water. They are therefore of particular value in the irritable bowel syndrome, in which intermittent diarrhoea and constipation may both occur, and in which they are often combined with drugs which have an antispasmodic effect on the large bowel (for example mebeverine and dicyclomine). They are also used to control the consistency of the stool in patients with an ileostomy. Their adverse effects and contra-indications have been discussed in section 25.4.1.

25.5.4 Miscellaneous drugs used in specific circumstances

In some forms of diarrhoea specific agents may be indicated. For example, anti-inflammatory drugs, such as indomethacin, may be of value in postirradiation enteritis. Cholestyramine binds bile acids in the gut and is therefore useful in treating diarrhoea due to bile acids (for example in Crohn's disease and post-vagotomy diarrhoea). Pancreatic enzymes may help in controlling diarrhoea due to pancreatic malabsorption.

25.6 Irritable bowel syndrome

The treatment of this common condition, in which abdominal pain is associated with intermittent diarrhoea and constipation in the absence of identifiable bowel pathology, is most unsatisfactory. In some cases bran (up to 30 g/d) or one of the bulk-forming agents (for example sterculia or ispaghula husk) may be of help in patients in whom constipation is a major feature. Antispasmodic drugs (for example mebeverine and alverine citrate) are also frequently used, and patients are more likely to respond when an antispasmodic drug is used in combination with a bulk-forming agent. The anticholinergic effect of a tricyclic antidepressant can also be useful. Peppermint oil is sometimes prescribed, but there is little evidence of its efficacy.

It has recently been shown that some patients benefit from the exclusion of certain foodstuffs from the diet, including wheat flour, dairy products, citrus fruits, tea, coffee, nuts, chocolates, and food additives and colourings. The majority of patients will react to 2–4 of these. Patients should be asked to try an exclusion diet for 2 weeks under the supervision of a dietician. If this works challenge with individual foods can be tried.

25.7 Gastrointestinal infections

The general principles of treating infections and the specific treatment of helminthic infestations, amoebiasis, and giardiasis are discussed in Chapter 22. Here we shall deal with other gastrointestinal infections.

In all cases of infective diarrhoea, especially during the acute phase, it is important to avoid dehydration. This may be achieved simply by increasing oral fluid intake, but in severe cases i.v. fluids may be required.

Rehydration in severe infective diarrhoea (for example in cholera) is best achieved using the oral rehydration solution recommended by the World Health Organization (WHO). It can be made up by adding to 1 L of water the following constituents: sodium chloride 3.5 g, sodium bicarbonate 2.5 g, potassium chloride 1.5 g, and glucose 20 g or sucrose 40 g. Absorption of the fluid and electrolytes in this solution is enhanced by the glucose, even in severe diarrhoea. If the solution cannot be taken orally it should be given by nasogastric tube. If dehydration is severe an i.v. infusion of an appropriate electrolyte solution may be used. Whether the oral or i.v. route is chosen care must always be taken not to cause fluid overload. Oral salt and sugar solutions in water (salt 1 level teaspoon per litre and sugar 8 level teaspoons per litre) plus some source of potassium (for example orange juice) can be used as alternatives in an emergency.

25.7.1 Specific infections

(a) Traveller's diarrhoea

There is no specific therapy for traveller's diarrhoea, and symptomatic relief, for example with codeine phosphate, is all that is required.

(b) Shigellosis

Acute *Shigella* infections are usually self-limiting and require no therapy besides oral fluids. Antibiotics should not be used, because of the danger of producing resistant organisms. However, in severe cases, or in cases which are prolonged, antibiotics may be necessary, and the choice depends on local bacterial sensitivities. If the organism is sensitive to sulphonamides then sulphadiazine or co-trimoxazole, for example, may be used. If not, the best choice is usually ampicillin or in penicillin-sensitive patients a quinolone, such as ciprofloxacin. Five days' treatment is usually sufficient.

(c) *Salmonella* infections

(i) Typhoid fever

In typhoid antibiotic therapy is indicated, the first choice being chloramphenicol. It is given in a dosage of 50 mg/kg/d in divided doses for 2 weeks. Children need larger dosages than adults (100 mg/kg/d), but these high dosages should not be used in neonates (see p. 139). The oral route is usually adequate, but i.v. therapy can be given to patients who cannot take oral therapy. Do not give chloramphenicol i.m. unless both oral and i.v. routes are unsuitable: absorption does occur after i.m. injection, but it is variable and erratic.

When the organism is resistant to chloramphenicol, amoxycillin (1 g six-hourly orally) or co-trimoxazole (two tablets 12-hourly orally) may be given instead for 2 weeks.

If there are complications, such as meningitis, osteomyelitis, or abscesses, treatment may have to be continued in high dosages for longer than 2 weeks.

A small percentage of patients will relapse about 2 weeks after adequate antibiotic therapy, and will require another course of antibiotics. The choice is the same as before, but the decision will depend on the sensitivity of the organism, which may have altered. A small percentage of patients who recover go on to become chronic carriers, continuing to excrete the organism in the stool or urine, and often harbouring a growth of organisms in the gall-bladder. Chronic carriers are asymptomatic but spread the infection. Eradication of organisms can be difficult but may sometimes be achieved by a course of amoxycillin (1 g q.d.s. plus probenecid for 3 months). If there is also chronic biliary disease cholecystectomy may be required, followed by oral amoxycillin for a month, although organisms may persist in the biliary tree. Chloramphenicol is of no value in these cases, since it does not penetrate the gall-bladder.

(ii) *Salmonella* gastroenteritis

Treatment is by maintenance of fluid balance and symptomatic relief of vomiting and diarrhoea (for example with a phenothiazine and an opiate respectively). Antibiotics should not be used except if there is a bacteraemia or in patients with immune suppression. In such cases i.v. chloramphenicol should be used as for typhoid. The alternative is i.v. ampicillin. If the organism is resistant to both chloramphenicol and ampicillin then i.v. ciprofloxacin or oral co-trimoxazole may be used instead.

(d) Cholera

There is no specific antibiotic therapy for cholera, since it is due to an exotoxin produced by the *Vibrio*, and the most important aspect of therapy is to maintain fluid balance by oral or i.v. replacement of the large volumes of fluid lost via the bowel (up to 20 L per day). The WHO rehydration solution, which is best for this purpose, is detailed at the beginning of this section. None the less, there is some evidence that antibiotics may shorten the duration of the disease, and all patients should be given tetracycline (500 mg q.d.s. orally) or co-trimoxazole (two tablets b.d. orally). Cholera vaccine should also be used during an epidemic to try to contain the spread of the disease.

(e) *Clostridium difficile*

The syndrome known as antibiotic-associated pseudomembranous colitis is due to a superinfection of the large bowel by *Clostridium difficile* in patients who have taken broad-spectrum antibiotics. It occurs most commonly with clindamycin or lincomycin, but has also been reported with ampicillin, amoxycillin, cephalosporins, and co-trimoxazole, and with metronidazole in combination with aminoglycoside antibiotics.

In mild cases withdrawal of the antibiotic and fluid replacement may be sufficient, but in more severe cases vancomycin should be given (125 mg q.d.s. for 1–2 weeks). If vancomycin is ineffective metronidazole (500 mg t.d.s) is an alternative, and bacitracin and tetracycline have also been reported to be effective. Relapse occurs in about 15–20 per cent of cases within 4–21 d and should be treated with vancomycin. Antidiarrhoeal opiates should not be used because of the risk of acute colonic dilatation.

(f) *Campylobacter* enteritis

This is probably the most common cause of infective diarrhoea in the UK, accounting for about 10–15 per cent of cases. It is usually self-limiting, lasting only a few days, but severe cases may need treatment with erythromycin or a tetracycline.

(g) *Yersinia* enteritis

This is usually self-limiting and needs no treatment. In severe cases a tetracycline or co-trimoxazole should be used.

(h) Tuberculosis

Treatment of gastrointestinal tuberculosis is carried out on the same principles as for pulmonary tuberculosis (see Chapter 24). Treatment should be given for a year. If there is obstruction or fistula formation, surgery will be necessary.

(i) Viral infections

No specific therapy is indicated. Supportive therapy with fluid replacement and symptomatic relief of diarrhoea if prolonged are sufficient.

25.8 Ulcerative colitis

The drugs used in the treatment of ulcerative colitis are listed in Table 25.7.

25.8.1 The mechanisms of action of drugs used in the treatment of ulcerative colitis

(a) Sulphasalazine and its analogues

Sulphasalazine is a chemical compound of a salicylate, 5-aminosalicylic acid, and a sulphonamide,

∎ **Table 25.7** Drugs used in the treatment of ulcerative colitis

---

1. *Acute attack*
   Corticosteroids (for example prednisolone, p. 584)
   Aminosalicylates (p. 688)

2. *Prevention of recurrence*
   Aminosalicylates
      Mesalazine
      Olsalazine
      Sulphasalazine

3. *Chronic active ulcerative colitis*
   Aminosalicylates
   Corticosteroids
   Azathioprine (p. 651)

---

sulphapyridine, joined by a nitrogen bond. Sulphasalazine is poorly absorbed after oral administration and is hydrolysed to its two components by bacteria in the large bowel. Although the mechanism of action of sulphasalazine is not known it has been shown that its therapeutic effect is due to the salicylate component. This may be related to the anti-inflammatory properties of salicylates, mediated via inhibition of prostaglandin synthesis, or perhaps by some action on interferon receptors in the large bowel. The adverse effects of sulphasalazine (including headache, nausea, skin rashes, and reversible impairment of male fertility) are mainly due to the sulphonamide.

In recent years two alternatives to sulphasalazine have become available, mesalazine and olsalazine. They are more expensive than sulphasalazine but have fewer adverse effects. They may be used in patients who are known to be allergic to sulphonamides or in those who do not tolerate sulphasalazine, or in men trying to start a family.

Mesalazine is the name which has been given to 5-aminosalicylic acid. It is well absorbed from the gut, and so it is prepared in special formulations which prevent absorption before the drug reaches the large bowel. The dose is 1.2–2.4 g daily in divided doses. Alternatively it can be given by enema (100 mL at bedtime). Olsalazine is a compound of two molecules of mesalazine joined by a nitrogen bond. Like sulphasalazine it is poorly absorbed and passes to the large bowel, where it is hydrolysed by gut bacteria to mesalazine. The dose in an acute attack is 1–3 g daily orally in divided doses, and in maintenance 0.5 g b.d.

Mesalazine is generally well tolerated. Olsalazine occasionally causes diarrhoea severe enough to warrant stopping therapy; the risk of diarrhoea can be reduced by gradually increasing the dose over a few days at the start of therapy and if the drug is taken with food. Both mesalazine and olsalazine may also cause asthma in salicylate-sensitive individuals (see p. 111).

(b) Corticosteroids and immunosuppressive drugs

Corticosteroids presumably act in ulcerative colitis by virtue of their anti-inflammatory effects and azathioprine by its immunosuppressive effects.

25.8.2 Acute severe ulcerative colitis

This is characterized by severe diarrhoea, blood, mucus, and pus in the stool, fever, tachycardia, anaemia, and a raised erythrocyte sedimentation rate. Patients with acute severe ulcerative colitis should be treated in hospital. The following are the important points of management.

(a) Fluid and electrolytes

At first no food or oral fluids should be given. Intravenous infusion of fluids and electrolytes (for example potassium) should be used to replace losses. Plasma or albumin infusions may be required to treat hypoalbuminaemia, and blood transfusion to treat anaemia.

(b) Corticosteroids

Corticosteroids have been found to be of value in the treatment of an acute attack of ulcerative colitis. They may act by suppressing the inflammatory and immunological responses which occur in ulcerative colitis (see Chapter 36). They should be given both i.v. and rectally: hydrocortisone 100 mg q.d.s. i.v. and hydrocortisone enemas (100 mL) 100 mg b.d.

(c) Antibiotics

Antibiotics were used in the first effective regimens for the treatment of acute severe ulcerative colitis, on the supposition that the normal bowel flora may be more pathogenic when the bowel is inflamed. However, more recently controlled trials have suggested that an antibiotic adds nothing to the treatment outlined above, unless specifically indicated.

The above regimen will lead to improvement in about 75 per cent of cases. In those who get worse or who do not improve within 5 d colectomy will be necessary. In those who respond, oral fluids and a light diet can be introduced after 5 days and oral steroids (prednisolone 40 mg daily) can be given instead of i.v. steroids. Steroid enemas (for example prednisolone 20 mg in 100 mL) should be continued and sulphasalazine (1 g b.d. orally) or one of its analogues should be started. In patients who develop constipation as remission occurs a bulk laxative will help. The dosage of oral prednisolone should be tailed off and withdrawn over approximately 2 months. If full remission occurs it will also be possible to withdraw the steroid enemas. However, sulphasalazine or one of its analogues should be continued indefinitely, since they reduce the risk of relapse, which steroids do not. In a few patients in whom active disease continues chronically, steroid enemas or even oral steroids may need to be continued (see chronic ulcerative colitis below).

25.8.3 Mild or moderate acute attacks of ulcerative colitis

A distinction should be drawn between proctitis and more extensive disease, since the treatments are different.

Ulcerative proctitis (diagnosed when the upper limit of inflammation can be seen at sigmoidoscopy) is treated by steroid enemas (for example prednisolone 20 mg in 100 mL, preferably in a foam formulation given at night) and sulphasalazine or one of its analogues (sulphasalazine 1 g b.d.; mesalazine 1.2–2.4 g daily in divided doses; olsalazine 1–3 g daily orally in divided doses). In patients who do not settle with this treatment, mesalazine enemas may help. In resistant cases oral steroids may be required and rarely surgery may be necessary.

Mild disease extending beyond the rectum is treated with oral prednisolone 20 mg daily, steroid retention enemas, and oral sulphasalazine for 1 month. The steroid is withdrawn over the next month, the retention enemas are stopped, and the sulphasalazine is continued indefinitely. Moderate disease (more than four stools daily) is treated in the same way, except that a higher dose of prednisolone (40 mg) is used. A typical regimen would be 40 mg daily for 1 week, 30 mg daily for 1 week, and 20 mg daily for the next month; if improvement is sustained the dosage can be reduced to withdrawal over the next few weeks.

25.8.4 Chronic ulcerative colitis

Chronic ulcerative colitis in remission usually requires only treatment with regular sulphasalazine or one of its analogues. Patients should also be given a supply of prednisolone enemas to use at the first signs of relapse.

A few patients have chronic active ulcerative colitis and require continuous treatment with daily prednisolone enemas and in some cases oral prednisolone. Azathioprine may be added to this regimen in some cases with good effect. Occasionally chronic active ulcerative colitis will not respond to medical therapy and surgery will be required.

25.9 Crohn's disease

Corticosteroids may be useful in an acute attack of Crohn's disease. They can be given orally or intravenously for ileal or colonic disease or rectally for left-sided colonic disease.

Sulphasalazine (1 g b.d.) may be helpful for active colonic disease, but is less effective than corticosteroids. It is probably not helpful if there is pure ileal disease.

Azathioprine is generally reserved for those who have a poor response to steroids or in whom steroids have caused serious adverse effects. In a dose of 2.5 mg/kg/d it may reduce steroid requirements.

Metronidazole (20 mg/kg/d orally) has been used for short-term treatment of acute symptoms and it has similar efficacy to sulphasalazine. It can be useful for patients who have peri-anal or colonic disease. An alternative is ciprofloxacin (250–750 mg b.d.). Specific deficiencies due to malabsorption and diarrhoea should be treated as indicated (for example with potassium, folic acid, iron, vitamin B_{12}, and vitamin D). Diarrhoea, due to malabsorption of bile acids, may respond to cholestyramine.

For patients who have active disease unresponsive to medical therapy, or who develop strictures of the bowel, surgery is indicated. However, in contrast to ulcerative colitis, in which colectomy cures the disease, the incidence of recurrence of Crohn's disease after surgery is high.

25.10 Drugs and the liver

25.10.1 The effects of drugs on bilirubin metabolism and liver function

Drugs can cause hyperbilirubinaemia by altering bilirubin metabolism. They can also cause liver damage directly or by biliary obstruction (cholestasis).

(a) Drugs which alter bilirubin metabolism

(i) By haemolysis

Drugs may cause hyperbilirubinaemia through haemolysis (see Chapter 28). Because bilirubin conjugation is saturable this leads to an increase in the concentration of circulating unconjugated bilirubin. There is thus jaundice without impairment of liver function. Since unconjugated bilirubin is not excreted in the urine this is sometimes known as 'acholuric jaundice'. Drugs which can cause haemolysis are listed in Table 26.9.

(ii) By displacement of bilirubin from plasma proteins

Drugs such as salicylates and sulphonamides can displace bilirubin from plasma albumin, causing an increase in the concentration of circulating unbound bilirubin. This is of importance in the fetus and neonate, since the unbound bilirubin enters the brain and can cause kernicterus (see p. 155).

(b) Drugs causing hepatocellular damage

Some drugs can cause hepatocellular damage, resulting in different clinical syndromes, including acute hepatitis, chronic active hepatitis, hepatic cirrhosis, and hepatic tumours. The commonly implicated drugs are listed in Table 25.8. The following examples illustrate some specific drug-related hepatic problems.

(i) Paracetamol

The liver damage associated with paracetamol overdose is due to the formation of a hepatotoxic metabolite (see Fig. 35.1). Therapeutic doses of paracetamol are 95 per cent metabolized to conjugates of sulphate and glucuronide, and the rest to a reactive intermediate, which is detoxified by conjugation with glutathione. In overdose the sulphate and glucuronide conjugation pathways are saturated, and more drug is converted to the reactive intermediate. The glutathione available for its detoxification is rapidly depleted, and the metabolite accumulates and binds covalently to liver cell proteins, causing irreversible damage.

■ **Table 25.8**   Drugs which can cause liver damage

---

1. *Acute hepatocellular damage*

   Non-dose-related
   Antituberculous drugs
      Ethionamide
      Isoniazid
      PAS
      Pyrazinamide
      Rifampicin
   Carbamazepine
   Dantrolene
   Halothane
   Imidazoles (for example ketoconazole)
   Ibuprofen
   Indomethacin
   Methoxyflurane
   Methyldopa
   Monoamine oxidase inhibitors
   Nitrofurantoin
   Penicillamine
   Phenobarbitone
   Phenylbutazone
   Phenytoin
   Propylthiouracil
   Quinidine
   Sulphonamides
   Tricyclic antidepressants
   Valproate

   Dose-related
   Alcohol
   Amiodarone
   Azathioprine
   Chlorambucil
   Hydrocarbons (for example glue sniffing)
   Iron salts (overdose)
   Mercaptopurine
   Methotrexate
   Paracetamol (overdose)
   Salicylates
   Tetracyclines (large i.v. doses)

2. *Intrahepatic cholestasis*

   Non-dose-related
   Antithyroid drugs
      Carbimazole
      Methimazole
      Methylthiouracil
   Benzodiazepines
   Clavulanic acid
   Dextropropoxyphene
   Erythromycin salts
   Gold salts
   Imidazoles (for example ketoconazole)
   Penicillamine
   Phenothiazines
   Phenylbutazone
   Sulphonylureas
      Chlorpropamide
      Glibenclamide
      Tolbutamide
   Tricyclic antidepressants
      Amitriptyline
      Iprindole
      Imipramine

   Dose-related
   Anabolic steroids
      Methyltestosterone
      Norethandrolone
   Azathioprine
   Mercaptopurine
   Oestrogens

3. *Cirrhosis*
   Alcohol
   Methotrexate

4. *Chronic active hepatitis*
   Dantrolene
   Isoniazid
   Methyldopa
   Nitrofurantoin
   Oxyphenisatin

5. *Hepatic tumours (benign and malignant)*
   Anabolic steroids
   Oestrogens (combined oral contraceptive)

6. *Gallstones*
   Clofibrate
   Oestrogens

Liver damage can be prevented by providing glutathione-like substances, such as acetylcysteine, so that the reactive metabolite can be removed by conjugation and the liver cell can be protected (see Chapter 35).

(ii) Isoniazid

Long-term treatment with isoniazid causes liver enzymes to rise in most patients and liver damage in about 15 per cent of patients; a small number may develop chronic active hepatitis. Liver damage is caused by a metabolite. Isoniazid is mostly acetylated to acetylisoniazid, which is in turn converted to acetylhydrazine. Acetylhydrazine is thought to be converted to a reactive metabolite, which binds covalently to liver proteins, causing damage. Although it was originally thought that fast acetylators (see Chapter 8) were more likely to develop liver damage due to isoniazid, this finding has not been confirmed. Since acetylhydrazine is itself detoxified by the same N-acetyl-transferase, acetylator status may not play a part in the pathogenesis of isoniazid hepatotoxicity.

(c) Drugs causing intrahepatic cholestasis

The drugs which cause intrahepatic cholestasis are listed in Table 25.8. A drug well recognized for its association with intrahepatic cholestasis is chlorpromazine, which causes a hypersensitivity reaction in about 0.5 per cent of patients. The reaction starts within 1–4 weeks of beginning treatment and is accompanied by fever, chills, itching, nausea, and vomiting. There may be eosinophilia. The liver damage is usually reversible on withdrawal, but full recovery may take several weeks or months. It has been suggested that, in common with other hypersensitivity reactions involving the liver, it is due to conjugation of the drug or a metabolite with liver cell proteins, and that this hapten–protein complex is antigenic, provoking attack by lymphocytes and the production of antibody.

(d) Drugs associated with an increased risk of gallstones

The incidence of gallstones is increased by oral contraceptives or clofibrate. This may lead to obstructive jaundice.

25.10.2 The effects of impaired liver function on drug elimination and action

A list of drugs which should be avoided or used with care in patients with liver disease is given in Table 25.9. Drug use may be affected in such patients for several different reasons.

(a) Pharmacokinetics altered

(i) Hepatic clearance reduced

If a drug is metabolized in the liver, reduced metabolism and accumulation with toxicity may occur in liver failure. The functional capacity of the liver is large, and chronic impairment of liver function usually has to be considerable before there are important changes in drug clearance. However, hepatic drug clearance may be reduced in acute hepatitis, in hepatic congestion due to

■ Table 25.9 Drugs to be avoided or used with care in patients with liver disease

---

1. *Pharmacokinetics altered*
   (a) Hepatic clearance reduced
       Chloramphenicol
       Clindamycin
       Isoniazid
       Drugs with a high hepatic extraction ratio (see Table 3.6)
   (b) Biliary clearance reduced
       Fusidic acid
       Rifampicin
   (c) Reduced binding to plasma proteins
       Phenytoin
       Warfarin

2. *Pharmacodynamics altered*
   (a) Drugs which inhibit clotting factor synthesis
       Oral anticoagulants
   (b) Drugs whose adverse effects are enhanced
       Biguanides (lactic acidosis)
       Chloramphenicol (bone-marrow suppression)
       Cimetidine (confusional states)
       Methyldopa (idiosyncratic reactions)
       Niridazole (CNS toxicity)
       Non-steroidal anti-inflammatory drugs (gastrointestinal bleeding)
       Sulphonylureas (hypoglycaemia)

3. *Drugs which contribute to the pathophysiology of liver disease*
   (a) Hepatotoxic drugs (see Table 25.8)
   (b) Drugs which contain a lot of sodium
       Some antacids
       Sodium salts of penicillins
   (c) Drugs which cause sodium and water retention
       Carbenoxolone
       Corticosteroids
       Non-steroidal anti-inflammatory drugs
   (d) Drugs which cause potassium loss
       Carbenoxolone
       Corticosteroids
       Thiazide and loop diuretics (may also precipitate encephalopathy)
   (e) Drugs which may precipitate hepatic encephalopathy
       Lithium
       Opioid analgesics
       Sedatives and hypnotics
       Potassium-wasting diuretics

---

cardiac failure, and if there is intrahepatic arteriovenous shunting.

In contrast to renal failure (see Chapters 3 and 26) there is no easy way of calculating changes in dosage required in patients with impairment of hepatic function, partly because there is no clear-cut test of hepatic drug-metabolizing capacity, even by a single metabolic route, comparable to the creatinine clearance in renal failure, and partly because the the clearance of a drug by the liver is due not only to its metabolism but also to transport into the bile and excretion of bile. Dosages of drugs which are metabolized by the liver therefore have to be altered, where possible, according to the therapeutic response, and with careful clinical monitoring for signs of toxicity, particularly if the clinical response is hard to measure.

For drugs which have a high hepatic extraction ratio and a large first-pass metabolism by the liver (see Chapter 3 and Table 3.6), hepatic impairment may increase the systemic availability of the drug, thus reducing oral dosage requirements. In such cases i.v. dosage requirements may be unaltered. For example, oral dosages of chlormethiazole may need to be reduced in liver disease because of reduced systemic availability, but i.v. dosages are not altered.

(ii) Biliary clearance reduced

Biliary excretion is quantitatively important for very few drugs, but dosage requirements of rifampicin and fusidic acid may be affected by biliary obstruction.

(iii) Decreased binding to plasma albumin

If there is hypoalbuminaemia below 25 g/L the binding of drugs to plasma albumin will be reduced. The most important example of a drug which may be affected by changes in plasma protein binding is phenytoin. For a discussion of the relevance of this effect see Chapter 10.

(b) Pharmacodynamics altered

The effects of the oral anticoagulants are increased in liver disease because of impaired synthesis of clotting factors. In addition there is a miscellany of drugs whose adverse effects are increased in liver disease (see Table 25.9).

(c) Drugs which contribute to the pathology of liver disease

(i) Fluid and electrolyte balance

In patients with portal hypertension, oedema, and ascites, drugs which contain sodium or which cause sodium and water retention (see Table 25.9) may worsen the condition. If there is secondary hyperaldosteronism drugs which cause potassium loss are more likely to cause hypokalaemia, and that in turn may lead to hepatic encephalopathy.

(ii) Drugs which may precipitate hepatic encephalopathy

Many drugs with central nervous depressant actions (for example phenothiazines, opiates, lithium, antihistamines) may precipitate hepatic encephalopathy (Table 25.9). Chlormethiazole (in reduced oral dosages) or a benzodiazepine which is not metabolized and which has a relatively short half-time (see Table 31.3) are relatively safe if a hypnotic is required.

An excessively brisk diuresis may precipitate hepatic encephalopathy, so care must be taken when prescribing diuretics, particularly the potent loop diuretics, such as frusemide or bumetanide, in patients with liver disease.

25.11 Drug therapy in the treatment of chronic liver disease

25.11.1 Oedema and ascites

Retention of sodium and water occurs in chronic liver disease for a variety of reasons: hypoalbuminaemia reduces the colloid oncotic pressure of the plasma, leading to transudation of fluid; portal hypertension also causes transudation of fluid, because of increased hydrostatic pressure in the splanchnic veins; reduced renal blood flow due to the reduced intravascular volume leads to increased renal sodium retention, and this is partly mediated by increased aldosterone production.

The management of hepatic oedema and ascites is with a low-salt diet and diuretics. Usually moderate salt restriction (to 80 mmol/d) is all that can be achieved, by advising patients not to add salt to their food. Despite recent concerns about its safety, based on observations of tumours in animals, spironolactone (100–400 mg/d) is still the drug of choice, since it is an aldosterone antagonist. If it is not fully effective on its own, spironolactone may be combined with a loop diuretic such as frusemide, but care must be taken not to produce too brisk a diuresis, because of the risk of precipitating acute electrolyte disturbances and hepatic encephalopathy. Therapy should be carefully monitored by daily weighing and weight loss should be no greater than 0.5 kg/d in ascites alone or 1 kg/d if there is peripheral oedema as well. The urinary sodium:potassium ratio during effective therapy should be greater than 1.0.

If hypokalaemia does not respond to spironolactone additional potassium supplements may be required (see Chapter 26).

In resistant ascites large-volume paracentesis is safe and effective; it should be combined with an intravenous infusion of albumin.

25.11.2 Hepatic encephalopathy

The pathogenesis of hepatic encephalopathy in chronic liver failure is not fully understood. It is known that there is retention of nitrogenous toxins, such as ammonia, and an imbalance of amino acids with an increase in the concentrations of circulating aromatic amino acids and a reduction in branched-chain amino acids. How these changes might cause hepatic encephalopathy is not known, but there is evidence that central neurotransmitter function may be altered, with a reduction in brain noradrenaline and dopamine, an increase in brain 5-hydroxytryptamine, and perhaps an increase in GABA function. These changes might occur secondary to alterations in the transport of amino acids into the brain.

The treatment of acute hepatic encephalopathy is aimed at: (1) reducing the absorption of the nitrogenous breakdown products of dietary protein or the protein derived from blood after a gastrointestinal haemorrhage, since these are the source of most of the nitrogen-containing toxins in hepatic encephalopathy, and (2) reducing or eliminating any precipitating factors, for example by withholding diuretics, by treating infections, or by treating gastrointestinal bleeding and consequent hypovolaemia. Protein intake should be reduced to 20 g/d or less, and calories should be provided in the form of carbohydrate. The lower bowel should be evacuated using oral lactulose (30 mL t.d.s.). Oral neomycin should also be given (1–2 g orally q.d.s.). It acts by reducing the production of gut-derived toxins by gastro-intestinal bacteria. It may also cause a small reduction in dietary protein absorption.

In chronic hepatic encephalopathy the protein intake should be increased to the maximum tolerated (usually about 50 g/d) and lactulose should be given in a dosage of 30 mL t.d.s. orally, increasing if necessary to a maximum total of 200 mL daily. The dosage should be titrated according to the stools, which should be soft in consistency and two or three in number per day. Lactulose may act by altering bacterial metabolism in the colon, with reduced production of ammonia, or by reducing colonic transit time.

25.11.3 Acute bleeding from gastro-oesophageal varices

Acute variceal bleeding is a medical emergency. Blood losses should be replaced immediately, preferably with fresh whole blood; central venous pressure monitoring may be required to assess volume requirements. Fresh frozen plasma should be given to replace deficient clotting factors and vitamin K_1 (phytomenadione, 10 mg slowly i.v.) to stimulate their production.

The diagnosis should be confirmed as soon as possible by endoscopy. If the bleeding has stopped, sclerotherapy (i.e. injection of the varicose vessels with a sclerosant) should be performed. If there is active bleeding, measures should be taken to control it, using either sclerotherapy, oesophageal tamponade with a Sengstaken tube, or reduction of portal pressure by splanchnic vasoconstriction with intravenous vasopressin or its analogue terlipressin. Sclerotherapy, if available, is the treatment of choice, since oesophageal tamponade and vasopressin are temporizing measures only, and the patient will eventually require sclerotherapy or, if bleeding continues, oesophageal transection.

Vasopressin is given by i.v. infusion over 20 min in a dose of 20 i.u. in 100 mL of 5 per cent dextrose; this can be repeated at 4-hourly intervals if required. Its adverse effects are facial pallor, intestinal colic, and defaecation, and these are signs of pharmacological efficacy. More seriously it can cause coronary arterial constriction and myocardial infarction. Terlipressin is given in a single i.v. dose of 2 mg, which can be repeated every 4–6 h until bleeding stops or to a maximum of four doses. It has a longer duration of action than vasopressin and fewer adverse effects.

The long-term management of oesophageal varices which have previously bled is with sclerotherapy. H_2 antagonists and β-adrenoceptor antagonists have been used to prevent bleeding, but the H_2 antagonists are ineffective and β-blockers, despite the encouraging results of some trials, have not yet found a place in treatment.

The treatment of varices which have not bled is problematic. There is little evidence that sclerotherapy reduces the risk of variceal bleeding or improves mortality. However, evidence is emerging that β-adrenoceptor antagonists may be helpful in the primary prevention of bleeding.

25.11.4 Chronic active hepatitis

Corticosteroids are of value in treating the autoimmune form of chronic active hepatitis and may act by immunosuppression (see Chapter 36) and they prevent progression to cirrhosis. A typical regimen would be prednisolone 60 mg daily orally, reducing over a period of a few weeks to a maintenance dose of 10–15 mg daily. In those who need higher dosages, or those in whom severe adverse effects occur, the dosage of prednisolone may be reduced by adding azathioprine. Alpha-interferon is beginning to find a place in the treatment of chronic active hepatitis due to hepatitis B and non-A non-B hepatitis.

25.11.5 Pruritus in jaundice

Jaundice due to chronic cholestatic liver disease is often accompanied by pruritus. Cholestyramine acts by binding bile acids in the gut and preventing their reabsorption via the ileum. It is given in a dosage of 12–24 g daily orally and may give symptomatic relief. However, it is of no value if there is complete biliary obstruction, since in that case there will be no excretion of bile acids.

25.12 Drug treatment of gallstones

In developed countries about 80 per cent of gallstones are pure cholesterol stones or stones containing mostly cholesterol. The rest are pigment stones or mixed stones containing calcium. Only cholesterol stones are susceptible to drug therapy.

The pathogenesis of cholesterol stones is incompletely understood. It is partly due to supersaturation of cholesterol in the bile with cholesterol precipitation, but other factors must operate, since gallstones do not always occur in people whose bile is supersaturated with cholesterol. There are several factors which lead to increased cholesterol content in bile, for example obesity, pregnancy, and drugs such as clofibrate and oestrogens. Reduced bile salt absorption in ileal disease (for example in Crohn's disease) also causes an increase in biliary cholesterol both in proportion to the other constituents (one of which is bile salts) and in absolute amounts, since bile salts normally inhibit cholesterol synthesis.

Cholesterol stones may therefore be treated with bile acids. They inhibit cholesterol production and increase the proportion of bile salts in the bile, thereby reducing the proportional content of cholesterol. Stone formation is halted and with long-term treatment dissolution occurs. Chenodeoxycholic acid (10–15 mg/kg/d) and its epimer ursodeoxycholic acid (8–10 mg/kg/d) are used. They need to be given for at least 3 months to allow even the smallest stones to dissolve. The larger the stone the longer dissolution takes, and treatment may have to be continued for up to 2 years. Because the time taken to dissolve a stone is proportional to the square of its radius, very large stones (over 20 mm in diameter) are not treated in this way. For stones less than 10 mm in diameter 6 months treatment will usually be enough.

The recurrence rate after dissolution is high (70 per cent in 5 years) and repeated treatment may be needed. For this and other reasons medical treatment of gallstones is restricted to certain patients.

1. Patients with radiolucent stones.
2. Those with few or no symptoms. It is better to treat symptomatic patients surgically.
3. Those in whom surgery is contra-indicated for any reason.
4. Those who do not have a contra-indication to bile acid treatment. This excludes from treat-

ment patients with biliary obstruction, a non-functioning gall-bladder, ileal disease with poor absorption of bile acids, patients with peptic ulceration, and pregnant women.

The major adverse effect of the cholic acids is diarrhoea, less so with ursodeoxycholic acid than chenodeoxycholic acid. It occurs in about a third of patients and there is some tolerance with long-term treatment. Lipid-lowering drugs (see Chapter 27) and drugs which increase the biliary excretion of cholesterol (for example oestrogens) oppose the therapeutic effects of the cholic acids.

26 Drugs and the kidney and the drug therapy of renal, urinary tract, and prostatic disorders

Co-author: J.D. Firth

26.1 Diuretic therapy

26.1.1 Mechanisms of action of diuretics in relation to disease

The main uses of diuretics are in the treatment of oedema due to cardiac failure, renal disease (the nephrotic syndrome and chronic renal failure approaching end stage), and cirrhosis of the liver, and in the treatment of hypertension (particularly the thiazides). The use of the diuretics in the practical management of these conditions is discussed under the relevant disease headings. Here we shall present a broad view of diuretic action and use. Details about important members of each class of diuretics can be found in the Pharmacopoeia.

There are important differences between the actions of different diuretics, which can be exploited in their therapeutic use. The various diuretics used are listed in Table 26.1 and the main sites of action of the various classes of diuretic and some qualitative differences between their effects are shown in Table 26.2. Their sites of action in the nephron are shown in Fig. 26.1.

26.1.2 The clinical importance of the differences in action between diuretics

(a) Efficacy and maximal diuretic effect

If a large brisk diuresis is required (for example in acute left ventricular failure) then one would use a loop diuretic, such as frusemide or bumetan-ide. The loop diuretics are also called 'high-ceiling' diuretics, because they have a high maximal efficacy compared with the thiazide and other diuretics (see p. 53 and Fig. 4.5) and are capable of achieving at least a 2.5 times greater sodium and water diuresis than the thiazides. They also act much more quickly. They also act as venodilators, which is probably why they act so quickly in the relief of acute left ventricular failure. Thiazides produce a smaller diuresis, and it is usually spread out over a longer period of time. In patients with mild cardiac failure the milder diuretic effect of the thiazides may be more acceptable to the patient. A fierce diuresis, with frequent passages of large volumes of urine, can be quite uncomfortable, particularly for old people. In addition, in old women there may be the problem of incontinence, which is made much worse by diuretics, and in old men with benign hypertrophy of the prostate acute large volume diuresis may precipitate acute retention of the urine.

(b) Antihypertensive effect of diuretics

There is no doubt that the thiazides are just as effective as the loop diuretics as antihypertensive drugs, and possibly more effective. The mechanism of action of the thiazide diuretics in hypertension is still undecided, but one or more of three mechanisms may be involved.

1. A sodium diuresis, producing reduced intracellular sodium concentrations within vascular smooth muscle cells and reduced reactivity of vascular smooth muscle muscle to noradrenaline released from sympathetic

■ **Table 26.1** Diuretics

1. *Thiazides* (*Benzothiadiazines*; p. 695)
   Bendrofluazide
   Hydrochlorothiazide
   Cyclopenthiazide
   Other thiazides include benzthiazide, chlorothiazide, hydroflumethiazide, methyclothiazide, and polythiazide.
   Other sulphonamide diuretics with similar actions and adverse effects to the thiazides include chlorthalidone, metolazone, quinethazone, and xipamide. Mefruside is related to frusemide but in action more closely resembles the thiazides.

2. *Loop diuretics*
   Bumetanide (p. 566)
   Ethacrynic acid
   Frusemide (p. 608)

3. *Potassium-sparing diuretics*
   Amiloride (p. 551)
   Triamterene (p. 697)
   Aldosterone antagonists
     Spironolactone (p. 687)
     Potassium canrenoate (p. 687)

4. *Osmotic diuretics*
   Mannitol

5. *Carbonic anhydrase inhibitors*
   Acetazolamide (p. 537)

6. *Examples of combinations of diuretics with potassium*
   (i) Thiazides + potassium chloride
        Bendrofluazide 2.5 mg + potassium 7.7 mmol (Centyl K®)
   (ii) Loop diuretics + potassium chloride
        Bumetanide 500 μg + potassium 7.7 mmol (Burinex K®)
        Frusemide 20 mg + potassium 10 mmol (Lasikal®)
        Frusemide 40 mg + potassium 8 mmol (Diumide-K Continus®)

7. Examples of combinations of thiazide or loop diuretics with potassium-sparing diuretics
   (i) Thiazides + potassium-sparing diuretics
        Benzthiazide 25 mg + triamterene 50 mg (Dytide®)
        Hydrochlorothiazide 50 mg + amiloride 5 mg (co-amilozide 5/50; Amilco®;
          Hypertane 50®; Moduretic®; Normetic®)
        Hydrochlorothiazide 25 mg + triamterene 50 mg (Dyazide®; Triamco®)
        Hydroflumethiazide 50 mg + spironolactone 50 mg (Aldactide 50®)
   (ii) Loop diuretics + potassium-sparing diuretics
        Frusemide 20 mg + spironolactone 50 mg (Lasilactone®)
        Frusemide 40 mg + amiloride 5 mg (co-amilofruse 5/40; Frumil®; Lasoride®)

■ **Table 26.2** Pharmacological comparison of diuretics

Diuretic	Site of action	Urinary excretion				Potency on Na$^+$ excretion	Potency as diuretic
		Na$^+$	K$^+$	Cl$^-$	HCO$_3^-$		
Thiazide diuretics	Cortical segment; early part of distal tubule	↑	↑	↑	↓	+ +	+ +
Loop diuretics	Medullary segment; ascending limb of the loop of Henle	↑	↑	↑	↓ or ⇔	+ + +	+ + +
Potassium-sparing diuretics	Distal tubule	↑	↓	⇔	↑	+	+
Aldosterone antagonists	Distal tubule	↑	↓	⇔	↑	+*	+*
Mannitol	Throughout tubule (depends on osmotic load)	↑	⇔	↑	↑	+	+ + +
Carbonic anhydrase inhibitors	Proximal tubule	↑	↑↑	⇔	↑	+	+

*Na$^+$ excretion and diuresis are more marked when there is significant secondary hyperaldosteronism (for example oedema due to cirrhosis of the liver).
Symbols: ↑ = increased; ↓ = reduced; ⇔ = unchanged.

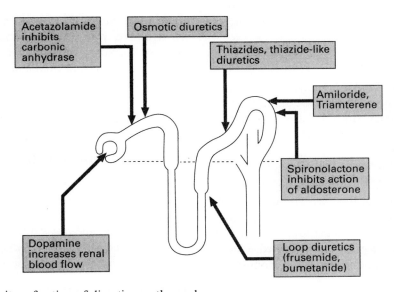

■ **Fig. 26.1** The sites of action of diuretics on the nephron.

nerve-endings and possibly other vasoconstrictors.
2. Haemodynamic changes consequent upon an initial hypovolaemia produced by diuresis.

3. A direct vasodilating action on arterioles. Diazoxide, which is a thiazide, is a vasodilator which reduces peripheral resistance and lowers the blood pressure, despite the fact that it

produces sodium retention. This vasodilator action may be produced by increased potassium flux through potassium channels.

In the treatment of hypertension thiazide diuretics are preferred to loop diuretics or any of the other classes of diuretics.

(c) Effects on potassium balance

Both the thiazide and the loop diuretics produce potassium loss, and, in contrast to the difference in their relative effects on sodium and water diuresis, their effects on potassium are roughly equipotent. There are certain circumstances in which this loss may be excessive, in which case it may be dangerous, and replacement therapy or the administration of a potassium-sparing diuretic becomes necessary (see section 26.2). If the plasma potassium concentration is below 3.5 mmol/L or if it is below 4.0 mmol/L and there is evidence of total body potassium depletion (for example alkalosis, electrocardiogram changes) then steps should be taken to replenish body stores and to prevent further loss.

The following are guidelines to potassium conservation and replacement during diuretic therapy.

(i) Digoxin therapy

Active measures should be taken to conserve potassium in patients in cardiac failure taking digoxin and diuretics, since the effects of digoxin are potentiated by potassium depletion.

(ii) Secondary hyperaldosteronism

If there is secondary hyperaldosteronism, for example in cirrhosis of the liver with oedema and ascites, thiazide or loop diuretics may produce significant potassium depletion. Potassium-sparing diuretics are generally indicated. Plasma potassium concentrations should be monitored.

(iii) Old people

Old people are particularly liable to develop potassium depletion with thiazide and loop diuretics. Malnutrition increases the risk. Many physicians routinely use a potassium-sparing diuretic with the thiazide or loop diuretics in old people in order to avoid this complication.

(iv) Intercurrent illness

Intercurrent illness during diuretic therapy is not unusual and may produce severe potassium depletion. Vomiting and diarrhoea are common causes.

(v) Drugs

Laxatives increase potassium loss from the bowel. Corticosteroids may cause sodium and water retention, particularly in old people, and diuretics may be required. However, they also cause potassium loss, which may exacerbate that produced by diuretics, and potassium-sparing diuretics or potassium supplements may therefore be required.

Conversely, potassium supplements must sometimes be avoided because of an increased risk of hyperkalaemia. This is most important in patients with renal impairment, and monitoring of plasma potassium concentrations is necessary when treating such patients with diuretics. It can be very difficult to predict exactly what effects diuretics will have on the plasma potassium concentration in patients with renal impairment.

In most circumstances, other than those outlined above, routine potassium supplements or potassium-sparing diuretics are not required, for example in uncomplicated essential hypertension or mild cardiac failure.

26.1.3 The choice of agents for repletion and conservation of potassium during diuretic therapy

If there is potassium depletion then separate potassium supplements must be given in doses sufficient to replace losses. If there is no potassium depletion, and it is felt that measures should be taken to conserve the body's potassium stores, then there are several choices:

(1) potassium supplements as separate formulations;

(2) potassium supplements in combination tablets with a diuretic;

(3) a combination of a potassium-wasting diuretic with a potassium-sparing diuretic as separate formulations;

(4) a combination of a potassium-wasting diuretic with a potassium-sparing diuretic in a single formulation.

Examples of the types of combination tablets which are available are given in the Pharmacopoeia.

(a) Potassium supplements

If it is decided to give potassium chloride, it should be given as separate tablets rather than combination formulations, for the following reasons. The normal dietary intake of potassium is about 50 mmol/d, which is balanced by urinary excretion of 50 mmol/d. The usual daily dose of a thiazide or loop diuretic when given acutely causes an additional urinary potassium loss of about 20 mmol/d. However, more potassium than this will be lost in the treatment of severe oedema, and supplements of about 48 mmol of potassium chloride per day (for example 2 tablets of Slow-K® t.d.s.) may be required. Since most combination formulations of diuretics with potassium chloride contain 8 mmol of potassium and half the usual dose of diuretic, a full dose of diuretic will provide only 16 mmol of potassium a day, which may well be insufficient. Thus, in the treatment of oedema and in heart failure, combination formulations of diuretics with potassium chloride are too inflexible for a correct diuretic/potassium balance to be achieved and probably provide too little potassium.

In the treatment of uncomplicated essential hypertension with thiazide diuretics potassium supplements are usually not required and combination diuretic/potassium tablets are a needless expense. Thus, there is little place for combination tablets of diuretics and potassium chloride. If potassium is to be given in order to prevent potassium depletion it should be given as separate tablets. However, it should also be remembered that potassium tablets are difficult for patients to take: slow-release potassium tablets may be difficult to swallow and many people find effervescent tablets nauseating. As a result compliance is often poor. For this reason potassium-sparing diuretics are in general preferable if prevention of potassium loss is required.

(b) Potassium-sparing diuretics

Potassium-sparing diuretics have several advantages over potassium supplements. Firstly, they conserve potassium rather than replacing it. For example, in patients with hepatic cirrhosis urinary potassium excretion simply increases to match extra potassium given in the form of potassium chloride. Secondly, they also have magnesium-sparing properties and will therefore prevent magnesium depletion due to thiazide and loop diuretics. Thirdly, they have some diuretic effect of their own and will thus supplement the diuretic actions of the potassium-wasting diuretics. Fourthly, they are easier to take.

Potassium-sparing diuretics are best given in separate formulations, to allow flexibility of dosage, although if a patient's potassium balance is stable and if there is a combination formulation which contains suitable doses of the diuretics being used, it may be simpler to prescribe such a formulation.

Care must be taken not to cause hyperkalaemia with potassium-sparing diuretics. They should almost never be used in conjunction with potassium supplements and extra care must be taken if they are used in conjunction with angiotensin converting enzyme inhibitors, such as enalapril, which are also potassium-sparing. Amiloride and triamterene should never be used in patients with renal failure, in whom potassium retention is common, and spironolactone should only be used in such patients if there is evidence of secondary hyperaldosteronism.

26.1.4 Resistance to potassium-wasting diuretics

Various factors in oedematous states may make it difficult to achieve an adequate diuresis with thiazide or loop diuretics.

(a) Secondary hyperaldosteronism

Secondary hyperaldosteronism becomes a significant factor late in cardiac failure, may sometimes be significant in the nephrotic syndrome, and is particularly important in hepatic cirrhosis. Spironolactone may therefore be helpful in controlling oedema in all of these conditions. Secondary hyperaldosteronism also occurs as a compensatory response to the diuresis produced by thiazide and loop diuretics themselves.

In late-stage cardiac failure and the nephrotic syndrome resistance to diuretics can sometimes be overcome by adding spironolactone. However, in hepatic cirrhosis spironolactone is generally used on its own, because it is very effective and because care must be taken with the potassium-wasting diuretics, which readily cause sodium and potassium depletion and hepatic encephalopathy.

(b) Lowered renal blood flow

Generally when renal blood flow falls there is increased proximal tubular reabsorption of sodium. In addition, because diuretics generally act from the luminal side of the nephron, reduced access of diuretics to their sites of action in the renal tubule mitigates their effects. In severe cardiac failure reduced renal blood flow is probably the most common mechanism whereby oedema becomes resistant to diuretic therapy. This resistance can sometimes be overcome by bed rest, or by increasing cardiac output with positive inotropic drugs, or by renal arteriolar vasodilatation with dopamine.

(c) Renal failure

One of the complications to avoid in renal failure is sodium and water overload, and it can be very difficult to get rid of sodium and water by diuresis in patients with renal failure and a low glomerular filtration rate. The reasons for this are not entirely clear. However, it may be related to poor entry of diuretics into the urine in renal failure, partly because of reduced renal blood flow and partly because in renal failure organic acids accumulate and block the transport of diuretics into the urine. Large doses of frusemide (for example 0.5–2 g orally or i.v.) can overcome this problem, but care must be taken to avoid ototoxicity, which is a risk with large doses of frusemide. In these circumstances if frusemide is given i.v. it should be given by infusion at a rate no greater than 4 mg/min.

(d) Decreased absorption due to oedema of the bowel wall

In severe congestive cardiac failure there may sometimes be poor absorption of frusemide and thiazide diuretics, and therefore a poor response. In patients who fail to respond to oral diuretics it is always worth giving a small dose of frusemide (20–40 mg) intravenously to see if this will overcome apparent resistance. If it does and the heart failure improves oral therapy may later become effective. Sometimes in these patients a better response may be obtained if the frusemide is given by slow infusion at a rate of 4 mg/min rather than by bolus injection. The reasons for this are not clear. As an alternative to i.v. frusemide, oral bumetanide, which is better absorbed, may prove effective in some cases.

In refractory cases metolazone (2.5–10 mg daily) should be considered. Metolazone is a thiazide-like diuretic which acts all along the nephron. It is very potent and sometimes causes a massive diuresis. It can therefore cause dehydration and hypovolaemia and its use is best left to specialists. Patients should weigh themselves daily and stop treatment if their weight loss exceeds 0.5 kg/d.

26.1.5 Adverse effects of diuretics

The common adverse effects of the diuretics are listed in Table 26.3.

■ **Table 26.3** Adverse effects of diuretics

Thiazide, thiazide-like, and loop diuretics
  Hyponatraemia (sodium depletion)
  Hypovolaemia (volume depletion)
  Raised blood urea
  Hypokalaemia (potassium depletion) and
    alkalosis
  Hypomagnesaemia (magnesium depletion)
  Hyperuricaemia and gout
  Carbohydrate intolerance (more with
    thiazides)
  Erectile impotence

Frusemide and ethacrynic acid (high-dose)
  Ototoxicity

Bumetanide
  Myalgia

Potassium-sparing diuretics
  Risk of hyperkalaemia

Spironolactone
  Risk of hyperkalaemia
  Dyspepsia, peptic ulceration
  Painful gynaecomastia (particularly in cirrhosis)

26.1.6 Drug interactions with diuretics

Indomethacin, possibly because of actions on renal prostaglandins, inhibits the diuretic effect of frusemide.

Drugs which promote sodium reabsorption, for example corticosteroids and oestrogens, antagonize the effects of diuretics.

Drugs which promote potassium excretion, for example corticosteroids, purgatives, and amphotericin B, may act additively with the thiazide and loop diuretics to produce serious potassium depletion.

Conversely, potassium-sparing diuretics and potassium supplements may produce serious hyperkalaemia if they are used together or in combination with angiotensin converting inhibitors, such as enalapril, particularly if there is a degree of renal impairment.

The potassium depletion produced by the thiazide diuretics and loop diuretics may significantly enhance the actions of the cardiac glycosides and cause digitalis toxicity. It may also impair the action of the class I antiarrhythmic drugs.

The combination of gentamicin and frusemide is more nephrotoxic than either alone. If a loop diuretic is required in a patient receiving gentamicin use bumetanide, which carries a lower risk of eighth nerve damage.

26.2 Potassium depletion

The causes of potassium depletion are listed in Table 26.4. The treatment of diuretic-induced potassium depletion is replacement using potassium chloride, either orally (as elixir, effervescent tablets, or slow-release tablets, according to patient preference), or sometimes by i.v. infusion. It is important to use the chloride salt, since potassium depletion is invariably accompanied by chloride depletion, and if that is not corrected the extra potassium will not be retained by the kidney.

The slow-release formulations of potassium chloride now available uncommonly cause serious adverse effects, although anorexia, nausea, and vomiting are not uncommon. Oesophageal ulceration occasionally occurs because of hold-

■ **Table 26.4** Causes of potassium depletion and hypokalaemia

1. *Drug-induced*
   Corticosteroids
   Carbenoxolone
   Diuretics
   Insulin in diabetic ketoacidosis
   Laxatives (chronic abuse)

2. *Gastrointestinal loss*
   Vomiting
   Diarrhoea
   Malabsorption (for example coeliac disease)

3. *Renal loss*
   Tubular damage (for example during the diuretic phase of acute tubular necrosis)

4. *Increased adrenal gland activity*
   Cushing's syndrome
   Primary and secondary hyperaldosteronism

5. *Old age*
   Usually there are several factors in the elderly who present with potassium depletion: malnutrition, poor dietary potassium intake, vomiting, diarrhoea, and drugs are common causes.

up of sustained-release potassium chloride tablets in the oesophagus. This has been reported in patients with mitral stenosis and a large left atrium, which presses on the oesophagus. However, in old patients tablets may readily adhere to the oesophageal mucosa, even in the absence of narrowing, and patients should be advised to wash down their tablets with a glass of water. Small intestinal ulcers occur rarely. As an alternative to slow-release formulations patients may be given an effervescent formulation or an elixir, although these formulations frequently cause anorexia, nausea, and vomiting. Oral replacement of potassium loss has the obvious hazard of going too far and producing hyperkalaemia.

When potassium depletion is severe, or if the patient is unable to take oral formulations, i.v. administration is necessary. Take great care with the i.v. administration of potassium salts, because too rapid infusion may cause hyperkalaemia and a fatal cardiac arrhythmia. Potassium salts should never be injected as a bolus, but should be given by infusion at a rate of 10 mmol/h, unless depletion is very severe (for example in diabetic ketoacidosis), when a rate of up to 20 mmol/h is acceptable, provided there is careful monitoring of the plasma potassium concentration and the electrocardiogram (looking for T wave peaking with hyperkalaemia). Usually not more than 120 mmol of potassium should be given per day. If you add potassium to fluid in an infusion bottle (for example saline) make sure that the solution is thoroughly mixed before infusion. Potassium salts should never be added to blood, blood products, mannitol, or solutions of lipids or amino acids (see p. 123).

Very great care must be taken when giving i.v. potassium to patients with renal impairment, because of the greatly increased risk of dangerous hyperkalaemia.

26.3 Hyperkalaemia

The causes of hyperkalaemia are listed in Table 26.5. When plasma potassium concentrations reach 6.5 mmol/L peaked T waves on the electrocardiogram usually develop. As the concentration rises to 7–8 mmol/L the PR interval becomes prolonged, the P wave disappears, and

■ **Table 26.5** Causes of hyperkalaemia

---

1. *Drug-induced*
   Potassium supplements
   Potassium-sparing diuretics
   ACE inhibitors

2. *Reduced renal mass*
   Acute and chronic renal failure

3. *Reduced adrenal gland activity*
   Hypoaldosteronism (Addison's disease)

4. *Shifts across cell membranes from inside to outside*
   Acidosis
   Cell destruction (for example rhabdomyolysis, haemolysis, tumour lysis, burns)
   Diabetic ketoacidosis
   Hyperkalaemic periodic paralysis
   Massive blood transfusion

---

the QRS complex widens. These electrocardiogram signs are the best guide to serious hyperkalaemia.

26.3.1 The treatment of hyperkalaemia

Wherever possible the primary cause of the hyperkalaemia should be treated.

When hyperkalaemia is severe. i.e. when there are electrocardiogram signs more severe than T wave peaking (usually when the plasma potassium concentration is over 7.0 mmol/L), calcium gluconate should be given (10–30 mL of a 10 per cent solution i.v. over 5 min), preferably with electrocardiogram monitoring. This treatment should be used with great caution in patients taking cardiac glycosides, since calcium salts given intravenously may precipitate digitalis toxicity. Calcium acts by reducing cardiac membrane excitability and thus prevents potassium-induced arrhythmias. However, it does not affect the hyperkalaemia itself, and its effects are therefore only temporary,

To lower the plasma potassium concentration insulin should be given (20 i.u. of soluble insulin i.v. over 15–30 min). Insulin shifts potassium into cells and thus lowers the extracellular potassium concentration. Glucose is given at the same time (100 mL of a 50 per cent solution) to prevent hypoglycaemia. Sodium bicarbonate is also given (50–100 mL of an 8.4 per cent solution, i.e. 50–100 mmol, i.v. over 15–30 min). This will correct acidosis if present and help to shift potassium into cells. Care should be taken in renal failure not to overload with sodium and thus increase extracellular fluid volume. The hypokalaemic effect of sodium bicarbonate occurs within an hour and lasts several hours.

If the plasma potassium concentration is between 5.5 and 6.5 mmol/L the above measures are not required. Instead more gentle lowering of the plasma potassium concentration can be achieved with the sodium salt of the ion-exchange resin polystyrene sulphonate (Resonium A®) (15 g 3–4 times daily orally, or rectally as a retention enema). The sodium on the resin exchanges with potassium, which is thus removed from the body as the resin is expelled rectally. However, this exchange of ions may produce sodium overload, and if this is a danger in patients with heart failure then calcium polystyrene sulphonate (Calcium Resonium®) should be used instead. Since the ion exchange resins cause constipation a laxative such as lactulose should also be given.

The most common cause of hyperkalaemia is renal failure, in which case these measures are all only temporarily effective, unless renal function can be rapidly restored. After the treatment of hyperkalaemia in patients with renal failure they should be referred to a renal unit for further management.

26.4 The place of drugs in the management of acute renal failure

Drugs have only a small part to play in the management of acute renal failure.

26.4.1 Diuretics and dopamine in acute tubular necrosis

There is some evidence that frusemide and/or mannitol may prevent or lessen the degree of acute tubular necrosis if they are given before or very soon after a potentially causative event, for example an episode of significant renal hypoperfusion.

Once acute tubular necrosis is established frusemide may produce a flow of urine in some patients without altering blood urea or creatinine concentrations. However, the establishment of urine flow can help the management of plasma potassium concentrations and intravascular volume problems.

In some circumstances there may be uncertainty about the central venous pressure, and it may not be known if the patient is or is not hypovolaemic and whether oliguria is due to hypoperfusion. If there are other clear physical signs of hypovolaemia, for example postural hypotension, a fluid challenge should be given, in the form of 1 L of isotonic saline given rapidly, with the patient under continuous observation. If clinical observation does not enable an unequivocal decision to be made about a patient's

intravascular volume, a central venous pressure line should be inserted for direct measurement of the venous pressure.

In hypovolaemic states, and sometimes despite adequate volume replacement, oliguria persists, even though the syndrome of acute tubular necrosis is not established. In some patients a low dose of dopamine given by i.v. infusion can produce renal arteriolar vasodilatation and increased urine flow. The addition of frusemide i.v. can increase urine flow even more.

However, great care needs to be taken in using diuretics in cases of this sort, and specialist advice should always be sought if possible. The dangers are as follows.

(a) High-dose intravenous frusemide

High-dose i.v. frusemide may be ototoxic, and it must be given by slow infusion (see below). If gentamicin is also being used, as may be the case in renal failure due to Gram-negative septicaemia, its ototoxic effects will be potentiated by frusemide.

(b) Dopamine infusion i.v.

Too high a dose can produce renal vasoconstriction and worsen acute tubular necrosis.

In acute renal failure therefore:

1. Monitor central venous pressure if the intention is to use diuretic therapy in any patient with suspected, incipient, or established acute renal failure due to acute tubular necrosis.

2. Resist the temptation to increase the dose of dopamine if a low dose is ineffective.

3. Do not rely on diuretic therapy to prevent or reverse oliguria in acute tubular necrosis and do not delay dialysis if it is otherwise indicated.

4. Use bumetanide if you have to give a loop diuretic to a patient to whom you are also giving an aminoglycoside antibiotic.

The dosage regimens of frusemide and dopamine used in acute renal failure are as follows:

(i) High-dose frusemide

For the first dose frusemide 250 mg/25 mL is diluted in 225 mL of sodium chloride injection BP, and this solution is given at a rate of no more than 4 mg/min. If fluid overload may be a problem the frusemide may instead be given in its original volume via an infusion pump. If urine volume does not increase to 40–50 mL/h with this first infusion, give double the amount at the same rate (i.e. 500 mg at 4 mg/min). If again there is no response give a third dose of 1000 mg. If there is still no response dialysis will be required.

(ii) Dopamine

Dopamine can be particularly useful in the incipient stage of acute renal failure, when a renal vasodilating dose of 1–5 micrograms/kg/min together with diuretics may reverse oliguria.

26.4.2 Drug treatment of hyperkalaemia in acute renal failure

See the section on hyperkalaemia above.

26.4.3 The use of antibiotics in renal failure

In patients who are seriously ill with renal failure there is a temptation to use drugs to treat various symptoms and complications. However, it is important to consider drug dosages very carefully, because many drugs are cleared by the kidney, and the risks of dose-related adverse effects are considerable. Furthermore, many drugs may be directly nephrotoxic. Problems with drugs in renal failure are dealt with in section 26.11, but because antibiotics have a special place in acute renal failure we shall deal with them here. Special attention must be paid to antibiotics in acute renal failure for four reasons.

1. Acute septicaemia may cause acute renal failure.
2. Patients with acute renal failure are particularly prone to secondary infection.
3. Some antibiotics may cause or worsen acute renal failure.
4. The handling of several antibiotics is considerably changed by renal failure, thus predisposing to adverse reactions.

The antibiotics to which particular attention must be paid are listed in Table 26.6.

26.4.4 The use of other drugs in renal failure

For drugs which are eliminated mostly by the kidneys, dosages will need to be altered in renal failure. The methods for adjusting dosages of drugs in these circumstances are discussed in Chapter 6 (pp. 70–3). Certain drugs which ought to be avoided in renal failure are listed in Table 26.6.

26.5 The place of drugs in the management of chronic renal failure

There is a restricted place for drugs in the management of chronic renal failure. While chronic dialysis or renal transplantation will solve many of the metabolic problems of renal failure, hypertension, anaemia, and bone disease (with hyperparathyroidism) still pose problems.

26.5.1 Hypertension

The treatment of hypertension in chronic renal failure should be as outlined in Chapter 23, with three provisos.

Firstly, diuretics are ineffective when the glomerular filtration rate falls below 20 mL/min.

Secondly, the angiotensin converting enzyme (ACE) inhibitors, such as captopril and enalapril, are particularly effective in hypertension in chronic renal failure and should be among the first choices. However, they should not be used in patients with renal artery stenosis, in whom they can make renal function worse. This is because in a kidney whose perfusion is low due to impaired blood supply, glomerular capillary pressure is maintained by increased renin and angiotensin production. Local inhibition of the production of angiotensin then reduces the glomerular capillary hydrostatic pressure and the filtration rate in the affected kidney.

Because the only worthwhile investigation for renal artery stenosis is renal angiography, which cannot be carried out on all patients with hypertension, it is reasonable to start treatment with an ACE inhibitor in patients with renal hypertension, provided that renal function is checked 2–3

▌ **Table 26.6**   Drugs which can cause renal damage and/or which can accumulate in renal failure

Drug	Type of renal damage (if nephrotoxic)	Hazards of excess accumulation	Comments
1. *Antibiotics*			
Aminoglycosides	Renal tubular necrosis	Ototoxicity; further renal damage	Reduce dosages; monitor plasma concentrations
Amphotericin B	Renal tubular necrosis		Common; dose-related
Nitrofurantoin	Renal tubular necrosis	Peripheral neuropathy	Avoid
Penicillins	Interstitial nephritis	Convulsions, haemolytic anaemia	Reduce large dosages (normal dosages not affected)
Quinolones	Renal tubular obstruction		Due to crystalluria (rare); hydrate well
Sulphonamides	Renal tubular obstruction		Due to crystalluria (rare with modern drugs)
	Interstitial nephritis		Reduce dosages (or avoid)
Tetracyclines		Toxicity causes nausea, vomiting, and diarrhoea; dehydration then causes further renal damage; increased uraemia also due to an antianabolic effect	Avoid in renal failure and old people; use doxycycline instead
Vancomycin (i.v.)	Interstitial nephritis	Ototoxicity	Reduce dosages
2. *Other drugs (avoid or use in reduced dosages)*			
ACE inhibitors		Hyperkalaemia	
p-aminosalicylic acid (PAS)		Potentiates acidosis; increased risk of GI bleeding	
Chlorpropamide		Hypoglycaemic effect cumulative and prolonged	
Nitrofurantoin		Peripheral neuropathy	
Phenformin		Lactic acidosis, ketosis, and hyperuricaemia	
Potassium		Hyperkalaemia	
Potassium-sparing diuretics		Hyperkalaemia	
Non-steroidal anti-inflammatory drugs		Reduced glomerular filtration rate	

days and 2–3 weeks afterwards. If renal function has not deteriorated treatment can be continued. In such cases it is also important to monitor plasma potassium concentrations in patients with renal failure who are given ACE inhibitors, because of their effect in inhibiting aldosterone secretion and thus retaining potassium.

Thirdly, the effects of the α_1-adrenoceptor antagonists, for example prazosin, will be enhanced by a reduced intravascular volume. These drugs should not be used in patients who are water- or sodium-depleted.

26.5.2 The management of calcium, phosphate, and vitamin D problems in chronic renal failure

To set the background for a rational approach to treatment, a simple understanding of the effects of chronic renal failure on calcium and phosphate metabolism is helpful, and this is illustrated in Fig. 26.2.

(a) Treatment of phosphate retention

The hyperphosphataemia of chronic renal failure is treated with agents which bind phosphate in the gut lumen and prevent its absorption. Formulations of calcium carbonate are preferred, in dosages of 2.5–9.0 g/d, depending on response. Calcium carbonate should be taken with meals, since it is otherwise ineffective. It can cause hypercalcaemia, which is the factor which usually limits dosage. Aluminium hydroxide (30 mL after meals) is also effective, but it cannot be used in long-term treatment because of encephalopathy, anaemia, and bone disease. It may be used in the short-term treatment of hyperphosphataemia which does not respond to calcium carbonate.

The adverse effects of calcium supplements are ectopic calcification, the production of pseudogout, and hypercalcaemia.

(b) Vitamin D derivatives

Renal osteodystrophy in chronic renal failure is resistant to conventional forms of vitamin D, since it is due to defective activation of 25-

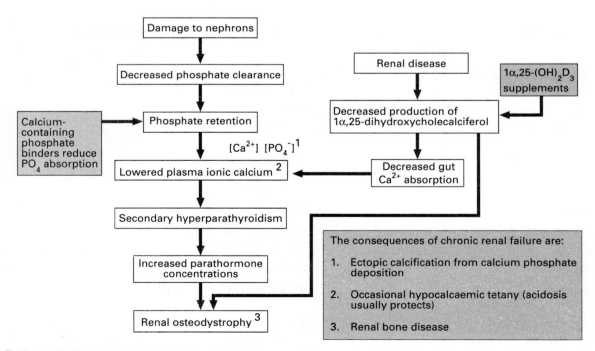

■ **Fig. 26.2** The effects of chronic renal failure on calcium and phosphate metabolism and the sites and mechanisms of action of drugs used to treat those effects.

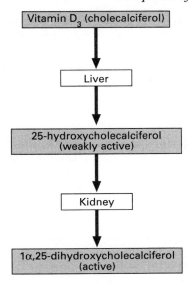

Orally administered 1α-hydroxycholecalciferol undergoes rapid conversion to 1α,25-dihydroxycholecalciferol in the liver.

■ **Fig. 26.3** The metabolic activation of vitamin D and of 1α-hydroxycholecalciferol (see also Fig. P9, p. 706).

hydroxycholecalciferol to 1α,25-dihydroxychole-calciferol, which normally takes place in the kidney (Fig. 26.3). Treatment is therefore with 1α-hydroxycholecalciferol (alfacalcidol) or 1α,25-dihydroxycholecalciferol (calcitriol).

The initial dose of alfacalcidol is usually 0.25–1 microgram orally daily. The initial dose of calcitriol is 1 microgram orally daily, increasing according to response. Most patients will respond to daily doses of 1 microgram of alfacalcidol or 2–3 micrograms of calcitriol, although sometimes higher dosages may be needed. When these vitamin D derivatives are used plasma calcium concentrations should be monitored at least weekly during the early stages of treatment to avoid hypercalcaemia and monthly when treatment is stable.

26.5.3 Anaemia

The identification of erythropoietin and its subsequent preparation by genetic engineering in bacteria has revolutionized the treatment of anaemia in chronic renal failure. Erythropoietin is given i.v. or s.c. in a dosage varying from 15 to 500 units/kg three times a week. The exact dose in an individual must be carefully titrated according to response.

Erythropoietin is probably more effective subcutaneously than intravenously, and this may allow considerable savings in costs. The major adverse effect of erythropoietin is an increase in blood viscosity, which can result in increased blood pressure, and vascular thrombosis. Epileptic fits resembling those which have been described in hypertensive encephalopathy have also been described. It reduces the rate of dialysis clearance, and in patients on long-term dialysis it may be necessary to adjust the dialysis schedule in order to compensate.

26.5.4 Changes in drug action in renal failure

(a) Pharmacokinetic

In renal failure a reduction in the clearance of drugs which are mostly cleared by the kidney results in reduced dosage requirements of those drugs. The ways in which such dosage changes may be calculated are discussed in Chapter 6.

In addition, protein binding of acidic drugs may be reduced in renal failure, probably because of a reduction in the affinity of the drug-binding sites on plasma albumin. The consequences of this are discussed in Chapter 10. The binding of basic drugs is not altered in renal failure.

(b) Pharmacodynamic

The actions of some drugs on the tissues may be altered in renal failure. The following are examples of this.

The brain may be more sensitive than usual to the CNS depressant effects of tranquillizers, sedatives, and opiate analgesics. However, renal failure has to be quite advanced for this to happen.

In renal failure the control of body fluid volumes may be disturbed, and if for any reason patients are hypovolaemic they become very sensitive to hypotensive agents, particularly α-adrenoceptor antagonists and the ACE inhibitors.

Patients with uraemia have an increased tendency to bleed. The effects of anticoagulants may therefore be enhanced and aspirin and other non-steroidal anti-inflammatory drugs are more liable to produce significant gastrointestinal bleeding.

Drugs which cause sodium retention, (for example non-steroidal anti-inflammatory drugs) may produce fluid overload, oedema, and heart failure.

Hyperkalaemia is often a consequence of renal failure. The additional effects of potassium-sparing diuretics, potassium supplements, and ACE inhibitors have been discussed above (see p. 348).

Finally, patients in renal failure may be more sensitive to the effects of acetylcholinesterase inhibitors, such as neostigmine, because of reduced cholinesterase activity.

26.6 The drug treatment of glomerulonephritis

Certain drugs, particularly penicillamine, gold salts, and captopril, have been implicated in some cases of glomerulonephritis. They should be withdrawn if such an association is suspected. Similarly, any other primary causative factor, for example a tumour or infection, should be treated appropriately.

Diuretics (see p. 343) may be needed for peripheral oedema in the nephrotic syndrome. Should these fail to work orally, intravenous diuretics, perhaps combined with infusions of salt-poor albumin, may prove effective.

The specific drug treatment of glomerulonephritis is generally disappointing. Too few controlled clinical trials have been performed in most cases to show definite efficacy. However, in a few cases there is good evidence to support the use of drug therapy, which will usually be undertaken by specialists; these include minimal-change glomerulonephritis, lupus-related nephritis, Goodpasture's syndrome, and some forms of vasculitis. In other forms of nephritis there is no effective specific therapy.

26.6.1 Minimal-change glomerulonephritis

Corticosteroids are of value in minimal change disease, and cyclosporin or cyclophosphamide may be used in some refractory cases. Remission in minimal change nephritis can be obtained with prednisolone, 1 mg/kg body weight daily for children, or in adults 60 mg daily, given for 3 weeks. A diuresis usually occurs at about the tenth day of treatment. After 3 weeks the dosage is usually reduced to 0.3 mg/kg body weight daily and continued for 3–6 months. There are various sorts of corticosteroid regimen advocated and local specialist advice should be sought. About 95 per cent of children respond and 45 per cent become free of proteinuria. About 70 per cent of adults respond, but 55 per cent relapse. If relapses cannot be controlled with prednisolone, or if steroid toxicity is a problem, cyclosporin or cyclophosphamide may be tried for 6–12 weeks. Cyclosporin is given in an initial dosage of 6–10 mg/kg/d, aiming to produce whole-blood steady-state concentrations of 100–200 ng/mL (radioimmunoassay), then adjusting the dosage as required to maintain that concentration. Cyclophosphamide is given in a dosage of 2 mg/kg body weight daily.

26.6.2 Lupus-related glomerulonephritis

Corticosteroids with azathioprine or cyclophosphamide may be effective in some types of lupus-related disease.

26.6.3 Goodpasture's syndrome and necrotizing vasculitis

High-dose corticosteroids/cyclophosphamide/plasmapheresis (in varying combinations) may be helpful in anti-glomerular basement disease (Goodpasture's syndrome) and in some forms of necrotizing vasculitis or rapidly progressing glomerulonephritis (for example Wegener's granulomatosis).

26.6.4 Acute post-streptococcal glomerulonephritis

Acute post-streptococcal glomerulonephritis is a form of acute proliferative glomerulonephritis. Oral phenoxymethylpenicillin treatment is indicated, to eradicate Group A haemolytic streptococci. Sodium and protein restriction may be necessary and hypertension should be treated as necessary. Other drugs do not influence the course of the renal pathology.

26.6.5 Diffuse mesangiocapillary (membranoproliferative) glomerulonephritis

Corticosteroids and immunosuppressive therapy are used but are of unproven efficacy.

26.6.6 Membranous glomerulonephritis

The nephrotic syndrome and hypertension should be treated as detailed elsewhere. Similar immuno-suppressive regimens are used as in rapidly progressive glomerulonephritis; the results are not conclusive.

26.7 Drugs in the treatment of urinary tract infection

The general principles of antibiotic therapy are outlined in Chapter 22. The clinical problems of urinary tract infection include the following:

> urethritis
> cystitis
> acute and chronic pyelonephritis
> prostatitis
> asymptomatic bacteriuria
> recurrent urinary tract infection.

The commonest infective organism in uncomplic-ated cases of urinary tract infection is *E. coli* (about 80 per cent of cases). When there is recurrent infection or when there are other com-plicating factors, such as surgical instrumentation or catheterization, other organisms, such as *Proteus* (very common), *Klebsiella*, *Enterobacter*, *Pseudomonas aeruginosa*, *Staphylococcus aureus*, and enterococci, may be responsible.

The following practical points should be noted.

1. Establish the diagnosis of urinary tract infec-tion by urinary microscopic examination and by sending a urine specimen for culture and sensitivity testing, if indicated.

2. After treatment is complete, check for cure by a repeat examination and culture of the urine.

3. One attack of lower urinary tract infection in a man and more than two attacks in a woman are signals to investigate the urinary tract for underlying pathology in the urethra, bladder, ureters, kidneys, or prostate.

26.7.1 Uncomplicated infections of the lower urinary tract

If the infection at first sight appears to be uncom-plicated by other abnormalities of the bladder, ureters, or kidneys, assume that the infection is due to *E. coli*.

For cystitis the choices are generally:

> co-trimoxazole or trimethoprim
> amoxycillin or co-amoxiclav
> ciprofloxacin

The duration of therapy is usually about a week, but a single dose of amoxycillin 3 g may cure uncomplicated lower urinary tract infection.

26.7.2 Acute pyelonephritis

(a) In hospital

The choices are generally:

> first: ampicillin, amoxycillin, or co-amoxiclav
> second: ciprofloxacin.
> third: gentamicin (in combination with ampicillin)

Parenteral antibiotic therapy is often necessary because of nausea and vomiting.

(b) In domiciliary practice

Amoxycillin, co-trimoxazole, or ciprofloxacin are the usual choices. If the infection is severe genta-micin can be given i.m., but in that case it is generally better to treat the infection in hospital. The duration of therapy is 1–2 weeks. The choice of antibiotic for the total course of therapy will depend crucially on the results of the pretreat-ment culture.

24.7.3 Recurrent pyelonephritis

Antibiotic therapy of exacerbations of pyelo-nephritis will depend on the infecting organism and the factors rendering the urinary tract prone to infection (for example anatomical abnormalities, bladder dysfunction, stones). Suppressive or prophylactic therapy is dealt with below.

26.7.4 Recurrent urinary tract infection

In women with normal urinary tracts who suffer recurrent urinary tract infections (often associated with sexual intercourse) in whom simple measures (such as pre- and post-coital micturition and the application of an antiseptic cream to the periurethral area) do not prevent attacks, prophylaxis may be tried for 6 months followed by reassessment. The choices are co-trimoxazole (one tablet each night), nitrofurantoin (50 mg each night), or ciprofloxacin (250 mg every night).

If there are irremediable abnormalities of the urinary tract associated with recurrent symptomatic urinary tract infections, similar therapy may be indicated for even longer, with periodic reassessments. Resistance of infecting organisms often occurs and may be anticipated by the prescription of antibiotics in rotation, for example one month of co-trimoxazole, followed by one month of nitrofurantoin, followed by one month of ciprofloxacin, and so on.

26.7.5 Asymptomatic bacteriuria

If there is no structural or functional neurological abnormality of the urinary tract in a young woman then treatment is not indicated. Asymptomatic bacteriuria should be treated with the appropriate antibiotic in pregnancy, in which symptomatic urinary tract infections frequently complicate asymptomatic bacteriuria.

The management of asymptomatic bacteriuria in old people is difficult. If it is truly asymptomatic, if the patient is fit, well, and mobile, and if there are not associated urinary tract abnormalities, treatment is probably unnecessary. However, if there is incontinence or increased frequency of micturition, or if the patient is ill and has to be in bed or resting for long periods of time (during which florid infection may occur), then probably the appropriate antibiotics should be given.

26.7.6 Urinary tract infection in pregnancy

The problem of treating urinary tract infection in pregnancy is common. What drugs are safe?

One should avoid co-trimoxazole, because of the risk of teratogenicity and kernicterus if used in late pregnancy, gentamicin, because of the risk of fetal ototoxicity, tetracyclines, because of discolouration of teeth and interference with bone growth in the fetus, and the quinolones, because of evidence from animal studies that they may cause fetal arthropathy.

The penicillins and probably the cephalosporins are safe in pregnancy, but the safety of clavulanic acid (in co-amoxiclav) has not been established.

26.7.7 Urinary infections and catheterization

Generally, prophylactic antibiotics in catheterized patients, particularly those with long-term catheters, do little to prevent urinary tract infections and lead to problems with resistant organisms. Antibiotic therapy should be limited to the treatment of acute infections.

26.7.8 Genitourinary tuberculosis

The drug treatment of genitourinary tuberculosis is undertaken on similar principles to that of pulmonary tuberculosis (Chapter 24). The following regimen has been found to be effective in the majority of cases:

> rifampicin 600 mg o.d. orally;
> isoniazid 300 mg o.d. orally (with pyridoxine);
> ethambutol 25 mg/kg o.d. orally for 2 months followed by 15 mg/kg o.d. orally.

This regimen should be continued for 2 years (i.e. longer than in pulmonary tuberculosis).

Corticosteroids (for example prednisolone 20 mg o.d.) may be of value in relieving ureteric strictures, but surgical intervention may be necessary, as it may be in other aspects of genitourinary tuberculosis.

26.8 Drug treatment of urinary calculi

If possible the primary cause of the urinary calculi should be treated, for example the resection of a parathyroid adenoma or the treatment of a primary cause of hypercalcaemia (see p. 377). Modern methods of dealing with stones using ultrasonic lithotripsy and keyhole surgery are very effective in dealing with renal calculi. Drug treatment is limited to the relief of the symptoms of acute renal colic due to a calculus and to measures taken to prevent the formation of stones.

26.8.1 Renal colic

For pain give pethidine 100 mg i.m., morphine 10 mg s.c. or i.m., or diamorphine 5 mg s.c. or i.m. Since the narcotic analgesics can cause ureteric spasm, atropine should also be given (0.3–0.6 mg s.c.). Avoid pethidine in renal failure. Recent evidence suggests that diclofenac, 75 mg i.m. followed by a further dose 30 min later, may be as effective as pethidine.

26.8.2 Prevention of stone formation

(a) Calcium oxalate and apatite stones with hypercalciuria

A high fluid intake is essential and should be sufficient to maintain a urine output of 2.5–3.5 L/d. Calcium in the diet should be restricted, as should oxalate in cases of intestinal oxalosis. A thiazide diuretic, such as bendrofluazide 5 mg o.d., reduces renal tubular calcium excretion. Sodium cellulose phosphate, 12–15 g daily, reduces dietary calcium absorption from the gut. If calcium stone-formers have high uric acid excretion, alkalinization of the urine (see below) and allopurinol may be helpful.

(b) Uric acid stones

Avoid excess purines in the diet and ensure a high fluid intake. Maintain an alkaline urine, keeping urinary pH at around 8.0, for example with potassium citrate mixture 10 mL t.d.s. Excess alkalinization may result in calcium stone formation, so care must be taken, and in many patients a high fluid intake and allopurinol will suffice. The treatment of gout is discussed on p. 420.

(c) Cystinuria

Ensure a high fluid intake (3–5 L/d) and alkalinize the urine with either potassium citrate

mixture, as above, or sodium bicarbonate 12 g daily, keeping the urine pH over 8.0. If a high fluid intake and alkalinization of the urine are ineffective give penicillamine 250 mg t.d.s. to a maximum of 500 mg q.d.s.

26.9 Drugs and the urinary bladder: the treatment of incontinence, detrusor instability, and enuresis

As the bladder fills, stretching of its wall initiates afferent nerve impulses, which pass to the cerebral cortex and result in the sensation of wanting to pass urine. At the act of micturition parasympathetic activity results in contraction of the detrusor muscle and co-ordinated urethral sphincter relaxation, and urine is passed.

Old people are particularly prone to symptoms of increased frequency of micturition, urgency of micturition, incontinence, suprapubic bladder pain, and urethral pain. These symptoms may be associated with bladder disease, such as inflammation due to infection or neurological disease. 'Detrusor instability' is the term used to describe involuntary contraction of the bladder without evidence of pathology.

Sometimes symptoms of this kind can be exacerbated by diuretics, hypnotics, and tranquillizers, withdrawal of which may help. However, often the bladder symptoms can be very disturbing to the patient and difficult to control. Attempts have therefore been made to control bladder irritability medically by inhibiting parasympathetic drive to the bladder with antimuscarinic drugs, although this has not been altogether successful, because of generalized atropinic adverse effects. Nevertheless, drugs with anticholinergic actions can bring relief in some old patients who suffer from distressing increase of frequency of micturition and incontinence, particularly at night, and in whom urinary tract infection and other urinary abnormalities have been investigated and treated. In some cases mechanical methods of treatment may be preferred (for example pads, cystoplasty, and artificial sphincters).

The muscarinic antagonists commonly used to treat increased urinary frequency and incontinence are propantheline, oxybutinin, and flavoxate. There is little to choose between these compounds, which have similar therapeutic and adverse effects. The usual dosages are propantheline 15–30 mg b.d. or t.d.s., oxybutinin 5 mg 2–4 times a day, and flavoxate 200 mg t.d.s. The benefit:risk ratio is low for these drugs, and unacceptable anticholinergic adverse effects, particularly in old people, are common. They should never be used in patients with urinary outflow tract obstruction or glaucoma. (Emepromium, previously widely used, is no longer available in the UK; terodiline, which was useful in some cases because of its additional calcium antagonist action, has been withdrawn from the market because it caused cardiac arrhythmias.)

Recently the α_1-adrenoceptor antagonists prazosin and indoramin have been found to reduce increased urinary frequency and the symptoms of outflow tract obstruction in benign prostatic hypertrophy. Increased sympathetic tone increases these symptoms, presumably through contraction of the smooth muscle in the bladder and urethra. Prazosin is given in a dosage of 500 micrograms b.d. initially (taking care to avoid severe hypotension with the first dose, see p. 543) followed by 1–2 mg daily. Indoramin is given in a dosage of 20 mg b.d.

In postmenopausal women with stress incontinence associated with urethral atrophy low-dose oestrogen (for example conjugated oestrogens 0.625–1.25 mg o.d) may help. In children the problem of nocturnal enuresis is often treated with tricyclic antidepressants. The results are good but therapy is limited by adverse effects, including behavioural disorders. These drugs have also been used for their anticholinergic properties in incontinence in old people.

26.10 Drug therapy of tumours of the kidney

Under this heading we shall deal only with nephroblastoma (Wilms' tumour).

26.10.1 Nephroblastoma

Nephroblastoma is the second most common abdominal malignant tumour in infants and children after neuroblastoma. The peak incidence is at 3–4 y. Five to ten per cent are bilateral. About 38 per cent have pulmonary metastases by the time of diagnosis, and some of those will have liver secondaries as well.

There are three approaches to treatment: surgical removal, post-operative radiotherapy if there is local spread, and adjuvant chemotherapy. With this combined approach 80 per cent of children are free of the disease at 2 years. Chemotherapy is usually with actinomycin D and vincristine (see cancer chemotherapy, Chapter 36).

26.11 Drug therapy of prostatic disease

26.11.1 Benign prostatic hyperplasia

Surgery is the treatment of choice for benign prostatic hyperplasia. In those who are awaiting surgery a trial of medical therapy may be justified. α_1-adrenoceptor antagonists act by relaxing the prostatic muscle. They include prazosin (in an initial dose of 0.5 mg at night followed by 0.5 mg b.d. for 2–7 nights, increasing the dosage to a maximum of 2 mg b.d. as required) and indoramin (initially 20 mg b.d. increasing to a maximum of 100 mg daily in divided doses). Both can cause hypotension, dry mouth, and nasal congestion.

Attempts to reduce the size of the prostate with luteinizing-hormone-releasing hormone (LHRH) analogues, oestrogens, or antiandrogens have been limited by the adverse effects of these drugs. Since the trophic action of testosterone on the prostate is mediated by its active metabolite 5-α-dihydrotestosterone, which is produced by a local enzyme called 5-α-reductase, the reductase inhibitor finasteride promises to have a specific action in reducing prostatic size. However, despite early encouraging results, it is not yet clear what role this drug will have in the treatment of prostatic hyperplasia.

26.11.2 Carcinoma of the prostate

Controversy surrounds the choice of surgery, radiotherapy, and/or medical (hormonal or cytotoxic) treatment for the various stages of prostatic carcinoma.

Hormonal manipulation, in which the aim is to lower blood testosterone concentrations, is an option in patients whose tumours have extended outside the capsule of the gland but without distant metastases; however, it is more commonly used in patients with distant spread. Some surgeons still practice orchidectomy and some still use stilboestrol. However, stilboestrol treatment of non-metastatic, non-symptomatic prostatic carcinoma does not prolong life and may in fact shorten it by increasing the likelihood of cardiovascular disease. When it is used for treating symptomatic prostatic carcinoma (for example bone pain from metastases) its adverse effects are gynaecomastia, loss of libido, sodium and water retention with oedema and cardiac failure, and nausea and vomiting.

Increasingly, therefore, gonadotrophin-releasing hormone (LHRH) analogues (buserelin and gonadorelin) are being used, with or without initial adjunctive therapy wtih antiandrogens. It may seem paradoxical to treat a testosterone-dependent tumour with substances which will increase the release of testosterone. Indeed, when the LHRH agonists are begun, the initial rise in plasma testosterone concentration may exacerbate the symptoms of metastatic disease and cause worsening bone pain and occasionally spinal cord compression from vertebral metastases or ureteric obstruction from tumour surrounding the ureters. For this reason, antiandrogens (cyproterone acetate or flutamide) may be used in the early stages of treatment with the LHRH analogues, either before starting treatment or when antiandrogen therapy is indicated symptomatically. For example, some would give cyproterone acetate 100 mg t.d.s. orally for a week before and one month after the start of therapy with the LHRH analogues.

However, after initial stimulation of testosterone secretion there is down-regulation of pituitary LHRH receptors during long-term therapy, and this results in inhibition of the release of LH and a reduction in testosterone secretion. Some androgen continues to be secreted by the adrenal gland and for this reason some surgeons are beginning to use LHRH analogues combined with an androgen antagonist during long-term therapy, in order to reduce androgen production as much as possible.

Goserelin acetate has a half-time of several hours. It is given as a depot injection of 3.6 mg into the subcutaneous fat of the anterior abdominal wall every 28 d.

In contrast, buserelin acetate has a half-time of a few minutes. It is given initially in a dose of 0.5 mg subcutaneously 8-hourly for 7 d and then intranasally (one 100 microgram spray to each nostril) 6 times a day during maintenance therapy. Depot formulations of buserelin are currently being developed.

Apart from the adverse effects mentioned above during initial therapy, the LHRH analogues may cause breast swelling and tenderness, hot flushes, and loss of libido.

26.11.3 Prostatitis

The penetration into the prostate of antibiotics active against Gram-negative organisms is generally poor. Therapy is usually begun with co-trimoxazole until the results of prostatic fluid culture and sensitivity are known. Ciprofloxacin is an alternative. Treatment should be continued for 4 weeks. Suppressive therapy is sometimes necessary with co-trimoxazole (one tablet each night) or nitrofurantoin (100 mg each night).

26.12 Drug-induced renal damage

Drugs may cause impairment of renal function in two ways: direct renal damage or changes in renal function and indirect damage via effects on blood supply.

26.12.1 Direct renal damage and changes in renal function

The drugs which can cause direct renal damage and their sites of action in the kidney are shown in Fig. 26.4. The figure also shows the sites of action of some drugs which alter renal function; for example, lithium can cause diabetes insipidus by inhibiting the action of antidiuretic hormone

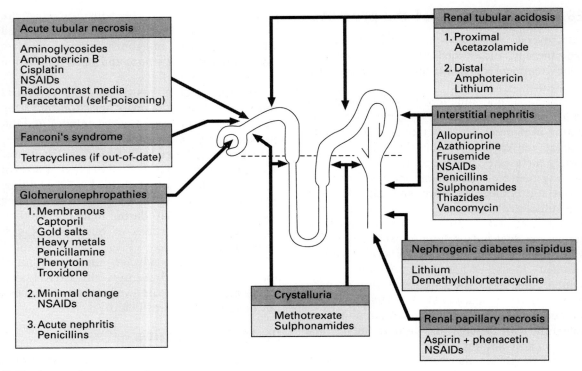

■ Fig. 26.4 The adverse effects of drugs on the kidney.

(ADH) on the collecting ducts. The specific problems that can be caused by antibiotics, discussed under the management of acute renal failure, are listed in Table 26.6.

26.12.2 Indirect damage via effects on blood supply

Drugs which cause vasculitis may affect the kidneys. These include amphotericin B and, through hypersensitivity, the penicillins and sulphonamides.

Drugs which cause intravascular haemolysis (see Table 28.9) may cause haemoglobinuria to a sufficient degree to cause acute renal failure. Vascular thrombosis, for example due to antifibrinolytic drugs, such as ε-aminocaproic acid, may cause renal failure if it involves the renal vessels.

26.13 Drugs and dialysis

The factors which determine the extent to which a drug is removed from the body during dialysis

relate to the characteristics of the drug, of the patient, and (for haemodialysis) of the equipment.

26.13.1 Characteristics of the drug

(a) Molecular weight

The larger the drug molecule the lower will be its rate of clearance by dialysis. The dialysis of a drug with a molecular weight less than 500 daltons depends in turn on the effective membrane surface area and the rate of flow of blood and dialysate. For drugs with molecular weights above 500 daltons only the membrane surface area is important.

(b) Water solubility

Poorly water-soluble drugs are poorly dialysed, since dialysis fluids are aqueous. For example, glutethimide, which has a low molecular weight is none the less not well dialysed, being poorly water-soluble.

(c) Protein binding

Drugs which are highly protein bound are poorly cleared by dialysis, since the rate of transfer across the dialysis membrane is proportional to the concentration gradient between unbound drug in the plasma and drug in the dialysis fluid. For example, propranolol is highly protein bound and is poorly removed by dialysis, even though its molecular weight is low.

(d) Apparent volume of distribution

If a drug is extensively bound in body tissues then even if it passes readily across dialysis membranes there may be little of the total drug removed from the body. For example, digoxin is poorly removed by dialysis because it is so extensively distributed to body tissues.

(e) The usual route of drug clearance

If a drug is mostly eliminated by hepatic metabolism at a rate of clearance appreciably greater than the rate of dialysis clearance then dialysis will affect total clearance only to a small extent.

26.13.2 Characteristics of the patient

Only one patient characteristic is important, that of body weight. Total clearance of a drug by the body's normal mechanisms is proportional to body weight, but dialysis clearance is constant for a given piece of equipment. It follows that the smaller the patient the greater will be the contribution to total body clearance of dialysis.

26.13.3 Characteristics of the haemodialysis equipment

(a) The membrane

As the surface area and porosity of the membrane increase, so does the rate of clearance of the drug. Because the peritoneal membrane has different characteristics to haemodialysis membranes some drugs are removed by peritoneal dialysis but not by haemodialysis and vice versa (see Table 26.7).

(b) The rate of flow of dialysis fluid

The importance of the rate of flow of dialysis fluid for drugs with a low molecular weight is discussed above.

▌ **Table 26.7** Drugs for which dialysis may be expected to remove significant quantities from the body

Aminoglycosides (HP)	Meprobamate (HP)
Amoxycillin (H)	Methaqualone (H)
Ampicillin (H)	Methotrexate (H)
Azathioprine (H)	Methyldopa (HP)
Carbenicillin (H)	Metronidazole (H)
Cephalosporins (most) (HP)	Nitrofurantoin (H)
Chloral hydrate derivatives* (HP)	Nitroprusside (HP)
Colistimethate (P)	Nortriptyline (P)
Co-trimoxazole (H)	Paracetamol (H)
Cyclophosphamide (H)	Pentazocine (H)
Diazoxide (HP)	Phenobarbitone* (HP)
Diphenhydramine (H)	Phenytoin* (H)
Ethambutol (HP)	Primidone (H)
5-Fluorocytosine (HP)	Procainamide (H)
5-Fluorouracil (H)	Quinidine (H)
Gallamine (HP)	Quinine (H)
Isoniazid (HP)	Salicylates* (HP)
Lithium* (HP)	Sulphonamides* (HP)

H = haemodialysis; P = peritoneal dialysis.
*Dialysis may be useful in cases of self-poisoning with these drugs and in severe cases of self-poisoning with ethanol, methanol, bromides, fluorides, and mushrooms.

26.13.4 The clinical significance of dialysis of drugs

The relevance of dialysis to drug therapy has four aspects.

1. Routine dialysis may cause loss of drugs from the body, with subsequent loss of therapeutic effects.
2. Routine dialysis may cause changes in the body's physiology, for example changes in fluid and electrolyte balance, which may alter the response to the drug.
3. Drugs may alter the kinetics of dialysis.
4. Dialysis may be useful in hastening the elimination of drugs from the body after self-poisoning.

(a) Loss of therapeutic effect

A list of drugs which are significantly affected by dialysis is given in Table 26.7. However, it is not always possible to predict the extent or rate of removal of a drug by dialysis, because of differences in dialysis equipment and because there is relatively little information from formal studies of individual drugs.

However, if one knows that a drug is likely to be lost from the body during dialysis, one should monitor treatment closely to try to determine how to adjust dosages (see Chapter 7). For example, one would measure plasma gentamicin concentrations to determine how much extra gentamicin to give during or after a dialysis.

(b) Changes in fluid and electrolyte balance

It is important to avoid potassium depletion in patients taking cardiac glycosides or class I antiarrhythmic drugs (see p. 346).

(c) Alteration of dialysis kinetics

Drugs which alter peripheral blood flow, for example vasodilators such as hydralazine, or vasoconstrictors such as adrenoceptor agonists, may alter the rate of clearance of drugs by dialysis.

(d) Treatment of self-poisoning by dialysis

This is dealt with for the relevant drugs in Chapter 35.

27 The drug therapy of endocrine and metabolic disorders

Co-author: R. M. Hillson

27.1 Disorders of the pituitary gland

27.1.1 Hypopituitarism

Reduced function of the anterior pituitary gland results in underactivity of the organs which are normally stimulated by the pituitary trophic hormones, of which the most important are ACTH (the adrenocorticotrophic hormone, corticotrophin) and TSH (thyroid stimulating hormone). In children growth hormone deficiency is also important. Gonadotrophin deficiency, although not directly life-threatening, can cause much misery and requires treatment.

(a) ACTH deficiency

For adrenal insufficiency secondary to hypopituitarism it is usual to use a glucocorticoid which also has some mineralocorticoid activity, such as hydrocortisone 20–30 mg orally. In order to mimic diurnal variation in the normal daily production of endogenous corticosteroids, the total dose should be divided into two doses, two-thirds to be taken in the morning and one-third in the evening. Occasionally it may also be necessary to use a mineralocorticoid, in which case one would use 9-α-fluorohydrocortisone (fludrocortisone) 50–200 micrograms orally o.d.

If there is severe acute hypopituitarism (so-called 'pituitary apoplexy') i.v. hydrocortisone should be used in the same dosages as described below for acute adrenocortical insufficiency.

(b) TSH deficiency

Hypothyroidism secondary to hypopituitarism is treated in exactly the same way as primary hypothyroidism (see p. 371). However, it is important to note that when hypothyroidism is due to hypopituitarism corticosteroid replacement must be undertaken before thyroid replacement, or at least concurrently, since thyroid replacement alone may precipitate acute adrenal insufficiency in these patients.

(c) Gonadotrophin deficiency

In hypopituitarism the sex steroid hormones are used to achieve or maintain sexual maturity. If fertility is a problem one uses gonadotrophins.

Gonadal steroids are discussed in detail in the Pharmacopoeia (p. 678). In a man testosterone is used. In a woman with a uterus an oestrogen must be used with a progestogen (for example oestradiol or conjugated oestrogens plus norgestrel). In a woman who has had a hysterectomy an oestrogen can be used alone, since there is no risk of endometrial carcinoma. Oestrogen cream may ameliorate atrophic vaginitis. These hormonal replacement therapies must not be used for contraception. In children the use of gonadal steroids should be delayed until full skeletal growth has occurred, since they cause epiphyseal fusion and stunting of growth. The uses and dosages of the gonadotrophins are discussed in the Pharmacopoeia.

(d) Growth hormone deficiency

In children with hypopituitarism whose epiphyses have not fused human growth hormone is used. Growth hormone of human origin (hGH or somatotrophin) has been replaced by a peptide of the same amino acid sequence prepared by genetic engineering in bacteria (somatropin). The dosage of somatropin is 0.1 units/kg/d s.c. or

0.5–0.7 units/kg/week in two or three divided doses i.m.

The adverse effects of growth hormone are antibody formation and lipoatrophy at the site of injection. The latter can be minimized by using a different site of injection every time, as in the treatment of diabetes mellitus with insulin. Glucose tolerance may be worsened by growth hormone, and patients with diabetes mellitus may need to change the dosages of their hypoglycaemic drugs. Excessive growth occurs only if large dosages are given for long periods of time.

(e) Infertility

The treatment of infertility with hormones of the anterior pituitary and anti-oestrogens is discussed in Chapter 12.

27.1.2 Pituitary overactivity

(a) ACTH

Increased pituitary ACTH production is dealt with under adrenocortical hyperactivity (p. 369).

(b) Gigantism and acromegaly

These conditions arise from increased growth hormone production, usually due to a pituitary adenoma. Surgical removal of the tumour is the definitive treatment, and may be supplemented by radiotherapy. If surgery is not possible, or if growth hormone hypersecretion persists after surgery, bromocriptine may be used to reduce growth hormone secretion (see the Pharmacopoeia, p. 598).

(c) Hyperprolactinaemia

Hyperprolactinaemia may be due to a variety of causes, including drugs (see Table 27.1), some of which are treatable. For example, drug-induced hyperprolactinaemia resolves on withdrawing the drug, but if that is not possible or desirable then bromocriptine can be used. Bromocriptine should also be used when treatment of the primary abnormality is not possible or when hyperprolactinaemia is due to an adenoma which has not extended outside the *sella turcica*. For larger prolactin-secreting tumours surgical removal is indicated with or without radiotherapy. Bromocriptine is then used post-operatively to reduce circulating prolactin concentrations, which often

∎ **Table 27.1**   Factors affecting prolactin secretion

1. *Causes of hyperprolactinaemia*
   Prolactin-secreting pituitary adenoma
   Other endocrine abnormalities
     Destructive lesions of the hypothalamus and
       pituitary stalk
     Primary hypothyroidism
   Drugs
     Dopamine receptor antagonists
       Butyrophenones
       Domperidone
       Metoclopramide
       Phenothiazines
       Sulpiride
       Thioxanthenes
     Inhibitors of dopamine synthesis
       Benserazide
       Carbidopa
       Methyldopa
     5-HT reuptake inhibitors
       Tricyclic antidepressants
       Fluvoxamine
     Histamine (H_2) receptor antagonists
     Oestrogens
     Reserpine
   Chest wall lesions
   Chronic breast stimulation
   Herpes zoster
   Trauma and surgery
   Ectopic prolactin production

2. *Drugs which inhibit prolactin secretion*
   Dopamine receptor agonists
     Apomorphine
     Bromocriptine
     L-dopa
     Lisuride
     Pergolide
   Drugs which stimulate dopamine release or
     block its reuptake
     Amphetamines
     Methylphenidate
     Nomifensine
   5-HT receptor antagonists
     Methysergide
   GABAmimetics
     Sodium valproate
   Cholinoceptor antagonists
     Atropine
   Cholinesterase inhibitors
     Neostigmine
     Physostigmine

remain high. In patients with large prolactinomas in whom surgery is not possible bromocriptine can be used to reduce the size of the tumour and to counteract hyperprolactinaemia. Some also use bromocriptine routinely before surgical removal of a prolactinoma in order to shrink it and make surgical removal of a large tumour easier.

Reduction of the plasma prolactin concentration improves fertility, but despite evidence of its safety in a large number of pregnancies, there is still concern about the safety of bromocriptine in pregnancy. Barrier contraception should therefore be advised until regular menses return. If a period is missed, early pregnancy can be detected using plasma human chorionic gonadotrophin (HCG) measurement. Pregnancy may cause enlargement of a pituitary adenoma, and careful supervision will be necessary in such cases.

27.1.3 Diabetes insipidus

Water reabsorption in the distal renal tubule is controlled by secretion of antidiuretic hormone (ADH or vasopressin) in the posterior pituitary (the neurohypophysis), and this in turn is mainly controlled by plasma osmolality. When plasma osmolality falls below 280 mosm/L ADH secretion is switched off and a diuresis occurs. Above this threshold there is a linear increase in ADH secretion with increasing osmolality. Diabetes insipidus occurs either when there is failure of secretion of ADH from the neurohypophysis (cranial diabetes insipidus) or when neurohypophyseal ADH production is adequate but the kidney fails to respond (nephrogenic diabetes insipidus).

(a) Mechanisms of action of drugs used to treat diabetes insipidus

ADH and its analogues act by increasing the permeability of the renal tubule to water, thus enhancing water reabsorption.

The thiazide diuretics have a paradoxical effect in reducing the urine flow rate in diabetes insipidus. They probably act by causing sodium depletion, which leads to increased water reabsorption in the proximal tubule. Increased dietary sodium intake prevents the therapeutic effects of diuretics, and patients should be instructed to limit their intake of salt when using diuretics for diabetes insipidus. The main use of the thiazide diuretics is in the nephrogenic form of diabetes insipidus, but they can also be used in the cranial form if there is only partial deficiency of ADH.

Chlorpropamide, clofibrate, and carbamazepine act by increasing ADH release from the pituitary. They are therefore ineffective in nephrogenic diabetes insipidus, in which ADH secretion is increased, and they are generally not used in cranial diabetes insipidus because of their adverse effects.

(b) Practical aspects of the treatment of cranial and nephrogenic diabetes insipidus

(i) Cranial diabetes insipidus

Cranial diabetes insipidus is usually idiopathic, but it may be genetic or due to trauma, a tumour, an infection, or a vascular abnormality. However, the treatment is the same whatever the cause. Mild cranial diabetes insipidus (urine output less than 4 L/d) may not need treatment, although a thiazide diuretic (for example hydrochlorothiazide 50–100 mg o.d. or chlorothiazide 0.5–1.0 g o.d.) may be useful to reduce urine output if required.

In other cases, desmopressin is the treatment of choice, since it has a longer duration of action than other forms of ADH and since it is relatively selective for the V_2 subtype of vasopressin receptor it has much less of a constricting effect on vascular and other smooth muscle. It is given nasally by atomized spray containing 10 micrograms/spray or by instillation of a solution of 100 micrograms/mL. The patient should be given clear instructions on how to use the nasal spray or intranasal tube, since improper use will result in a poor response to therapy. The dosage of desmopressin must be tailored to each individual's requirements according to the clinical response. Start with a single dose of 10 micrograms intranasally in the evening. The antidiuretic effect should come on within an hour and last at least 8 h. If the antidiuretic effect is not maintained during the next day an extra dose will be required in the morning and perhaps another in the afternoon. The dosage should then be titrated according to response, aiming to use the smallest total daily dose which results in a daily urine output of 2 L. Usual maintenance dosages are 10–20 micrograms b.d. or t.d.s. If a patient cannot take desmopressin nasally (for example at times of operations) it can be given i.m. It has a longer duration of action by this route and can be given once daily (1–2 micrograms). Overdosage of desmopressin causes water intoxication.

When cranial diabetes insipidus can be expected to be transient (for example in association with an acute head injury) i.m. desmopressin or vasopressin or intranasal desmopressin as appropriate may be used temporarily. Intranasal lypressin is an alternative to desmopressin, but it has a much shorter duration of action.

(ii) Nephrogenic diabetes insipidus

Nephrogenic diabetes insipidus has a variety of causes, including congenital, drugs (for example lithium or demethylchlortetracycline), and chronic renal disease. Because pituitary function is normal there is hypersecretion of endogenous ADH and exogenously administered ADH analogues are therefore ineffective. The underlying cause should be treated. If further treatment is required give a thiazide diuretic (for example hydrochlorothiazide 50–100 mg orally o.d.). Remember to take care when using thiazide diuretics in patients who are also taking lithium (see p. 132).

27.2 Disorders of the adrenal gland

27.2.1. Primary adrenocortical insufficiency

(a) Chronic adrenocortical insufficiency

Chronic adrenocortical insufficiency due to primary disease of the adrenal cortex (Addison's disease) requires treatment with a glucocorticoid and a mineralocorticoid. The dose of the glucocorticoid should be split into two parts, two-thirds to be given in the morning and one-third in the evening, in order to mimic the normal diurnal variation in secretion. Hydrocortisone

(20 mg in the morning and 10 mg in the evening) is the glucocorticoid of choice; cortisone (12.5–37.5 mg orally daily) is less well absorbed. Despite the mineralocorticoid actions of hydrocortisone and cortisone, most patients also require fludrocortisone (50–300 mg orally o.d.). In contrast, patients with adrenocortical insufficiency secondary to pituitary ACTH deficiency often do not require fludrocortisone.

At times of stress (for example during acute infections or at times of operation) corticosteroid requirements increase and replacement dosages of corticosteroids should therefore be doubled temporarily in order to avoid acute adrenocortical insufficiency. If oral therapy cannot be taken then i.m. or i.v. hydrocortisone (300 mg per day) should be used instead.

Patients with chronic adrenocortical insufficiency should carry a steroid card (see Fig. 36.2) or wear some form of identification (for example a bracelet or locket) containing information about their condition. They should also be warned that in the event of an acute stress (for example an acute infection, a major dental procedure) they should immediately both double the dose of corticosteroid and seek medical advice. For emergency treatment patients and their relatives should be given a supply of hydrocortisone, needles, and syringes and should be taught how to give an intramuscular injection during any illness involving vomiting.

(b) Acute adrenocortical insufficiency

An Addisonian crisis is a medical emergency requiring immediate treatment. Salt, water, and glucose should be replaced using i.v. dextrose (5 per cent) plus isotonic saline. The usual fluid requirement is about 4 L in the first 24 h, 2 L being given during the first 4 h. Subsequent fluid requirements are less and can be judged by the previous day's urinary output, adding 500 mL for 'insensible' losses (for example in sweat, perspiration, and faeces). Hydrocortisone (100 mg i.v.) should be given immediately, and at the same time oral therapy with either cortisone acetate or hydrocortisone should be started, beginning with a high dose (for example 50 mg of hydrocortisone 6-hourly) and reducing over the next few days to a maintenance dosage according to requirements. If oral therapy is not possible continue with i.v. or i.m. hydrocortisone 6-hourly until it is.

27.2.2 Adrenocortical hyperactivity

Adrenocortical hyperactivity is known as Cushing's disease when it is due to hypersecretion of ACTH by a pituitary adenoma and Cushing's syndrome when it is due to any other cause. The different causes are listed in Table 27.2. The sites of action of drugs which affect steroid biosynthesis are shown in Fig. 27.1.

Where possible the lesion causing adrenocortical hyperactivity should be removed surgically; this applies to primary adrenal tumours, pituitary tumours, and primary tumours producing ectopic ACTH. The following specific drug treatments are also appropriate.

(a) Adrenal adenoma

Metyrapone is given for a few weeks or months before surgical removal of an adenoma, in order to inhibit corticosteroid synthesis and thus reduce the risks of surgery by correcting the metabolic abnormalities associated with Cushing's syndrome. The dosage of metyrapone is 1–4 g daily orally in divided doses. The dosage should be titrated in order to keep the mean plasma cortisol concentration at around 350 nmol/L. The hirsutism in women which is associated with Cushing's syndrome may be made worse during this therapy, since the androgenic precursors of hydrocortisone accumulate (Fig. 27.1), and patients should be reassured. After surgical removal replacement

■ **Table 27.2** Causes of adrenocortical hyperactivity

1. *Primary*
   Adrenocortical adenoma
   Adrenocortical carcinoma

2. *Secondary*
   Pituitary adenoma (Cushing's disease)
   Drug-induced (ACTH or corticosteroids)
   Ectopic ACTH secretion (for example bronchogenic carcinoma)

corticosteroid therapy will be required for up to 2 years.

(b) Adrenal carcinoma

If surgical removal of an adrenal carcinoma is not possible or is incomplete the cytotoxic drug mitotane (o,p-DDD), which is relatively selective for cells of the adrenal cortex, may be used in conjunction with radiotherapy. The dose of mitotane is 4–6 g/d orally. Mitotane very commonly causes nausea and vomiting and often causes somnolence, lethargy, and skin rashes. However, these are dose-related effects, which can be reduced by using low dosages and by supplementing treatment with either metyrapone or aminoglutethimide, both of which reduce adrenal corticosteroid production (Fig. 27.1).

(c) Pituitary adenoma

Surgical removal of a pituitary ACTH-secreting adenoma is the treatment of choice. If this is not possible pituitary irradiation followed by bilateral adrenalectomy is indicated. Pituitary irradiation is necessary in order to reduce the risk of Nelson's syndrome, enlargement of the pituitary adenoma after bilateral adrenalectomy. 'Chemical adrenalectomy' with aminoglutethimide is an alternative in patients who cannot have an operation. Glucocorticoid and mineralocorticoid replacement therapy will be necessary in both cases and thyroid and sex hormone replacement may also be necessary.

(d) Ectopic ACTH production

Removal of the ACTH-producing tumour is curative if complete. Otherwise treatment with metyrapone or aminoglutethimide will help reduce corticosteroid production, as may bilateral adrenalectomy.

27.2.3 Primary hyperaldosteronism

Primary hyperaldosteronism (Conn's syndrome) may be due either to an adrenal adenoma secreting aldosterone or less commonly to bilateral adrenal hyperplasia. For an adenoma surgical removal is the treatment of choice and the aldosterone antagonist spironolactone should be given before the operation in order to normalize the plasma potassium concentration. If surgery

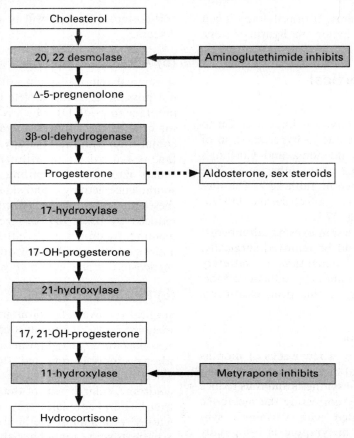

■ **Fig. 27.1.** The effects of aminoglutethimide and metyrapone on steroid hormone biosynthesis.

is not possible, or in bilateral adrenal hyperplasia, in which surgery is contra-indicated, spironolactone is generally used. Antihypertensive drugs may also be required and the potassium-retaining effect of the ACE inhibitors makes them first choice.

27.2.4 Phaeochromocytoma

Surgical removal of a phaeochromocytoma is the treatment of choice. Drugs are used either in relation to surgery or to control the blood pressure in patients in whom surgery is not possible or has not proved successful, or in disseminated malignant phaeochromocytoma. For a few days before surgery patients should be treated with a combination of α- and β-adrenoceptor antagonists, for example phenoxybenzamine (0.5 mg/kg in two divided doses) plus propranolol (40 mg orally t.d.s.), whether or not they are hypertens-

ive, in order to ensure complete α- and β-blockade at the time of operation. Treatment with the β-adrenoceptor antagonist should be started only after full α-blockade has been achieved, otherwise severe hypertension may occur, because of inhibition of skeletal muscle vasodilatation.

For anaesthesia methoxyflurane and enflurane are the inhalational anaesthetics of choice. During surgery phentolamine and noradrenaline should be immediately available for control of the blood pressure. Severe hypertension can be treated with i.v. phentolamine 1–5 mg as required. Tachycardias and ventricular ectopic arrhythmias can be treated with i.v. propranolol 0.5–1 mg as required. If the blood pressure falls after removal of the tumour it should be maintained with i.v. noradrenaline. If hypertension persists post-operatively it may be treated with a β-adrenoceptor antagonist.

For patients in whom surgery is not possible or has failed medical management may be achieved with a combination of α- and β-adrenoceptor antagonists as described above for pre-operative management. In cases which are resistant to this approach an alternative is α-methyl-*p*-tyrosine, which inhibits catecholamine biosynthesis in the tumour.

27.3 Disorders of the thyroid gland

27.3.1 Hypothyroidism

The treatment of hypothyroidism is the same whatever the cause. In the absence of heart disease it is usual to start treatment with a low dose of thyroxine (50 micrograms orally o.d.). The dosage can then be increased at 6-week intervals in increments of 50 micrograms until the serum T_4 (and the TSH in primary hypothyroidism) is normal. The usual maintenance dosage of thyroxine is 100–200 micrograms orally o.d. In patients with heart disease it is best to start with a lower daily dose of thyroxine, say 25 micrograms, or in severe cases 10 micrograms. This is because treating hypothyroidism too quickly in such cases may lead to severe angina pectoris or myocardial infarction, heart failure, or cardiac arrhythmias. In a few cases it may prove impossible to restore thyroid function completely to normal without incurring severe angina. Low initial doses should also be used in old people.

Rarely hypothyroidism may present as myxoedema coma, which is a medical emergency. The principles of treatment are to give thyroid hormone and hydrocortisone, and to treat hypothermia, dehydration, hyponatraemia, hypercapnia, and infection.

In myxoedema coma the thyroid hormone of choice is tri-iodothyronine (liothyronine), which has a shorter duration of action than thyroxine. The dosage is 50 micrograms i.v. at first then 25 micrograms 8-hourly until improvement occurs. Most physicians also give hydrocortisone i.v. in dosages of 100–300 mg/d, although its efficacy is unproven. The rationale for its use is that the 'hypothyroid' adrenal cortex cannot supply the amount of steroid necessary for the increase in metabolism produced by replacement thyroid hormone. A corticosteroid will in any case be required if hypothyroidism is due to pituitary failure rather than primary thyroid disease. When the acute problem has resolved oral thyroxine can be substituted for liothyronine.

27.3.2 Hyperthyroidism

(a) Mechanisms of action of drugs which affect thyroid function

The mechanisms of action of drugs which affect thyroid function are illustrated in Fig. 27.2. The thionamides (carbimazole, its active metabolite methimazole, and propylthiouracil) act by inhibition of the oxidation of iodate, of the iodination of tyrosine, and of coupling of the iodotyrosines to form the thyronines T_3 and T_4. Propylthiouracil also inhibits the conversion of T_4 to the active T_3 in the plasma. These drugs are used in the long-term management of hyperthyroidism and to prepare patients for thyroid surgery.

Iodine acts by inhibiting the release of T_3 and T_4 from the thyroid into the plasma. In this way it very rapidly reduces thyroid function and it is used to treat thyrotoxic crisis ('thyroid storm'). Radioactive iodine acts by destroying functioning thyroid cells.

Potassium perchlorate acts by inhibiting the uptake of iodine by the thyroid.

The β-adrenoceptor antagonists rapidly relieve the acute symptoms of hyperthyroidism, principally by blocking the β-adrenergic effects of the sympathetic nervous system. They also inhibit the peripheral conversion of T_4 to T_3.

(b) The practical management of hyperthyroidism

The acute symptoms of hyperthyroidism (tachycardia, tremor, anxiety, and restlessness) can be rapidly controlled using a non-selective β-adrenoceptor antagonist, such as propranolol. Initial dosages should be relatively high, say 40 mg orally t.d.s. or q.d.s., since the metabolism of propranolol is accelerated in hyperthyroidism. If the acute symptoms are not relieved within 24–48 h increase the dosage. Exophthalmos is not affected by β-adrenoceptor antagonists. Pro-

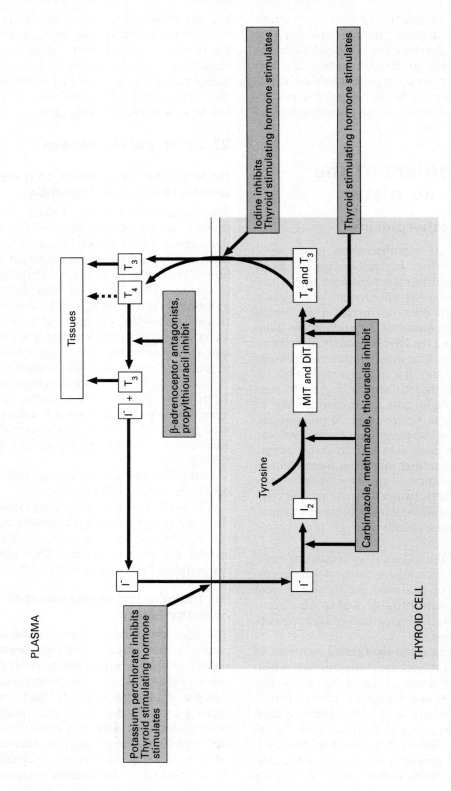

∎ **Fig. 27.2.** The effects of drugs on thyroid hormone metabolism. MIT, monoiodotyrosine; DIT, diiodotyrosine.

pranolol is also of value in treating atrial fibrillation in hyperthyroidism, and is often used in combination with digitalis (see p. 282). In patients with heart failure a β-adrenoceptor antagonist may be used cautiously, but it should be combined with digitalis and, if necessary, diuretics. For the contra-indications to the β-adrenoceptor antagonists see the Pharmacopoeia (p. 544).

Treatment with propranolol should be continued until thyroid function has been made normal with other treatment and then withdrawn gradually.

The long-term treatment of hyperthyroidism involves three options: antithyroid drugs, radioactive iodine (^{131}I), and surgery. It is usual in most patients to start with antithyroid drugs, reserving radio-iodine for those cases in which drug therapy fails. However, if there is a single adenoma, a large goitre, or evidence of local compression one would choose surgery or radio-iodine if surgery were contra-indicated.

(i) Drug therapy

The full effects of drug therapy take several weeks to occur. Carbimazole (in the UK) or methimazole (in the USA) are the drugs of choice. The initial dosages are 10–20 mg orally t.d.s., continuing until the patient is euthyroid. The therapeutic effects start to become noticeable after 1–2 weeks and are complete after 4–8 weeks. The dosage is then reduced gradually to a daily oral maintenance dose, usually 5–15 mg. Some use an alternative form of therapy known as 'block and replace', in which carbimazole (45 mg daily) is given for 12–24 months with thyroxine (150 micrograms daily initially then adjusted as for hypothyroidism). This approach may improve compliance and fewer follow-up visits are required.

If carbimazole has unwanted effects, such as skin rashes or neutropenia, propylthiouracil may be used instead in a dosage of 300–450 mg orally o.d. Although propylthiouracil can also cause skin rashes and neutropenia, as well as other blood dyscrasias, cross-reactivity with carbimazole or methimazole is uncommon. The 'block and replace' approach can also be used with propylthiouracil.

If drug therapy is effective it should be continued for at least 12–24 months and then withdrawn. After withdrawal the rate of relapse is high, being about 50 per cent in the first 2 years, with a small continuing rate of relapse thereafter, most occurring within 4 years. For this reason all patients should be seen regularly even after treatment has been withdrawn. If relapses occur repeated courses of drug therapy may be given, but in such cases, or in patients in whom serious adverse effects have occurred, surgery or radio-iodine treatment may be preferred. If hyperthyroidism is associated with a goitre its size may increase during treatment and this may warrant surgical intervention.

The important adverse effect shared by all the antithyroid drugs is neutropenia. It is uncommon and reversible but potentially fatal, and patients should be warned to stop taking the drug immediately if they develop a fever or a sore throat and to consult a doctor for a full blood count. Routine blood counts are not helpful, since neutropenia occurs rapidly and without warning with these drugs. The risk reduces with increasing duration of therapy. The treatment of neutropenia is discussed in Chapter 28.

(ii) Radioactive iodine (^{131}I)

Treatment with radioactive iodine is always curative if a large enough dose is used. However, there are several disadvantages to its use. Firstly, it is better reserved for men over 40 years of age and post-menopausal women. This is mainly because of the risk of gonadal irradiation (there being little evidence that therapeutic radio-iodine is associated with an increased risk of leukaemia or other malignancies in later life). Radio-iodine should not be used in pregnancy nor in breast-feeding women. Secondly, there is a high incidence of hypothyroidism after radio-iodine treatment: about 15 per cent of patients are hypothyroid within 2 years and about 60 per cent within 20 years.

If radio-iodine is to be used, the signs and symptoms of thyroid activity should first be controlled as well as possible with antithyroid drugs and propranolol, since radio-iodine may cause thyroid storm.

There is no simple way to calculate the optimum dose of radio-iodine for an individual, so one starts with a therapeutic dose which carries a minimal chance of causing hypothyroidism. Calculations based on thyroid size and on tests of ^{131}I uptake by the thyroid are imprecise, but give some guidance to the first dose that may be tried. The usual dose which one would use to attempt to cure hyperthyroidism without causing subsequent hypothyroidism is 80 microcuries/g of thyroid (the normal thyroid gland weighs 20 g), and this can be corrected upwards if the 24 h ^{131}I uptake is known (for example doubled if the uptake is only 50 per cent). Some patients will require a second dose to effect a cure and a few will require more than two doses. However, the full effects of a single dose of radio-iodine take 6 months to occur and repeat doses should not be considered for that period of time. During this time symptoms can be controlled with propranolol and antithyroid drugs may be needed for a while.

Because of the continuing risk of hypothyroidism, follow-up should be indefinite after radioiodine. Some therefore prefer to give a large dose of radio-iodine (for example 15 mCi) and start replacement treatment immediately with thyroxine. In cases of toxic multinodular goitre larger doses, 30–60 mCi, are required to produce the same effect.

(iii) Surgery

Where there is a single toxic adenoma surgical removal is the treatment of choice. Surgery is also appropriate if there is a large goitre, and for those in whom repeated drug treatment has failed and radio-iodine is undesirable (i.e. premenopausal women and men under 40 years). Subtotal thyroidectomy is curative in the majority of cases, but there is a small relapse rate of about 10 per cent overall. Hypothyroidism after operation is quite common, occurring in about 30 per cent of cases in 10 years.

It is important to relieve the symptoms and signs of hyperthyroidism before surgery. This can be done by giving carbimazole 30–60 mg orally per day for 8 weeks followed by iodine for 2 weeks (as Lugol's aqueous iodine solution, containing iodine 5 per cent and potassium iodide 10 per cent, total iodine 130 mg/mL, 0.1–0.3 mL orally t.d.s.). In patients in whom antithyroid drugs have caused serious adverse effects propranolol can be used instead, but it must be remembered that propranolol does not cause remission, but merely controls some of the effects of hyperthyroidism.

(c) Special problems in hyperthyroidism

(i) Inflammatory thyroid disease

Hyperthyroidism presenting as part of an acute inflammatory thyroiditis may be treated symptomatically with propranolol until the condition settles, and no further treatment is then usually necessary. In some cases resolution may be hastened by the use of prednisolone. If the thyroiditis is painful aspirin or another non-steroidal anti-inflammatory drug will help. Follow-up is required to monitor for hypothyroidism.

(ii) Drug-induced hyperthyroidism

The drugs which can cause hyperthyroidism are discussed in the next section. If withdrawal of the drug is not possible carbimazole may be used. If there is a poor response then it is worth trying potassium perchlorate, 1 g/d, particularly in cases attributable to iodine (for example in amiodarone). In some cases prednisolone has been reported to be effective.

(iii) Pregnancy

Radio-iodine should not be used in pregnancy nor during breast-feeding, and pregnancy should be avoided for at least 3 months after a dose of radio-iodine. An antithyroid drug should therefore be used in these circumstances, but since all cross the placenta and can cause fetal goitre or hypothyroidism, low dosages should be used (preferably less than 30 mg/d of carbimazole or methimazole or 300 mg/d of propylthiouracil), in order to produce normal thyroid function, monitoring progress frequently with free hormone assay if possible. Treatment should usually be withdrawn about 4 weeks before term and reintroduced after delivery in normal dosages. If the patient insists on breast-feeding, propylthiouracil, which does not enter breast milk to any great extent, should be used.

(iv) Thyrotoxic eye disease

Ophthalmopathy may improve with treatment of hyperthyroidism. In severe exophthalmos there may be difficulty in closing the eyes, with consequent drying and corneal ulceration. In such cases 'artificial tears' (1 per cent methylcellulose) can help. Guanethidine eyedrops (5 per cent, applied 1–2 times daily) may help to reduce periorbital and eyelid oedema.

In very severe cases a short course of high-dosage steroid therapy (for example prednisolone 60 mg o.d., tapering off after a few days) may be successful. Otherwise surgical treatment may be necessary.

(v) Thyrotoxic crisis ('thyroid storm')

Thyrotoxic crisis is a medical emergency requiring immediate treatment. It may occur after partial thyroidectomy if the patient has not been properly prepared by preoperative treatment of the thyrotoxicosis (see above) or if hyperthyroidism is not recognized in a patient undergoing any form of surgery. It may also be precipitated by radio-iodine, infection, myocardial infarction, thromboembolic disease, or other severe stresses of illness.

A β-adrenoceptor antagonist should be given parenterally at first, for example propranolol 0.5–2.0 mg i.v. 6-hourly, followed by oral therapy when signs and symptoms have subsided. Anti-thyroid drugs should be given in high dosages orally or by nasogastric tube if required, for example carbimazole 60–120 mg or propylthiouracil 600–1200 mg per day. Iodine should also be given to inhibit the release of thyroid hormone. Sodium iopodate (500 mg/day orally), if available, is better than Lugol's aqueous iodine solution (0.3 mL t.d.s.), since it also inhibits the peripheral conversion of T_4 to T_3. The iodine should be given 1 h after starting i.v. carbimazole or propylthiouracil.

Corticosteroids (for example hydrocortisone 100 mg i.v. q.d.s. or dexamethasone orally or i.v. 2 mg q.d.s.) are given to inhibit the peripheral conversion of T_4 to T_3. Complications should be treated as required, for example dehydration with i.v. fluids and hyperpyrexia by direct cooling and with i.m. chlorpromazine if there is also a need for sedation. As the patient gets better all this treatment can be withdrawn gradually except the carbimazole, which should be continued in normal doses.

27.3.3 Non-toxic goitre

If non-toxic goitre is associated with iodine deficiency it may be reversed by replacement therapy, for example with Lugol's iodine, although nowadays this is not often the case and most patients do not require treatment. However, if there are symptoms from the enlarged gland, such as dysphagia due to oesophageal compression, medical or surgical treatment should be offered. Medical treatment should be with thyroxine, in an initial daily dose of 50 micrograms, increasing in increments of 50 micrograms at monthly intervals to 100–200 micrograms per day. If this is ineffective partial thyroidectomy may be required.

27.3.4 Drugs and thyroid function

Drugs can interact with thyroid function in four ways.

(a) Thyroid function tests

Some drugs alter thyroid function tests in the absence of thyroid disease (Table 27.3).

(b) Drug-induced thyroid disease

Some drugs can cause hypothyroidism or hyperthyroidism. Drugs which cause hypothyroidism also frequently produce a goitre, because TSH secretion by the pituitary increases in response to the reduction in thyroid hormone secretion. Some important examples of drugs which can cause thyroid disease are given in Table 27.3.

(c) Altered pharmacokinetics of drugs in thyroid disease

Thyroid disease can alter the disposition and elimination of some drugs.

(i) Distribution

The apparent volume of distribution of digoxin is altered in thyroid disease, being increased in hyperthyroidism and reduced in hypothyroidism. The resultant changes in plasma digoxin concentrations after loading doses may partly explain resistance to digoxin in hyperthyroidism and increased sensitivity in hypothyroidism.

(ii) Metabolism

Important examples of drugs whose metabolism is increased in hyperthyroidism are methimazole (and hence carbimazole), the β-adrenoceptor antagonists propranolol and practolol, and hydro-

■ **Table 27.3** The effects of drugs on thyroid function tests and on thyroid function

---

1. *Drugs which interfere with thyroid function tests*
   (a) Increased thyroid binding globulin (increased T_4)
       Oestrogens and oral contraceptives
   (b) Decreased thyroid binding globulin (decreased T_4)
       Androgens
       Phenylbutazone
       Phenytoin
       Salicylates
   (c) Decreased serum T_3
       Amiodarone
       Carbamazepine
       Phenobarbitone
       Phenytoin
   (d) Increased serum T_4
       Amiodarone
       Orphenadrine

2. *Drugs which can cause hypothyroidism*
   Aminoglutethimide
   Amiodarone
   Antithyroid drugs
   Lithium
   Phenylbutazone
   Sulphonamides
   Sulphonylureas (chlorpropamide, tolbutamide)

3. *Drugs which can cause hyperthyroidism*
   Amiodarone
   Iodides
   Thyroxine

---

cortisone. The metabolism of propranolol is reduced in hypothyroidism.

(iii) Renal elimination

Glomerular filtration rate is increased in hyperthyroidism and reduced in hypothyroidism. One would therefore expect changes in the clearance of drugs which are mostly excreted by the kidneys. This has been shown for digoxin.

(d) Altered pharmacodynamic effects of drugs in thyroid disease

Thyroid disease can alter the pharmacodynamic effects of some drugs. The pharmacological effects of cardiac glycosides are increased in hypothyroidism and reduced in hyperthyroidism, independently of the pharmacokinetic changes mentioned above.

The prothrombin time is prolonged in hyperthyroidism and shortened in hypothyroidism, perhaps because of altered catabolism of clotting factors. This leads to reduced requirements of warfarin in hyperthyroidism and increased requirements in hypothyroidism. Always be guided by the prothrombin time.

27.4 Disorders of calcium metabolism

27.4.1. Hypocalcaemia

The main causes of hypocalcaemia are listed in Table 27.4. The dosages of vitamin D analogues and of calcium salts which are used in the treatment of these conditions are given in the Pharmacopoeia (pp. 705 and 571 respectively).

The aims of treatment in hypocalcaemia are to maintain the plasma calcium concentration within the reference range and to avoid hypercalcaemia. Measurements of plasma calcium concentrations should be made as often as is necessary to achieve these aims. The reference range for plasma or serum calcium concentrations is 2.25–2.75 mmol/L if the albumin concentration is 40 g/L. If the albumin concentration is not 40 g/L the measured calcium concentration should be corrected by adding or subtracting 0.025 mmol/L for every g/L of serum albumin concentration below or above 40 g/L respectively; for example, if the measured serum calcium was 2.35 mmol/L and the serum albumin was 36 g/L, one would add 0.1 mmol/L (i.e. 4×0.025) to the measured value to get the corrected value, i.e. 2.45 mmol/L.

(a) Hypoparathyroidism

Hypoparathyroidism responds readily to 1α-hydroxycholecalciferol (alfacalcidol), which is converted to the active 1α,25-dihydroxycholecalciferol (calcitriol) in the liver (see Fig. 26.3). Alternatively one can use calcitriol itself, or dihydrotachysterol. Vitamin D (for example

■ **Table 27.4** Causes of disorders of calcium metabolism

---

1. *Hypocalcaemia*
   Hypoparathyroidism
   Vitamin D deficiency
   Renal osteodystrophy (see Chapter 26)
   Congenital rickets
       X-linked dominant (vitamin D-resistant)
       Autosomal recessive (1α,25-
          dihydroxycholecalciferol responsive)
       Autosomal recessive (1α,25-
          dihydroxycholecalciferol resistant)
   Acute pancreatitis
   Magnesium deficiency

2. *Hypercalcaemia*
   Endocrine
       Hyperparathyroidism*
       Hyperthyroidism
       Adrenocortical insufficiency
       Phaeochromocytoma
   Malignancy*
       Multiple myeloma
       Metastatic bone disease
       Non-metastatic hormone-secreting tumours
   Drugs
       Calcium
       Thiazide diuretics
       Vitamin A analogues
       Vitamin D analogues
   Sarcoidosis
   Tuberculosis
   Immobilization
   Acute renal failure
   Familial hypocalciuric hypercalcaemia

---

*These are the common causes of hypercalcaemia; the rest are rare.

calciferol) can also be used, but very high dosages are required and the onset of action is very slow. Daily doses are 1–2 micrograms of alfacalcidol and 0.5–2 micrograms of calcitriol. Calcium supplements are usually also given, since lack of parathyroid hormone reduces calcium absorption and increases urinary calcium loss.

(b) Malabsorption

Alfacalcidol is usually indicated, since very high dosages of vitamin D are required and dosage requirements vary enormously. Oral calcium supplements are also given.

(c) Nutritional hypocalcaemia

Nutritional rickets, nutritional osteomalacia, and osteomalacia of pregnancy respond to ordinary dosages of vitamin D.

(d) Anticonvulsant-induced osteomalacia

Since anticonvulsant-induced osteomalacia is probably due to diversion of the relatively inactive precursors of 1α,25-dihydroxycholecalciferol it can be treated with alfacalcidol.

(e) Hypocalcaemic tetany

Hypocalcaemic tetany should be treated with calcium gluconate, 10–20 mL of a 10 per cent solution given slowly i.v.

27.4.2 Hypercalcaemia

The causes of hypercalcaemia are listed in Table 27.4.

(a) The emergency treatment of severe symptomatic hypercalcaemia

The emergency treatment of severe hypercalcaemia consists firstly of i.v. fluid replacement with saline and added potassium chloride (see p. 349); several litres may be needed to make good the deficit (4–8 L/d in the first few days). When one is sure that fluid replacement is proceeding adequately one may add i.v. frusemide to increase calcium excretion. If these measures are insufficient then one may try a bisphosphonate, calcitonin, or plicamycin, and of these a bisphosphonate is the first choice. (Calcitonin and the bisphosphonates are also used in the treatment of Paget's disease of bone (see p. 425).)

The bisphosphonates (for example disodium pamidronate and disodium etidronate) inhibit the growth and dissolution of hydroxyapatite crystals and retard bone resorption and formation. They are particularly useful in treating hypercalcaemia due to malignancies. Pamidronate is given in a single slow infusion of 15–60 mg. Etidronate is given by i.v. infusion of 7.5 mg/kg over at least 2 h on 3 successive days.

Calcitonin inhibits osteoclast activity and reduces the renal tubular reabsorption of calcium.

It is given i.v. and has a rapid but short-lasting effect in hypercalcaemia. It is particularly effective in cases in which there is an increased turnover of bony calcium, for example Paget's disease and hyperthyroidism. It may also be of value in hypercalcaemia due to malignancy, vitamin D intoxication, and hyperparathyroidism. For dosages and adverse effects see the Pharmacopoeia (p. 568).

Plicamycin is a cytotoxic drug which in low doses has a specific effect on osteoclasts and blocks calcium resorption. In a dosage of 25 micrograms/kg/d on three or four consecutive days it can reduce plasma calcium concentrations to normal. Plicamycin is a local irritant and causes inflammation if it leaks outside a vein; it should be infused into a large vein in 1 L of 5 per cent dextrose over 6 h. Nausea and vomiting are common and it can also cause bleeding, liver damage, and renal damage.

(b) Drug therapy of chronic hypercalcaemia

Where possible the underlying cause should be treated, for example parathyroidectomy for a parathyroid adenoma. Patients who are to have a parathyroidectomy are prone to the postoperative complications of hypocalcaemia. This can usually be prevented by giving alfacalcidol or calcitriol for 2 d before and for 1–2 weeks after the operation. However, sometimes calcium gluconate i.v. may also be required.

If it is not possible to treat the underlying cause of hypercalcaemia drugs can be used to produce symptomatic relief, i.e. to lower the plasma calcium concentration without altering the underlying cause. Oral corticosteroids are effective in reducing the plasma calcium concentration in patients with sarcoidosis, multiple myeloma, and vitamin D intoxication. Prednisolone may be used in the usual way (see Chapter 36), starting with 30–60 mg orally per day. The response to corticosteroids is slow, taking about 2 weeks.

If corticosteroids are ineffective or not applicable, dietary calcium restriction should be tried and sodium cellulose phosphate, which chelates calcium in the gut, can be given in an oral dosage of 5 g t.d.s. with meals. It may cause diarrhoea and is contra-indicated in patients with renal failure and cardiac failure.

27.5 Diabetes mellitus

27.5.1 Mechanisms of action of drugs used in the treatment of diabetes mellitus

The drugs used in the treatment of diabetes mellitus are listed in Table 27.5.

∎ **Table 27.5**   Drugs used in the treatment of diabetes mellitus

1. *Insulin* (p. 617)
   - (a) Short-acting
     Soluble insulin
     Neutral insulin
   - (b) Intermediate-acting
     Semilente (insulin zinc suspension, amorphous)
     Isophane
     Globin zinc
     Biphasic (mixtures)
   - (b) Long-acting
     Ultralente (insulin zinc suspension, crystalline)
     Lente (insulin zinc suspension, mixed amorphous/crystalline)
     Protamine zinc insulin

2. *Sulphonylureas* (p. 691)
   - (a) Short half-time
     Glipizide
     Glymidine
     Tolbutamide
   - (b) Intermediate half-time
     Glibenclamide
     Glibornuride
     Gliclazide
   - (c) Long half-time
     Chlorpropamide
     Gliquidone

3. *Biguanides*
   Metformin (p. 631)

(a) Insulin

Insulin has several different effects on the metabolism of carbohydrates, fats, and proteins through its actions on specific cell membrane receptors. It promotes glucose uptake and utilization in fat and muscle, increases hepatic glycogen formation, and inhibits hepatic gluconeogenesis. It also inhibits lipolysis and increases protein synthesis.

(b) Sulphonylureas

The sulphonylureas act principally by stimulating insulin secretion and release by the pancreas, probably acting by inhibiting cellular potassium efflux through ATP-sensitive potassium channels, which are linked to insulin secretion. They may also have some long-term effects by increasing the numbers of insulin receptors on cell membranes. They are therefore of no value in treating patients who are severely insulin deficient.

(c) Biguanides

The biguanides have several actions, including inhibition of hepatic gluconeogenesis and an increase in peripheral glucose utilization due to increased sensitivity to insulin. They may also inhibit intestinal glucose absorption.

27.5.2 The practical management of the different acute clinical presentations of diabetes mellitus

(a) Acute ketotic hyperglycaemia

This is a medical emergency requiring immediate treatment. The aims are as follows:

(1) to correct dehydration with *fluid*;

(2) to lower the blood glucose concentration to normal with *insulin*;

(3) to correct acidosis, if severe, using *bicarbonate*;

(4) to maintain *potassium* balance;

(5) to treat underlying associated factors (for example infection).

A regimen of treatment is summarized in Table 27.6. Although treatment should be initiated promptly, the aim is to restore fluid and electrolyte balance over a period of days rather than hours. Abrupt changes are dangerous.

(i) Intravenous fluids and electrolytes

Patients with diabetic ketoacidosis have the following deficits: fluid 5–11 L; sodium 300–700 mmol; potassium 200–700 mmol. These deficits should be corrected as follows:

Isotonic saline should be given by continuous i.v. infusion of 5 L over the first 6.5 h (see Table 27.6), and then at a rate of 500 mL 4-hourly until the blood glucose concentration falls to 10–16 mmol/L when one should switch to 10 per cent dextrose. Adjust the infusion rate according to the central venous pressure in old patients, in patients with shock, and in patients with cardiac or renal disease.

Potassium balance should be judged by plasma potassium concentration measurements and changes in the electrocardiogram. Measure the plasma potassium concentration initially and at least 4-hourly. The result must be available within 15 min for it to be of use in management. Despite the total potassium deficit the initial potassium concentration is often 6 mmol/L or more, since potassium moves from the cells into the plasma. This hyperkalaemia can usually be detected by peaked T waves on the electrocardiogram or in more severe cases by widening of the QRS complex, which merges with the T wave, and loss of both R and P waves. However, insulin drives potassium into cells and causes hypokalaemia. So, if the electrocardiogram shows no evidence of hyperkalaemia or if the plasma potassium is known to be below 6 mmol/L, add 20 mmol of potassium to the first litre of saline. If the initial potassium concentration is 6 mmol/L or more, or if there is electrocardiogram evidence of hyperkalaemia, wait until the potassium has fallen below 6 mmol/L before infusing potassium. Then adjust the rate of infusion according to the plasma potassium concentration (for example if it is 5.0–5.9 mmol/L give 13 mmol/h; if 4.0–4.9 mmol/L give 20 mmol/h; if 3.0–3.9 give 26 mmol/h; if 2.0–2.9 give 39 mmol/h).

(ii) Insulin

Give an i.v. loading dose of soluble insulin (10 i.u.), then give soluble or neutral soluble insulin by continuous i.v. infusion or, if i.v. infusion is

∎ **Table 27.6**   A summary of the treatment of acute ketoacidotic hyperglycaemia

1. *Fluid*
   Isotonic saline:
     1 L in the first 30 min
     1 L in the next hour
     1 L in the next hour
     1 L in the next 2 h
     1 L in the next 2 h
     500 mL 4-hourly thereafter
   Change to 10 per cent dextrose when blood glucose is 10–16 mmol/L

2. *Potassium*

Plasma potassium concentration	Potassium dosage
>6.0 mmol/L	none
5.0–5.9 mmol/L	13 mmol/h
4.0–4.9 mmol/L	20 mmol/h
3.0–3.9 mmol/L	26 mmol/h
2.0–2.9 mmol/L	39 mmol/h
<2.0 mmol/L	50 mmol/h

3. *Insulin*
   (a) 6 i.u./h by continuous i.v. infusion
       Reduce to 2 i.u./h when blood glucose is 10–16 mmol/L
         or use an i.v. sliding scale (see Table 27.7)
   or
   (b) 6 i.u. hourly by i.m. injection after an initial dose of 20 i.u.
       Reduce to 12 i.u. 4-hourly s.c. when blood glucose is 10–16 mmol/L
       (Do not give s.c. or i.m. insulin to patients in shock)

4. *Sodium bicarbonate*
   (a) If arterial pH < 7.0 and patient extremely ill: 300 mL of a 1.26 per cent solution

5. *Other measures*
   Nasogastric tube if patient unconscious
   Bladder catheter if urine not passed within 4 h
   Antibiotics as required for infection
   Oxygen if P_AO_2 below 10 kPa

6. *Monitoring*
   Blood glucose: initially and hourly thereafter
   Plasma potassium: initially and 4-hourly thereafter; if potassium needs to be given at a rate greater than
       26 mmol/L it should be monitored in an intensive care unit
   Arterial pH: initially and again after bicarbonate or if the patient remains unwell
   ECG: continuously if possible during potassium infusion
   CVP: In old patients and in patients with shock or cardiac disease
   General clinical state (pulse, blood pressure, respiration, conscious level): hourly at first

not possible, in repeated doses i.m. By i.v. infusion the rate is 6 i.u./h, reducing to 2 i.u./h when the blood glucose concentration falls to 10–16 mmol/L. By repeated i.m. injection the dose is 20 i.u. initially, followed by 6 i.u. every hour, reducing to 12 i.u. s.c. 4-hourly when the blood glucose concentration falls to 10–16 mmol/L.

If the blood glucose concentration does not begin to fall within 2 h of starting insulin, and the infusion line and insulin pump have been checked and are working, the dosage by i.v. infusion should be doubled. If i.m. insulin has been used, intermittent i.v. therapy can be tried instead. Insulin administration in this way should be continued until the arterial pH is normal.

(iii) Acidosis

Acidosis will resolve without specific treatment if the deficits of insulin, fluid, and electrolytes are restored and if oxygenation is adequate. The use of 8.4 per cent sodium bicarbonate in ketoacidosis has been linked with cerebral oedema, and it should be reserved for patients in whom cardiac arrest appears imminent or has already occurred. A 1.26 per cent solution of sodium bicarbonate (50 mL, i.e. 50 mmol) may be used to correct acidosis if the blood pH is below 7.0 and the patient is very ill.

(iv) Other measures

Nasogastric tube Because diabetic ketoacidosis causes gastric dilatation a nasogastric tube should be passed if there is impairment of consciousness, to reduce the risk of vomiting and aspiration.

Bladder catheterization This should be done after 4 h if the patient has not passed urine.

Antibiotics Antibiotics should be used appropriately (see Chapter 22) for proven or suspected infection.

Oxygen Some patients become hypoxic and 60 per cent oxygen should be given if the P_AO_2 falls below 10 kPa (see p. 301).

(v) Treatment after the acute phase

The long-term treatment of diabetes mellitus in an individual will depend on how much, if any, endogenous insulin the patient can make. However, because the occurrence of ketoacidosis usually indicates severe insulin deficiency, most patients who present in this way will require long-term insulin therapy.

There are two broad approaches to determining insulin dosage requirements after the acute stage: one is to give 6-hourly subcutaneous doses of a short-acting insulin according to a sliding scale, converting later to twice daily insulin; the other is to give twice-daily subcutaneous insulin straight away.

An example of a sliding scale is shown in Table 27.7, and it is used as follows. Measure the glucose concentration in the urine or preferably in the capillary blood four times a day (usually just before meals) and give the dose of insulin appropriate to the concentration. On the following day increase all the doses (except the lowest) by 4 units if the mean blood glucose concentration during the previous day was greater than

■ **Table 27.7** Examples of sliding scales of insulin doses for the treatment of diabetes mellitus when dosage requirements are not known

Blood glucose (mmol/L)	Dose of soluble or neutral insulin (i.u./h)
1. *Intravenous, continuous*	
<4.0	None
4.0–5.9	0.5
6.0–7.9	1.0
8.0–9.9	1.5
10.0–12.9	2.0
13.0–15.9	2.5
16.0–18.9	4.0
19.0–23.0	5.5
>23.0	7.0
2. *Subcutaneous, intermittent*	
<6.7	4
6.7	8
10.0	12
13.3	16
22.2	20

In the continuous intravenous regimen changes in the infusion rate of insulin should be based on hourly measurements of the blood glucose concentration.

In the intermittent subcutaneous regimen insulin is given four times a day. The scale should be revised according to the previous day's measurements (see text for details).

10–13 mmol/L. The eventual maintenance dosage is calculated from the total effective insulin dosage in a day. Alternatively, in patients who were previously taking oral hypoglycaemic drugs or who may be anticipated to respond to oral therapy, an oral hypoglycaemic drug can be started as soon as they are eating, and the insulin can be gradually withdrawn. The main problem with the sliding-scale method is that it causes peaks and troughs in the blood glucose concentration, because only a short-acting insulin is used. However, it is easy to use and those who are not experienced in the management of diabetes may find it helpful in working out patients' initial daily insulin dosage requirements.

In the other approach, one guesses the total amount of insulin the patient will need and gives it as a twice-daily subcutaneous injection of a short-acting and intermediate- or long-acting insulin (see the types of regimen described below). If the blood glucose concentrations between dosages are over 16 mmol/L an extra single dose of a short-acting insulin can be given subcutaneously. Alternatively, the transition can be smoothed by the use of a sliding scale to top up the twice daily doses. For patients who were previously taking insulin, their previous dosage, or one slightly higher than before, can be restarted in this way as soon as they are eating normally. This method allows a more rapid return to normal for the patient.

(b) Non-ketotic hyperglycaemia

This condition is sometimes called 'hyperosmolar coma', but the term is misleading, since the plasma osmolality is also increased in ketoacidosis and the patient is not necessarily comatose. The important features here are the relative absence of ketones and the frequent occurrence of hypernatraemia (plasma sodium concentration over 150 mmol/L).

The treatment of non-ketotic hyperglycaemia is along the same lines as for ketoacidotic hyperglycaemia, but there are some important differences.

(i) Fluid replacement

If there is hypernatraemia there is a temptation to give half-normal (i.e. half-isotonic, 75 mmol/L) saline rapidly. However, to do so carries the risk of cerebral oedema, because of excessive intravascular sodium dilution. None the less, it is desirable to lower the plasma sodium concentration. A rational approach to this problem is to start as for ketoacidosis, by replenishing the intravascular volume with isotonic saline for the first 3 h and then if there is still hypernatraemia, to continue with half-normal saline until the plasma sodium concentration falls below 150 mmol/L.

(ii) Insulin doses

Non-ketotic patients require less insulin than ketotic patients. However, this does not pose a problem with the regimens described above, which involve a low-dose i.v. infusion or low doses given by repeated i.m. injection. If regular blood glucose concentration measurements are made, the dose of insulin can be reduced at the appropriate time (i.e. when the blood glucose concentration falls to 10–16 mmol/L). Most of these patients will not require insulin after treatment of the acute phase and they should be switched to oral hypoglycaemic drugs or even diet alone (see below).

(iii) Arterial thrombosis

Patients with non-ketotic hyperglycaemia have a high risk of arterial thrombosis. They should all be given prophylactic heparin, at least subcutaneously (5000 i.u. t.d.s.), and many would use full doses of i.v. heparin (see Chapter 23, p. 299)

(iv) Precipitating factors

Diuretics and phenytoin are sometimes the precipitating factors in non-ketotic hyperglycaemia. If that is so they should be withdrawn.

(c) Acute hypoglycaemia

The symptoms of acute hypoglycaemia are dizziness, indecision, clumisness, slow thinking, sweating, palpitation, a feeling of hunger, and tingling around the mouth. The treatment of acute hypoglycaemia in an unconscious patient is either with glucagon (1 mg i.m., repeated if necessary) or with dextrose (50 mL of a 50 per cent solution i.v. into a large vein, because of the risk of venous thrombosis) repeated if necessary. In severe cases or in hypoglycaemia due to sulphonylurea overdose it may be necessary to use a continuous intravenous infusion of 10 per cent dextrose to maintain the blood glucose concentration within the reference range. It may take two days for the risk of recurrent hypoglycaemia to recede in patients taking sulphonylureas.

Since glucagon is easier to inject than dextrose, it is suitable for use by patients' relatives if acute hypoglycaemia occurs at home. However, it has a slower onset of action than dextrose and the latter would be preferred in hospital. Furthermore, if glucagon is used extra dextrose must also be given, since glucagon acts by mobilizing glycogen.

In a conscious patient with symptoms of hypoglycaemia all activities should be stopped and quickly absorbed dextrose should be given orally (for example as a sugary drink or sweet or as a soluble dextrose tablet), followed by a meal or a snack. All diabetics and their immediate family should be taught to recognize the signs and symptoms of hypoglycaemia, so that immediate treatment can be given when necessary.

It is important to note that a single bout of hypoglycaemia may be followed for 24–36 h by poor diabetic control with high blood glucose concentrations. However, one should not increase insulin doses during that time, and indeed it is often necessary to *reduce* insulin doses in order to avoid recurrence of hypoglycaemia.

27.5.3 The long-term treatment of diabetes mellitus

The treatment of diabetes mellitus takes three forms: diet alone, diet plus oral hypoglycaemic drugs, or diet plus insulin.

The aim of treatment is to control blood glucose concentrations within reasonable limits, avoiding both hyperglycaemia and hypoglycaemia. Since it is believed that good control of blood glucose concentrations will reduce the incidence of the long-term complications of diabetes mellitus, it is thought desirable to keep blood glucose concentrations below 10 mmol/L and preferably between 4 and 8 mmol/L. For this reason patients should monitor their own therapy at home, at least by measuring glucose concentrations in the urine or better still in capillary blood. Monitoring of blood glucose and HbA_{1c} concentrations in diabetes is discussed below.

(a) Diet

All patients with diabetes mellitus should be given advice about diet. If the patient is overweight calories should be restricted so that weight may be lost, but even in patients whose weight is ideal it is desirable to alter the balance of the types of food they eat.

Dietary management in diabetes is complicated, and a detailed discussion is beyond our scope. However, some simple principles apply.

1. Advice should be tailored to the individual's own habits and abilities. This is particularly important in old people, who may find it totally impractical to alter the habits of a lifetime and who may not be able to afford to do so.

2. Dietary fat intake, particularly animal fat, should be reduced in favour of carbohydrate. Cholesterol intake should be reduced to under 300 mg/d.

3. It is not simply the *quantity* of carbohydrate which a diabetic patient takes but the *rapidity with which it is absorbed* which is important. If carbohydrate is rapidly absorbed there will be high peak blood glucose concentrations, which may cause increased glycosylation of tissue proteins and hence tissue damage. Slowly-absorbed carbohydrate will lead to a smoother pattern of lower blood glucose concentrations, despite the same carbohydrate intake. This principle is discussed in Chapter 3 and illustrated in Fig. 3.1. Rapidly-absorbed carbohydrates (for example sugary drinks) should be reserved for hypoglycaemic emergencies or vigorous exercise. Foods containing slowly-absorbed carbohydrates include pulses (for example beans, lentils), bread, potatoes, rice, cereals, and pasta.

4. The frequency of meals is important for the diabetic patient. Small frequent meals help to reduce the fluctuations in blood glucose concentrations.

5. Foods with a high fibre ('roughage') content, such as pulses, raw vegetables, wholemeal bread, and bran (as cereals or bran supplements), are also recommended, since they slow down the absorption of carbohydrates.

6. Artificial sweeteners (for example aspartame, saccharin, or cyclamate) should be used in

place of glucose or fructose. Sorbitol is also suitable, but its use is limited by diarrhoea.

(b) Oral hypoglycaemic drugs

For older diabetic patients (those with maturity-onset or so-called type II diabetes) oral hypoglycaemic drugs are usually sufficient. The choice lies between the sulphonylureas and the biguanide metformin. Metformin should be used in over-weight patients, since it tends to help them lose weight while the sulphonylureas tend to make them gain weight. However, although many diabetic patients are overweight, some physicians start with a sulphonylurea, perhaps because they have a greater maximal efficacy than metformin. None the less, metformin may be preferred in those in whom hypoglycaemia may be an unacceptable risk (for example professional drivers). It is also used to augment the effects of the sulphonylureas.

(i) Sulphonylureas

None of the sulphonylureas is clearly preferable to the others, although there are differences among them.

Glibenclamide (2.5–20 mg daily in one or two divided doses) is currently the most commonly used, but as many as one in three patients taking it experience hypoglycaemia, which can be fatal. Although it has a relatively short half-time in the blood, its pharmacological effect is more prolonged, as it is concentrated in the islet cells, thereby potentially lowering the blood glucose for 24 h or so after a single dose.

Chlorpropamide (250–500 mg o.d.) also has a long duration of action (over 24 h), but it is less likely to cause hypoglycaemia than glibenclamide, although when it does it can last for several days. Its other unwanted effects (for example hyponatraemia and alcohol-associated flushing) have led to its being used less often nowadays.

Tolbutamide (500 mg t.d.s.) is a short-acting hypoglycaemic drug with a duration of action of 3–6 h. For this reason it is useful in old people, although they may find the large tablet hard to swallow.

Glipizide (2.5–30 mg in one or two divided doses) is short-acting (for about 4 h) at low doses and longer acting (up to about 12 h) at higher

doses. It may be more effective than the other sulphonylureas, but it is more expensive.

Gliclazide (40–160 mg once daily) (duration of action 6–12 h) is an effective alternative to glibenclamide, and since it may be safer it is gradually replacing it in some centres. It also has a theoretical advantage over the other sulphonylureas in that it reduces platelet aggregability, although it is not clear whether this effect confers any long-term benefit.

There is evidence that prolonged exposure to sulphonylureas may desensitize the pancreatic beta cells to their effects, and for this reason even the shorter acting drugs are nowadays generally given only once a day or divided into two doses if hypoglycaemia is a problem.

Of all the sulphonylureas, gliclazide and gliquidone appear to be the safest to use in patients with renal impairment, although care should be taken in monitoring blood sugar concentrations particularly during the early stages of treatment and if renal function changes. In patients with severe renal impairment insulin should be used. The sulphonylureas should be used with caution in patients with severe hepatic impairment, who should preferably be treated with insulin.

(ii) Metformin

Metformin (500–1500 mg daily) is usually added to augment the effects of the sulphonylureas at a late stage of treatment. It may cause troublesome diarrhoea, which may be permanent if very high dosages are used. Tolerance may also occur. Metformin should never be used in patients with renal impairment or hypoxia, because of the risk of lactic acidosis.

Drug interactions with oral hypoglycaemic drugs are important. They are listed in Table 27.8, as are drug interactions with insulin.

Patients who take oral hypoglycaemic drugs should be instructed to monitor their progress by glucose testing and general self-assessment as carefully as those who are taking insulin, since the risks of long-term tissue damage are serious in all cases.

If the combination of adequate diet with a sulphonylurea and metformin fails to control the blood glucose concentration satisfactorily (as it will in about 10 per cent of patients with type II diabetes) insulin should be introduced promptly.

■ **Table 27.8** Important drug interactions with hypoglycaemic drugs

Object drug(s)	Precipitant drug(s)	Effect of the interaction
All sulphonylureas and insulin	Diabetogenic drugs (corticosteroids, diazoxide, frusemide, thiazides, thyroid hormones)	Reduced hypoglycaemic effect
All sulphonylureas and insulin	β-Adrenoceptor antagonists (β_1-selective drugs may be safer)	(a) Increased hypoglycaemic effect (b) Inhibition of the signs and symptoms of hypoglycaemia (except sweating)
All sulphonylureas and insulin	Monoamine oxidase inhibitors	Increased hypoglycaemic effect
Tolbutamide, chlorpropamide, glibenclamide	Phenylbutazone	Inhibition of metabolism or renal excretion, i.e. increased hypoglycaemic effect
Tolbutamide	Rifampicin	Enhanced metabolism, i.e. reduced hypoglycaemic effect
Tolbutamide	Salicylates, chloral derivatives, sulphinpyrazone, sulphonamides	Protein-binding displacement, i.e. temporarily increased hypoglycaemic effect (see Chapter 10)
Alcohol	Chlorpropamide	Flushing (see also alcohol in the Pharmacopoeia)

(c) Insulin

Insulin is essential for young (juvenile-onset or so-called type I) diabetics and for older diabetics in whom oral therapy has become inadequate; it may also be required in some forms of secondary diabetes, during pregnancy, and when there is serious concurrent disease.

(i) Starting insulin therapy

There is no standard calculation which will establish the correct starting dose of insulin for an individual. The usual daily dose is around 0.5 i.u. per kg body weight, but in general larger dosages are needed for overweight people, those who take no regular exercise, those with concurrent illnesses, very high blood glucose concentrations, and ketosis, or those who are also taking corticosteroids. Smaller dosages are needed for slim people, those who exercise regularly, and those who have some residual insulin production (for example those in whom oral hypoglycaemic drugs are only just inadequate). Dosages above 1 i.u. per kg suggest insulin resistance, the cause of which should be investigated. The important causes of insulin resistance are listed in Table 27.9.

The total daily dosage is divided by the rule of thirds: two-thirds before breakfast, one third before the evening meal; at each time of administration two-thirds intermediate- or long-acting insulin one-third short-acting. Then the dosages are fine-tuned using the finger-prick blood glucose measurement as a guide (see below). If the patient is in hospital the starting dose can be higher than in a patient beginning treatment at home (an increasing trend, using the expertise of specialist diabetes nurses). For example, for a young 70 kg man in hospital one might start with 36 i.u. of insulin per day, given as 24 i.u. before breakfast and 12 i.u. before the evening meal. If he were at home one would start with 12 i.u. in the morning and 6 i.u. in the evening and gradually increase the dose as required. The daily requirements often rise as a patient's appetite returns after the acute presentation, fall during the so-called 'honeymoon' period (when the last few beta cells in the pancreas recover sufficiently from acute ketoacidosis to produce insulin), and

■ **Table 27.9** Some causes of insulin resistance

1. *Poor diabetic control*
   Diabetic ketoacidosis
   Persistently high blood glucose concentrations

2. *Intercurrent events*
   Puberty
   Pregnancy
   Infection
   Myocardial infarction
   Major injury or surgery

3. *Drugs*
   Steroid excess

4. *Inherited resistance syndromes*

5. *Other disorders*
   Obesity
   Acromegaly
   Rare immunological disorders

then rise again as endogenous insulin production finally stops.

(ii) Long-term insulin therapy

Insulin treatment must be tailored to suit the patient. If a regimen fails to control the blood glucose or causes the patient difficulties it should be changed; if the patient cannot accept the treatment it rarely works. It is important for patients to know their treatment goals. For example, a pregnant diabetic woman should aim to have a fasting blood glucose level below 5 mmol/L and a random glucose level below 7 mmol/L. In contrast, an old woman living alone should never have a blood glucose level below 6 mmol/L but should avoid too many above 11 mmol/L.

Combinations of insulins of different durations of action are used in providing good control of the blood glucose concentration throughout the day. The following are common examples.

(i) An intermediate-acting insulin plus a short-acting insulin given together in the morning and evening

With this type of regimen the day can be considered to be split into four parts. The periods immediately after the injections (i.e. the morning and the evening) are controlled by the short-acting insulin and the other two periods (i.e. the afternoon and the night) by the intermediate-acting insulin. The 70 kg man cited above might start off taking 8 i.u. of soluble plus 12 i.u. of isophane insulin in the morning and 4 i.u. of soluble plus 8 i.u. of isophane in the evening. He could then adjust the doses of the individual components according to the blood glucose concentration at different times of the day. He would take three main meals and three snacks a day at regular times.

(ii) An intermediate- or long-acting insulin at bedtime and injections of a short-acting insulin before each meal

In this regimen the long-acting insulin provides a continuous background of insulin in the circulation, giving cover overnight and for a variable period during the next day; the short-acting insulin provides control of the fluctuations in blood glucose concentrations which can occur after meals.

In this regimen half the total daily requirement is given as the short-acting insulin. It is a flexible regimen, but it relies on frequent finger-prick blood glucose measurements for optimal control. It allows patients to maintain good control while varying their meal times and the amount they eat. It may also allow them to omit daytime snacks, but the bedtime snack should never be omitted by patients taking insulin, since it protects them from nocturnal hypoglycaemia. Using this regimen our patient might take 18 i.u. of ultralente insulin at 10 p.m. and 6 i.u. of soluble insulin before each main meal.

(iii) A long-acting insulin in the morning plus a short-acting insulin in the morning and evening

This is a variant of the previous regimen, which is slightly less flexible, because of the peak effect of the long-acting insulin occurs during the day rather than the night, but it may mean fewer injections during the day. Examples of this type of regimen are lente or ultralente insulin in the morning plus soluble insulin the morning and evening.

(iv) A long-acting insulin in the morning with or without a short-acting insulin in the morning only

This is a variant of (iii), in which the evening dose of short-acting insulin is omitted. It rarely achieves normal blood glucose concentrations throughout the day. However, it can be used for patients in whom the evening blood glucose concentration is not high enough to make an extra dose of short-acting insulin absolutely necessary, and it is particularly useful for patients (for example old people) who prefer only one injection a day. Examples of this type of regimen are lente or ultralente insulin plus soluble insulin in the morning. In a few patients even the single dose of the short-acting insulin may be unnecessary.

In Table 27.10 are shown the ways in which the dosages of the insulins used in these regimens can be changed in patients who are able to monitor their blood or urine glucose concentrations at the appropriate times. It is usual when altering insulin doses to make alterations of no more than 4 units at a time.

27.5.4 Some practical aspects of diabetes care

All patients should have rapid access to support, both by telephone and in person, for example from the specialist diabetes nurse.

(a) Essential information for patients

All patients with diabetes mellitus treated with drugs should:

(1) know what hypoglycaemia is and how to treat it.

(2) carry a diabetic card at all times.

(3) carry glucose (dextrose) or sugar (sucrose) at all times.

(4) exercise care when driving or operating machinery or when in other hazardous circumstances; insulin-treated diabetics should avoid such activities during the first week of treatment; in the UK all patients should inform the Driver and Vehicle Licencing Centre that they are diabetic; insurance companies regard diabetes as a material fact of which they should be informed.

■ **Table 27.10** Guidelines for altering insulin dosages according to blood glucose concentrations

| *Example 1:* | morning: isophane + soluble |
| | evening: isophane + soluble |

Poor control (for example blood glucose under 4 mmol/L or over 10 mmol/L):	Alter dose of:
before breakfast*	p.m. isophane
before lunch	a.m. soluble
before evening meal	a.m. isophane
before bed	p.m. soluble

| *Example 2:* | morning: ultralente + soluble |
| | evening: soluble |

Poor control (for example blood glucose under 4 mmol/L or over 10 mmol/L):	Alter dose of:
before breakfast*	ultralente
before lunch	a.m. soluble
before bed	p.m. soluble

*Remember that hyperglycaemia or excess glycosuria before breakfast may be a rebound response to nocturnal *hypoglycaemia*, in which case the relevant insulin dose should not be increased. A careful history may elucidate symptoms of nocturnal hypoglycaemia (for example a drenching overnight sweat or disturbed dreams).
The blood glucose should be over 6 mmol/L at bedtime.
It is usual to adjust insulin doses only if the blood glucose is consistently too low or too high (for example for 3 d)

(b) Monitoring therapy

Individual insulin dosage requirements vary enormously, but the majority of patients are controlled with total daily doses of between 20 and 60 units. All patients who are capable of doing so, or their relatives or carers, should learn how to adjust their insulin doses in response to changes in blood or urine glucose concentration (see Table 27.10), food intake, exercise, and illness. Some patients also learn how to alter the dosages of their oral hypoglycaemic drugs within the safe dosage range.

At intervals a nurse or doctor should check patients' long-term glycaemic control, by reviewing their blood glucose measurements and by measuring HbA$_{1c}$ at least once a year.

(i) Urine glucose testing

Urine glucose measurement provides an indirect measure of glycaemia and is less useful than finger-prick glucose testing. It is inaccurate, since the renal threshold for glucose elimination varies from individual to individual. Thus, glycosuria may be absent even when the blood glucose concentration is increased; conversely, glycosuria can occur when the blood glucose is normal, because of a low renal threshold. However, some patients cannot do finger-prick tests, and in those cases urine-testing strips may be used. Clinitest® tablets are now obsolete.

(ii) Finger-prick blood glucose testing

Measurement of the blood glucose concentration by finger-prick testing is the method of choice. There are several types of finger-pricking lancets and automatic devices available, and patients should be given the opportunity to find the one which is most comfortable and practical for them. The finger to be pricked should be clean, warm, and dry, and it is usual to use the fingers of the non-dominant hand. Although patients may use their own devices repeatedly, nurses and doctors should discard immediately after use any equipment which punctures or contacts the patient's skin, in order to avoid the risk of transmission of hepatitis or HIV and of injury to others. There is now available a finger-pricking device in which the lancet automatically retracts into a disposable platform, and this makes contamination or injury virtually impossible.

The blood can be tested by any one of a variety of reagent strips and measuring devices available commercially. However, if the manufacturers' instructions are not followed precisely, these systems are useless and may be dangerously misleading. The following are the important points to note.

1. The strips must be in date and dry.
2. Timing, if required, should be precise, using a watch with a second-hand.
3. Wiping or blotting of the blood, if required, should be performed with the correct material.
4. The results can be read by eye, provided vision (including colour vision) is adequate; many diabetics with eye disease have difficulties with this.

There are two types of reading meter available: reflectance meters, which detect the colour on the strip and convert it into a glucose concentration reading, and biosensors, which convert the difference between the electrical signals from a glucose oxidase pad and a reference pad on the strip into a digital reading. Biosensor technology has revolutionized blood glucose monitoring, since there is no need for wiping or blotting and an accurate result is available within 30 s, if the user has followed the instructions correctly.

Ideally during long-term therapy blood glucose concentrations should always be in single figures (i.e. below 10 mmol/L). The targets at which one would aim are shown in Table 27.11. At first, insulin-treated patients should test their blood before each meal, before bed, and occasionally at between 1 a.m. and 3 a.m. if possible. Some continue to do this in the long term; others reduce the frequency to once or twice a day, varying the time of day, or to a profile of four times a day on one day a week. It is also sensible to check the blood before bed every night if there is any suggestion of nocturnal hypoglycaemia; in insulin-treated patients the blood glucose concentration at bed-time should be at least 6 mmol/L. In unusual circumstances or during illness, testing should be increased to at least four times a day. If the blood glucose concentration is over 16 mmol/L the urine should be tested for ketones; extra fast-acting insulin should be given and if ketones are present in medium or large amounts,

▮ **Table 27.11** Targets for blood glucose and plasma lipid concentrations in the treatment of diabetes mellitus

Measure	Ideal	Acceptable
Blood glucose (mmol/L):		
Fasting	4.0–6.7	<7.8
After eating	4.0–8.0	<10.0
Urine glucose (per cent)	0	<0.5
Cholesterol (mmol/L):		
Total	<5.2	<6.5
HDL>	>0.9	>0.9
Fasting triglycerides (mmol/L)	<1.7	<2.3

or if the patient feels ill or is vomiting or has diarrhoea, help should be sought immediately. Some patients are prone to develop ketoacidosis rapidly, and this course of action may be needed at a blood glucose concentration lower than 16 mmol/L.

Patients taking oral hypoglycaemic drugs or diet alone should test their blood four times daily to start with. Once stable, testing can be limited to a fasting sample and one taken 2 h after the largest meal of the day. The frequency of testing should be increased in unusual circumstances or illness, as for insulin-treated patients.

(iii) Glycosylated haemoglobin measurement

The amount of HbA_{1c} as a percentage of total haemoglobin is a useful measure of the degree of glycaemia during the 4–6 weeks before the sample was taken. However, it may be difficult to interpret in patients with haemolysis or with haemoglobinopathies.

(c) Formulations of insulin

The different types of insulin formulation are listed in the Pharmacopoeia. Three forms of insulin are available: bovine, porcine, and human. Human insulin is produced in two ways: by enzymatic modification of porcine insulin and by the introduction of human insulin genes into *E. coli* or yeasts. Bovine insulin is slightly more immunogenic than porcine and human insulins. There is no important difference between porcine insulin and the two types of human insulin in terms of efficacy, but there is some evidence that human insulin is more rapidly absorbed after subcutaneous injection and that patients who take human insulins may be less aware of hypoglycaemia when it occurs; the mechanism of this is not understood. Currently 80 per cent of insulin-treated patients in the UK use human insulin.

Fast-acting (soluble or neutral) insulin is clear, like water. It is the only insulin which can be injected intravenously and intramuscularly as well as subcutaneously. All other insulins are cloudy, because of the ways in which they have been modified to alter their absorption rates. Cloudy insulins can only be given subcutaneously. If a clear insulin becomes cloudy it has become contaminated and must be discarded.

(d) Insulin injections

Patients should be carefully instructed in how to fill the insulin syringe accurately and how to give a subcutaneous injection properly. It is important to avoid intracutaneous injection (which will result in poor diabetic control and tissue damage at the site of injection) and intramuscular injection (which will result in hypoglycaemia due to quick absorption of insulin). The introduction of the insulin 'pen', using insulin cartridges with easy selection of dosages, has eliminated many of the problems associated with insulin injections. This method of injection often makes repeated daily injections more acceptable to the patient. Disposable syringes are marketed for one-time use only, although some patients re-use them for up to at least a week or change the needle more often if it becomes too blunt. Used needles and syringes must be carefully disposed of (for example in a special 'sharps' container or by using a needle clipper) to avoid injuries and illicit use.

Any two different insulins may be mixed in the same syringe. If a clear insulin is to be drawn into the same syringe as a cloudy insulin the former should be drawn up first in order to prevent contamination. The resulting mixture should be injected immediately, since some forms of long-acting insulin (those which contain zinc or protamine) modify the short-acting insulins chemically.

The availability of some formulations of insulins in fixed proportions means that a new diabetic patient can start treatment easily without having to learn how to mix insulins at first. A practical regimen is twice-daily injections of a mixture of 30 per cent soluble insulin with 70 per cent isophane (for example Humulin M3® or Mixtard® insulin). The disadvantage of this is the lack of flexibility in adjusting the doses of the individual insulins.

(e) Sites of injection

The usual sites of self-injection are the skin over the thighs, upper buttocks, and abdomen, but the arms may also be used if a nurse or relative is giving the injection. Whatever site is chosen it is important to use a different site each time (for example first the left thigh, then the right thigh, then the lower left quadrant of the abdomen, etc.). Absorption is faster from the arms and abdomen than from the thighs or buttocks and a few patients may find that they have to avoid certain injection sites if the differences are great enough to be detected clinically. If the muscles underlying the injection site are exercised the rate of absorption is further increased.

(f) Recognition of hypoglycaemia

Most insulin-treated patients and some on oral hypoglycaemic drugs will sooner or later experience an attack of hypoglycaemia, and they (and their relatives) should learn to recognize the signs and symptoms, so that prompt treatment may be instituted when necessary. For this reason some doctors deliberately subject insulin-treated patients to acute hypoglycaemia in hospital as a demonstration. If a patient is taking a β-adrenoceptor antagonist the usual signs of hypoglycaemia (see p. 382) may be masked, although sweating is usually preserved, since it is mediated by sympathetic cholinergic transmission.

(g) Prevention of complications

Patients should be told about the importance of good blood glucose control in preventing the long-term complications of diabetes mellitus. They should also be warned about the dangers of injury to the feet, which can result in ischaemic damage and in severe cases may lead to the need for amputation. Old patients and those with peripheral vascular disease should be advised to attend a chiropodist regularly. All diabetic patients should be advised not to smoke.

On the physician's part, regular checks of the blood pressure, the urine for protein, and the optic fundi are important for the early detection of treatable complications. Hypertension in the diabetic should be vigorously treated, since there is evidence that this reduces the extent of long-term renal damage.

27.5.5 Special circumstances in the treatment of diabetes mellitus

(a) Intercurrent infections

Insulin dosage requirements increase during infection. Patients should be educated in two important aspects of their treatment at such times (for example during a bout of influenza).

1. During infections they should increase their dosages of insulin as indicated by blood and urine tests (for example using the method outlined in Table 27.10).

2. If they are vomiting or not eating they will still need some insulin to maintain normal metabolism, and total insulin requirements may be reduced or increased. For example, a patient who takes ultralente insulin in the morning with once- or twice-daily soluble insulin would continue to take the ultralente and adjust the doses of soluble insulin according to the blood glucose concentration.

(b) Operations

(i) Elective surgery

Diabetic patients who are to have planned operations requiring general anaesthesia should ideally be first on the operating list in the morning. In all cases their usual treatment should be omitted on the day of the operation.

During long operations a continuous i.v. infusion of insulin and potassium should be given as 3 units/h of soluble insulin with 2 mmol/h of potassium chloride in 10 per cent dextrose, 100 mL/h (i.e. 15 units of insulin and 10 mmol of potassium in 500 mL of dextrose given over 5 h). An alternative method is to give the 10 per cent dextrose and potassium as described but to give separate intravenous injections of insulin according to a sliding scale (see Table 27.7) with hourly blood glucose measurements; this allows more flexible glucose control.

Patients using long-acting insulins should ideally be changed to short- and intermediate-acting insulins on the day before surgery. Patients who had a dose of long-acting insulin on the day before surgery may need an extra dose of dextrose (10–20 g i.v.) before the operation. Patients with poor blood glucose control should be admitted early for proper control with short- and intermediate-acting insulins before surgery.

Post-operative hyperglycaemia should be controlled using an i.v. or s.c. sliding-scale of the types shown in Table 27.7 until patients are once more eating and can be given their usual dose of oral hypoglycaemic drug or insulin.

(ii) Emergency operations

When diabetic control is required during an emergency operation careful hourly measurements of blood glucose should be made. Good control can usually be achieved by giving a low-dose continuous infusion of soluble insulin and potassium with 10 per cent dextrose, as described above, provided that care is taken to check the blood glucose concentration hourly.

(c) Pregnancy

Good control of diabetes during pregnancy improves the outcome for the fetus. The aim should be to control the fasting blood glucose concentration within the reference range (3.5–5.0 mmol/L), and random glucose concentrations should be below 7 mmol/L. This should be achieved with a regimen of short-acting plus intermediate- or long-acting insulins (see section 27.5.3.(c) regimens (i) or (ii)).

Monitoring should be by regular blood glucose concentration measurements, and not by urine measurements, since the threshold for renal excretion of glucose changes during pregnancy. The treatment of diabetes in pregnancy is discussed in more detail in Chapter 12 (p. 156).

27.6 Disorders of lipid metabolism

27.6.1 Mechanisms of action of drugs which lower plasma lipid concentrations

Plasma lipids comprise a group of compounds which includes cholesterol, triglycerides, phospholipids, and free fatty acids. Because these compounds are relatively insoluble in water they are found in the plasma either as lipoproteins or (in the case of free fatty acids) bound to albumin.

The usual method of classifying plasma lipoproteins relates to their densities: HDL, LDL, and VLDL (high-density, low-density, and very low-density lipoproteins respectively), and chylomicrons (of a density similar to VLDL). The lipid and protein contents of these lipoproteins are shown in Table 27.12.

The main functions of the lipoproteins are as follows:

chylomicrons: the transport of exogenous (i.e. dietary) triglycerides;
VLDL: the transport of endogenous triglycerides;
LDL: the transport of cholesterol to the tissues;
HDL: the transport of cholesterol out of the tissues.

The mechanisms of action of drugs used to lower plasma lipid concentrations are shown in Fig. 27.3 in relation to a simplified scheme of lipid metabolism. The drugs are listed in Table 27.13, and the effects they have on circulating lipids and lipoproteins are shown in Table 27.14.

(a) Exchange resins

The exchange resins cholestyramine and colestipol sequester bile acids in the gut, thus reducing their reabsorption after biliary excretion. This removes feedback inhibition of the conversion of bile acids to cholesterol, LDL receptors are stimulated, and cholesterol metabolism increases. Thus, plasma concentrations of cholesterol and LDL fall. The exchange resins increase HDL concentrations by an unknown mechanism. They do not change plasma triglyceride concentrations or may even increase them slightly by increasing VLDL.

(b) Fibrates

The fibrates (clofibrate, bezafibrate, fenofibrate, and gemfibrizol) reduce hepatic cholesterol synthesis and the secretion of VLDL into the blood. As a result the plasma concentrations of cholesterol and VLDL fall. The fibrates also reduce plasma concentrations of triglycerides and LDL and increase HDL concentrations by unknown mechanisms. LDL receptor numbers increase. The fibrates increase cholesterol excretion in the bile and thus predispose to cholesterol gallstones.

(c) HMG CoA reductase inhibitors

The HMG CoA reductase inhibitors (simvastatin, lovastatin, and pravastatin) inhibit the rate-limiting enzyme in cholesterol synthesis in the liver, hydroxymethylglutaryl coenzyme A (HMG

■ **Table 27.12** The lipid and protein contents of various lipoproteins

	Content (per cent)			
	HDL	**LDL**	**VLDL**	**Chylomicrons**
Triglycerides	5	8	50	85
Cholesterol				
esterified	15	40	15	3
non-esterified	3	10	7	3
Phospholipid	27	22	18	7
Protein	50	20	10	2

■ **Table 27.13** Lipid-lowering drugs

1. *Exchange resins* (p. 581)
   Cholestyramine
   Colestipol

2. *Fibrates* (p. 605)
   Bezafibrate
   Clofibrate
   Fenofibrate
   Gemfibrizol

3. *HMG CoA reductase inhibitors* (p. 614)
   Lovastatin
   Pravastatin
   Simvastatin

4. *Nicotinic acid and analogues*
   Acipimox
   Nicofuranose
   Nicotinic acid

5. *Others*
   Neomycin
   Probucol

CoA) reductase. Plasma concentrations of cholesterol and LDL thus fall and LDL receptor numbers increase. There are also small falls in plasma triglycerides and VLDL. HDL concentrations are increased by an unknown mechanism.

(d) Nicotinic acid and related compounds

Nicotinic acid and the related compounds nicofuranose and acipimox inhibit the synthesis and secretion of VLDL, inhibit the synthesis of LDL, and inhibit lipolysis. They reduce plasma concentrations of cholesterol, triglycerides, VLDL, and LDL, and increase HDL.

(e) Other drugs

Other drugs which have been used for their lipid-lowering effects include probucol and neomycin. Probucol is an antioxidant which reduces the oxidation of LDL and the secretion of VLDL. It also increases the excretion of bile acids. It lowers the plasma concentrations of cholesterol and VLDL. However, it also lowers HDL, which may not be helpful. Neomycin precipitates cholesterol in the gut, thus preventing its absorption. It therefore acts like cholestyramine.

27.6.2 The management of disorders of lipid metabolism

Because of the evidence that accumulation of lipids in vascular tissue is an important early step in the development of arterial atheroma, and because of the epidemiological evidence relating increased plasma lipid concentrations to an increased risk of coronary heart disease, it has been thought that the use of lipid-lowering manoeuvres might be of value in either the primary or secondary prevention of coronary artery disease. These ideas have been bolstered by the results of clinical intervention studies, predominantly in middle-aged men, in which dietary or drug treatment has been shown to reduce the frequency of events related to coronary heart disease: a 1 per cent reduction in serum cholesterol concentration is associated with a 2 per cent

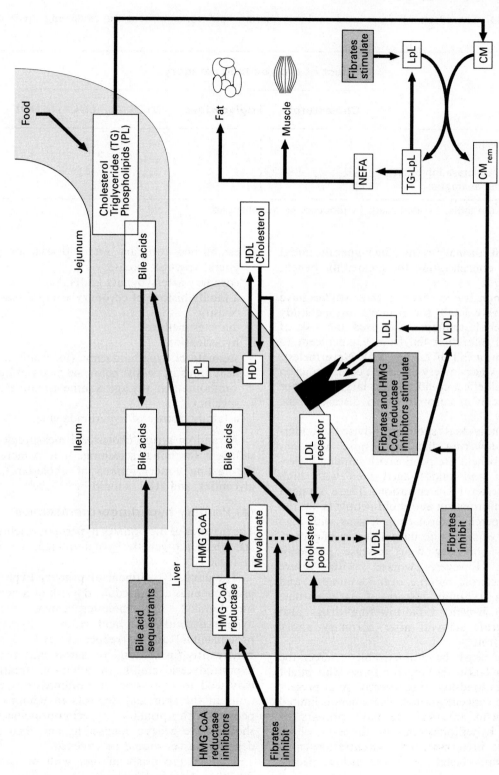

■ **Fig. 27.3.** The effects of drugs on lipid metabolism.

■ **Table 27.14** The effects of drugs used to lower plasma lipid concentrations on circulating lipids and lipoproteins

Drug	Effect of drug on lipid category				
	Cholesterol	Triglycerides	VLDL	LDL	HDL
Exchange resins	↓↓	↑	⇔	↓↓	↑
Fibrates	↓	↓↓↓	↓↓↓	↓	↑↑
HMG CoA reductase inhibitors	↓↓↓	↓	↓↓↓	↓↓↓	↑
Nicotinic acid analogues	↓	↓↓↓	↓	↓	↑

Symbols in the table: ↑ = increased; ↓ = reduced; ⇔ = unchanged

reduction in coronary events; the higher the initial cholesterol concentration the greater the benefit of lowering it.

The demonstrated effects in these studies have been relatively small: for example, in one study in which cholestyramine was used the risk of myocardial infarction fell from 9.8 per cent to 8.1 per cent, a fall of 1.7 per cent. Nevertheless, because coronary artery disease is common, even such a small effect could make a large difference to the burden of coronary heart disease in the community.

Which individuals should be advised to undertake lipid-lowering therapy? Those who undoubtedly benefit are people with familial hyperlipidaemias and middle-aged men with high serum cholesterol concentrations. There is a need for more information about old people (since the risk of hypercholesterolaemia lessens with age) and about women (who have a degree of protection from coronary heart disease premenopausally). However, women with severe hypercholesterolaemia (i.e. over 7.8 mmol/L) and those with a family history of early cardiac disease do benefit. Lipid-lowering drugs also improve graft survival after coronary artery bypass grafting.

It would clearly be impracticable to screen the whole population looking for those who might benefit from lipid-lowering therapy, so at present serum lipid concentration measurement is limited to those who are likely to have primary or secondary hyperlipidaemias or those in whom a reduction in serum lipid concentrations may be particularly beneficial. These include people with:

established coronary artery disease or peripheral vascular disease;
coronary artery bypass grafts;
a family history of coronary artery disease;
obesity;
diabetes mellitus;
hypertension;
stigmata of hyperlipidaemia (for example corneal arcus in people below 40 years of age or xanthomata at any age; xanthelasmata are less specific);
a family history of hyperlipidaemia.

A random serum cholesterol measurement is sufficient for initial screening. If it is increased the fasting concentrations of cholesterol, triglycerides, and HDL should be checked.

(a) Primary hyperlipoproteinaemias

The features of the primary hyperlipoproteinaemias, which are genetically determined, are listed in Table 27.15.

The aims of treatment of primary hyperlipoproteinaemias are to reduce the risk of atheroma (in familial hypercholesterolaemia, familial hypertriglyceridaemia, and remnant hyperlipoproteinaemia) and to reduce the risk of acute pancreatitis (in chylomicronaemia and familial hypertriglyceridaemia). In addition, treatment may lead to regression of xanthomatous eruptions in the skin and deposits in tendons. All people with primary hyperlipoproteinaemias should have genetic counselling and their first-degree relatives should be screened.

Treatment consists of diet with or without drugs, as described below.

∎ **Table 27.15** The main features of the primary hyperlipidaemias

Type	Cholesterol	Triglycerides	Increased lipoproteins	WHO type
Polygenic hypercholesterolaemia	↑	⇔	LDL	IIa
Familial hypercholesterolaemia**	↑↑↑	⇔	LDL	IIa, IIb
Familial combined hyperlipidaemia*	↑	↑	LDL, VLDL	IIa, IIb, IV
Remnant hyperlipoproteinaemia*	↑↑	↑↑	LDL, CM	III
Familial hypertriglyceridaemia†	↑	↑↑↑	VLDL, CM	IV, V
Chylomicronaemia†	↑	↑↑↑	VLDL, CM	I, V

*Increased (**greatly increased) risk of coronary artery disease.
†Increased risk of pancreatitis.
↑ = increased.

(b) Secondary hyperlipoproteinaemias

Hyperlipoproteinaemias, particularly hypertriglyceridaemia, may occur secondary to the effects of a variety of drugs and diseases (see Table 27.16). Treatment in these cases should be by treatment of the primary condition or withdrawal of the offending drug. Lipid-lowering drugs should not be used unless the plasma lipid concentrations remain high.

(c) General approaches to lowering plasma lipid concentrations

Hyperlipidaemias should never be treated in isolation from other risk factors. Smokers should be advised to stop smoking and those who do not exercise regularly should be encouraged to do so. The causes of secondary hyperlipidaemias (Table 27.16) should be treated. Obese people should be advised on how to lose weight by reducing their total caloric intake (see section 27.7).

If there is hypercholesterolaemia a weight-reducing cholesterol-lowering diet should be recommended. A simple diet of fat restriction consists of reducing total fat intake to 30 per cent of total calories, reducing saturated fat intake to less than 10 per cent of total calories, and reducing daily cholesterol intake to 100 mg per 1000 calories. If there is obesity total calories should be restricted (see section 27.7). These diets should contain at least 30 g of fibre per day. If the cholesterol is not within acceptable limits within 6 weeks of diet, a more rigorous dietary approach may be adopted, in which saturated fat

∎ **Table 27.16** Some causes of secondary hyperlipoproteinaemias

1. *Hypertriglyceridaemia*
   Diabetes mellitus
   Obesity
   Alcoholism
   Chronic renal failure
   Chronic liver disease
     Cholestasis
     Cholelithiasis
     Hepatocellular disease
     Hepatoma
   Drugs
     Oestrogens

2. *Hypertriglyceridaemia with hypercholesterolaemia*
   Diabetes mellitus
   Hypothyroidism
   Nephrotic syndrome
   Renal transplantation

3. *Hypertriglyceridaemia with reduced HDL*
   Non-selective β-adrenoceptor antagonists
   Norgestrel
   Isotretinoin (vitamin A analogue)

intake is reduced further and daily cholesterol intake is reduced to less than 200 mg in total. If this is ineffective or unacceptable, or if there is hypertriglyceridaemia, lipid-lowering drugs should be used.

(d) The use of drugs in lowering plasma lipid concentrations

All lipid-lowering drugs have adverse effects, the risks of which must be balanced against the potential benefits of treatment. Since many patients are asymptomatic this must be carefully explained. Every effort should be made to reduce the plasma lipid concentrations by non-pharmacological means and to reduce other risk factors before giving lipid-lowering drugs. The bile acid sequestrants are the first-line drugs and the second-line drugs are the fibrates, the HMG CoA reductase inhibitors, and the nicotinic acid derivatives.

(i) Bile acid sequestrants

The bile acid sequestrants cholestyramine and colestipol are still generally used as first-line treatment for pure hypercholesterolaemia, since experience with them is long and since they have few major adverse effects. Furthermore, they are currently the only drugs used in hyperlipidaemic children and pregnant women. However, they are inconvenient to take and can cause uncomfortable adverse effects, such as abdominal gripes, wind, and constipation. They should be introduced gently, starting with half a sachet daily in fruit juice (cholestyramine 2 g) or sprinkled on muesli (colestipol 2.5 g) at breakfast time for a week, then increasing the dose gradually (cholestyramine 12–24 g, colestipol 15–30 g, both in two to four divided doses). Questran® contains sugar and so Questran A®, which contains aspartame, is recommended. Other drugs should be taken either 1 h before or 4 h after a dose of a bile acid sequestrant. In some patients who have taken large doses for many years folate and fat-soluble vitamin deficiencies may occur and replacement therapy will be required. As mentioned above, the bile acid sequestrants should not be used if there is hypertriglyceridaemia.

(ii) Fibrates

Gemfibrozil (300–600 mg b.d.) is the only fibrate whose lipid-lowering effect has been shown to be associated with both a reduction in the frequency of coronary events (in middle-aged men) and few adverse effects during long-term use. Other fibrates include bezafibrate (200 mg t.d.s. or 400 mg at night) and fenofibrate (200–400 mg daily in divided doses). Clofibrate (1.5–2.0 g daily in divided doses) predisposes to gallstones and can only be used in patients who have had a cholecystectomy.

The fibrates commonly cause nausea and abdominal discomfort. They may occasionally cause a myositis-like syndrome with raised muscle enzymes; the risk of this is increased if they are combined with the HMG CoA reductase inhibitors, and this combination should not be used. They can occasionally cause erectile impotence. The fibrates are highly protein bound and this may be reduced in renal impairment. This is particularly important for clofibrate, whose protein binding is saturable at high doses in the therapeutic range. Fibrates should therefore be used with care in patients with renal impairment. Clofibrate may increase the plasma cholesterol in patients with primary biliary cirrhosis.

(iii) HMG CoA reductase inhibitors

The HMG CoA reductase inhibitors are very effective in lowering plasma cholesterol concentrations, but their long-term safety has not been established. They are ineffective in homozygous familial hypercholesterolaemia, in which LDL receptors are absent. Simvastatin and pravastatin (both 10–40 mg daily) are best given at night, when cholesterol synthesis is at its peak. They can cause a wide variety of gastrointestinal complaints, and their main adverse effect is a reversible myopathy. Abnormal liver function tests have been reported, and liver function tests should be made before starting treatment and regularly thereafter. In animals they may cause cataracts and although these have not been reported yet in humans, yearly examination of the lenses is recommended. They should not be used in combination with the fibrates (see above).

(iv) Nicotinic acid derivatives

If other drugs are ineffective nicotinic acid, nicofuranose, or acipimox may be added. Acipimox (up to 1200 mg daily in divided doses with meals) is quite well tolerated. Dosages of nicotinic acid should be low to start with because it can cause severe flushing, dizziness, and palpitation due to vasodilatation in the early stages of treatment. Start with 100- 300 mg orally t.d.s. and increase gradually over 2–4 weeks to 1–2 g t.d.s. The dosage of nicofuranose is 0.5–1 g t.d.s.

(v) Others

Probucol should be used with caution in people with ischaemic heart disease, since it can cause ventricular arrhythmias associated with prolongation of the QT interval. It is slowly cleared from the body and premenopausal women must take contraceptive precautions during treatment and for 6 months after stopping.

Omega-3 marine triglycerides are sometimes used in the treatment of hypertriglyceridaemia (5 capsules or 5 mL twice daily with food). They can cause nausea and belching.

(e) The practical management of hyperlipidaemias

The type of treatment one uses depends on the plasma cholesterol and triglyceride concentrations. Suggested drug regimens for patients with different patterns of lipid abnormalities are listed in Table 27.17.

(i) Cholesterol 5.2–6.5 mmol/L

Mild hypercholesterolaemia should be treated with diet alone.

▐ **Table 27.17** Suggested lipid-lowering drugs for patients with different profiles of serum lipid concentrations

Increased lipid	Drug(s)
Cholesterol alone	1. Bile acid sequestrant 2. Fibrate or HMG CoA reductase inhibitor*
Cholesterol and triglyceride	Fibrate or Nicotinic acid derivative
Triglyceride alone	Fibrate or Nicotinic acid derivative or Omega-3 marine triglycerides

*The bile acid sequestrants may be combined with the fibrates or with the HMG CoA reductase inhibitors, but the fibrates and the HMG CoA reductase inhibitors should not be combined with each other.

(ii) Cholesterol 6.6–7.8 mmol/L

In moderate hypercholesterolaemia begin with simple diet and progress if necessary to a more rigorous form. If the cholesterol does not fall drugs may be considered for patients with coronary artery disease or symptomatic peripheral vascular disease or for those with two other risk factors.

(iii) Cholesterol over 7.8 mmol/L

In severe hypercholesterolaemia begin with simple diet and progress if necessary to a more rigorous form. If the cholesterol does not fall and all possible steps have been taken to treat the causes of secondary hyperlipidaemia (see Table 27.16) drugs should be used. Treatment should be most vigorous in patients with familial hyperlipoproteinaemias, those with a family history of early death due to coronary heart disease, and those with a very low HDL concentration.

(iv) Triglycerides 2.3–5.6 mmol/L

This should be treated with diet and the patient should be advised to reduce alcohol and sugar intake. An increased concentration of triglycerides may sway the balance towards drug treatment in patients with a low HDL concentration and a cholesterol concentration which stays above 6.5 mmol/L despite diet. The bile acid sequestrants should not be used to treat hypertriglyceridaemia, since they may cause an increase in plasma triglycerides.

(v) Triglycerides over 5.6 mmol/L

Severe hypertriglyceridaemia carries an increased risk of pancreatitis and should be treated vigorously. Start with diet and advise total abstinence from alcohol and a large reduction in sugar intake. If the cholesterol is over 6.5 mmol/L with a low HDL concentration use lipid-lowering drugs (but not bile acid sequestrants).

27.7 The management of obesity

Obesity should be managed by treating any identifiable causes and by diet. There should rarely be any need for drugs. Treatable causes include hypothyroidism, Cushing's syndrome, and other rarer disorders.

Patients' dietary intake and habits should be assessed and they should be advised to eat a low calorie (usually 1000 calorie), low fat, low sugar diet. Very low calorie diets are potentially dangerous, but occasionally a 600 calorie diet may be appropriate under medical and biochemical supervision, taking care to avoid vitamin and mineral deficiencies and hyperuricaemia. Total starvation is not recommended, because of the morbidity which occurs during refeeding.

If vigorous dietary effort has failed to produce the desired weight loss, the appetite suppressant dexfenfluramine (d-fenfluramine) may be used under medical supervision as an adjunct to continued dietary effort. Dexfenfluramine acts by stimulating the release of 5-HT and inhibiting its re-uptake, and it lacks the amphetamine-like properties of the racemic mixture fenfluramine (l-fenfluramine plus d-fenfluramine), which are due to l-fenfluramine. In an oral dosage of 15 mg b.d. dexfenfluramine reduces appetite and can help a patient to lose weight if used in conjunction with diet. However, it should not be used for more than 3 months and is not a substitute for proper dietary control of weight. It should not be used in individuals with a history of a mental disorder or of drug or alcohol abuse or in patients taking MAO inhibitors. It may potentiate the effects of antihypertensive, antidiabetic, or sedative drugs.

28 The drug therapy of blood disorders

Co-author: M. E. Haines

28.1 Anaemias

28.1.1 Iron deficiency anaemia

The aims in treating iron deficiency anaemia are to remove the cause and to increase red cell mass by giving iron. The main causes of iron deficiency anaemia are listed in Table 28.1.

Iron may be given orally or parenterally, and in almost all patients the oral route is satisfactory. Iron in oral formulations is in the ferrous form, since that is the form in which iron is absorbed, mostly from the upper jejunum. Normal dietary iron absorption is 1–2 mg from a dietary intake of 10–20 mg, balancing the daily losses, which are mainly from sloughing of cells from the gastrointestinal tract and skin and from urinary losses. If there is iron loss in excess of daily intake gastrointestinal iron absorption increases. For example, during menstruation dietary absorption increases to 2–3 mg/d. However, the maximum possible daily intake is usually no more than 4 mg, and if this is not sufficient to compensate for losses iron deficiency will result.

The total body iron deficit may be roughly calculated from the following equation:

$$\text{iron deficit (mg)} = \text{Hb deficit (g/dL)}$$
$$\times \text{body weight (kg)} \times 0.65 \text{ (dL/kg)} \times 3.4 \text{ (mg/g)}$$

This equation derives from the fact that the normal blood volume is 65 mL/kg (i.e. 0.65 dL/kg) and the amount of iron in 1 g of haemoglobin is 3.4 mg. Thus, in a 70 kg man with a haemoglobin of 8 g/dL (normal 15.5) the estimated deficit would be:

$$(15.5 - 8.0) \times 70 \times 0.65 \times 3.4 = 1160 \text{ mg}.$$

Since the normal total body iron content is 3–5 g, such a deficit would be a major one.

(a) The choice of an oral iron formulation

The following types of iron formulations are available for oral administration:

(1) ferrous salts in fluid formulations, ordinary tablets and capsules, and slow-release tablets and capsules;

(2) formulations which contain both a ferrous salt and folic acid (for use in pregnancy);

■ **Table 28.1** Causes of iron deficiency anaemia

---

1. *Chronic blood loss*
   Gastrointestinal
   Disease of the gastrointestinal tract (for example hiatus hernia, peptic ulcer, carcinoma of the large bowel, intestinal parasites)
   Drug-induced (for example aspirin and other non-steroidal anti-inflammatory drugs; see Table 29.1)
   Menstrual (over 80 mL/cycle = 46 mg iron)
   Recurrent haemoptysis (for example vascular abnormalities, pulmonary haemosiderosis)

2. *Increased requirements*
   Pregnancy
   Treatment of megaloblastic anaemia

3. *Malabsorption*
   Malabsorption syndromes
   Post-gastrectomy

4. *Dietary deficiency*

---

(3) formulations which contain both a ferrous salt and a wide variety of vitamins and minerals.

The ranges of amounts of iron available in unit dosage forms of these formulations are given in Table 28.2.

The total daily dose of elemental iron should usually be 150–300 mg. Dose for dose there is no difference among the different available salts, so that one's choice of formulation is dictated by three things: efficacy, patient acceptability, and cost.

(i) Efficacy

The efficacy of an iron formulation depends on how much of its iron content is released at its main site of absorption in the upper part of the small intestine. In this respect ordinary tablets or capsules are preferable, since iron absorption from slow-release formulations may be very variable (for example in patients with gastrointestinal hurry).

(ii) Patient acceptability

Two main factors influence patient acceptability of ferrous formulations: adverse effects, particularly gastrointestinal disturbances (for example nausea, abdominal discomfort, diarrhoea, or constipation) and the frequency of administration (once-a-day therapy is more likely to be acceptable than thrice-a-day therapy). These factors may lead patients to prefer slow-release formulations, despite their disadvantages (mentioned above).

(iii) Cost

Here the ordinary tablets and capsules are to be preferred, slow-release and fluid formulations being generally more expensive.

■ **Table 28.2**   A summary of the elemental iron content of a variety of iron formulations

Type of formulation	Ferrous salts available	Range of elemental iron content (mg/dose*)	Comments
1. *Iron alone*			
(a) Elixirs and mixtures	Sulphate, fumarate, succinate, and glycine sulphate	12–100	
(b) Tablets and capsules	Sulphate, fumarate, gluconate	35–150	
(c) Slow-release formulations	Sulphate, fumarate, and glycine sulphate	47–110	
2. *Iron + folic acid*			
(a) Tablets and capsules	Sulphate, fumarate, gluconate, and glycine sulphate	30–110	Folic acid 350–5000 micrograms
(b) Slow-release formulations	Sulphate	47–110	Folic acid 300–500 micrograms
3. *Iron + minerals/vitamins*			
(b) Tablets and capsules	Sulphate and fumarate	5–100	Most contain vitamin C and members of the vitamin B complex. A few contain folic acid
(c) Slow-release formulations	Sulphate	47–105	

* One tablet, one capsule, or 5 mL of fluid.

Initially therefore start treatment with an ordinary formulation, such as ferrous sulphate tablets 200 mg (= 60 mg of elemental iron) t.d.s. If the patient complains of gastrointestinal disturbances reduce the dosage to 200 mg b.d. Alternatively a change to ferrous gluconate or ferrous fumarate may help. If the symptoms persist one may be forced to switch to a slow-release formulation. The problem of failure to respond to treatment is dealt with below.

In the prevention of iron deficiency anaemia in pregnancy it is customary to give a formulation which contains not only a ferrous salt but also folic acid, which prevents the megaloblastic anaemia of pregnancy. The choice of formulation here can be made almost entirely on grounds of cost, since in this case the ordinary tablets and capsules can be given once a day and generally do not cause adverse effects. Total iron requirements during pregnancy amount to about 3–4 mg/d. This requires a minimum daily intake of 30 mg of elemental iron, and this is provided by all the available iron/folic acid formulations (Table 28.2). Folate requirements in pregnancy are increased by four to ten times, but normal requirements are so low (about 100 micrograms per day) that only a small daily dose is required. Therefore, most iron/folic acid formulations contain folic acid in excess of requirements (Table 28.2). The special use of high dosages of folic acid in preventing neural tube defects is mentioned elsewhere (p. 158)

In a patient with established iron deficiency adequate replacement should result, after a delay of a few days, in an increase in haemoglobin of 0.1–0.2 g/dL per day (i.e. about 1 g/dL per week). Although treatment may be stopped when the haemoglobin is normal it is often continued for longer (up to 6 months) to provide some extra reserve. Long-term treatment will be necessary if the underlying cause cannot be remedied.

(b) Failure to respond to oral iron

If a patient's anaemia fails to respond to oral iron several possibilities must be considered.

(i) Pharmaceutical

If the patient is taking a slow-release formulation absorption may not be adequate. A switch to an ordinary formulation or to an elixir may help. Conversely, if poor compliance is suspected in a patient taking an ordinary formulation a switch to a once-a-day slow-release formulation may help.

(ii) Pharmacokinetic

Absorption of iron may be reduced in malabsorptive states, and this may affect medicinal iron as well as dietary iron. Malabsorption of dietary iron due to achlorhydria is due to a failure to convert dietary ferric salts to the ferrous form and therefore does not affect the absorption of medicinal iron.

(iii) Excessive loss

Continued loss of iron through heavy blood loss may outstrip the rate at which replacement iron can be given. An increase in dosage, if tolerated, may help (although one should not neglect to treat the underlying cause). However, in such cases blood transfusion or parenteral iron may be necessary.

(iv) Wrong diagnosis

Hypochromic anaemia may be due to causes other than iron deficiency. If the diagnosis is not in doubt and manipulation of the oral regimen fails to produce a therapeutic response parenteral iron should be considered.

(c) Parenteral iron therapy

Parenteral iron should be used only if there is failure to respond to oral therapy in the following circumstances:

(1) excessive adverse effects from oral iron or poor compliance;

(2) malabsorption of oral iron;

(3) continued loss when the underlying cause cannot be remedied (in some cases intermittent blood transfusion may be sufficient).

Two parenteral iron formulations are available: iron dextran and iron sorbitol. Iron dextran may be given i.m. and i.v. However, the occasional occurrence of severe allergic reactions after i.v. infusion dictates that the i.v. route be used rarely and with caution. Iron sorbitol may only be given i.m.

The administration of parenteral iron is discussed in the Pharmacopoeia (p. 620)

28.1.2 Anaemia due to deficiency of vitamin B$_{12}$ or folate

The main causes of megaloblastic anaemia are given in Table 28.3. If eradication of the underlying cause is not possible long-term treatment with vitamin B$_{12}$ and/or folic acid will be necessary.

(a) Pernicious anaemia

Pernicious anaemia is due to deficient production of intrinsic factor by parietal cells in the stomach,

■ **Table 28.3** Causes of megaloblastic anaemia

1. *Vitamin B$_{12}$ deficiency*
   - (a) Malabsorption
     - Gastric causes
     - Pernicious anaemia
     - Gastrectomy
     - Intestinal causes
     - Stagnation
     - Tropical sprue
     - Ileal resection and Crohn's disease
     - Fish tapeworm (*Diphyllobothrium latum*)
   - (b) Inadequate intake
     - Strict vegetarianism (Veganism)

2. *Folate deficiency*
   - (a) Inadequate intake
     - Dietary insufficiency; predisposing factors include old age. alcoholism, and scurvy
   - (b) Malabsorption
     - Coeliac disease
     - Dermatitis herpetiformis with malabsorption
     - Tropical sprue
   - (c) Increased demands
     - Pregnancy and lactation
     - Haemolytic anaemias
     - Malignancy and chronic inflammatory diseases
   - (d) Drugs
     - Anticonvulsants (for example phenytoin, barbiturates)
     - Dihydrofolate reductase inhibitors (for example pyrimethamine, trimethoprim, triamterene, methotrexate)

since intrinsic factor is necessary for the absorption of vitamin B$_{12}$ in the ileum. Daily requirements of vitamin B$_{12}$ are 1–2 micrograms and total body stores are 2000–5000 micrograms. Initially therefore one gives large doses of vitamin B$_{12}$ in order to replenish body stores. Thereafter it is sufficient to give large doses intermittently at long intervals.

Vitamin B$_{12}$ is the term used for several different cobalamins. Hydroxocobalamin is now the treatment of choice for vitamin B$_{12}$ deficiency and it is converted in the body to adenosylcobalamin. In pernicious anaemia it is given in a dosage of 1000 micrograms i.m. every 2–3 d to a total of six doses, followed by a single injection of 1000 micrograms every 3 months for life.

The response to initial therapy with hydroxocobalamin is very rapid, and the reticulocyte count starts to rise within 3 or 4 d, reaching a peak in 6–8 d, and gradually returning to normal in 2–3 weeks. The height of the reticulocyte response depends on the severity of the anaemia; in severe cases it may reach 40–50 per cent. The haemoglobin should return to normal within 5–6 weeks, as should platelet and white cell counts, which are often low in pernicious anaemia.

If red cell production during treatment is very fast, iron stores may be depleted due to excessive demands. If iron deficiency results during treatment of pernicious anaemia, or if you suspect that body iron stores may already be depleted (for example in a woman with heavy menstrual periods) treatment with oral iron should be given (for example ferrous sulphate 200 mg b.d.).

In pernicious anaemia therapy with folic acid is not necessary. Indeed, if folic acid alone is inadvertently given to a patient with pernicious anaemia the neurological effects of vitamin B$_{12}$ deficiency may be precipitated or exacerbated. This emphasizes the need to make an accurate diagnosis in a case of megaloblastic anaemia.

Blood transfusion is rarely required in pernicious anaemia and should be reserved for those with a haemoglobin below 4 g/dL and evidence of tissue hypoxia, when even the rapid response to hydroxocobalamin would not be fast enough, for example in patients with severe congestive cardiac failure, angina pectoris, or evidence of cerebral hypoxia.

(b) Other causes of vitamin B$_{12}$ deficiency

The treatment of vitamin B$_{12}$ deficiency due to causes other than pernicious anaemia is in most cases the same as for pernicious anaemia, but if the cause can be found and remedied (for example antibiotic therapy and surgery to remedy bacterial overgrowth in blind gastrointestinal loops) hydroxocobalamin therapy need be continued for only so long as is required to return the haemoglobin to normal.

(c) Folate deficiency

Total body folate stores are about 5 mg and daily requirements of folic acid are about 100–200 micrograms, a value which is not greatly exceeded by dietary intake. In pregnancy folic acid requirements may increase up to tenfold and folic acid supplements should be given to prevent megaloblastic anaemia (see iron deficiency above).

In other conditions associated with folate deficiency the usual dosage of folic acid is 10–20 mg o.d. orally for a week or two, followed by an oral maintenance dosage of 5 mg o.d. These dosages will be suitable in all cases of megaloblastic anaemia due to folate deficiency (Table 28.3) except those due to dihydrofolate reductase inhibitors, since they inhibit the conversion of folic acid to its active metabolites. In such cases folinic acid may be used instead, 15 mg orally o.d.

28.2 Myeloproliferative disorders

The myeloproliferative disorders include polycythaemia rubra vera, myelofibrosis, chronic granulocytic leukaemia, and essential thrombocythaemia. They are grouped together because they are regarded as being a continuum of disorders. For example, patients with polycythaemia may go on to develop myelofibrosis or acute myeloblastic leukaemia.

28.2.1 Polycythaemia rubra vera

In polycythaemia rubra vera there is an increase in circulating red cell mass with an increase in the numbers of circulating white cells and platelets. This form of polycythaemia must be distinguished from other forms, such as those secondary to chronic hypoxia or to abnormal erythropoietin production by a tumour or a renal abnormality.

The aim of treatment of polycythaemia rubra vera is to reduce the numbers of circulating red cells and platelets. Three forms of treatment are available: venesection, radioactive phosphorus (^{32}P), and alkylating agents (for example busulphan). In addition to these, most patients will require treatment of hyperuricaemia (for example with allopurinol 300 mg orally o.d.).

(a) Venesection

Venesection is effective in reducing red cell mass and in some cases may be all the treatment that is required. However, venesection does not reduce the numbers of circulating platelets and does not alter the risk of thromboembolism. ^{32}P and busulphan can be used to reduce the numbers of red cells and platelets, thus reducing the risk of thromboembolism, but there is then an increased risk of other complications, particularly haemorrhage (perhaps due to abnormal platelet function). There is also a risk of leukaemia with busulphan and ^{32}P treatment.

The aim of venesection should be to reduce the haematocrit to between 45 and 50 per cent. Iron deficiency will eventually occur, since 200 mg of iron are removed with every 500 mL of blood, but iron treatment should be given only if there are symptoms of iron deficiency (i.e. a sore tongue and angular stomatitis).

(b) Busulphan

Because of the risk of adverse effects busulphan should be reserved for short courses of treatment in patients with very high platelet counts (above 800×10^9/L). It is given in an initial dosage of 4–6 mg orally o.d., reducing to 2 mg o.d. when the platelet count is reduced by 50 per cent. Treatment can be withdrawn when the platelet count falls below 250×10^9/L. The adverse effects of busulphan are given in the Pharmacopoeia (p. 566).

(c) Radioactive phosphorus (^{32}P)

^{32}P may be used instead of busulphan in patients with very high platelet counts (above 800×10^9/L) if short-term treatment with busulphan is ineffective. It is given in a single dose of 3–5 mCi (111–185 MBq) i.v. One dose will be effective in well over half of all patients, but some may need a second dose (2–3 mCi; 74–111 MBq) at 8–12 weeks. ^{32}P is particularly useful in producing long-term control in old people, reducing their need to attend hospital too frequently.

28.2.2 Myelofibrosis

Myelofibrosis results in anaemia, splenomegaly, and hepatomegaly. Bleeding may occur because of thrombocytopenia, gout because of hyperuricaemia, and anaemia both because of haemorrhage and because of ineffective erythropoiesis due to folate deficiency.

Treatment is usually symptomatic and may be limited to blood transfusion to keep the haemoglobin at or above 9 g/dL. Busulphan or hydroxyurea may also be used, especially if there is symptomatic splenomegaly (with abdominal swelling and pain or discomfort). Busulphan is given in a dosage of 2–4 mg orally o.d. for 3–4 weeks, followed by 2 mg two to three times a week. The blood count should be monitored regularly. If hydroxyurea is used it is begun in a dosage of 500 mg daily and the dosage is increased according to white cell and platelet counts and the response of the splenomegaly.

Allopurinol may be used to treat hyperuricaemia. Ineffective erythropoiesis may be countered by treating folate deficiency.

28.2.3 Thrombocythaemia

Thrombocythaemia may occur in isolation ('essential thrombocythaemia') or secondary to one of the other myeloproliferative disorders. It should be treated with ^{32}P as for polycythaemia, or if that fails with busulphan 2–4 mg/d or hydroxyurea 1–2 g/d.

28.2.4 Chronic granulocytic leukaemia

In chronic granulocytic leukaemia the aim of drug therapy is to treat symptoms, since current drug therapy does not prolong survival. Reduction of the circulating load of neoplastic cells and of spleen size produces symptomatic relief, and this can be achieved with busulphan or hydroxy-

urea. One recommended regimen is to give 4–6 mg orally o.d. until the white cell count is 10×10^9/L, then to withhold treatment until the count is 25×10^9/L, and then to repeat the busulphan. As an alternative one may use hydroxyurea (0.5–2.0 g orally o.d.), particularly in patients who develop pulmonary fibrosis or thrombocytopenia on busulphan. Since it is cleared unchanged by the kidneys dosages should be reduced in renal failure. Its major adverse effects are those of all other cytotoxic drugs (see p. 512).

The major difference between busulphan and hydroxyurea is that the effects of the former persist after a course of therapy, while the latter must be given as long-term therapy since withdrawing it will result in an increase in white cell count.

Hyperuricaemia may be treated with allopurinol, which should also be used to prevent hyperuricaemia when cytotoxic drugs are used.

In patients in whom cytotoxic drugs are contra-indicated (for example in pregnancy) or in those in whom very high white cell counts are causing adverse effects, a rapid reduction in white cell count may be achieved with a cell separator.

For young patients bone-marrow transplantation will produce a cure in up to 70 per cent of cases. It should be offered to those under 50 years who have an HLA identical sibling; otherwise efforts should be made to find a donor for an unrelated bone-marrow transplant.

When chronic granulocytic leukaemia becomes acute it should be treated according to whether it is an acute myeloid or lymphoid leukaemia (see below).

28.3 Lymphoproliferative disorders

The term 'lymphoproliferative disorders' is used to describe the group of malignancies which arise from lymphatic tissues. These disorders include chronic lymphocytic leukaemia and the lymphomas (Hodgkin's and non-Hodgkin's lymphomas).

28.3.1 Chronic lymphoid leukaemias

The chronic lymphoid leukaemias include chronic lymphocytic leukaemias (B-cell and T-cell), prolymphocytic leukaemia, and hairy cell leukaemia. B-cell chronic lymphocytic leukaemia is the commonest.

In contrast to acute lymphoblastic leukaemia, chronic lymphocytic leukaemia almost always affects the middle-aged and elderly and often needs no drug treatment. When treatment is given it is with the aim of reducing the total body load of lymphocytes, and this should be done only in patients who have evidence of a marked increase in the numbers of lymphocytes in the bone-marrow and who develop anaemia, thrombocytopenia, and neutropenia, or in patients who have substantial lymph node or splenic enlargement. The overall prognosis is not improved by drug therapy, but symptomatic treatment, if judiciously used, can improve the quality of life.

Chlorambucil is the usual initial treatment, either as continuous low-dose therapy (2–4 mg orally o.d.) or as high-dose intermittent therapy (20 mg/m^2) for 2–3 days. Improvement will occur in over 50 per cent of cases. Cyclophosphamide, 1–2 mg/kg/d, is an alternative.

In patients with auto-immune thrombocytopenia or haemolytic anaemia a short course of prednisolone may be used (60 mg daily initially, tailing off to a maintenance dosage as improvement occurs). Prednisolone should also be used

before starting chlorambucil in patients who present with features of bone-marrow suppression. Large masses of lymph nodes may need treatment with radiotherapy and splenomegaly may need splenectomy.

28.3.2 Hodgkin's lymphoma

The approach to the patient with Hodgkin's lymphoma depends on the stage of the disease, as outlined in Table 28.4. The reason for staging is that the prognosis in stages I and IIA is very good with the use of irradiation only, while in stages IIIB and IV the prognosis is not as good and chemotherapy is required. The treatment of stages IIB and IIIA is controversial: some use radiotherapy alone, some add chemotherapy, and some use chemotherapy followed by radiotherapy to the sites of the original disease.

There are several different suitable drug regimens for the treatment of Hodgkin's lymphoma The so-called 'MOPP' regimen, outlined in Chapter 36 (p. 515) produces remission in about 60–80 per cent of cases, usually by the third to sixth course. There is little evidence that maintenance therapy thereafter improves survival. The 5 y survival rate is about 50–70 per cent. In stage IVB disease regimens which alternate MOPP with

■ **Table 28.4** Therapeutic approaches to Hodgkin's lymphoma based on staging (the Ann Arbor modification of the Rye system)

Stage*	Definition	Therapy
I	Disease limited to one group of lymph nodes or to a single non-lymphatic site	Irradiation of affected sites
II	Disease limited to more than one group of nodes, with or without localized non-lymphatic involvement, all on one side of the diaphragm only	Irradiation of affected sites
III	Involvement of nodes and/or spleen on both sides of the diaphragm, with or without localized non-lymphatic involvement	See text
IV	Disseminated disease	Chemotherapy

*The stages are subdivided into types A (asymptomatic) and B (symptomatic, i.e. weight loss, fever, night sweats).

ABVD (adriamycin, bleomycin, vinblastine, and dacarbazine) may produce initial remission rates of about 90 per cent.

28.3.3 Non-Hodgkin's lymphoma

In contrast to Hodgkin's lymphoma the non-Hodgkin's lymphomas have a relatively poor prognosis. They may be classified clinically in a similar fashion to Hodgkin's lymphoma, but there is no clear-cut allied therapeutic strategy, mainly because most patients have stage III or IV disease at the time of presentation. Histological classification is therefore used as a guide to treatment. The non-Hodgkin's lymphomas may be classified histologically as being of low grade, intermediate grade, or high grade, depending on the cell type, size, and distribution.

Low-grade non-Hodgkin's lymphomas have a good prognosis but are generally not curable, although in the rare case presenting in stage I they may be cured by radiotherapy. For other stages no treatment is usually necessary, unless there are symptoms or a large tumour mass, in which case chlorambucil should be used (10 mg/d orally for 2 weeks, stopped for 2 weeks, then repeated until a response occurs). This treatment is associated with remission rates of over 60 per cent.

Most high-grade lymphomas are disseminated at the time of diagnosis and are treated by combination chemotherapy, with a response rate of about 60–70 per cent. A typical example of a combined chemotherapeutic regimen is the 'CHOP' combination, which is given in a cycle which is repeated every 3 weeks to a total of six courses:

C = cyclophosphamide 750 mg/m^2 i.v. on day 1;

H = hydroxydaunomycin (doxorubicin) 50 mg/m^2 i.v. on day 1;

O = Oncovin® (vincristine) 1.4 mg/m^2 i.v. on day 1;

P = prednisolone 25 mg q.d.s. orally on days 1–5.

Lymphoblastic lymphomas can be treated in a similar fashion to acute lymphoblastic leukaemia (see below).

28.4 Acute leukaemias

The principles of cancer chemotherapy are discussed in Chapter 36 and here we shall discuss some aspects of the particular management of acute myeloid and lymphoid leukaemias, although it is beyond the scope of this book to discuss these specialized problems in detail.

28.4.1 Acute myeloid leukaemia

The term 'acute myeloid leukaemia' encompasses several varieties of leukaemia, including monocytic, myelomonocytic, and promyelocytic leukaemia, depending on the particular myeloid cell line predominantly involved.

The aims of treatment are to use drugs firstly to produce a complete haematological remission and then to prevent a relapse. Typical induction therapy would involve the use of three drugs, such as daunorubicin (50 mg/m^2 i.v. for 3 d), cytosine arabinoside (100 mg/m^2 by i.v. infusion b.d.), and 6-thioguanine (100 mg/m^2 orally b.d. for 10 d). Remission is achieved in 70 per cent of cases after one course and may be higher after a second course. Therapy to prevent relapse will then consist of other cytotoxic drugs, including mitoxantrone and etoposide. Other methods of maintaining remission include allogenic and autologous bone-marrow transplantation. Supportive therapy is facilitated by the use of indwelling central lines (such as a Hickman catheter) for giving chemotherapeutic drugs, blood products, and antibiotics.

The adverse effects of cytotoxic drugs are outlined in Chapter 36. In acute myeloid leukaemia anaemia is particularly dangerous when it is associated with thrombocytopenia, and these should be treated with blood and platelet transfusions. However, care should be taken in patients with high blast cell counts, which can lead to hyperviscosity and cerebral infarction. Platelet transfusion should be given if there is bleeding, in the presence of sepsis, or in anticipation of a fall in platelet count due to chemotherapy. Allopurinol should be used to treat and prevent hyperuricaemia.

28.4.2 Acute lymphoblastic leukaemia

The aims of treating acute lymphoblastic leukaemia, which mostly affects young adults and children, are to induce a haematological remission, to maintain that remission, and to eradicate leukaemia cells from the CNS or to prevent their invasion there. Examples of two regimens used are given in Chapter 36.

(a) Induction of remission

Remission is commonly obtained with daunorubicin, vincristine, prednisolone, and asparaginase.

(b) Treatment of the CNS

Radiotherapy and intrathecal methotrexate are used, often in combination, because systemically administered drugs do not eradicate leukaemia cells from the CNS. In some centres high-dose methotrexate alone is used, since long-term adverse effects have been attributed to cranial irradiation.

(c) Maintenance of remission

Maintenance therapy is with monthly vincristine and prednisolone, together with weekly methotrexate and daily mercaptopurine. The dosages of methotrexate and mercaptopurine are titrated to the neutrophil count and maintenance therapy is continued for 2 years. Remember that if allopurinol is used to treat hyperuricaemia the dosage of mercaptopurine must be reduced (see p. 128).

28.5 Monoclonal gammopathies

The monoclonal gammopathies comprise a group of conditions which includes multiple myeloma, plasmacytomas, Waldenstrom's macroglobulinaemia, heavy chain disease, and primary amyloidosis.

28.5.1 Multiple myeloma

In multiple myeloma there is neoplastic infiltration of plasma cells. This results in anaemia, lytic bone lesions, hypercalcaemia, renal failure, and an increased susceptibility to infection. Patients can be classified into those with small, intermediate, or large tumour cell masses, on the basis of haematological, biochemical, and radiological findings (Table 28.5). This classification allows one to assess the prognosis before treatment and

to assess the response to chemotherapy. The aims of treatment are to induce a remission, to maintain that remission, and to treat the complications of the disease.

(a) Induction of remission

Melphalan is a conventional effective therapy for myeloma. A typical regimen is $7 \, mg/m^2$ orally o.d. given for 4 d and repeated at intervals of 3–4 weeks. Weekly cyclophosphamide i.v. is an alternative to melphalan.

The dosage of melphalan can be altered depending on the response or the occurrence of toxicity. The dosage should be reduced if the white cell count falls below $4.5 \times 10^9/L$ or if the platelet count falls below $100 \times 10^9/L$. Treatment should be withdrawn if the counts fall below $3 \times 10^9/L$ or $75 \times 10^9/L$ respectively. Therapy should also be monitored by regular measurement of haemoglobin, serum calcium (if increased), serum IgG and IgA, and urinary excretion of light chains.

One can expect remission in about 50 per cent of cases, irrespective of the tumour cell mass before treatment.

(b) Maintenance of remission

If improvement occurs with induction therapy (a fall to below 50 per cent in the concentration of serum myeloma protein from the pre-treatment value) maintenance therapy should be continued using melphalan and prednisolone in intermittent courses as before. For those with a small tumour cell mass treatment should be given for 1 year, but patients with a large tumour cell mass may require treatment for longer.

Dosages of melphalan should be reduced in patients with renal failure in proportion to the creatinine clearance.

Survival time in multiple myeloma depends on the time spent in remission. Patients with a small tumour cell mass who respond to therapy have a median survival time of 40–46 months, while those with a large tumour cell mass and who are unresponsive have a median survival time of 9–14 months.

Regimens of combination chemotherapy (for example the so-called ABCM regimen: adriamycin (doxorubicin), BCNU (carmustine), cyclophosphamide, and melphalan) have recently been

■ **Table 28.5** Prediction of tumour mass in multiple myeloma

	Small tumour mass	Large tumour mass
Haemoglobin	Over 10 g/dL	Below 8.5 g/dL
Serum calcium*	Below 3 mmol/L	Over 3 mmol/L
Immunoglobulins	IgG below 50 g/L	IgG over 70 g/L
	or	or
	IgA below 30 g/L	IgA over 50 g/L
Bone X-ray	Normal or one lesion	Many lesions
	All of the above = low tumour mass†	Any of the above = high tumour mass†

*Corrected for serum albumin:
  corrected calcium (mmol/L) = measured calcium + (0.025 × (40 − albumin in g/L))
†Patients who do not fulfil either of these criteria are classified as having an intermediate tumour mass.

shown to be more effective than melphalan alone. The combination of vincristine with doxorubicin and high-dose prednisolone is also effective and is useful when there is renal impairment, since melphalan and some of the active metabolites of carmustine are eliminated via the kidneys.

(c) Treatment of complications

(i) Hypercalcaemia

Hypercalcaemia usually responds to vigorous rehydration with oral fluids or intravenous saline, prednisolone, and treatment of the underlying myeloma. Frusemide can be used to increase urinary calcium excretion, although care must be taken to avoid dehydration through its diuretic action. Bisphosphonates both i.v. and orally may also be of help (see p. 377). In some patients plicamycin may be of value when other methods fail (see p. 378). However, plicamycin should not be used in patients with thrombocytopenia, since it may impair clotting factor synthesis, increasing the likelihood of bleeding. In such patients or if plicamycin is ineffective calcitonin may be of value.

(ii) Bone pain

Symptomatic relief of bone pain may be achieved with local radiotherapy. If there is bony involvement with hypercalcaemia, bone formation may be encouraged by the use of sodium fluoride (50 mg orally b.d.) with calcium carbonate (1 g orally q.d.s.).

(iii) Hyperuricaemia

Hyperuricaemia should be treated with allopurinol. Allopurinol should also be given 2 d before starting chemotherapy and continued during it in order to prevent drug-induced hyperuricaemia.

(iv) Hyperviscosity

Increased plasma viscosity, especially in IgA myeloma, may cause visual defects, changes in mental state, neurological deficits, or haemorrhage. It should be treated by encouraging a high fluid intake and, if severe, with plasmapheresis.

(v) Renal impairment

Dehydration must be avoided. If renal failure occurs dialysis may be necessary.

(vi) Infections

Patients with multiple myeloma are more susceptible to infections, because of impaired white cell function and reduced amounts of normal immunoglobulins. If there is any evidence of infection specimens should be taken for culture and aggressive antibacterial therapy should be started immediately (see below).

28.5.2 Waldenström's macroglobulinaemia

Waldenström's macroglobulinaemia is a slowly progressing low-grade lymphoma characterized by the secretion of an IgM paraprotein. The increase in IgM concentrations can lead to a marked increase in blood viscosity which can give rise to the hyperviscosity syndrome, the acute effects of which may require correction by plasmapheresis. The plasma concentration of paraprotein can be reduced with drugs such as chlorambucil, leading to improvement in bone-marrow function.

28.6 Drug-induced blood dyscrasias

Drugs can cause selective thrombocytopenia, selective leucopenia (usually neutropenia or so-called agranulocytosis), or pancytopenia, in which all the formed elements of the blood are affected. They can also cause haemolytic anaemia. Virtually any drug can cause any of these adverse effects, but some do it more commonly than others, and they are listed in Tables 28.6–28.9.

28.6.1 Prevention of blood dyscrasias

Before using a drug which carries a relatively high risk of causing a blood dyscrasia the relative benefit:risk ratio must be assessed. For example, in the treatment of some infections (for example *Haemophilus influenzae* meningitis and typhoid fever) chloramphenicol remains the drug of first choice, because these diseases are serious and chloramphenicol is considerably more effective than other drugs. However, for other infections alternative antibiotics may be equally good or better and the risk of neutropenia less than with chloramphenicol.

In the treatment of malignancies the risk of pancytopenia has to be set against the potential benefit. It may be difficult to assess the benefit:risk ratios for various cytotoxic drug combination schedules and treatment decisions in the indi-

■ **Table 28.6** Drugs which can cause pancytopenia*

Antibiotics
  Chloramphenicol
  Isoniazid
  Sulphonamides
  Streptomycin
Anticonvulsants
  Hydantoins (for example phenytoin)
  Succinimides (for example ethosuximide)
  Primidone
  Troxidone
Antimalarial drugs
  Pyrimethamine
  Antirheumatic drugs
  Colchicine
  Gold salts
  Indomethacin
  Penicillamine
  Phenylbutazone and oxyphenbutazone
Antithyroid drugs
  Carbimazole and methimazole
  Potassium perchlorate
  Thiouracils
Cytotoxic and immunosuppressive drugs
  (see Table 35.2)
Oral hypoglycaemic drugs
  Chlorpropamide
  Tolbutamide
Psychotropic drugs
  Meprobamate
  Mianserin
  Phenothiazines (for example chlorpromazine)
  Tricyclic antidepressants (for example amitriptyline)
Others
  Acetazolamide

*These drugs can also cause selective neutropenia or thrombocytopenia

vidual often have to be based on the results of formal clinical trials in the population.

28.6.2 Identification of patients at risk

It is generally not possible to identify the patients who are most at risk, but those with a history of drug allergy or of a previous blood dyscrasia should be monitored closely. Any drug known

■ **Table 28.7** Drugs which can cause selective neutropenia

Drugs which can also cause pancytopenia
(Table 28.6)
Amodiaquine
Antihistamines
Captopril
Metronidazole
Mianserin
Para-aminosalicylic acid
Phenindione
Sulphasalazine
Thiacetazone

■ **Table 28.8** Drugs which can cause selective thrombocytopenia

Drugs which can also cause pancytopenia
(Table 28.6)
Carbamazepine
Chloroquine
Digitoxin*
Mepacrine
Meprobamate
Methyldopa*
Quinidine*
Quinine*
Rifampicin*
Salicylates*
Tetracyclines
Thiazide diuretics

*These drugs may cause thrombocytopenia by a direct effect on circulating platelets, similar to that caused by apronal (Sedormid®), rather than by an effect on the bone-marrow (see Chapter 9, p. 111).

to have caused a blood dyscrasia in a patient should not be given to that patient again.

28.6.3 Monitoring for blood dyscrasias

Patients should be warned of the possibility of a blood dyscrasia when the risk is very high and they should be educated about the warning signs: general malaise, fever, a sore mouth or throat, signs of bruising, haemorrhage (for example nose bleeds), and skin rashes.

Regular monitoring of blood counts is necessary for drugs which cause dose-dependent inhibition of marrow function, for example cytotoxic drugs. It is of less value for other drugs, since the blood dyscrasia may occur suddenly. A pre-dose full blood count should be done before starting treatment with a high-risk drug (for example chloramphenicol, phenylbutazone) and at regular intervals during therapy.

28.6.4 Treatment of blood dyscrasias

With cytotoxic drugs careful monitoring of the blood count will allow anticipation of blood dyscrasias and appropriate adjustment of dosages. However, if overtreatment with a cytotoxic drug inadvertently occurs, or if a non-dose-related blood dyscrasia occurs unexpectedly, the suspected drug or drugs should be withdrawn immediately. Unfortunately there are no tests which will identify the causative drug in an unexpected case, and all drugs must be suspected.

(a) Anaemia

Treat anaemia by transfusion to bring the haemoglobin above 12 g/dL. Transfusion should be repeated if the haemoglobin falls to 9 g/dL.

(b) Thrombocytopenia

If thrombocytopenia results in haemorrhage blood losses should be replaced by transfusion. Platelet transfusion may sometimes be necessary to help the patient over an acute haemorrhagic crisis. Drugs which can cause gastrointestinal bleeding should be avoided or withdrawn. In patients in whom platelet damage is associated with antibody production a short course of a corticosteroid may help.

(c) Neutropenia

It is important to prevent infection in patients with neutropenia and to treat infections vigorously when they occur. Infections in these patients are usually due to the organisms which they themselves carry and the risk of such infections can be reduced by scrupulous hygiene. A typical

▮ **Table 28.9** Drugs which can cause haemolytic anaemia

---

1. *Immune (i.e. due to the combination of drug hapten with antibody)*
   Cephalosporins
   Quinidine
   Quinine
   Penicillins
   Stibophen
   Sulphonamides

2. *Autoimmune (i.e. due to an antibody directed against the red cell membrane)*
   L-dopa
   Mefenamic acid
   Methyldopa
   Phenacetin

3. *In association with glucose-6-phosphate dehydrogenase (G6PD) deficiency*
   See Table 8.1

4. *Through altered red cell metabolism (effects enhanced by G6PD deficiency)*
   Dapsone
   Phenacetin

---

approach in the patient with neutropenia involves daily washing or bathing, regular shampooing with a disinfectant such as chlorhexidine, daily hydrogen peroxide and nystatin mouthwashes, the application of nystatin cream to armpits and groins, and the use of an antibiotic spray (for example framycetin) to eradicate nasal *Staphylococcus aureus*.

The use of sophisticated techniques for 'reverse barrier nursing' has not been shown to be of value in preventing infection, but it is common to nurse patients in single rooms and to have as few people as possible concerned with their regular care, in order to reduce the chance of the transfer of organisms.

When infection occurs it should be identified as quickly as possible by clinical examination, and by culture of blood, sputum, urine, and any obviously infected lesions. Antibacterial drugs should be given immediately without waiting for the results of culture. The antibiotics chosen should, in combination, be effective in treating both Gram-positive and Gram-negative organisms, particularly *Staph. aureus*, *Pseudomonas* spp., *E. coli*, and *Proteus* spp. One recommended

combination is gentamicin (80 mg i.m. or i.v. 6-hourly, adjusting the dose according to renal function) plus a penicillin with antipseudomonal activity, such as piperacillin (200–300 mg/kg/d in divided doses by i.v. infusion).

Particular care should be taken with indwelling lines, in which infections are common, especially with *Staph. epidermidis*, for which vancomycin would be the treatment of choice.

Fungal infections may be prevented using oral fluconazole or nystatin and nystatin pessaries.

In patients whose infection does not respond to first-line antimicrobial therapy and in whom there is persistent fever for up to two days without a formal identification of the infecting organism, a change to two other broad-spectrum antibiotics, one of which should be vancomycin, would be a reasonable strategy.

Continuing fever, prolonged neutropenia, and failure to respond to second-line antibiotics, warrants the empirical use of intravenous amphotericin, on the assumption that there is a fungal infection.

Various drugs have been used to try to accelerate recovery of bone-marrow function, but none has proven efficacy. The most promising agents currently are the cloned colony-stimulating factors (GCSF, GMCSF, etc), which have been shown to reduce the duration of neutropenia after chemotherapy.

28.7 Complications of blood transfusion

We shall not deal in detail with blood transfusion, but a few points are worth making in relation to the prevention and treatment of its complications (listed in Table 28.10).

28.7.1 Immune reactions

Immune reactions to blood products are not uncommon, despite careful cross-matching, and the most serious is when incompatible blood is transfused. When any transfusion reaction occurs, stop the transfusion immediately and replace the i.v. giving-set, but continue infusing with saline in order to maintain access to the circulation. Check that the correctly labelled blood was being given for that patient and send the packet of blood to the laboratory for repeat cross-matching. If the wrong blood has been given make sure that another patient is not also at risk because of a mix-up. Send blood and urine samples to the laboratory for the diagnosis of acute haemolysis. If haemolysis has occurred specialist management of shock, renal failure, and disseminated intravascular coagulation may be required. It is most important to maintain renal blood flow in such cases by giving i.v. frusemide 40–80 mg initially, making sure at the same time that the patient remains well hydrated.

Febrile reactions are the commonest problem in transfusion, and are most commonly due to antibodies against white cells and need no specific treatment. Reactions consisting of urticaria and itching occur within minutes and can be treated satisfactorily with an antihistamine (see p. 523) and hydrocortisone 100 mg i.v. Recurrent allergic reactions to blood can be ameliorated by the prophylactic use of an antihistamine. See also the treatment of anaphylactic shock (p. 524).

28.7.2 Circulatory overload

Circulatory overload causing cardiac failure in patients with a normal intravascular volume is avoidable by giving frusemide 20 mg i.v. just before each unit of blood or packed cells. If cardiac failure occurs the transfusion should be stopped and frusemide given i.v. Other treatment of left ventricular failure may sometimes be necessary (see p. 291).

28.7.3 Complications of massive transfusion

In patients who require large volumes of blood hyperkalaemia, hypocalcaemia, hypothermia, and bleeding may occur.

Hyperkalaemia may occur because potassium in the red cells of citrated blood used in transfusion leaks into the plasma. Children and patients with renal failure must be carefully monitored in order to avoid this complication.

Hypocalcaemia may occur because of sequestration of calcium by citrate. Calcium gluconate should be given (10 mL of a 10 per cent solution i.v.).

■ **Table 28.10** Complications of blood transfusion

1. *Immediate*
   (a) Complications of any transfusion
       Acute allergic reactions
       Haemolysis
       Fever
       Anaphylaxis
       Air embolism
       Circulatory overload
       Infections causing acute septicaemia
       Hyperkalaemia
   (b) Complications of massive transfusion
       Hypocalcaemia (due to excess citrate)
       Hypothermia
       Coagulation defects due to dilution of clotting factors

2. *Delayed*
   Infections, particularly hepatitis and AIDS
   Iron overload (transfusion siderosis)
   Delayed hypersensitivity
   Delayed haemolytic reactions

Hypothermia may occur because of the transfusion of a large amount of blood which has been stored at 4°C. It can be avoided by warming the blood before transfusion, but care must be taken during warming not to cause haemolysis by overheating.

Bleeding may occur because of dilution of clotting factors and platelets, which can be replaced by an infusion of fresh frozen plasma and platelets.

28.7.4 Transfusion siderosis

In patients who are given large amounts of blood repeatedly (for example in thalassaemia) iron overload may occur. When the total body load of iron is greater than 0.7 g/kg it causes damage to the tissues in which it is deposited, analogous to the tissue damage found in haemochromatosis. This can result in failure of growth in children, hepatic and cardiac failure, and sometimes endocrine disorders (for example diabetes mellitus, hypoparathyroidism).

Treatment is with desferrioxamine, as outlined in the Pharmacopoeia (p. 594). Vitamin C (100–200 mg orally o.d.) is given with desferrioxamine to enhance its therapeutic effect.

28.8 Blood substitutes

Colloidal solutions can be given instead of plasma or blood when hypovolaemia is a problem, for example in burns or shock or while waiting for blood after acute blood loss. They are of three types: dextrans, gelatins, and hydroxyethyl starch. They are not of value if there is also protein depletion, when plasma should be used.

28.8.1 Dextrans

Dextrans are polymers of glucose available in mixtures of different molecular weights. The available formulations have average osmotically-active molecular weights of about 20 000 daltons (dextran 40), 35 000 daltons (dextran 70), and 55 000 daltons (dextran 110). The half-time of these dextrans is about 12 h.

Dextran 70 is the plasma substitute of choice when small volumes are required. However, in large amounts it may cause bleeding, by inhibiting platelet aggregation, enhancing fibrinolysis, and depleting factor VIII.

Cross-matching of blood cannot be done after dextran has been infused. Mild allergic reactions are common and occasionally serious reactions can occur.

Because of its effects on coagulation dextran 40 is sometimes used in the prophylaxis of venous thrombosis (see p. 297)

28.8.2 Gelatins

Partially degraded gelatin is available as succinylated gelatin and polygeline, which have a lower average molecular weight than dextran 70 (about 24 000 daltons) and a shorter half-time (about 5 h).

Gelatins are used in the short-term replacement of fluid losses during surgery and can be given in large volumes, since they do not affect coagulation. Allergic reactions are uncommon. Polygeline contains much more calcium than succinylated gelatin and this can cause clotting if it is mixed with citrated blood or fresh frozen plasma.

Hydroxyethyl starch

Hydroxyethyl starch has an average molecular weight of 70 000 daltons and a very long half-time (about 17 d). It is expensive and has no particular advantages over dextrans and gelatins. It occasionally causes acute allergic reactions.

29 The drug therapy of disorders of bones and joints

Co-author: A. G. Mowat

29.1 Arthritis

Under this heading we shall consider the therapy of non-infective inflammatory arthritis, particularly rheumatoid arthritis and its variants, including arthritic involvement in connective tissue diseases, such as systemic lupus erythematosus, the therapy of osteoarthritis, of ankylosing spondylitis and related disorders, of soft tissue rheumatism, and of gout.

Drug treatment in these conditions can be considered in two parts.

1. Control of symptoms by analgesics and non-steroidal anti-inflammatory drugs.

2. Special measures in inflammatory arthritis, aimed at controlling the disease process, using gold salts, penicillamine, chloroquine, sulphasalazine, or azathioprine. Systemic corticosteroids are now used only infrequently in rheumatoid arthritis.

29.1.1 Mechanisms of action of non-steroidal anti-inflammatory drugs in relation to arthritis

So many non-steroidal anti-inflammatory drugs are on the market that the choice is bewildering. In the list given in Table 29.1 most of the non-steroidal anti-inflammatory drugs available are listed and many are discussed in the Pharmacopoeia (pp. 653, 669, 677). The student should be familiar with those asterisked in the Table.

There are two aspects of the actions of the non-steroidal anti-inflammatory drugs to consider: their analgesic effects and their anti-inflammatory effects. The analgesic effects of these drugs come on quickly and go away within a few hours. In contrast, their anti-inflammatory effects come on over a few days and require regular and repeated dosage.

Non-steroidal anti-inflammatory drugs inhibit the conversion of arachidonic acid to cyclic endoperoxides by inhibiting the enzyme cyclooxygenase, and this results in reduced production of prostaglandins such as PGE_2 and prostacyclin (Fig. 29.1). Many of the actions of the non-steroidal anti-inflammatory drugs, both therapeutic and adverse, are probably brought about through this action.

Non-steroidal anti-inflammatory drugs probably produce at least some of their anti-inflammatory effects by inhibition of prostaglandin synthesis. Prostaglandins are normally released in inflammatory responses. They are involved in the production of hyperalgesia, erythema, and exudation, and their effects are synergistic with the effects of other inflammatory mediators. As the inflammatory reaction is controlled this pharmacological effect results in a reduction in pain, tenderness, swelling, and temperature, reduced stiffness, and increased movement and strength of movement in the affected joints.

Inhibition of prostaglandin synthesis is also responsible for the gastrointestinal mucosal damage, peptic erosions and ulcers, and gastrointestinal bleeding associated with the non-steroidal anti-inflammatory drugs. Misoprostol, a prostaglandin analogue, can prevent these effects when given with the non-steroidal anti-inflammatory drugs, although it should not be used routinely in all patients taking these drugs (see p. 326).

▮ **Table 29.1** Non-steroidal anti-inflammatory drugs

1. *Salicylates* (p. 677)
   Aspirin*
   Benorylate
   Choline magnesium trisalicylate
   Diflunisal
   Aloxiprin
   Salsalate

2. *Arylalkanoic acids* (p. 653)
   (a) Acetic acid derivatives
       Diclofenac
       Etodolac
       Indomethacin*
       Sulindac
       Acemetacin
       Tiaprofenic acid
       Tolmetin
   (b) Propionic acid derivatives
       Fenoprofen
       Flurbiprofen
       Ibuprofen*
       Ketoprofen
       Naproxen*
   (c) Butyric acid derivatives
       Fenbufen
       Nabumetone

3. *Anthranilic acids* (p.653)
   Mefenamic acid

4. *Pyrazolones* (p. 669)
   Azapropazone
   Phenylbutazone
       (ankylosing spondylitis only)

5. *Oxicams*
   Piroxicam
   Tenoxicam

*Drugs with which the student should be familiar.

The bleeding tendency produced by non-steroidal anti-inflammatory drugs is also caused by inhibition of platelet cyclo-oxygenase. Reduced production of thromboxane interferes with platelet aggregation and there is an increased bleeding tendency, which adds to the dangers of peptic erosion.

29.1.2 The clinical use of non-steroidal anti-inflammatory drugs

In mild rheumatoid arthritis or osteoarthritis and early in the disease all that may be needed to control symptoms is intermittent analgesia with mild analgesics.

When symptoms become more severe and are not controlled by simple analgesics non-steroidal anti-inflammatory drugs are given.

In using anti-inflammatory drugs it is important to recognize that there is a great deal of variability in patients' responses to different drugs. Patients should be educated to recognize a clinical response, and should know about the common adverse effects of the non-steroidal anti-inflammatory drugs. For many patients complete control of daytime and night-time pain, the total relief of morning stiffness, and the return of full function is an unrealistic hope, but a trial of three or four different drugs from different chemical groupings (see Table 29.1) over an 8-week period is not unreasonable when trying to establish effective therapy in an individual with chronic disease.

There are different therapeutic fashions in various parts of the world as regards first and subsequent choices of these drugs in the treatment of arthritis. While in the USA there are many proponents of aspirin (600–900 mg q.d.s.) as first choice, in the UK many rheumatologists feel that these dosages of aspirin carry an unacceptably high risk of adverse effects, and they prefer to start treatment with an arylalkanoic acid derivative, such as ibuprofen or naproxen, which have a lower incidence of adverse effects. Alternative first choices might be diclofenac, fenoprofen, flurbiprofen, or sulindac.

If one starts with, say, an arylalkanoic acid derivative and if in an adequate dosage one's first choice does not appear to be working well within 2–3 weeks a switch to another drug is indicated, even a drug of the same class, for example from naproxen to flurbiprofen. Many rheumatologists will back up the daytime choice if necessary with indomethacin 100 mg at night, giving slow-release formulations or suppositories if adverse effects prove a nuisance. This improves morning stiffness and relieves overnight pain, which can be very distressing.

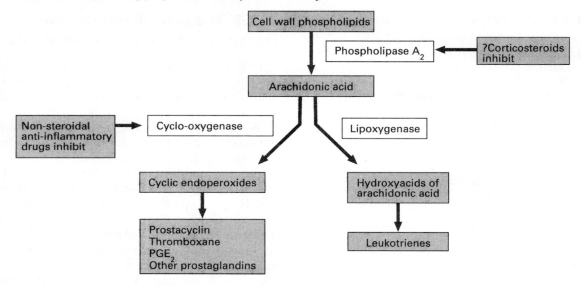

■ **Fig. 29.1** Biosynthetic pathways of leukotrienes and prostaglandins, and the mechanisms of actions of drugs which inhibit their production.

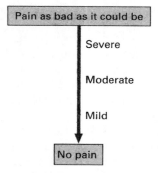

■ **Fig. 29.2** A visual analogue scale used in rating severity of pain. When descriptive terms such as 'severe', 'moderate', and 'mild' are included it is called a graphic rating scale. The line is usually 10 cm long to allow ease of measurement of the point marked by the patient. A vertical format may produce more reliable results than a horizontal one. (Adapted from Huskisson (1974). *Lancet* **ii**, 1127–31, with permission.)

Many patients with rheumatoid arthritis or osteoarthritis may also need, in addition to their non-steroidal anti-inflammatory drug therapy, a further supply of a drug to be used specifically as an analgesic, for example paracetamol, co-codamol, or co-proxamol. Some patients find

that a small dose of aspirin, in addition to their other non-steroidal anti-inflammatory drug therapy, is effective as an acute analgesic, while others 'top up' with an extra dose of their non-steroidal anti-inflammatory drug, which can produce extra analgesia for a time.

The duration of treatment depends on the disease. In osteoarthritis there may be short-term symptoms from one or two joints, in which case treatment can be withdrawn after a few weeks. On the other hand, if the affected joints cause chronic pain, stiffness, and functional disability, prolonged treatment may be necessary. In such cases physical treatments and surgery may also be required.

In rheumatoid arthritis an acute flare-up may require only short-term treatment with a non-steroidal anti-inflammatory drug. However, if the disease is chronically active long-term therapy will be needed. If the disease is active and causing serious symptoms and disability after 6 months of what is thought to be optimal therapy, disease-modifying drugs may be necessary (see below), although before considering such therapy other measures should be considered, such as intra-articular steroids and orthopaedic procedures for problem joints.

Monitoring the effects of anti-inflammatory drugs is difficult, but may be helped by the use of a visual analogue scale, such as that shown in Fig. 29.2.

29.1.3 Mechanisms of action of disease-modifying drugs in rheumatoid arthritis

Certain drugs seem able not simply to relieve the symptoms of rheumatoid arthritis, but actually to alter the course of the disease. These drugs are listed in Table 29.2.

(a) Penicillamine

Although penicillamine has many known actions, none convincingly explains its therapeutic effect in rheumatoid arthritis. Its actions include chelation of metals, alteration of cross-linkage of collagen, alteration in the production of some immunoglobulins, a reduction in the concentrations of circulating immune complexes, suppression of lymphocyte stimulation by some agents, and enhancement of neutrophil chemotaxis.

(b) Gold salts

Gold salts are taken up by macrophages. They inhibit phagocytosis and lysosomal enzyme activity. Cell-mediated immune reactions are suppressed. In rheumatoid arthritis gold salts reduce the concentrations of rheumatoid factor and immunoglobulins. However, none of these actions adequately explains their therapeutic

■ **Table 29.2** Drugs which may modify the disease process in rheumatoid arthritis

---

Chloroquine (p. 580)
Corticosteroids (p. 584)
Gold salts (p. 610)
    Sodium aurothiomalate
    Auranofin
Immunosuppressive drugs
    Azathioprine (p. 561)
    Cyclophosphamide (p. 590)
    Cyclosporin (p. 591)
    Methotrexate (p. 632)
Penicillamine (p. 657)
Sulphasalazine (p. 688)

---

effects. Nor are the mechanisms clear whereby gold salts produce their adverse effects.

(c) Chloroquine

The basis of the action of chloroquine in arthritis is also very poorly understood. Among its effects it may have a direct anti-inflammatory action by stabilizing lysosomes, thereby inhibiting the release of lysosomal enzymes and preventing their inflammatory effects.

(c) Sulphasalazine

The mechanism of action of sulphasalazine in rheumatoid arthritis is not known, although it does have immunosuppressive actions. The sulphapyridine rather than the salicylate seems to be the active component (contrast ulcerative colitis, see p. 333).

(d) Corticosteroids and immunosuppressive drugs

These drugs presumably act by virtue of their immunosuppressive and anti-inflammatory actions. However, as with other disease-modifying drugs in rheumatoid arthritis, their exact mechanisms of action are unknown. Among the immunosuppressive drugs which have been used in rheumatoid arthritis are azathioprine, methotrexate, cyclophosphamide, and cyclosporin.

For further discussion of immunosuppressive drugs see Chapter 37.

29.1.4 The clinical use of disease-modifying drugs in rheumatoid arthritis

The disease-modifying drugs are toxic. One must therefore have good reasons for using them and should generally seek specialist advice before doing so. The indications for disease-modifying drugs in rheumatoid arthritis are when non-steroidal anti-inflammatory drugs have been used for 6 months without ameliorating severe disease or when there is progressive disease with deformities, erosions, and worsening disabilities. Extra-articular manifestations of disease, such as nodules, neuropathy, skin ulcers, and purpuric rashes, may also be indications.

The first choice usually lies between penicillamine and gold salts. Chloroquine and sulphasalazine are alternatives.

(a) Penicillamine

Penicillamine is effective in about 60 per cent of patients within 8–12 weeks of treatment and in about 70 per cent within 6 months. Joint swelling is reduced and nodules disappear. The erythrocyte sedimentation rate (e.s.r.) and rheumatoid factor fall. In adults one would start with 250 mg daily orally, increasing after 4–6 weeks to 500 mg daily. Some patients may require 750 mg or 1 g daily.

The high incidence and serious nature of the adverse effects of penicillamine, some of which are dose-related, limit its usefulness (Table 29.3). About 60 per cent of patients will experience adverse effects and about 30 per cent will withdraw from treatment as a result. Because of these adverse effects clinical supervision of patients should include a monthly blood count (including platelets), examination of the urine for protein, and monitoring of renal function.

■ **Table 29.3** Adverse effects of penicillamine

Adverse effect	Comment
Anorexia and nausea	Often resolves; do not reduce dosage
Loss of taste	Transient; resolves on continuation
Morbilliform rash	Occurs early; reduce or stop therapy; may rechallenge starting with low dosage
Pemphigus-like rash	Late onset; stop drug
Mouth· ulcers	Stop drug
Thrombocytopeniau	Stop drug if platelet count below 50×10^9/L
Pancytopenia	Stop drug
Proteinuria	Observe carefully; monitor 24 h urinary protein and check renal function; not always necessary to stop therapy
Nephrotic syndrome	Stop drug

If the patient tolerates penicillamine well it should be continued at the lowest effective dosage for as long as the arthritis remains active.

(b) Gold salts

Like penicillamine the therapeutic effects of gold salts develop slowly, reaching a maximum after about 4–6 months of therapy. Up to 50 per cent of patients respond. Gold is given i.m. as sodium aurothiomalate or orally as auranofin.

(i) Intramuscular gold

If the i.m. route is to be used a 10 mg test dose must first be given to exclude hypersensitivity and this is followed by 50 mg i.m. weekly until a response occurs. If the disease is controlled the interval between doses can be lengthened to 2 weeks or longer, a change in dosage interval being undertaken only every 3 months, because of the time it takes for the effect of an increase or decrease in dosage to be reflected in the clinical state. If there is no response after a total of 1000 mg has been given (i.e. treatment for about 20 weeks) i.m. gold should be discontinued. If there is a response treatment with monthly injections should be continued while the arthritis persists and for 5 years after complete remission. It is important to monitor carefully for adverse effects on the kidneys (i.e. proteinuria) and on the blood.

(ii) Oral gold

Auranofin is given in a dose of 6 mg/d in one or two doses, increasing after 3 months to 9 mg/d for a further 3 months if there is no response. Oral gold has fewer adverse effects than parenteral gold but is also less effective.

Gold salts cause adverse effects similar to those of penicillamine, and careful supervision in the same way, with monitoring of blood and urine, is necessary. Rashes occur in about 30 per cent of patients and can lead to exfoliative dermatitis, so that when a rash occurs treatment is usually stopped. As with penicillamine, thrombocytopenia, neutropenia, and pancytopenia can occur, and since they are potentially fatal treatment must be stopped. Proteinuria and the nephrotic syndrome also occur and require withdrawal of treatment. With oral gold diarrhoea is the most common adverse effect.

(c) Chloroquine

Chloroquine has the same sort of clinical effects as penicillamine and gold salts, and is an alternative to them for patients with less severe rheumatoid arthritis in whom the response to non-steroidal anti-inflammatory drugs is suboptimal. It is also used in systemic and discoid lupus erythematosus. It does not prevent progression of bony erosions.

The main drawback of chloroquine is its ocular toxicity, leading to progressive loss of vision, due to a retinopathy, the incidence of which increases if the dosage exceeds 250 mg daily for longer than one year. Any patient taking chloroquine should have a full ophthalmological examination once a year.

The recommended dosage of chloroquine base is 150 mg daily (equivalent to 150 mg of chloroquine phosphate and 200 mg of chloroquine sulphate). Some use chloroquine for 10 months of the year with 2 months rest. Hydroxychloroquine has fewer adverse effects than chloroquine, apart from retinopathy, and it is given in a dosage of 400 mg daily.

(d) Sulphasalazine

Sulphasalazine is effective in up to about 70 per cent of patients after 1 year. It is given in a usual maintenance dosage of 2–3 g/d. Adverse effects, mainly nausea, vomiting, and rashes, occur in about 25 per cent, but can be minimized by the gradual introduction of enteric-coated tablets over a period of 4 weeks. A clinical response may be expected within 4–8 weeks.

(e) Corticosteroids

The general anti-inflammatory and immuno-suppressive actions of corticosteroids are dealt with in Chapter 37.

In relation to rheumatoid arthritis it is important to note that:

1. Corticosteroids may suppress inflammation, but they do not alter the course of the disease.

2. The dosages required to suppress inflammation almost always produce Cushing's syndrome with all its serious implications.

3. The adverse effects of corticosteroids can cause as much suffering as the disease.

4. Once having initiated corticosteroid therapy it is very difficult to withdraw it.

The general rule therefore is to avoid the use of corticosteroids in the treatment of rheumatoid arthritis. With extreme care, and keeping in mind all the points above, there may occasionally be a case for their use, as for example when non-steroidal anti-inflammatory drugs have been unsuccessful in old people. Then an acute attack of rheumatoid arthritis can be controlled with small doses of prednisolone (not more than 5.0–7.5 mg daily), gradually reducing to complete withdrawal over a few months. Such treatment should be instituted only by a specialist rheumatologist. Corticosteroids may also be required for the treatment of some extra-articular problems, for example vasculitis, pneumonitis.

Intra-articular corticosteroids have a special place in active rheumatoid arthritis, being used to relieve symptoms confined to one or two joints. However, joint damage may occur with repeated injections and so care must be taken.

(f) Immunosuppressive drugs

Immunosuppressive drugs (which are discussed in Chapter 37) have a slow onset of action, like penicillamine and gold salts. Generally they are not used until both penicillamine and gold salts have been tried, and only when the disease is severe.

Azathioprine is used in a dosage of 1.5 mg/kg/d (usual adult dosage 100 mg/d). Marrow suppression, infection, nausea, vomiting, and diarrhoea are its major adverse effects. Full blood counts should be checked every month.

Methotrexate is being increasingly used in rheumatoid arthritis by specialist rheumatologists, although it is not yet licensed for this purpose in the UK. The dosage is 7.5–10 mg orally in several divided doses over a period of 12 h once a week. The response rate appears to be higher than with other disease modifying drugs, but there is a high risk of serious adverse effects, including pancytopenia, stomatitis, nausea, vomiting, diarrhoea, and renal impairment. Careful monitoring should pick these up and they are usually reversible if methotrexate is withdrawn early, but there remains concern about liver and lung toxicity (cirrhosis and pulmonary fibrosis). There may also be a place for folic acid supplements taken 3 d after the methotrexate to limit some of these adverse effects.

29.2 Gout and hyperuricaemia

29.2.1 Mechanisms of action of drugs used in the treatment of gout and hyperuricaemia

The drugs used in the treatment of gout and hyperuricaemia are listed in Table 29.4 and their mechanisms of action are shown in Fig. 29.3.

(a) Acute attacks of gout

(i) Non-steroidal anti-inflammatory drugs

The drugs in this group which are used in the treatment of acute attacks of gout (see Table 29.1) have effects similar to their effects in rheumatoid arthritis.

(ii) Colchicine

Colchicine is concentrated by leucocytes, within which it binds to microtubular protein. This is thought to cause inhibition of the migration of leucocytes into the areas in which sodium mono-urate crystals are deposited in the acute gouty attack, thereby reducing the inflammatory response.

∎ **Table 29.4** Drugs used in the treatment of gout and hyperuricaemia

---

1. *Acute attacks of gout*
   Non-steroidal anti-inflammatory drugs, for example indomethacin (see Table 29.1)
   Colchicine (p. 583)

2. *Long-term control of gout or hyperuricaemia*
   Allopurinol (p. 550)
   Probenecid (p. 666)
   Sulphinpyrazone (p. 689)

(b) Long-term control of gout and hyperuricaemia

(i) Allopurinol

Allopurinol inhibits the formation of uric acid from precursor xanthines by inhibition of the enzyme xanthine oxidase. The precursors are more soluble than uric acid and are readily excreted by the kidneys. Allopurinol is not effective in the treatment of an acute attack of gout, but is used to prevent attacks of gout and to prevent deposition of urate crystals in the kidney, thus preventing gouty nephropathy. It also prevents the deposition of urate crystals in other soft tissues. It thereby prevents the formation of gouty tophi and can cause their disappearance.

(ii) Probenecid and sulphinpyrazone

These drugs inhibit the active reabsorption of uric acid in the proximal tubule (see Fig. 29.4) and thus increase its urinary excretion.

29.2.2 The treatment of acute gout

First-choice treatment for a patient with acute gout is now a non-steroidal anti-inflammatory drug, such as indomethacin or naproxen. One would give indomethacin in an initial dose of 50–100 mg orally and continue with 50 mg every 4–6 h until the symptoms subsided, continuing then with lower dosages at longer intervals for about a week (for example 25 mg t.d.s.). Naproxen would be given in an initial dose of 750 mg followed by 250 mg every 8 h until the attack subsided.

Colchicine is effective and specific in acute gout, but it is not easy to use optimally and it causes gastrointestinal toxicity. It is therefore not now the treatment of first choice in acute gout. If it is used it should be started as early as possible in an acute attack, since it becomes less effective the longer the attack has gone on. The initial dose is 1 mg, followed by 500 micrograms every 2 h until the pain is relieved or vomiting or diarrhoea occurs. No more than a total of 10 mg should be given in a single course and a course should not be repeated within 3 d.

Systemic corticosteroids have no place in the treatment of acute gout, but in certain circum-

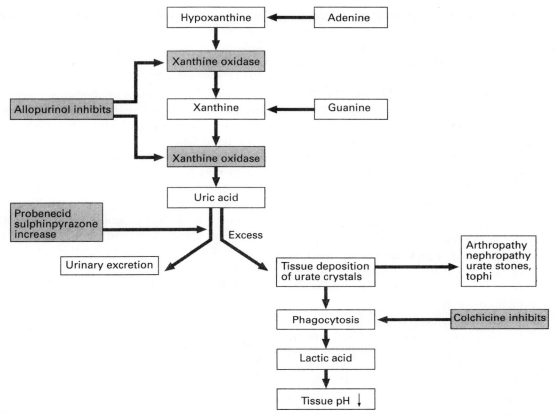

■ **Fig. 29.3** The pathophysiology of gout and the sites and mechanisms of action of drugs used in its treatment.

stances, for example in post-operative gout, or when the above therapy is ineffective, ACTH (corticotrophin) is effective (80 i.u. i.m. repeated the next day or after 2 d as necessary). Rebound gout may occur on stopping treatment and colchicine should be given to prevent this (0.5 mg t.d.s. for one week).

29.2.3 Treatment of threatened attacks

Patients who suffer from gout may have acute attacks, despite the preventive treatment described below. Such attacks may be aborted by the early and judicious use of a non-steroidal anti-inflammatory drug, such as indomethacin 25–50 mg 6-hourly for a few doses. In such cases treatment should be started at the onset of symptoms which the patient recognizes as being prodromal.

29.2.4 The long-term management of gout

In any patient with gout it is important to recognize that there may be associated conditions that need treatment or advice. These include hyperlipidaemia, obesity, hypertension, and excess alcohol intake. In a patient with hyperuricaemia (serum or plasma uric acid concentration over 0.42 mmol/L in adult men or 0.36 mmol/L in women) therapy to lower the uric acid concentration should be considered:

(1) if there have been acute attacks of gout;

(2) if there are tophi;

(3) if there is evidence of renal failure;

(4) if in the absence of signs or symptoms of gout there is a family history of gout and possible complications, for example renal failure and hypertension.

Allopurinol is the treatment of choice for asymptomatic gout, when treatment is indicated (i.e. case (4) above). The choice of drug in the treatment of symptomatic gout lies between allopurinol, which blocks the production of uric acid, and one of the uricosuric drugs (probenecid or sulphinpyrazone), which promote the excretion of uric acid. In both cases the aim is to lower plasma concentrations of uric acid.

Ideally one should measure not only serum uric acid concentrations, but also the urinary uric acid excretion rate. Then a rational choice of treatment can be made as follows:

1. If the serum uric acid is high and the 24 h urinary excretion of uric acid is consistently increased (on a restricted purine diet) to above 3.6 mmol/d then the patient is an over-producer of uric acid and allopurinol is the treatment of choice.

2. If the serum uric acid is high but the 24 h urinary excretion of uric acid is consistently lower than 2.4 mmol/d then there is reduced excretion of uric acid and a uricosuric drug may be preferred. Note, however, that uricosuric drugs are contra-indicated in nephrolithiasis.

(a) Allopurinol

Despite the theoretical considerations outlined above, allopurinol is now probably the treatment of choice in all cases. The initial dosage is 300 mg o.d. orally. The serum uric acid concentration should be checked after 3 months and the dose of allopurinol may then have to be adjusted accordingly. The usual maintenance dosage is 200–600 mg o.d. and it is likely that treatment will be life-long. Note that during the start of therapy with allopurinol acute attacks of gout may occur. For this reason colchicine 0.5 mg b.d. or a non-steroidal anti-inflammatory drug, such as indomethacin 25–50 mg b.d., should also be given for the first month or two. Allopurinol should not be started within 3 weeks of an acute attack of gout, as it may precipitate another attack.

The commonest adverse effect of allopurinol is rash, which may necessitate a switch to a uricosuric drug. The ampicillin/amoxycillin rash (see p. 111) is more likely to occur when a patient is also taking allopurinol. Dosages of allopurinol should be reduced in patients with severe renal failure.

(b) Uricosuric drugs

If patients are intolerant of allopurinol, probenecid or sulphinpyrazone may be used, although they are relatively ineffective in patients with poor renal function.

Probenecid should be started in a low dosage, which may be gradually increased (for example 250 mg b.d. increasing to 500 mg b.d. after a week and then to 2 g daily in divided doses over the next few weeks) depending on the effect on the serum uric acid concentration. When the uric acid concentration has been satisfactorily lowered it may be possible to reduce the dosage of probenecid and still keep the uric acid concentration within the reference range.

Sulphinpyrazone is an alternative to probenecid. It is given in an initial dosage of 100–200 mg/d in divided doses, increasing to 600 mg/d and then reducing to a maintenance dosage according to serum uric acid concentrations.

Uricosuric drugs should not be given within 3 weeks of an acute attack of gout. Their initial use should be accompanied by prophylactic therapy against an acute attack, using either colchicine or a non-steroidal anti-inflammatory drug, as for allopurinol (see above).

During the first few weeks of therapy with uricosuric drugs it is necessary to ensure adequate clearance of the extra urinary load of uric acid and to avoid uric acid gravel. Fluid intake should therefore be at least 2 L/d and it may be necessary to alkalinize the urine by giving potassium citrate or sodium bicarbonate mixtures (see the *British National Formulary*) or by giving acetazolamide 250 mg daily at night.

Salicylates block the actions of the uricosuric drugs and this combination must therefore be avoided.

Uricosuric drug therapy is contra-indicated in patients with renal failure and in those who have, or have had, uric acid stones. It should also be avoided in those who have a high rate of uric acid excretion before drug treatment (over 3.6 mmol/d on a restricted purine diet).

Both probenecid and sulphinpyrazone may cause rashes, nausea, and vomiting. Rarely probenecid may cause the nephrotic syndrome.

(c) Uric acid stones

See Chapter 26 (p. 359).

29.2.5 Drugs which cause hyperuricaemia and gout

Certain drugs can cause hyperuricaemia and precipitate gout.

Loop diuretics and thiazide diuretics inhibit the distal tubular secretion of uric acid, as do salicylates in low dosages (Fig. 29.4). Diuretic therapy is the commonest cause of hyperuricaemia; it rarely causes acute gout, but tophi may be formed around previously damaged joints, particularly in the fingers.

Cytotoxic drugs cause overproduction of uric acid from cellular purines during the treatment of leukaemias and lymphomas because they increase the rate of cell death. Allopurinol is often given to prevent this, but note that allopuri-nol inhibits the metabolism of mercaptopurine and azathioprine, dosages of which should be reduced when allopurinol is given (see p. 128).

29.3 Musculoskeletal disorders caused by drugs

Muscle pain, joint pain, bone pain, and associated syndromes may be caused by drugs. Some of the more important associations are shown in Table 29.5.

29.4 Paget's disease of bone

The treatment of Paget's disease is undoubtedly the field of the specialist, but every patient being treated by a specialist is also under the continuing care of a general practitioner, who may have to evaluate problems and difficulties which arise from specialist treatment and to monitor the effects of that treatment.

29.4.1 Mechanisms of action of drugs used in the treatment of Paget's disease

In Paget's disease there is excessive osteoclastic activity which leads to resorption of bone. There is also, probably as a secondary response, an increase in bone formation by increased osteoblast activity. This pattern of bone destruction followed by bone formation occurs in an abnormal pattern of lamellar bone (woven bone). During the end stage of the disease osteoclastic activity falls, sclerosis predominates, and the disease becomes inactive.

While the disease is active and bone destruction and formation are increased the bone-marrow becomes fibrotic and the whole bone is very vascular. This increased vascularity may produce functional arteriovenous fistulae which increase cardiac output and may rarely cause cardiac failure.

The abnormality of bone formation in Paget's disease may also cause bone pain, deformity and

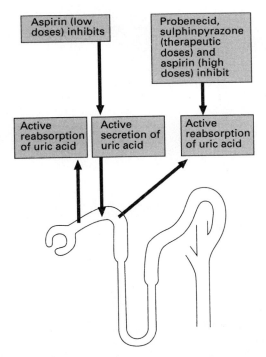

▪ **Fig. 29.4** Mechanisms of action of uricosuric drugs on uric acid secretion and reabsorption in the nephron.

■ Table 29.5 Musculoskeletal disorders induced by drugs

Disorder	Drugs associated
Arthritis and arthralgia	Amphotericin B
	β-Adrenoceptor antagonists
	Barbiturates
	Cimetidine
	Ethionamide
	Isoniazid
	Levamisole
	Pyrazinamide
	Quinidine
	Drug causing hypersensitivity reactions, for example sulphonamides
Lupus-like syndrome (with arthropathy)	Aminosalicylates
	Carbamazepine
	Chlorpromazine
	Ethosuximide
	Griseofulvin
	Hydralazine
	Isoniazid
	Methyldopa
	Methysergide
	Oral contraceptives
	Penicillamine
	Penicillin
	Phenylbutazone
	Phenytoin
	Primidone
	Reserpine
	Sulphonamides
	Tetracyclines
	Thiouracils
	Troxidone
Muscle pain and cramps	Carbenoxolone (reduced K^+)
	Cimetidine
	Clofibrate
	Corticosteroids
	Cytotoxic drugs
	Diuretics (reduced Na^+ and K^+)
	Lithium
	Oral contraceptives
	Penicillamine
	Purgatives (reduced Na^+ and K^+)
	Suxamethonium
	Terbutaline
Haemarthrosis	Anticoagulants
Osteoporosis	Corticosteroids
	Heparin (long-term)
	Methotrexate (long-term)
Osteomalacia	Aluminium hydroxide (long-term)
	Anticonvulsants (long-term)
	Bisphosphonates (see Paget's disease)
	Fluoride
Aseptic necrosis	Corticosteroids
Gout	Diuretics
	Cytotoxic drugs (see text)

enlargement of bones, fractures, osteosarcoma, and problems through pressure on nerves, such as the eighth cranial nerve, nerve roots, or the spinal cord.

Biochemically the increase in the rate of bone turnover leads to a raised serum alkaline phosphatase and increased urinary excretion of hydroxyproline. Serum calcium concentrations usually stay normal, but they can rise if there is prolonged bed-rest.

The drugs used in the treatment of Paget's disease are listed in Table 29.6.

(a) Calcitonin

Calcitonin reduces osteoclastic activity and inhibits bone resorption. This relieves pain. It rarely alters eighth nerve symptoms, but it can improve nerve root or spinal cord compression. It also reduces the vascularity of bone. During calcitonin therapy the serum alkaline phosphatase and the urinary excretion of hydroxyproline are reduced.

(b) Bisphosphonates

Bisphosphonates are pyrophosphate analogues, resistant to chemical and enzymatic degradation. They inhibit the growth and dissolution of hydroxyapatite crystals and retard bone resorption and formation, generally reducing bone turnover.

29.4.2 Treatment of Paget's disease

Treatment is not required in the majority of patients with Paget's disease, and when treatment is required for pain mild analgesics usually suffice. The indications for specific drug treatment (as opposed to analgesics only) in Paget's disease of bone are:

(1) severe bone pain;

(2) neurological complications;

(3) serious osteolytic lesions in weight-bearing bones;

(4) hypercalcaemia due to immobilization and rapid bone resorption;

(5) delayed union or non-union of fractures.

Evaluation of drug therapy is based on the clinical response, standardized radiological measurement techniques, and the serum alkaline phosphatase, urinary hydroxyproline, and serum calcium and phosphate if appropriate.

Calcitonin is expensive and has to be given by injection. However, it is still probably to be preferred to the bisphosphonates at present because

(1) we have more experience with it;

(2) it is better at relieving bone pain;

(3) the bisphosphonates do not regularly heal osteolytic lesions;

(4) if the dose of bisphosphonate is too high it may cause an increase in demineralization of bone and lead to osteomalacia.

Two forms of calcitonin are available, porcine and salmon. The latter is more suitable for long-term therapy, since antibodies form more readily in response to the former.

Salmon calcitonin (salcatonin) is given in a dosage of 100 units daily s.c., reducing after 2–3 months to 50 units three times a week. The corresponding dosages of porcine calcitonin can be calculated on the basis that 50 units of salcatonin equal 80 units of porcine calcitonin. If there is no improvement in pain after 6–8 weeks stop the calcitonin. If there is improvement continue for a year, stop therapy, and if symptoms recur start again. There are no hard and fast rules about long-term treatment, and each patient must be treated individually.

The adverse effects of calcitonin are nausea, vomiting, diarrhoea, flushing, paraesthesiae, and an unpleasant taste in the mouth. The occurrence of these adverse effects is variable and there does not seem to be other serious toxicity.

■ **Table 29.6** Drugs used in the treatment of Paget's disease

Non-narcotic analgesics (see drug therapy of pain, Chapter 32)
Calcitonin (p. 568)
Bisphosphonates

The bisphosphonate disodium etidronate is given in a single daily oral dose of 5 mg/kg for up to 6 months and then withdrawn. Food should be avoided for 2 h before and after a dose to improve its absorption. Some advocate the higher dose of 10 mg/kg daily for 3 months, although demineralization is more likely at this dosage, with the risk of fracture. The adverse effects of etidronate are nausea and diarrhoea. In about 5 per cent of patients there may be an increase in bone pain during the first month or so of treatment. Because of demineralization there is an increased incidence of spontaneous fractures at higher dosages.

The effects of both calcitonin and the bisphosphonates on bone can be monitored biochemically by measuring the serum alkaline phosphatase.

Newer bisphosphonates, such as disodium pamidronate, may prove to be as effective as etidronate in the treatment of Paget's disease with less of a demineralizing effect. However, although pamidronate is available in the UK for the treatment of tumour-induced hypercalcaemia, it is not yet licensed for use in Paget's disease.

30 The drug therapy of neurological disorders

Co-author: P. K. Panegyres

30.1 Meningitis and encephalitis

The main organisms which cause meningitis are listed in Table 30.1, along with the drugs used in their treatment. The principles of treating infections are outlined in Chapter 22, but there are some additional points worth emphasizing in relation to meningitis.

30.1.1 Initial treatment

Start treatment as soon as blood and cerebrospinal fluid (CSF) specimens have been obtained. One should try to identify the infecting organism immediately by microscopic examination of a Gram-stained sample of centrifuged CSF, so that the appropriate antibiotic may be given. However, if the organism cannot be identified do not delay treatment pending the results of microbiological culture.

In children under the age of 6 years, in whom meningitis is likely to be due to *H. influenzae*, or in neonates, in whom it is likely to be due to *E. coli*, start with ampicillin and chloramphenicol or cefotaxime. Remember to use dosages of chloramphenicol appropriate for children (see p. 139).

In older children and adults the organism is likely to be a coccus, so start with benzylpenicillin (penicillin G) i.v. and wait for the results of bacterial culture for further guidance. If the patient is allergic to penicillin start with chloramphenicol i.v.

30.1.2 Route of administration

All antibiotics used in the treatment of acute meningitis, with the exception of co-trimoxazole and those used in the treatment of tuberculous meningitis, should be given intravenously. Use of the intrathecal route is unnecessary, since the drugs commonly used penetrate well into the CSF or do so when the meninges are inflamed (see Table 22.5).

30.1.3 Duration of treatment

Treatment should be continued for at least 5–7 d after the patient has become afebrile, and the repeat examination of the CSF should show only a few white blood cells (fewer than 50/mm^3). In pneumococcal meningitis continue for 14 d after the fever has remitted and for at least 3 weeks in infections with Gram-negative organisms, in which the rate of relapse is high.

30.1.4 Complications of meningitis

In addition to the usual general care of a severely ill patient (for example maintenance of fluid and electrolyte balance, and maintenance of a clear airway and prevention of aspiration in the comatose patient) particular complications may need specific treatment. Convulsions should be treated with i.v. diazepam, chlormethiazole, or phenytoin (see p. 435). Cerebral oedema may respond to i.v. mannitol (1 g/kg of a 20 per cent solution (i.e. 350 mL for a 70 kg patient) given over 20 min and repeated if necessary at 4–12 h intervals; maximum 200 g in 24 h); corticosteroids are not of proven value in treating cerebral oedema in adults with meningitis, but may be of use in children. Headache should be treated with simple analgesics, although in severe cases narcotic analgesics may be required.

▌ **Table 30.1** Treatment of bacterial and fungal meningitis

Organism	Treatment of choice	Alternative
Meningococcus (*N. meningitidis*)	Benzylpenicillin	Chloramphenicol
Pneumococcus (*Strep. pneumoniae*)	Benzylpenicillin	Chloramphenicol
H. influenzae	Ampicillin + chloramphenicol	Chloramphenicol alone
E. coli	Cefotaxime	Cefuroxime or a third-generation cephalosporin (see Table 22.1)
Staph. aureus	Benzylpenicillin + cloxacillin	Vancomycin
Salmonella spp.	Ampicillin	Chloramphenicol
M. tuberculosis	Rifampicin + isoniazid + ethambutol + pyrazinamide	As for pulmonary tuberculosis (see Table 24.5)
Listeria monocytogenes	Ampicillin + tobramycin	Chloramphenicol
Legionella pneumophila	Erythromycin	
Cryptococcus neoformans	Amphotericin B + flucytosine	
Toxoplasmosis	Sulphadiazine + pyrimethamine	

30.1.5 Prevention of meningitis

Patients with CSF rhinorrhoea or otorrhoea are at risk of meningitis, and should be treated prophylactically with penicillin V, 500 mg orally q.d.s., until the leak stops.

Close contacts of a case of meningococcal meningitis (i.e. close family, close friends, and schoolmates) should be given prophylactic antibiotics. The drug of choice is rifampicin (600 mg orally b.d. for 2 d). Minocycline (100 mg orally b.d. for 5 d) is an alternative. Sulphadiazine (1 g orally b.d. for 2 d) has also been used, particularly in developing countries, because it is less expensive, but unfortunately many strains of meningococcus (for example Groups A and B) are nowadays resistant to sulphonamides. Immunization with meningococcal vaccines is sometimes an alternative in epidemics of infection with some groups of meningococci, and provides immunity for about 3 years.

30.1.6 Tuberculous meningitis

The principles in treating tuberculous meningitis are the same as those for pulmonary tuberculosis (see Chapter 24). Fortunately, most antituberculous drugs penetrate the CSF well, the one exception being streptomycin. Treatment can start with rifampicin, isoniazid, pyrazinamide, and ethambutol for 2 months, continuing with rifampicin and isoniazid for a further 10 months. In developing countries a regimen of isoniazid, pyrazinamide, and streptomycin is a suitable alternative. Despite the relatively poor penetration of streptomycin into the CSF it is generally given i.m. and intrathecal administration is not recommended.

Corticosteroids are not usually required, but prednisolone (20–40 mg orally daily) may be used if there is spinal block, a raised intracranial pressure, neurological signs, or a high protein concentration in the CSF.

30.1.7 Herpes simplex encephalitis

Herpes simplex is the most common cause of fatal acute sporadic viral encephalitis. The herpes virus is a DNA virus of which there are two types; the type 1 form causes encephalitis. Untreated it has a high mortality and morbidity. It has a predilection for the temporal lobes, the limbic system, and the inferior frontal and parietal lobes.

Herpes simplex encephalitis presents with personality changes, memory loss, aphasia, and seizures. These may be associated with fever, lassitude, myalgia, and gastrointestinal upsets.

Acyclovir (see p. 240) is effective in reducing mortality and morbidity. It is given i.v. in a dose of 10 mg/kg 8-hourly for 10 d. It is usually tolerated without significant adverse effects, but may cause headache, rashes, gastrointestinal upsets, and impairment of hepatic and renal function.

30.1.8 Other forms of meningitis and encephalitis

Cryptococcus neoformans is one of the most common fungal organisms causing infection in the nervous system and it may present acutely. It should be treated with flucytosine (150 mg/kg i.v. daily) and amphotericin (5 mg i.v. daily, increasing to a total of 1.0 mg/kg/d; this dose may then be given every second day to a total of 2–3 g).

Amphotericin may cause renal, hepatic, haematological, and neurological toxicity (see the Pharmacopoeia). As an alternative, fluconazole is increasingly being used in the treatment of acute cryptococcal meningitis and to prevent relapse and in patients with AIDS.

Nervous system involvement in Legionnaires' disease should be treated with erythromycin (0.5–1.0 g i.v. every 6 h for 3 weeks).

Meningoencephalitis due to *Listeria monocytogenes*, which usually occurs in immunosuppressed patients, is treated with ampicillin (1 g i.v. every 4 h) and tobramycin (2.5 mg/kg i.v. 8-hourly).

Lyme disease meningoencephalitis, caused by *Borrelia burgdorferi*, is treated with benzylpenicillin (1.2 g i.v. daily for 10 days).

Toxoplasmosis, which may occur in patients with AIDS, is treated with sulphadiazine (4 g orally initially then 2–6 g daily) and pyrimethamine (100–200 mg initially then 25 mg daily). Leucovorin (2–10 mg daily) should be given to offset the effect of pyrimethamine on folate metabolism.

Rickettsial infections of the nervous system are treated with chloramphenicol or a tetracycline.

30.2 Parkinson's disease and Parkinsonism

Parkinson's disease was first described by Sir James Parkinson (1755–1824) in his classic text *Essay on Shaking Palsy* (1817).

Parkinson's disease is characterized by hypokinesia, rigidity, and tremor, and this syndrome is due to reduced dopamine function in the corpus striatum. When the syndrome occurs secondary to some identifiable cause it is called Parkinsonism.

In order to understand the treatment of Parkinson's disease and Parkinsonism it is necessary to understand their pathophysiology.

30.2.1 Idiopathic Parkinson's disease

In idiopathic Parkinson's disease there is degeneration of the dopamine-containing neurones in the substantia nigra. The reason for this degeneration is not known, but it has been suggested that it may be due to an acceleration of the normal ageing process in these neurones secondary to an environmental toxin. This hypothesis was formulated following the observation that the designer drug methylphenyltetrahydropyridine (MPTP), which was synthesized by an addict attempting to synthesize pethidine (meperidine) illegally, can cause a syndrome closely similar to Parkinson's disease in both man and animals, associated with degeneration of cells in the substantia nigra.

The effect of MPTP has been attributed to a toxic metabolite, MPP^+, which is formed by oxidation of MPTP via monoamine oxidase (MAO) in the brain, and which disturbs mitochondrial oxidative function. Since this discovery other neurotoxins with similar selective effects have been identified.

30.2.2 Secondary Parkinsonism

(a) After encephalitis lethargica

Parkinsonism which occurs after encephalitis is due to degeneration of dopamine-containing nigrostriatal fibres.

(b) Degenerative diseases of the CNS

Degenerative diseases of the brain, such as Wilson's disease (hepatolenticular degeneration), may involve the nigrostriatal tract and result in Parkinsonism.

(c) Toxins

Manganese and carbon monoxide poisoning may cause degeneration of dopamine-containing nigrostriatal fibres.

(d) Drugs

Neuroleptic drugs (for example phenothiazines, butyrophenones) and metoclopramide are dopamine receptor antagonists in the corpus striatum and reduce the functional activity of dopamine.

30.2.3 Mechanisms of action of anti-Parkinsonian drugs

All the causes of Parkinsonism enumerated above result in a reduction in the functional activity of striatal dopamine, either because of reduced synthesis of dopamine or antagonism of its effects at post-synaptic receptors. The corpus striatum is involved in modulating voluntary movements by an effect upon the function of the pyramidal tract motor system, although the exact connections are still unclear. This function of the striatum is inhibited by dopamine, released from dopamine-containing neurones in the nigrostriatal tract, and stimulated by acetylcholine, released from cholinergic neurones in the striatum and acting on muscarinic receptors. Anything which reduces dopaminergic function will result in Parkinsonism in a susceptible individual.

Drug treatment in Parkinson's disease and some forms of Parkinsonism is therefore aimed at increasing dopaminergic activity. Drug-induced and post-encephalitic Parkinsonism respond to treatment with anticholinergic drugs. The various drugs which are used are listed in Table 30.2.

(a) Drugs which enhance dopaminergic function

L-dopa acts by being metabolized to dopamine in the brain, but its adverse effects are mostly due to its conversion to dopamine in the periphery. Its action can therefore be enhanced by the concomitant administration of the dopa decarboxylase inhibitors, benserazide and carbidopa, which prevent its breakdown in the periphery but not in the brain. Thus, the co-administration of L-dopa with a dopa decarboxylase inhibitor allows lower dosages of L-dopa

■ **Table 30.2** Drugs used in the treatment of Parkinson's disease and Parkinsonism

---

1. *Acting through dopaminergic mechanisms*
   Levodopa (L-dopa) plus a peripheral decarboxylase inhibitor, such as carbidopa (Sinemet®) or benserazide (Madopar®) (p. 622)
   Dopamine receptor agonists
      Apomorphine
      Bromocriptine (p. 598)
      Lisuride
      Pergolide
   Amantadine
   Selegiline (p. 637)

2. *Acetylcholinoceptor antagonists (anticholinergic drugs)* (p. 538)
   Benzhexol
   Benztropine
   Biperiden
   Methixene
   Orphenadine
   Procyclidine

---

to be used. This means that less dopamine is formed in the periphery with fewer adverse effects, but enough dopamine is formed in the brain to produce a therapeutic effect.

Bromocriptine, lisuride, and apomorphine are agonists at dopamine receptors.

Amantadine acts by increasing dopamine release and inhibiting its re-uptake.

The MAO inhibitor selegiline enhances dopaminergic function by inhibiting the breakdown of dopamine. There are two isoenzymes of MAO, types A and B. Noradrenaline and 5-hydroxytryptamine are metabolized by type A MAO, while tyramine and dopamine are metabolized by both types A and B. Human brain, particularly the striatum, contains a preponderance of type B MAO. Selegiline selectively inhibits type B MAO and therefore inhibits the metabolism of dopamine in the striatum. However, selegiline is not associated with the 'cheese and wine' hypertensive reaction associated with conventional non-selective MAO inhibitors (see Chapter 10) for the following reasons.

1. Because type A MAO is still active when selegiline is given, noradrenaline is still metabolized in the periphery and sympathetic nerve-ending stores of noradrenaline do not increase.
2. Tyramine, which is the trigger of the hypertensive reaction, is a substrate of both type A and type B MAO and is therefore metabolized as it passes through the gut and liver.

Selegiline may also slow the rate of progression of Parkinson's disease by preventing the breakdown of substances such as MPTP to toxic derivatives.

(b) Drugs which reduce cholinergic function

The drugs which reduce cholinergic activity are all acetylcholine receptor antagonists.

30.2.4 Practical aspects of treatment

When Parkinson's disease is mild and not at all disabling, drugs are not required. However, there is currently a move, particularly in the USA, to prescribe selegiline at a very early stage in the disease in the hope of preventing further degeneration of nigrostriatal neurones thus slowing the progress of the disease. This is not yet a licensed indication for selegiline in the UK.

(a) L-dopa + a peripheral dopa decarboxylase inhibitor

As the illness progresses therapy with L-dopa plus a dopa decarboxylase inhibitor, either carbidopa or benserazide, becomes necessary. Two formulations are available in the UK: Sinemet® (levodopa plus carbidopa, also called co-careldopa) and Madopar® (levodopa plus benserazide, also called co-beneldopa).

The principle is to start with a low dosage, gradually increasing every 2–3 d (see the Pharmacopoeia for dosages, adverse effects, and interactions). Dosage requirements vary greatly and for each patient the dosage must be finely tuned in order to maximize the therapeutic benefit and minimize adverse effects.

There are several problems with long-term L-dopa therapy:

(i) Gradual ineffectiveness

L-dopa does not influence the progression and final outcome of Parkinson's disease. However, it does prolong survival, improve functional ability very markedly, and greatly enhance the quality of life. None the less, over a period of years in many cases L-dopa therapy becomes less effective, and with increasing dosages adverse effects increase.

(ii) 'Wearing-off' phenomenon

This phenomenon occurs when a patient notices the wearing off of the therapeutic effect as hypokinesia returns. This effect is usually related to falling plasma concentrations of L-dopa (and therefore by implication falling brain concentrations of dopamine) towards the end of a dosage interval. Some patients then benefit from shorter dosage intervals, although usually at the risk of increased dyskinetic reactions. Patients may also be helped by reducing their dietary protein intake, since the transport of L-dopa, which is an amino acid, both across the gut and into the brain, is inhibited by other amino acids.

(iii) 'On-off' phenomenon

This consists of a sudden loss of the anti-Parkinsonian effects of L-dopa with consequent rigidity and hypokinesia. The loss of effect occurs irregularly and may last for some hours. The switch 'on' is rapid and unrelated to the dosage of L-dopa. 'On-off' episodes may occur several times a day and can be very disabling.

(b) Bromocriptine and other dopamine agonists

If the problems posed by L-dopa (adverse effects, gradual ineffectiveness, or the on-off phenomenon) make it impossible to establish full and adequate dosages, bromocriptine may be added early on. Bromocriptine should be started in a dosage of 1.25 mg at night and gradually increased over a number of weeks to between 10 and 40 mg per day in divided doses taken with food.

Bromocriptine has a wide spectrum of adverse effects, among which hypotension, nausea, and psychotic reactions are not uncommon. It should be used with caution in people over 70 years of age.

Other dopamine receptor agonists, lisuride and pergolide, have been used instead of bromocriptine, but there is no evidence that either is to be preferred.

Recently the dopamine agonist apomorphine has been shown to be useful in patients with disabling 'on-off' phenomenon and 'end-of-dose' effect. It may be given by subcutaneous infusion or sublingually. It may cause nausea and vomiting, which can be prevented by domperidone.

(c) Selegiline

Through its action in prolonging the action of dopamine in the nigrostriatal tracts, selegiline has a number of effects which are helpful in the treatment of Parkinson's disease. It can be used to reduce the effective dosage of L-dopa, thus reducing its peripheral adverse effects and dyskinesias; it helps to smooth out the dose-related fluctuations in the anti-Parkinsonian effects of L-dopa; it is helpful in reducing the 'wearing-off' and 'on-off' effects encountered during long-term L-dopa therapy; and it may also prevent the progression of Parkinson's disease.

Selegiline is given orally in a dosage of 10 mg o.d. or 5 mg b.d. It is usually well tolerated, although it can occasionally cause hypotension, nausea, vomiting, confusion, and agitation. The incidence of adverse effects is less when selegiline and L-dopa are combined than when L-dopa is used alone.

(d) Amantadine

In mild Parkinsonism amantadine may also be effective. It is given in a dosage of 100 mg b.d. and an effect is usually seen within 3 d. If the disease remains mild its efficacy may persist, but as the disease progresses amantadine tends to become less effective. Its adverse effects include a dose-related livedo reticularis (a bluish mottling of the skin of the extremities), erythema and oedema of the ankles, insomnia, and hallucinations, particularly in old people.

(e) Anticholinergic drugs

Anticholinergic drugs may be useful in postencephalitic Parkinsonism and in drug-induced Parkinsonism, since in the latter the effects of dopamine agonists and L-dopa are blocked by dopamine receptor antagonists. In acute Par-

kinsonian crisis intravenous procyclidine (5 mg) or benztropine (2 mg) are effective. In patients taking long-term dopamine receptor antagonists it is better to reserve anticholinergic drugs for those in whom Parkinsonism is severe. Then procyclidine (2.5 mg t.d.s. orally) is preferred. Anticholinergic drugs mainly affect the tremor and rigidity of Parkinsonism and have little effect on hypokinesia. They are the treatment of choice in acute oculogyric crisis.

30.3 Epilepsy

An epileptic fit is caused by a paroxysmal disturbance of brain function, consequent upon a brief, unphysiological, synchronous discharge of neurones. An epileptic seizure may be either generalized (i.e. occurring throughout the brain) or partial (i.e. occurring in only one part of the brain).

Primary generalized seizures are of two types, tonic-clonic seizures (previously called 'grand mal') and absences (previously called 'petit mal'). In addition, generalized seizures may take the form of akinetic seizures, in which there is generalized loss of muscle power without loss of consciousness, or myoclonic seizures, in which there are multiple spasmodic muscle jerks.

Partial seizures may be either simple or complex. In simple partial seizures there is no loss of consciousness, while in complex partial seizures there is altered consciousness.

It is still unclear whether all generalized seizures result from a paroxysmal discharge of a focus of neurones with a subsequent rapid generalized spread of depolarization, or whether the discharge occurs synchronously throughout the brain. It is certainly the case that a seizure can begin partial and become generalized. Conversely, generalized seizures may be accompanied by EEG but not clinical evidence of focal origin. Both these types are known as secondarily generalized seizures.

30.3.1 Mechanisms of action of anticonvulsant drugs

Anticonvulsants act to prevent the spread of the neuronal excitation in epilepsy by mechanisms that are not fully understood, but which can be roughly divided into those which involve a stabilizing effect on excitable cell membranes and those which involve altered functional activity of neurotransmitters, which then act to inhibit the spread of seizure activity by blocking synaptic transmission.

Of the neurotransmitters which are affected by anticonvulsant drugs, the inhibitory transmitter γ-aminobutyric acid (GABA) is the chief. The benzodiazepines and the barbiturates enhance GABA function by interacting with GABA receptors at the $GABA_A$/benzodiazepine receptor complex. Valproate enhances GABA function by an unknown mechanism, but it may enhance GABA synthesis and/or release. Vigabatrine (γ-vinyl-GABA) increases GABA function by inhibition of GABA transaminase, which is responsible for the breakdown of GABA. It does this because it is structurally related to GABA and competes with it for the transaminase enzyme.

In Table 30.3 are listed the drugs used in the treatment of epilepsy with a summary of the currently favoured ideas about their mechanisms of action.

30.3.2 The practical use of anticonvulsants

(a) General principles

The classification of epilepsy discussed above bears no more than a purely empirical relationship to the effectiveness of anticonvulsant drugs.

This is not surprising, since the mechanisms of action at the functional neuronal level are largely unknown. However, some anticonvulsants have been shown to be effective in particular forms of epilepsy, and these are listed in the usual order in which they are generally chosen in each case in Table 30.4.

The aim of treatment is to suppress fits without impairing mental or motor function, and in children without producing behavioural disorders

■ **Table 30.4** Drugs of choice in the treatment of particular types of epilepsy

Type of epilepsy	Drugs of choice
Generalized tonic-clonic seizures (grand mal)	Phenytoin Carbamazepine Valproate Primidone Phenobarbitone
Generalized absences (petit mal)	Valproate Ethosuximide
Partial seizures (simple and complex)	Carbamazepine Phenytoin Primidone Phenobarbitone
Myoclonic seizures	Valproate Clonazepam
Grand mal + petit mal	Valproate Carbamazepine + ethosuximide

■ **Table 30.3** Drugs used in the treatment of epilepsy

Drug	Membrane effects	Neurotransmitter effects
Phenytoin (p. 663)	+	+ (5-HT)
Phenobarbitone (p. 662)	–	+ (GABA)
Primidone	–	+ (GABA)
Valproate (p. 700)	–	+ (?GABA)
Carbamazepine (p. 572)	+	?
Benzodiazepines (p. 564) (diazepam, clonazepam)	–	+ (GABA)
Ethosuximide	?	–
Paraldehyde	+	–?
Vigabatrin	–	+ (GABA)

which may result in difficulties at school. If possible therapy should be restricted to only one drug, and usually this is possible by careful attention to dosage. A second drug should be added only after individual drugs have failed to be effective in the presence of 'adequate' plasma concentrations (see Chapter 7) or if there are unacceptable adverse effects of the first drug or drugs of choice. Combined therapy may also be necessary in patients with more than one form of epilepsy (for example tonic-clonic seizures and absences).

All anticonvulsants have a fairly low therapeutic index, and it is therefore of paramount importance to tailor dosages carefully in the individual to try to maximize efficacy while minimizing adverse effects. As an aid to individualization of dosage regimens, plasma or serum drug concentrations may be measured if relevant and possible. The precise details of individual drug dosages can be found in the Pharmacopoeia, but in Table 30.5 are shown the usual adult dosages and therapeutic plasma concentration ranges and some indication of the usefulness of measuring

plasma concentrations in the practical management of epilepsy (see also Chapter 7).

For improved compliance once-a-day dosage is preferable, but this may not be possible in all cases, because of concentration-related adverse effects associated with the peak plasma concentrations which occur after a single large dose. However, most anticonvulsants can be given twice a day at most.

The dose-related adverse effects of the anticonvulsants are generally sedation, nystagmus, ataxia, and psychological changes, such as confusion, memory loss, and depression. Anticonvulsants may also cause mild mood changes and behavioural symptoms.

(b) Specific management of the individual

As an example, consider the details of starting treatment with phenytoin in an adult. One would start phenytoin in a dosage of 300 mg daily (in one dose at night or in two divided doses). After about two weeks steady-state plasma concentrations should have been reached in most cases and

■ **Table 30.5** Dosages and therapeutic plasma concentration ranges of different anticonvulsants

Drug	Usual adult dosage range at steady state after gradual introduction	Reported therapeutic plasma concentration range	Usefulness of measuring plasma concentrations
Carbamazepine	600–1200 mg daily	17–42 µmol/L (4–10 µg/mL)	Useful
Clonazepam	4–8 mg daily (in 3–4 divided doses)	41–285 µmol/L (13–90 µg/mL)	Usefulness unknown
Ethosuximide	1–2 g daily	284–710 µmol/L (40–100 µg/mL)	May be helpful, but base dosage more on clinical response
Phenobarbitone	90–180 mg daily	43–172 µmol/L (10–40 µg/mL)	Only moderately useful
Phenytoin	300–400 mg daily	40–80 µmol/L (10–20 µg/mL)	Must be measured to help to individualize dosages
Primidone	500–1000 mg daily	[Measure phenobarbitone]	Only moderately useful
Valproate	1000–1600 mg daily	350–700 µmol/L (50–100 µg/mL)	Not very useful
Vigabatrin	2–4 g daily	?	Usefulness unknown

the plasma concentration should be measured. If at that time the patient is fit-free there will be no reason to change the dosage. If not, the dosage may be increased, depending on the plasma phenytoin concentration, by either 25 mg/d or 50 mg/d and not more frequently than every 4 weeks (see p. 88). Once the patient becomes fit-free the dose of phenytoin may be continued, but one should watch carefully for signs of toxicity, since accumulation of phenytoin can sometimes occur over periods of more than 2–4 weeks.

The plasma phenytoin concentration can be used as a guide to help you to control therapy, but do not alter the dosage simply to obtain a particular plasma concentration. Rather adjust the dosage in order to make the patient fit-free while minimizing adverse effects. The following examples illustrate this principle.

1. If plasma concentrations on the initial dosage of 300 mg daily are in or even below the therapeutic range and the patient is free of fits and adverse effects do not alter the dosage.

2. If plasma concentrations are in the lower part of the therapeutic range (i.e. around 40–60 µmol/L) and the patient is free of toxicity but still having fits, increase the dosage so that the plasma concentration increases up to 80 µmol/L.

3. If plasma concentrations are in the upper part of the therapeutic range (i.e. around 80 µmol/L) and the patient is free of toxicity but still having fits, increase the dosage cautiously, since freedom from fits may occur in some patients only when the plasma phenytoin concentration is greater than 80 µmol/L. However, in such cases watch carefully for signs of toxicity.

Remember that in patients with reduced plasma protein binding of phenytoin (for example in renal failure or pregnancy) the unbound ('free') phenytoin concentration is greater than one would expect from the total phenytoin concentration measurement, and consequently the 'therapeutic range' of plasma concentrations is reduced (see Chapter 10 for a full discussion).

The principles of treating epilepsy with other drugs are similar to those for phenytoin, although

without the problem of saturable metabolism. Remember, however, that carbamazepine induces its own metabolism, and after a week or two of treatment plasma concentrations may fall without a change in dosage.

(c) Withdrawal of anticonvulsant therapy

In some individuals it may be possible to withdraw treatment after a period of time, although the decision on when and whether to do this is always difficult, particularly in those who want to drive, since their being allowed to do so depends on their being fit-free for a period of time (in the UK 2 years). Withdrawal should be considered only after the patient has been free of fits for at least 2 years, except in those with a history of recent onset, in which case 1 year may be acceptable. Drugs should be withdrawn slowly and only one drug at a time should be withdrawn. It is generally better not to withdraw therapy from patients with partial seizures or evidence of brain damage, in whom the risk of relapse is high. Before withdrawing treatment the implications must be discussed with the patient. Patients should be advised not to drive during and for 6–12 months after withdrawal.

30.3.3 Status epilepticus

Status epilepticus is potentially fatal and is a medical emergency requiring swift and effective treatment to minimize the risk of brain damage. It is essential to establish an airway and to have patients in a physical environment in which they cannot hurt themselves. These patients should be admitted to an intensive care unit and should be assessed by a neurologist.

(a) Diazepam

Methods of treating status epilepticus vary. We suggest using diazepam as a first choice, in the following way.

Ideally, diazepam should be given i.v. as an emulsion (Diazemuls®) in a dose of 10–20 mg over 3–6 min. The initial dose should be repeated in 30 min if necessary, and it can be followed by a continuous infusion of 100 micrograms/kg/h to a maximum of 30 mg/kg over 24 h.

Alternatively, some neurologists follow i.v. bolus doses of diazepam by an infusion of clonazepam, on the grounds that it has a longer duration of action and penetrates the brain better. The dose is 0.25 mg/h, increasing as required to 1 mg/h.

Slow i.v. injections and the insertion of i.v. lines can be difficult in a patient having a fit, and one may have to use the rectal route instead (diazepam 10–20 mg). This route of administration is also particularly helpful for emergency treatment in the home and can easily be used by a patient's relative.

If the fits do not respond to diazepam and clonazepam several choices are available.

(b) Chlormethiazole

Chlormethiazole is given by i.v. infusion of an 0.8 per cent solution (8 mg/mL), in an initial dose of 40–100 mL (320–800 mg), given over a period of 5–10 min to stop the convulsions, monitoring respiration carefully, particularly if following on diazepam. This is usually followed by 1–3 mL/min (8–24 mg/min) for 24 h, assuming respiratory and circulatory functions are well maintained, to ensure that the epileptic state has settled down.

(c) Phenytoin

Phenytoin may be given by slow intravenous infusion (13–18 mg/kg) at a rate of no more than 50 mg/min. Ideally the i.v. infusion of phenytoin should be carried out with cardiographic monitoring in case of cardiac arrhythmias.

(d) Barbiturates

In the USA i.v. barbiturates are frequently used. Phenobarbitone is injected at a rate of 50 mg/min i.v. to a total dose of 7 mg/kg (for example 500 mg infused over 10 min). If seizures continue after 30 min another 3 mg/kg can be given slowly i.v. Sodium amylobarbitone, 50 mg/min i.v., can also be used.

Barbiturates can cause respiratory depression and severe hypotension, and facilities for full resuscitation must be available. Ideally, by this stage the patient should be in an intensive care unit.

(e) Paraldehyde

Paraldehyde may be given i.v., but should be used only by those with experience. It can be very effective in terminating very resistant status epilepticus.

Paraldehyde for injection must be freshly prepared by dilution with 0.9 per cent sodium chloride to produce a 10 per cent (v/v) solution of paraldehyde. The total dose depends on the patient's response, but to start with it is infused at a rate of 1 mL/min for 10 min. This dose is repeated with each fit, to a total dose of not more than 100 mL in an hour. When seizures have stopped for 2 h a slow i.v. infusion of 5 mL of a 10 per cent solution is given.

Some still give paraldehyde i.m. and give 5 mL by deep i.m. injection into each buttock. However, this is unreliable and very painful and may cause sterile abscesses.

(f) Complete paralysis

In severe cases in which there is little or no response to drugs it is necessary to terminate status epilepticus by giving i.v. thiopentone, with or without muscle relaxants of the curare type. This requires the assistance of an anaesthetist.

<u>30.4</u> Migraine

In classical migraine there is a warning phase in which patients may know that an attack is going to occur soon: they may feel particularly well, their mood may alter, or they may feel listless or drowsy. Then the acute prodromal phase occurs, with neurological features, often visual, such as scintillating lights and visual scotomata, and less often hemiplegic and rarely hemisensory features. After 20–30 min the headache comes on. It usually begins in one spot behind an eye or in the temporal region and classically spreads unilaterally (the hemicrania which gives the disease its name), but the affected side can vary and it can become bilateral. The pain is often severe and throbbing. The patient feels awful and there is often photophobia, nausea, and vomiting. The episode usually lasts a few hours, but it can go on for a day or two. The further away from this classical description the symptoms of migraine become, the more difficult it is to diagnose, but paroxysmal headaches without prodromata are often called 'common migraine' or 'migrainous headaches'. It is always important to consider intracranial causes of such symptoms, for example tumours and vascular abnormalities such as aneurysms.

The cause of migraine is not known. There is most likely a paroxysmal disturbance of arterial calibre in the cerebral vessels, consisting of an initial vasoconstriction of intracranial vessels, causing cortical or brain-stem ischaemia (giving prodromal symptoms), followed by vasodilatation of the extracranial arteries in particular, which causes headache, apparently through stimulation of pain-mediating sensory nerve-endings in the arterial wall.

Exactly how these changes occur is still a mystery, but hypotheses abound. For example, dietary substances, for example tyramine (in chocolate and cheese) and alcohol, might release vasoactive substances (for example catecholamines, 5-hydroxytryptamine, kinins) from stores in platelets, nerve-endings, or other tissues, thus triggering an attack. It may also be that people who suffer migraine have altered reactivity of their blood vessels. In addition, any or all of these or other mechanisms may be subject to the influence of genetic determinants, sex hormones (as in premenstrual migraine and migraine caused by oral contraceptives), and psychosomatic factors.

30.4.1 Mechanisms of action of drugs used to treat migraine

The drugs used to treat migraine are listed in Table 30.6. It is difficult to propound the rationale of the therapy of migraine because of the lack of understanding of the cause of the illness and the mechanisms of action of some of the drugs. However, some of the actions of these drugs are clearly relevant to their use in migraine.

(a) Actions of drugs used in the acute attack

Analgesics and antiemetics used during an acute attack act by relieving symptoms. Antiemetic drugs may also hasten gastric emptying, which is slowed in migraine, and thus hasten the absorption of analgesics (see Fig. 10.1).

Ergotamine could act through one of several mechanisms. It is an α-adrenoceptor antagonist,

■ **Table 30.6** Drugs used in the treatment of migraine

1. *Treatment of an acute attack*
   Analgesics
     Aspirin (p. 677)
     Paracetamol (p. 657)
     Codeine (p. 641)
   Antiemetics
     Buclizine ⎱ both are antihistamines (H$_1$
     Cyclizine ⎰ receptor antagonists) (p. 559)
     Metoclopramide (p. 633)
   (There are several combination formulations of analgesics and antiemetics)

   Ergotamine
   Sumatriptan

2. *Prophylaxis*
   5-hydroxytryptamine (serotonin) antagonists
     Pizotifen (p. 664)
     Methysergide
   Other agents
     Propranolol (p. 544)
     Amitriptyline (p. 698)
     Cyproheptadine (p. 559)
     Naproxen (p. 653)
     Verapamil (p. 569)

a weak antagonist at 5-hydroxytryptamine (5-HT) receptors, and itself a direct vasoconstrictor. Any of these actions might modify the abnormal arterial vasoconstriction and vasodilatation thought to be operating in migraine.

Sumatriptan is an agonist at 5-HT receptors and mimics the effects of agonists at the receptor subtype known as 5-HT$_1$ receptors, which are mostly found in cranial blood vessels. It therefore causes vasoconstriction which is mostly limited to the carotid arterial circulation.

(b) Actions of drugs used in prophylaxis

The 5-HT receptor antagonists pizotifen and methysergide are thought to block the actions of 5-HT after its release from platelets and elsewhere. It is not known exactly how propranolol works, but apart from its β-blocking properties, which could interfere with a 'stress' response, it is also a 5-HT receptor antagonist.

30.4.2 The use of drugs in migraine

(a) The treatment of an acute attack

(i) Analgesics and antiemetics

Patients often find that during an acute attack of migraine they need to lie down in a quiet darkened room, and most find that an analgesic, with or without an antiemetic, is sufficient in the way of drug therapy.

The earlier analgesics can be given the better, and an analgesic taken during the warning or prodromal phases may prevent a headache altogether. Aspirin 600–900 mg or paracetamol 1–1.5 g every 4–6 h as necessary may be sufficient to see a patient through an attack.

Metoclopramide, 5–10 mg orally t.d.s., the first dose given as early as possible in an attack, relieves the nausea and helps speed the absorption of the analgesic. In a severe attack i.m. metoclopramide (10 mg) may be necessary.

Various proprietary formulations contain mixtures of an antiemetic and an analgesic (see for example the *British National Formulary*), and some patients find these suitable.

(ii) Ergotamine

Ergotamine is most effective when given early in an attack, preferably during the warning or prodromal phases. Because of unreliability of absorption (due to gastric stasis, vomiting, and the emetic action of ergotamine itself) ergotamine is best given sublingually, rectally, or by aerosol (see the Pharmacopoeia for dosages). If ergotamine is effective, competent patients may prefer to give themselves a subcutaneous or even an i.m. injection, especially if they have very severe migraine.

(iii) Sumatriptan

Sumatriptan should be given as soon as possible after the start of an attack. It is given in a dose of 6 mg subcutaneously, and this can be repeated after an hour; alternatively, it may be given orally (100 mg), but the onset of action is then delayed and may be prevented by vomiting. Sumatriptan is highly effective in the treatment of an acute attack of migraine but it is contra-indicated in patients with ischaemic heart disease or severe hypertension.

(b) Prophylaxis

The nature of migraine should be explained to patients and they should be reassured that the illness is not dangerous. In some cases the frequency of attacks can be reduced by simple measures. These include the identification of foods which precipitate an attack, and recognition, where relevant, of the role of alcohol or of the oral contraceptive. About 10–15 per cent of patients may benefit by avoiding specific foods. In patients who live unavoidably stressful lives relaxation techniques may help.

Drug treatment should generally be reserved for those whose attacks are more frequent than fortnightly.

(i) Pizotifen

In patients with frequent disabling attacks pizotifen (0.5–1.5 mg t.d.s) can be effective. It may cause drowsiness and interacts with alcohol, potentiating its effects on the brain. It also increases the appetite which may result in increased weight.

(ii) Propranolol

Propranolol (40–240 mg daily in divided doses) helps some patients.

(iii) Methysergide

In patients who do not respond to pizotifen or propranolol, methysergide can be tried in an initial dosage of 1 mg once at night, increasing to 1–2 mg b.d. or t.d.s.

The long-term use of methysergide may be associated with retroperitoneal fibrosis and occasionally fibrotic cardiac valvular disease. If effective it should be given in the minimum effective dose for 6 months at a time and then withdrawn for a month's 'drug holiday' before reinstitution. Patients should be asked to report any urinary symptoms or loin pain suggestive of retroperitoneal fibrosis.

Methysergide may also cause peripheral limb ischaemia (like ergotamine), hypotension, and oedema. Because of these serious adverse effects it should only be used by specialists.

(iv) Other drugs

Other drugs have been used from time to time. They include amitriptyline, cyproheptadine, naproxen, and verapamil.

30.5 Myasthenia gravis

Myasthenia gravis results, for reasons unknown, from the production of antibodies to nicotinic acetylcholine receptors in skeletal muscle. This causes blockade of the actions of acetylcholine, with symptoms and signs resembling the effects of curare, i.e. a competitive neuromuscular block. The clinical manifestations include weakness of the eye muscles (resulting in ptosis or diplopia) and difficulties in chewing, swallowing, and speaking. Proximal limb weakness is common and there may be distal limb weakness, with weak hands. There may also be respiratory muscle weakness. Characteristically the muscle weakness worsens as the muscles fatigue. The particular pattern of weaknesses and the way in which they fluctuate from day to day and from hour to hour are characteristic for the individual patient.

30.5.1 Mechanisms of action of drugs used in the treatment of myasthenia gravis

The drugs used in treating myasthenia gravis are listed in Table 30.7.

The cholinesterase inhibitors prevent the breakdown of acetylcholine by cholinesterase, and the concentration of acetylcholine at the neuromuscular junction increases, overcoming the effect of the inhibiting antibody.

Corticosteroids, such as prednisolone, presumably act by suppressing lymphocyte production of the acetylcholine receptor antibody.

Plasmapheresis is sometimes used in myasthenia to remove antibodies from the circulation and therefore reduce the degree of block.

30.5.2 The use of drugs in myasthenia gravis

(a) In diagnosis

(i) Edrophonium

Edrophonium is a cholinesterase inhibitor with a very short duration of action and it can be used in making the initial diagnosis of myasthenia gravis. It is particularly useful when the strength of weak facial muscles is being evaluated. Edrophonium can also be used in the differentiation of a myasthenic crisis (due to severe disease or too little cholinesterase inhibition) from a cholinergic crisis (due to too much cholinesterase inhibition and excess acetylcholine at the neuromuscular junction). Edrophonium will make a cholinergic crisis very transiently worse but it will greatly improve a myasthenic crisis. In making this differentiation it is crucial to observe the effect on the respiratory muscles, and in these circumstances the patient should be in an intensive care unit if possible.

Edrophonium should only be given in an intensive care unit. It is given i.v., usually in an initial dose of 2 mg. If there is no response within 30 seconds or if untoward effects occur give another 3 mg. If there is still no response give another 5 mg. Atropine (0.6–1.2 mg i.v.) should be given before edrophonium to prevent serious bradycardia.

(b) Treatment

(i) Neostigmine and pyridostigmine

The cholinesterase inhibitors are still used in mild cases of myasthenia gravis. The dosages of these drugs vary from patient to patient and must be tailored to the individual. They are similar in their efficacy, but there are some features which distinguish them.

▋ **Table 30.7** Drugs used in the treatment of myasthenia gravis

---

Acetylcholinesterase inhibitors (p. 539)
    Neostigmine
    Pyridostigmine
    Edrophonium (in diagnosis)
Immunosuppressive drugs
    Corticosteroids (p. 584)
    Azathioprine (p. 561)

---

1. The action of neostigmine after oral administration lasts 30–45 min, which is shorter than the duration of action of pyridostigmine.

2. Muscarinic adverse effects, particularly abdominal cramps, nausea, and diarrhoea, may be worse with neostigmine.

3. Some patients find that neostigmine gives a quicker and slightly greater improvement in muscle strength.

4. Pyridostigmine is sometimes more effective in bulbar muscle weakness.

Pyridostigmine is therefore usually preferred to neostigmine. It should be started in a dosage of 30–60 mg 6- to 8-hourly. The dosage may be increased by reducing the interval between doses, for example to 3-hourly during the day, or by increasing each individual dose. The usual total daily dose is 300–480 mg, taken in equally divided doses at 3- to 4-hourly intervals during the daytime. A total daily dose of over 480 mg is rarely well tolerated.

Neostigmine 15 mg is equivalent to pyridostigmine 60 mg. It is initially given in a dosage of 7.5–15 mg orally q.d.s., increasing to a usual total daily dose of 120 mg, taken in equally divided doses at 4-hourly intervals during the daytime.

At best the cholinesterase inhibitors restore muscle strength to around 80 per cent of normal, and there is no point in increasing dosages to try to achieve absolute normality, as this will result in unacceptable muscarinic adverse effects. If muscarinic effects occur they can sometimes be controlled by an antimuscarinic cholinoceptor antagonist, such as atropine (0.6 mg daily orally).

Parenteral formulations are available, and the dosages are much smaller parenterally than orally, because the drugs are poorly absorbed. Neostigmine 15 mg orally equals 1.5 mg i.m. and pyridostigmine 60 mg orally equals 2 mg i.m. Neostigmine can also be given subcutaneously.

Edrophonium can be used to test the adequacy of therapy with cholinesterase inhibitors. Edrophonium (2 mg i.v.) is given about 1 h after an oral dose of the cholinesterase inhibitor, when its action should be at a peak, and the patient's strength is tested before and after. If the strength improves significantly the dose of the oral cho-linesterase inhibitor may be increased. This should ideally be done in an intensive care unit.

(ii) Thymectomy

About 15 per cent of patients with myasthenia also have a thymoma. These patients respond well to treatment with prednisolone and azathioprine. Thymectomy is usually required to prevent or relieve obstruction, but it does not usually relieve the symptoms of myasthenia in these cases. Even if there is no thymoma the thymus is often structurally abnormal, and about 65 per cent of patients without a thymoma will respond favourably to thymectomy, 20–25 per cent having a complete remission and another 40 per cent having some improvement in symptoms. Thymectomy should particularly be considered in young patients.

(iii) Corticosteroids and azathioprine

In patients in whom myasthenia is limited to the ocular muscles prednisolone may be used initially instead of cholinesterase inhibitors or to replace them if they are ineffective. Prednisolone should be started in a low dose, such as 10 mg orally on alternate days, and this can be gradually increased in increments of 5 mg once a week to a total of 1.5 mg/kg on alternate days. For generalized myasthenia the patient should be admitted to hospital for steroid therapy. This departure from the usual method of using corticosteroids is because they may worsen myasthenia if large doses are given too quickly. When the disease is controlled the dosage of prednisolone can be reduced in the usual way (see p. 520). Short courses of prednisolone can also be helpful during transient bouts of deterioration.

In very severe cases of myasthenia, in patients with a thymoma, and in those without a thymoma who do not respond to thymectomy, the combination of prednisolone with azathioprine (2.5 mg/kg) can be very effective.

Plasmapheresis can be helpful in producing short-term improvement in patients with severe disease which is not responding well to prednisolone plus azathioprine.

(c) Treatment of crises

(i) Myasthenic crises

Often a myasthenic crisis co-exists with a cholinergic crisis. The management (ventilation, withdrawal of cholinesterase inhibitors, and sometimes plasma exchange) should be in an intensive care unit under the supervision of a neurologist.

In a myasthenic crisis the patient's oropharyngeal, laryngeal, and respiratory muscles may become so weak that it becomes impossible to maintain an adequate airway or respiratory movement. Various factors may precipitate a crisis, including infections, vigorous physical activity, and non-compliance with therapy. Certain drugs (listed in Table 30.8) may interact with the disease to cause a crisis, and myasthenic patients are exquisitely sensitive to competitive neuromuscular blocking agents, such as curare, but less sensitive to succinylcholine.

A myasthenic crisis can be diagnosed with the aid of edrophonium (see above) and treatment is by artificial ventilation. Patients in a true myasthenic crisis may be resistant to cholinesterase inhibitors, which are often withdrawn while ventilation and intensive care are given and reinstituted with good effect when the crisis has passed.

Plasmapheresis in such cases may restore responsiveness to cholinesterase inhibitors.

(ii) Cholinergic crises

Muscle fasciculation, pallor, sweating, small pupils, and excessive salivation are signs of excessive nicotinic and muscarinic cholinergic activity caused by overdose with cholinesterase inhibitors. The edrophonium test can be helpful in diagnosis (see above). Drug withdrawal is necessary and atropine may be used as an antidote.

■ **Table 30.8** Drugs which may worsen myasthenia gravis

Aminoglycoside antibiotics (for example gentamicin, streptomycin)
Antiarrhythmic drugs (lignocaine, procainamide)
β-Adrenoceptor antagonists (propranolol)
Phenothiazines
Phenytoin
Quinine and quinidine
Sedatives and hypnotics (for example barbiturates)

30.6 Muscle spasticity

Muscle spasticity occurs as a result of upper motor neurone lesions, and most commonly requires treatment in patients with spinal cord injuries and tumours, degenerative disease of the spinal cord, and multiple sclerosis. Spasticity can interfere markedly with remaining voluntary movement, and flexor spasms can be very painful.

30.6.1 Mechanisms of action of drugs used in the treatment of muscle spasticity

The drugs used in the treatment of muscle spasticity are listed in Table 30.9. Diazepam acts at the supraspinal and spinal cord levels by suppressing neuroneal transmission in polysynaptic more than monosynaptic reflex pathways. Whether this is due to its effect in enhancing GABA function is not known.

Baclofen is a GABA analogue which penetrates the CNS poorly. Its precise mechanism of action is unknown, but it is known to inhibit monosynaptic and polysynaptic neurotransmission at the level of the spinal cord.

Dantrolene is thought to act at the level of the skeletal muscle, inhibiting excitation–contraction coupling by reducing the amount of calcium released from the sarcoplasmic reticulum.

30.6.2 The use of drugs in the treatment of muscle spasticity

The drug therapy of muscle spasticity is generally only moderately effective and is limited by adverse effects.

■ **Table 30.9** Drugs used in the treatment of muscle spasticity

---

Diazepam (p. 564)
Baclofen (p. 563)
Dantrolene (p. 593)

(a) Diazepam

This is usually tried first, the dosage being limited by sedation and muscular hypotonia. The starting dosage of diazepam is usually 2–5 mg t.d.s. The dosage can be increased according to response in increments of 5 mg daily, and some patients tolerate 30–40 mg daily.

(b) Baclofen

Dosages of baclofen are started at 5 mg t.d.s. and increased to a maximum of 100 mg daily. Adverse effects include sedation, drowsiness, nausea, and hypotonia.

(c) Dantrolene

Dantrolene should be reserved for severely affected patients in whom there is none the less a realistic prospect of improvement. Initial dosages are 12.5–25 mg daily, increasing gradually at weekly intervals over a 4–7 week period to a maximum of 400 mg daily. If there is no worthwhile improvement after 6–7 weeks discontinue treatment.

Common adverse effects are drowsiness, muscle weakness, nausea, and vomiting. Liver function should be tested before dantrolene is given and 6 weeks after starting. Hepatic toxicity can be serious, and women over 30 y taking 300 mg or more daily seem most susceptible.

■ **Table 30.10** Causes of vertigo

1. *Vestibular disorders*
   Labyrinthine disease (inflammation, post-traumatic)
   Vestibular nerve or nucleus disease
     Neuronitis
     Tumours
     Drug toxicity
       Aminoglycoside antibiotics
       Frusemide
       Ethacrynic acid
   Menière's disease
   Benign positional vertigo

2. *Central neurological disorders*
   Brain-stem ischaemia
   Demyelinating disease (multiple sclerosis)
   Cerebellopontine angle tumours

3. *Systemic disease*
   Hypotension
   Vasculitis affecting the brain-stem

4. *Miscellaneous associations*
   Polycythaemia
   Diabetes mellitus
   Anaemia
   Dysproteinaemias

30.7 Vertigo

30.7.1 Mechanisms of action of drugs used in the treatment of vertigo

There are many causes of vertigo (see Table 30.10) but none of the drugs used in its treatment (listed in Table 30.11) acts on the causes. All of them interfere in one way or another with the labyrinthine or neuronal mechanisms by which the sensation of vertigo is mediated or appreciated and they therefore provide symptomatic relief only. The mechanisms whereby they do this are not known, although the following mechanisms have been proposed.

Antihistamines have been thought to act via their muscarinic blocking action, but there are also known to be histamine (H_1) receptors in the CNS and it is possible that the antihistamines act by blocking the central actions of histamine. It has also been suggested that they interfere with the functions of the vestibular nucleus and the reticular system.

Anticholinergic drugs, of which the use of hyoscine in motion sickness is the best example (discussed in Chapter 25, p. 321), presumably act by blocking muscarinic neurotransmission in the CNS.

Phenothiazines have antidopaminergic and anticholinergic activity and they may act at several points in the pathways which cause vertigo. It is worth noting that antihistamines and phenothiazines are also effective in the treatment of nausea, with or without vertigo.

▮ **Table 30.11** Drugs used in the treatment of vertigo

1. *Antihistamines (H₁ antagonists)* (p. 559)
   See list in Pharmacopoeia, but the following are favoured:
   Betahistine
   Buclizine
   Cinnarizine
   Cyclizine
   Dimenhydrinate

2. *Anticholinergic drugs* (p. 538)
   Hyoscine (scopolamine) (motion sickness)

3. *Tranquillizers*
   Diazepam (p. 564)

4. *Phenothiazines* (p. 645)
   Chlorpromazine
   Prochlorperazine
   Thiethylperazine

30.7.2 The use of drugs in the treatment of vertigo

(a) Acute severe vertigo associated with nausea and vomiting

Parenteral treatment is necessary because of vomiting. Prochlorperazine, 12.5 mg by deep intramuscular injection, may relieve the vertigo, nausea, and vomiting, allay the anxiety and distress, and sedate the patient. This may be followed by oral therapy. Note that old people are prone to extrapyramidal reactions with prochlorperazine, but phenothiazines should be used with caution in patients of all ages. If phenothiazines cause adverse effects a benzodiazepine (for example diazepam i.v. or rectally) may be a useful alternative.

(b) Moderate vertigo not associated with vomiting

Oral therapy with conventional doses of one of the antihistamines is usually sufficient.

In Ménière's disease drug therapy is complex. Because of the suggested excessive endolymph production in the labyrinth diuretic therapy is usually given. Antihistamines and anticholinergic drugs are also used.

30.8 Trigeminal neuralgia

Trigeminal neuralgia ('tic douloureux') is a disorder which is usually of unknown origin, but which sometimes accompanies multiple sclerosis. It causes attacks of intense pain in the distribution of the trigeminal nerve. The pain may be precipitated by touch, chewing, talking, or a cold wind. Patients may be able to identify trigger spots on the face, touching which causes an attack.

Carbamazepine is effective in relieving the symptoms of trigeminal neuralgia in a high proportion of cases, although high dosages are often required and about a third of patients may be unable to tolerate the consequent adverse effects, which include diplopia, ataxia, dizziness, and drowsiness. In a few patients a hypersensitivity reaction may occur, with skin rashes and rarely bone-marrow suppression.

▮ **Table 30.12** Drugs which may cause disorders of movement

1. *Tremor*
   B_2-adrenoceptor agonists (for example salbutamol)
   Lithium
   Xanthines

2. *Parkinsonism*
   Dopamine receptor antagonists
     Butyrophenones (for example haloperidol)
     Metoclopramide
     Phenothiazines (for example chlorpromazine)
     Thioxanthenes (for example flupenthixol)
   Reserpine

3. *Acute dystonias*
   Dopamine receptor antagonists
     Butyrophenones (for example haloperidol)
     Metoclopramide
     Phenothiazines (for example chlorpromazine)
     Thioxanthenes (for example flupenthixol)

4. *Akathisia and tardive dyskinesia*
   Dopamine receptor antagonists
     Butyrophenones (for example haloperidol)
     Phenothiazines (for example chlorpromazine)
     Thioxanthenes (for example flupenthixol)

One should begin carbamazepine therapy with a low dosage, say 100 mg t.d.s., increasing gradually over a period of weeks to a maximum of 1.6 g per day in divided doses. Most patients respond to 200 mg t.d.s. or q.d.s. Remember the phenomenon of autoinduction with carbamazepine (see p. 61) and be prepared to increase the dose if plasma concentrations (target range 25–50 μmol/mL) fall after a few weeks of steady-state therapy.

In cases in which carbamazepine is ineffective one may try baclofen (up to 20 mg t.d.s.), clonazepam (1–2 mg t.d.s.), or phenytoin (300 mg at night). In severe cases it may be necessary to lesion the trigeminal ganglion by phenol injection or radiofrequency rhizotomy, or to decompress or transect the trigeminal nerve.

30.9 Drug-induced movement disorders

Drugs which may cause disorders of movement are listed in Table 30.12.

31 The drug therapy of psychiatric disorders

Co-author: A. J. Wood

The groups of drugs used in psychiatric disorders are listed in Table 31.1. Although it is a formidable list, one can begin to learn something about the use of these groups of drugs by studying the representative members of each group listed in the right-hand column. These representative drugs may not be ideal for every patient, but they provide an introduction to each therapeutic class, upon which further experience can be built.

31.1 Mechanisms of action of drugs used in psychiatric disorders

Although it would be wrong to pretend that the mechanisms of action of any of the drugs used for treating psychiatric disorders are fully understood, it would also be wrong to suggest that nothing is known.

Research in neuropharmacology has revealed much about the pharmacological actions of psychotropic drugs, but there are problems in trying to relate the known pharmacological actions of psychotropic drugs to their therapeutic actions.

31.1.1 Hypnotics and anxiolytics

Benzodiazepines act at postsynaptic sites sensitive to the actions of GABA, where they enhance GABA function and thus cause increased inhibitory neurotransmission, which in turn leads to sedation and reduced anxiety.

The exact molecular interactions underlying this process are unknown, but it is a mechanism of great importance. Because there are specific binding sites for benzodiazepines in the brain, it has been proposed that there is an endogenous substance which normally binds to those sites and modulates GABA function; interference with this process might underlie both the symptoms of anxiety and changes in sleep pattern.

Chemicals have been identified, β-carbolines, which interact with specific benzodiazepine binding sites in the brain and cause a range of effects opposite to those of the benzodiazepines; these compounds cause anxiety and reduce sleep. Other endogenous substances which bind to benzodiazepine receptors have also been isolated from brain tissue and have been suggested to be naturally-occurring transmitters. It is thought that complex interactions between these endogenous transmitters and the benzodiazepine/GABA receptor complex, including adaptive changes in the receptor complex itself, might be one mechanism underlying the symptoms of anxiety.

Inhibitory GABA neurones are ubiquitous in the brain, and it is likely that the variety of clinical effects of the benzodiazepines reflects a range of possible interactions between GABA systems and other neurotransmitter pathways. One clue to the intermediate effector pathway in anxiety comes from the development of drugs, such as buspirone, gepirone, and ipsapirone, which are agonists at 5-HT_{1a} receptors and which are effective in the treatment of anxiety. This action implies that an effect of GABA on one or more of the 5-HT pathways in the brain might be important in the anxiolytic action of the benzodiazepines.

Subtypes of the GABA receptor have also been identified, and another possible explanation

■ **Table 31.1** Drugs used in the treatment of psychiatric disorders

Drug groups	Representative member
1. *Hypnotics*	
Benzodiazepines (p. 564)	Diazepam
Chlormethiazole (p. 579)	Chlormethiazole
Antihistamines (p. 559)	Promethazine (in children)
Chloral derivatives (p. 577)	Dichloralphenazone
2. *Anxiolytics*	
Benzodiazepines	Diazepam
β-adrenoceptor antagonists (p. 544)	Propranolol
3. *Antidepressants*	
Tricyclic antidepressants (p. 698)	Amitriptyline
Tetracyclic antidepressants	Maprotiline
Specific serotonin reuptake inhibitors	Paroxetine
Other reuptake inhibitors	Nomifensine
Monoamine oxidase inhibitors (p. 637)	Tranylcypromine
4. *Antipsychotic drugs*	
Phenothiazines (p. 645)	Chlorpromazine
Thioxanthenes (p. 645)	Trifluoperazine
Butyrophenones (p. 645)	Haloperidol
Others	Clozapine
5. *Lithium*	Lithium carbonate or citrate

for the range of clinical actions of the benzodiazepines lies in their interaction with different subtypes of GABA receptor.

31.1.2 Antidepressants

Most, although not all, of the tricyclic, tetracyclic, and other antidepressants inhibit the high affinity pump which takes up either noradrenaline or 5-HT from the synaptic cleft after their release. This reuptake process is the most important mechanism for terminating the actions of the monoamines. Some antidepressants are non-selective for the two monoamines, some inhibit noradrenaline uptake more than 5-HT uptake, some the reverse, and some are highly specific for 5-HT (the so-called 'specific serotonin reuptake inhibitors' or SSRIs) (see Table 31.2).

However, other antidepressant drugs, including iprindole and mianserin, do not block monoamine uptake at all. Thus, although there are good reasons for supposing that blockade of noradrenaline and/or 5-hydroxytryptamine uptake can somehow result in antidepressant activity, there may be other pharmacological routes to achieving the same antidepressant effect.

It is generally agreed that the antidepressants take 1–2 weeks to act, and this raises the possibility that adaptive pharmacological responses to the initial blockade of monoamine uptake are involved in the therapeutic action of the antidepressants. In experimental animals the long-term administration of tricyclic antidepressants leads to a reduction in the numbers of α_2-adrenoceptors, cortical β-adrenoceptors, and some 5-HT receptor functions, and to reduced activity of cortical noradrenaline-sensitive adenylate cyclase. Currently attention is being focused on these adaptive responses as a possible explanation for antidepressant activity. In this context it is interesting to note that mianserin, which is not a

■ **Table 31.2** Effects of antidepressants on monoamine reuptake

	Inhibition of uptake		
Drug	Noradrenaline	5-hydroxytryptamine	Dopamine
1. *Tricyclics*			
Amitriptyline	+ +	+ +	−
Desipramine	+ + +	+ +	−
Imipramine	+ +*	+	−
Nortriptyline	+ +	+	−
Iprindole	−	−	−
2. *Tetracyclics*			
Maprotiline	+ +	−	−
3. *Specific serotonin reuptake inhibitors*			
Fluoxetine	−	+ + +	−
Paroxetine	−	+ + +	−
4. *Others*			
Nomifensine	+ +	−	+

*Through its metabolite desipramine.

monoamine reuptake blocker, is an antagonist at α_2-adrenoceptors and 5-HT receptors, and this suggests that mianserin too has an effect on monoamine neurotransmission, albeit through a different mechanism of action.

In experimental animals, electroconvulsive shock, given in a manner similar to that in which electroconvulsive therapy is given to depressed patients, also has effects on monoamine neurotransmitters, some of which are similar to the effects of antidepressant drugs.

In addition, there is experimental evidence which shows that there is an abnormality of brain noradrenaline and 5-HT function in patients with depression, including studies on post-mortem brains of suicide patients and measurements of monoamine metabolites in the CSF. There are also changes in neuroendocrine responses to substances which alter the function of 5-HT receptors and adrenoceptors in depressed patients (for example reduced growth hormone responses to the α_2-adrenoceptor agonist clonidine in unipolar depression).

Many cyclic antidepressants also have anticholinergic and antihistaminic effects, but these are not thought to be linked to their antidepressant activity.

Monoamine oxidase (MAO) inhibitors inhibit the metabolism of noradrenaline, 5-HT, and dopamine. There is little doubt that they do this when given in adequate clinical dosages, and it is likely that the effective concentrations of brain monoamines rise as a result.

Presumably MAO inhibitors, by their effect on monoamine metabolism, and the cyclic antidepressants, by their effects on monoamine reuptake, both cause an increase in monoamine concentrations in the synaptic cleft, leading to common adaptive changes which result in the therapeutic antidepressant effect.

31.1.3 Lithium

There are several hypotheses concerning the mechanism of action of lithium in patients with affective illness.

The proposed effects of lithium are:

(1) that it 'stabilizes' neurotransmitter receptors against stimuli which cause upregulation and downregulation of receptor numbers;

(2) that it alters responses to receptor stimulation, and that it does this via effects on the second messenger systems which involve cyclic AMP and the polyphosphoinositides (see p. 47);

(3) that it increases the synthesis, turnover, and functional activity of brain 5-HT;

(4) that it alters certain aspects of neuronal membrane function by effects on sodium and potassium fluxes.

Which of these effects, if any, is responsible for the therapeutic effect of lithium is not known, but each hypothesis is backed by experimental evidence.

31.1.4 Antipsychotic drugs

It is believed that antipsychotic drugs act via antagonism of the actions of the neurotransmitter dopamine at its postsynaptic receptors, of which several subtypes have been identified in the brain.

The classical antipsychotic drugs, such as chlorpromazine and haloperidol, inhibit the action of dopamine on the postsynaptic dopamine receptors classified as D_2 receptors, but also to a lesser extent those classified as D_1. Indeed, although the various classical antipsychotic drugs have a range of pharmacological actions, for example α-adrenoceptor antagonism, histamine receptor antagonism, anticholinergic effects, and direct effects on membranes, the one feature they share is that of dopamine receptor blocking activity, and that is certainly the mechanism whereby they cause their Parkinsonian (extrapyramidal) adverse effects.

A novel type of drug, clozapine, is an antagonist at D_1 receptors with similar potency to the classical antipsychotic drugs, but it is much less potent at D_2 receptors and may also have some effect on D_4 receptors. Clozapine is an effective antipsychotic drug and causes fewer extrapyramidal adverse effects than the classical drugs.

There is furthermore some evidence which suggests that functional overactivity of dopamine may play a part in schizophrenia. For example, abuse of amphetamine, which causes release of dopamine in the brain, can lead to a paranoid psychotic state which can be indistinguishable from schizophrenia. However, no clear endogenous changes which incontrovertibly show an abnormality in the synthesis, turnover, or function of dopamine have so far been found in the schizophrenic brain which has not been exposed to neuroleptic drugs or in the CSF of patients with schizophrenia. It is therefore possible that the action of antipsychotic drugs in schizophrenia, which may be mediated by an effect on dopamine function, is only indirectly related to the primary neurochemical abnormality of the disorder.

As a parallel consider the actions of diuretics, whose beneficial effects in heart failure occur without any direct action of the drug on the primary site of disorder (the heart). The main site of action of diuretics is in the kidney, where they cause a sodium diuresis, preventing sodium retention brought about by poor renal perfusion and secondary hyperaldosteronism. By so doing they reduce blood volume, venous and pulmonary congestion, cardiac preload, and to some extent afterload, and the clinical state of heart failure improves.

By analogy it may well be that the abnormal brain function responsible for schizophrenia is 'channelled' through dopamine pathways in the brain and that the antipsychotic drugs, by their actions on dopamine receptors, block this 'channel' and modify the clinical manifestations of the disorder.

It is also known that antipsychotic drugs have long-term effects related to adaptive changes in the brain (see Chapter 4). These changes may be responsible for the adverse effect of tardive dyskinesia which antipsychotic drugs can cause (see below) and perhaps also for their therapeutic effects.

31.2 The use of drugs in the treatment of psychiatric disorders

It would not be appropriate here to enter into a discussion of the problems of psychiatric diagnosis, of the pros and cons of drug therapy versus psychotherapy in particular illnesses, or of the general role of psychotherapeutic and psychosocial interventions in the treatment of mental illness. Here we shall assume that diagnostic categories are appropriate, and we shall describe drug therapies which are known to be effective in those categories, the important issues surrounding their appropriate use, and their main adverse effects.

31.2.1 Insomnia

No currently available drug induces normal sleep, and all have drawbacks, such as tolerance, dependency, withdrawal reactions, and hangover effects. Thus, there is nothing which cures insomnia, i.e. which allows normal sleep without hangover, restores the normal sleep cycle, and maintains it after withdrawal.

Our understanding of sleep disorders is improving. We know, for instance, that somehow or other sleep is linked to circadian rhythms which depend on the function of biological clocks within the nuclei of the hypothalamus. The sleep EEG cycle has been described, with its alternating phases of slow-wave or non-rapid eye movement (non-REM) sleep and fast-wave or rapid eye movement (REM) sleep. These phases are thought to depend on the reciprocal functioning of aminergic inhibitory and cholinergic excitatory sets of neurones situated in the pontine brain stem. This improved understanding of the neuronal control of the sleep cycle has helped us to begin to understand the alterations in sleep which are produced by respiratory abnormalities, such as sleep apnoea, and by psychiatric disorders which may be associated with altered monoamine neurotransmission. However, it has not helped us to understand the mechanisms of action of the commonly used hypnotic drugs.

In recent years we have come to realize that hypnotic drugs have a pharmacological effect on sleep which is relatively short-lasting, and that the potential adverse effects of prolonged or casual administration of hypnotics can outweigh their therapeutic value. Thus, before prescribing hypnotic therapy one should consider the following points.

1. Is there an important reduction in the time and quality of sleep in this patient and is the patient's assessment of his or her sleep pattern accurate? These questions are important, because patients' assessment of the duration and quality of their sleep is highly subjective and because sleep requirements vary from individual to individual. For example, old people naturally sleep fewer hours at night than young people, partly because they tend to catnap during the day and partly because they may not actually need so many hours of sleep. Lying awake in the dark when the rest of the world is asleep can be unpleasant, and time seems to pass very slowly. This causes the patient to complain of insomnia and to seek help. Subjective feelings that their sleep has not been refreshing can also lead people to seek medical help, and whether or not one awakes from sleep feeling refreshed depends not only on the actual quality of a night's sleep, but also upon many factors in one's life, mood, and personality.

2. Is there a medical reason for poor sleep? Pain, depression, alcoholism, anxiety, stress, nocturia, itching, cough, and breathlessness can all affect sleep. In such cases treatment should be first directed at eliminating the primary cause rather than dealing symptomatically with the reported sleep disorder.

3. Particular care needs to be taken in old people when prescribing hypnotics, because their brains may be particularly sensitive to their effects, and because the half-times of the benzodiazepines (see Table 31.3) can be prolonged up to three-fold in old people. They may therefore become confused or ataxic while taking hypnotics, and may fall and injure themselves. Initial dosages of hypnotics in old people should be reduced.

4. Tolerance to the effects of hypnotic drugs occurs over a 2-week period. Most authorities now therefore recommend that hypnotic therapy should not be continued for longer than a week or two, because of the occurrence of dependence and the problem of withdrawal (see Chapter 34). Withdrawal can cause rebound insomnia, for which the patient again consults the doctor, who might be tempted to represcribe a hypnotic, and thus establish a vicious circle of withdrawal and represcription.

■ **Table 31.3** The mean half-times of some commonly used benzodiazeines

Drug	Half-time (h)
Clobazam*	20
Chlordiazepoxide*	24
Diazepam*	72
Flurazepam*	75
Loprazolam	9
Lorazepam	12
Lormetazepam	10
Nitrazepam	24
Oxazepam	12
Temazepam	10

*All these drugs are partly metabolized to active metabolites with long half-times (e.g desmethyldiazepam). Some of the benzodiazepines (for example clorazepate and prazepam) are completely metabolized to active metabolites with long half-times.

When it is decided to withdraw hypnotic therapy after prolonged use, the problem of withdrawal should be explained to the patient and a gradual reduction in dosage should be attempted. However, it is preferable to prevent dependence by limited prescribing in the first place, and when hypnotics are prescribed the patient should be told that it is important that therapy be of limited duration.

In practical terms, when one excludes those in whom sleep is perceived to be abnormal but is actually normal and those in whom a treatable underlying cause for insomnia can be found, one is left with a large group of patients who are justified in feeling that their sleep is inadequate. Amongst these, treatment with hypnotic drugs should be reserved for those with significant distress caused by what is a temporary problem in most cases.

The benzodiazepines are still the most commonly prescribed hypnotics, and the choice from among a large range of these drugs depends on their pharmacokinetics and the nature of the problem.

There is evidence that the benzodiazepines with relatively short half-times (see Table 31.3) and few or no active metabolites, such as tem-

azepam (10–30 mg) or oxazepam (15–25 mg), have less of a hangover effect and are less cumulative than say nitrazepam or diazepam. They may therefore be used as first choices in patients with simple insomnia.

In depressed patients with early morning wakening a sedative antidepressant, for example amitriptyline, given at night, may obviate the need for specific hypnotic therapy. However, if extra treatment is required a longer-acting benzodiazepine, such as diazepam (2–10 mg) or nitrazepam (5–10 mg), may help. On the other hand, if getting to sleep is a problem then shorter-acting compounds, such as temazepam (10–30 mg) or oxazepam (15–25 mg), would be preferred.

Hypnotic benzodiazepines should be taken 30 min before going to bed and dosages should be kept to the minimum necessary in all cases.

Chloral hydrate and dichloralphenazone are still sometimes used as hypnotics, especially in older people (see the Pharmacopoeia).

Barbiturates are no longer normally used as hypnotics in the UK, because of problems with tolerance and withdrawal.

31.2.2 Anxiety

Mild anxiety reactions to various social or family stresses are very common. Many people who complain of symptoms of anxiety will get better quickly, even if nothing is done. Simple supportive psychotherapy by the general practitioner, the passage of time, and the way in which the patient adapts to changed circumstances can all accelerate improvement. Anxiolytic therapy is therefore not needed for the majority of patients with mild symptoms. On the other hand, patients who have more severe symptoms or who fail to respond to simple supportive measures may benefit from anxiolytic drugs.

Benzodiazepines are still the most commonly prescribed drugs for the treatment of anxiety. Several are available, but there is little evidence that one is more effective than another. The treatment of anxiety with benzodiazepines should be limited to about 4 weeks, because of tolerance to their anxiolytic effects and because of the recognition that even short courses of benzodiazepines can lead to dependence and withdrawal symptoms. Withdrawal of benzodiazepines can lead to recurrence of the symptoms of anxiety, with dysphoria, tremor, sleeplessness, and occasionally psychotic reactions and convulsions. Problems during withdrawal may be less marked when drugs with long half-times are used for short periods of time.

Diazepam is a commonly prescribed anxiolytic in dosages of 2 mg t.d.s. in mild anxiety to 10 mg t.d.s. in more severe anxiety.

The azapyrone anxiolytic drugs (buspirone, gepirone, and ipsapirone) have actions different from those of the benzodiazepines. A symptomatic response to treatment may take up to 2 weeks and this should be explained to the patient. The azapyrones do not modify the symptoms of benzodiazepine withdrawal, and so they cannot be used as an immediate direct substitute for the benzodiazepines. However, their effects as sedatives and in slowing reaction times are much less marked than those of the benzodiazepines. They do not potentiate the central effects of alcohol or other psychotropic drugs and there is as yet no evidence of a withdrawal syndrome after discontinuation. Buspirone is given in an initial dosage of 5 mg b.d. increasing slowly to a daily maximum of 30–40 mg in 2 or 3 divided doses.

Patients with troublesome somatic symptoms in anxiety, for example palpitation, sweating, or tremor, may benefit from a non-selective β-adrenoceptor antagonist, such as propranolol (20–40 mg t.d.s.).

31.2.3 Depression

The problem of when to begin treating depression is highlighted by the fact that all trials of the effects of antidepressant drugs have shown that the placebo response rate is high (about 30 per cent), partly because depressive episodes are often self-limiting.

In the treatment of mild depression, drug therapy, apart from the symptomatic therapy of associated anxiety, as discussed above, has a minor role to play. However, in more severe depression, particularly that associated with biological disturbances, such as loss of appetite, constipation, early morning wakening, diurnal variation in mood, and psychomotor retardation, antidepressant drug therapy tends to be more

effective. There are no other good clinical predictors of responsiveness to antidepressant drugs.

(a) Tricyclic and tetracyclic antidepressants

The choice amongst cyclic antidepressant drugs is wide. The points to bear in mind are these:

1. Is the patient agitated? Is insomnia a problem? Is there a need for sedation? If so, an anxiolytic, sedative antidepressant, such as amitriptyline, may be prescribed.

2. Is lethargy and slowness a problem? If so, imipramine, which is less sedative than amitriptyline, may be used. Protriptyline, or one of the specific serotonin reuptake inhibitors (such as fluoxetine or paroxetine), which may be slightly stimulant, are suitable alternatives.

3. Is there likely to be a problem with cardiotoxicity, for example in patients with ischaemic heart disease? If so, consider one of the specific serotonin reuptake inhibitors, which affect the heart less than the tricyclic antidepressants.

4. Is there likely to be a problem with anticholinergic activity, for example in patients with glaucoma or prostatism? If so, consider lofepramine, a tricyclic antidepressant with less anticholinergic effects than others of this group, or a specific serotonin reuptake inhibitor.

Suicide is always a risk in patients with depression, and tricyclic antidepressant drug overdose can be particularly dangerous (see p. 496). For this reason one should prescribe only small amounts of an antidepressant at any time. Patients who are sufficiently depressed to require drug treatment should be seen frequently, in order to ensure that their depression is not worsening during the period before the drug begins to bring benefit and to assess their subsequent response to treatment.

Much has been made in the specialist literature of the use of plasma drug concentration measurements in monitoring and optimizing antidepressant drug therapy. Studies of the relationships between doses of antidepressants and their plasma concentrations have shown that for a given dose of antidepressant different patients will have remarkably different plasma drug concentrations, because of variability in the pharmacokinetics of the drugs (for example differences in hepatic metabolism). This is a situation in which plasma drug concentration measurement might in fact be useful (see p. 83). However, there is generally a poor relationship between the plasma drug concentration and the clinical antidepressant response, and this detracts from the value of monitoring antidepressant therapy in this way.

In carefully controlled studies of nortriptyline, low plasma nortriptyline concentrations are associated with a lack of response and intermediate concentrations with a good response. However, high concentrations are associated with a reduction in the therapeutic effect, and so the curve of plasma concentrations versus response looks like an inverted U (see Fig. 7.1). Studies with amitriptyline have shown either an inverted U curve or a linear relationship between response and dose. With imipramine the evidence is less clear, but the relationship may be linear.

However, there has not yet been a study to compare the outcome of antidepressant drug therapy with and without access to plasma drug concentration measurement; until that has been done we shall not know whether plasma concentration measurement is really helpful or not. The pharmacokinetics, adverse effects, drug interactions, and dosages of antidepressants are dealt with in the Pharmacopoeia. It is most important to recognize that the effective dosage in an individual is very variable, and that there is a latent period of about 2 weeks before the antidepressant effects of a given dosage regimen are seen, although an improvement in sleep may occur sooner. In contrast, adverse effects, particularly the anticholinergic effects of tricyclic antidepressants, occur much sooner than the antidepressant effect, and to some extent indicate the patient's tolerance of a given dosage.

As an example, consider the use of amitriptyline in the treatment of depression in an otherwise healthy 55-year-old woman. One would generally start with a low dosage and build up gradually, so that the patient can become tolerant of the adverse effects and excessive dosages can be avoided. Bedtime administration is recommended, since amitriptyline has sedative effects and aids sleep and since its peak adverse anticholinergic effects will occur during sleep. Some anxious, depressed patients find it preferable to spread out the dosage over the day, but most find bedtime administration preferable. Once-daily dosage is as effective as divided dosage, firstly because the half-times of these drugs are long (usually over 12 h), and secondly because the pharmacological action through which the therapeutic effect is mediated is probably not related to the moment-to-moment plasma drug concentration, but more to adaptive responses, which have a much longer half-time.

In an out-patient one would begin with 50 mg of amitriptyline at night and increase the daily dosage every 3 days by 25 mg, if tolerated, to a maximum initial total daily dose of 150 mg. Many patients will suffer anticholinergic effects at this dosage, and if the adverse effects are intolerable one would lower the total daily dose by 25 mg. In patients whose depression is resistant to conventional dosages of tricyclic antidepressants psychiatrists often use dosages which are higher than the published recommended ranges, if the patient can tolerate them, and some patients may benefit from this approach.

In old people initial dosages should be lower and increases in dosage should be undertaken more cautiously. For instance, with amitriptyline one would begin with 25 mg at night and increase as necessary every 2–3 d in increments of 10 mg. In this way one will pick up troublesome adverse effects early. Many old people will not tolerate more than 75 mg a day because of reduced clearance and increased pharmacodynamic sensitivity, particularly in relation to cardiotoxicity and hypotension. It is for this reason that drugs with fewer cardiac or anticholinergic adverse effects, such as lofepramine (140–210 mg daily in divided doses) or a specific serotonin reuptake inhibitor (for example fluoxetine 20 mg o.d.) are often preferred in old people.

In all patients treatment should be continued for 4–6 months after recovery at the dosage finally chosen. In first episodes of depression the dosage may then be gradually reduced over a few weeks and withdrawn. If there is a history of previous episodes of depression one should consider long-term prophylaxis using a dosage which is about half of the maximum dosage used in treating the acute depressive episode.

(b) Monoamine oxidase (MAO) inhibitors

Although they are effective antidepressants, the MAO inhibitors are not nowadays very popular, because of their potential to produce the hypertensive 'cheese reaction' and because of the risk of drug interactions. They therefore tend to be reserved for patients who have not responded to other antidepressant drugs and for those who are markedly phobic or hypochondriacal. They may also be useful for patients who have atypical somatic symptoms (hypersomnia and increased appetite with weight gain, as opposed to the more usual problems of poor sleep and loss of appetite). As with other antidepressants there is a latent period of about 2 weeks between starting treatment and the onset of therapeutic benefit.

The dosages, adverse effects, and interactions of MAO inhibitors are dealt with in the Pharmacopoeia, but the following important points should be remembered.

1. A hypertensive crisis may occur if a patient taking an MAO inhibitor also takes certain amine-containing foods, such as cheese, meat or yeast extracts, and unfresh poultry or game. All patients taking MAO inhibitors must be informed and educated about the risk of eating or drinking such foods (see Table 10.3).

2. Certain proprietary medicines, some of which may be bought at chemists' shops, contain sympathomimetic amines (for example decongestants for the relief of hay fever and the common cold). Such amines interact with MAO inhibitors in the same way as the amine-containing foods described above. Patients should be warned accordingly.

3. All patients taking an MAO inhibitor should be given a card (of the kind issued in the UK by the Department of Health) warning them of these dangers (see Fig. P7, p. 638).

31.2.4 Mania

The principles of treating mania lie in the use of antipsychotic (neuroleptic) drugs and possibly lithium in the acute phase, followed by maintenance therapy to prevent the recurrence of either manic or depressive episodes.

(a) Acute phase of mania

If the patient is very hyperactive parenteral doses of chlorpromazine or haloperidol may be needed and the i.m. route will generally be the most convenient. Once the patient is less active and more amenable, oral therapy with chlorpromazine, thioridazine, or haloperidol can be instituted. Dosages are listed in the Pharmacopoeia and must be tailored to the requirements of the individual. These drugs may produce a range of motor adverse effects, and as the manic phase comes under control extrapyramidal symptoms may require treatment with one of the anticholinergic anti-Parkinsonian drugs. Some of the anticholinergic drugs previously used in this context (for example benxhexol and benztropine) are now known to be abused by patients, because of the subjective 'high' which they give. Procyclidine seems to have less of an effect of this kind, and it is now widely used in the treatment of antipsychotic drug-induced movement disorders. It is given in an initial dosage of 2.5 mg t.d.s increasing to a usual maximum of 30 mg per day as required.

The acutely psychotic patient (whether manic or schizophrenic) may require very large doses of neuroleptic drugs, for reasons which are not understood. However, as the acute symptoms come under control the dosage of the antipsychotic drug can usually be gradually reduced.

The initiation of lithium therapy should generally be a specialist decision. Because lithium takes several days to reduce the acute symptoms of mania, it is usual to treat acute mania with antipsychotic (neuroleptic) drugs, and to reserve lithium for long-term prophylaxis, although occasionally a very mild episode may respond to lithium alone. Lithium is usually introduced once the symptoms of the acute illness have come under control with antipsychotic drugs.

Important aspects of lithium dosage, the formulations to use, and the monitoring of plasma lithium concentrations (necessary because of its low toxic:therapeutic ratio) are discussed in the Pharmacopoeia and in Chapter 7.

(b) The prophylaxis of manic-depressive disease

Manic-depressive disease is characterized by recurrent episodes of mania or depression, between which the patient may be quite well. The nature of these episodes is variable. Recurrent episodes of depression are most common (so-called 'unipolar illness'), but a mixture of manic and depressive episodes can occur (so-called 'bipolar illness'), as occasionally can recurrent manic episodes alone.

Whether or not lithium prophylaxis is indicated depends on the frequency of episodes of affective illness and their severity. Treatment may need to be continued indefinitely.

In bipolar illness, in which manic episodes occur, lithium is the preferred prophylactic agent. Lithium is also effective in the prevention of recurrent depressive episodes in unipolar illness, and here the choice is between lithium and tricyclic antidepressants. Whether or not one should use lithium or a tricyclic antidepressant in treating recurrent unipolar depression will depend on the patient's ability to tolerate the adverse effects of each type of drug and the psychiatrist's judgement of the benefit:risk ratio for that patient.

The dosages of lithium for prophylaxis, its adverse effects, and the importance of monitoring plasma concentrations are all discussed in the Pharmacopoeia and in Chapter 7.

The anticonvulsant drug carbamazepine is also used in the prophylaxis of bipolar illness, almost exclusively in specialist psychiatric clinics. It serves as a second-line drug in patients who do not respond to lithium, who cannot tolerate lithium, or in whom lithium is contra-indicated. In some patients with resistant bipolar illness a combination of lithium with carbamazepine may be effective. The plasma concentrations of carbamazepine which are associated with a therapeutic effect in bipolar depression are not the same as those which are associated with its anticonvulsant action, and the dosage of carbamazepine is usually monitored on the basis of the clinical response. The dosages and important adverse effects of carbamazepine are discussed in the Pharmacopoeia.

31.2.5 Schizophrenia

A brief description of schizophrenia is necessary for an understanding of the aims of drug therapy and of what is likely to be achieved by it.

Schizophrenia commonly first occurs during young adult life. Its onset may be insidious or acute. An acute attack may remit completely but may be followed by further acute attacks. After one or more acute episodes defects in personality and mental state may persist and these may gradually increase in severity.

Many patients who develop schizophrenia have normal premorbid personalities, while others have had more withdrawn, quiet, unsociable personalities.

Certain manifestations of schizophrenia are characteristic. Auditory hallucinations and delusions, often paranoid, are frequent. There may also be disorders of thought, in which patients may feel that their thoughts are being influenced or disrupted by outside forces, that thoughts are being inserted, withdrawn, or broadcast. Thinking is vague and unfocused and as a result communication can be difficult. Replies to questions do not constitute proper answers and can ramble on into irrelevancies. There may be a disturbance of affect: the schizophrenic is characteristically distant and lacking in warmth and rapport. Emotional responses may be incongruous: for example, the patient may suddenly laugh inappropriately at something serious or unfunny.

In addition to these psychological abnormalities there may also be abnormalities of posture and movement, of which catatonia is the most striking extreme example.

During the active phase of schizophrenia hallucinations, delusions, and other florid symptoms (so-called 'positive symptoms') tend to predominate. In the chronic phase there is increasing apathy and emotional blunting, with loss of motivation, poverty of speech, and loss of self-care ('negative symptoms').

In the treatment of this variable and complex psychiatric state drug treatment, although very important, is only one part of the overall therapeutic approach.

(a) The general effects of drug treatment in schizophrenia

Generally, antipsychotic treatment has a good effect on the positive symptoms of acute schizophrenia, i.e. hallucinations, delusions, and gross thought disorder. The negative symptoms, such as apathy and emotional passivity, are less responsive to treatment, although a new drug, clozapine (see below), may be more effective for those symptoms.

The acute phase of schizophrenia is more responsive than the chronic phase, but long-term antipsychotic drug therapy may help to prevent relapses and may have some effect in preventing or slowing the development of serious chronic negative symptoms in some patients.

Care should be taken during withdrawal of antipsychotic drugs, since relapse may occur, particularly if there are continuing psychosocial stresses, against which the antipsychotic drugs seem to have some protective effect.

The final outcome of drug treatment is variable. Good prognostic features include a normal premorbid personality, the occurrence of an acute illness, and catatonic features during the acute phase. Bad prognostic features include an abnormal premorbid personality, an insidious onset, and a preponderance of negative symptoms.

(b) The choice of drug in schizophrenia

Although there are differences in the overall spectrum of effects, both therapeutic and adverse, of the antipsychotic drugs, their essential therapeutic effects in schizophrenia are similar. Differences lie in the degree of sedation produced (good for the agitated patient), in the degree of quietening of the hyperactive state (good for the patient in acute florid schizophrenia), and in the risk of producing extrapyramidal and anticholinergic adverse effects. For example, chlorpromazine is sedative and is useful for violent, overactive, difficult patients who may become less disturbed without becoming stuporose. Haloperidol is also generally accepted as having a specific and useful effect in patients with marked hyperactivity. Haloperidol and trifluoperazine more frequently cause extrapyramidal adverse effects, while thioridazine and chlorpromazine do so less often.

Here we shall confine our discussion to chlorpromazine, haloperidol, and fluphenazine, whose use will illustrate many of the aspects of treatment.

In the acute phase the patient may be so disturbed that parenteral therapy is indicated. Chlorpromazine is usually given in a dosage of 50–100 mg i.m. every 6–8 h. However, when it is used in specialist psychiatric units, and especially for patients who are severely disturbed, larger and more frequent doses are often given initially and are titrated against the patient's clinical state. Chlorpromazine, probably because of its α-adrenoceptor blocking action, can produce profound hypotension when given parenterally and patients should, if possible, remain supine for 30–60 min after injection.

Haloperidol is a suitable alternative in the acute phase. Parenteral therapy may be required in dosages of 2–10 mg i.m. 6-hourly, although the effective dosage in an individual is variable and depends on the patient's clinical state.

When the most florid symptoms have settled down sufficiently, oral therapy may be started. Apart from great variability in the clearance rate of chlorpromazine and its metabolites from patient to patient there are also differences in the sensitivity of the schizophrenic state to the drug. Thus, it is necessary to be flexible in choosing dosages to match each patient's response. Effective oral dosages of chlorpromazine vary enormously, from a small dosage of 25 mg t.d.s., to a moderate dosage of 100 mg t.d.s., to huge dosages of 400 mg t.d.s. or more, which may be needed in very disturbed patients. The effective oral dosage range for haloperidol is similarly wide.

After the acute phase of the illness has come under control and stabilized long-term maintenance therapy may be desirable in order to reduce the risk of relapse. If oral therapy with chlorpromazine is continued, the dosage might be reduced, for example from 400 mg daily to 75 mg at night. However, sudden reductions in dosage are inadvisable, because of unpredictability of response and the risk of symptomatic relapse.

Long-term oral therapy can be unreliable because of poor compliance and sometimes uncertain systemic availability. For this reason intramuscular formulations have been developed which slowly release their drug from an intramuscular depot site over 1–3 weeks. These formulations can be substituted for chlorpromazine or haloperidol if they have been effective. One such formulation is fluphenazine decanoate in oil (Modecate®), which is given by deep intramuscular injection. Initially a test dose of 12.5 mg is given, followed, after an interval of 4–7 d, by 25 mg i.m. Injections are then usually given at intervals of 2–4 weeks, the exact dose and interval being determined by the individual response.

The routine of the depot injection clinic also serves to regularize the supervision and treatment of patients with schizophrenia, who are notoriously unpredictable in taking medicines.

(c) Resistant schizophrenia

In a few patients the standard antipsychotic drugs will be ineffective and other approaches may be tried. There is no consensus on what the next approach should be in such patients, and a variety of other treatments are used. These include electroconvulsive therapy (ECT) or the addition of a benzodiazepine or lithium to the standard antipsychotic treatment.

Recently, a novel dopamine antagonist, clozapine, has become available and is proving useful in resistant schizophrenia, although its use is limited by the serious adverse effect of neutropenia and by its tendency to cause seizures. Clozapine is an antagonist at dopamine receptors. However, in contrast to the classical antipsychotics, it is not very effective at the subtype of receptors known as D_2 and is more effective at D_1 and D_4 receptors. Clinically it is effective in the treatment of schizophrenia. In contrast to the classical antipsychotic drugs, it seems to have beneficial effects on the negative symptoms, and it is speculated that this may be related to an action on $5-HT_2$ receptors. It also has a lower risk of extrapyramidal adverse effects (see below). However, its licence in the UK currently restricts its use to specialists and only those who are registered with the special scheme which has been established for monitoring the white cell count regularly in order to minimize the risk of serious neutropenia. Any patient who is taking clozapine should not be given other drugs with a high risk of neutropenia (for example carbimazole).

(d) Adverse effects of antipsychotic drugs

The adverse effects of antipsychotic drugs are catalogued in the relevant sections of the Pharmacopoeia and are summarized in Table 31.4. The treatment of Parkinsonism and tardive dyskinesias can be problematic and further discussion is warranted here.

■ **Table 31.4** Adverse effects of antipsychotic drugs

Psychiatric	Sedation
	Depression
Extrapyramidal and motor	Acute dystonias
	Restlessness (akathisia)
	Parkinsonism
	Tardive dyskinesia
Autonomic	Hypotension
	Acute cholinergic effects
	Cardiac arrhythmias
Skin	Photosensitivity
Endocrine and metabolic	Weight gain
	Hyperprolactinaemia, galactorrhoea
	Gynaecomastia and loss of libido in men
Other	Hepatitis
	Blood dyscrasias (especially clozapine)
	Corneal and lens opacities (chlorpromazine)
	Retinal abnormalities (thioridazine)

(i) Parkinsonism

In most patients improvement can be obtained with one of the anti-Parkinsonian anticholinergic drugs, such as procyclidine. However, most authorities do not recommend the routine use of these drugs, but prefer to wait until the individual patient shows signs of needing them.

(ii) Tardive dyskinesia

After prolonged use the antipsychotic drugs can cause a disturbance of motor function, called tardive dyskinesia, which is characterized by orofacial grimacing and by chewing and athetoid (writhing) movements of the head, neck, and upper limbs. The pharmacological mechanism of this adverse effect is poorly understood, but studies in experimental animals have shown that long-term antipsychotic drug therapy causes an increase in the number of dopamine receptors in the basal ganglia, leading to overactivity of dopamine function, which is thought to be the cause of the abnormal movements, although other evidence points to an involvement of GABA pathways within the extrapyramidal motor system.

Tardive dyskinesia is exceedingly difficult to treat effectively. Anticholinergic drugs may worsen the symptoms and should be withdrawn. Very gradual reduction in antipsychotic drug dosages may be tried, although it may be difficult to strike a balance between controlling the psychosis and minimizing the tardive dyskinesia, which may sometimes be irreversible. However, if antipsychotic therapy can be withdrawn without relapse and without worsening the psychosis there may sometimes be a gradual improvement in the dyskinesia, and it may also subsequently become possible to restart antipsychotic drug therapy at a lower dosage. Conversely, sometimes withdrawal of the antipsychotic medication, even gradually, may worsen the tardive dyskinesia, and the former dosage of the drug must be given.

Medications which have been used to treat tardive dyskinesia include reserpine and tetrabenazine (which deplete dopamine), lithium (which may 'desensitize' dopamine receptors), benzodiazepines (which alter GABA neurotransmission in the extrapyramidal tracts), and various means of increasing acetylcholine activity by providing more choline, for example as lecithin. Unfortunately, none of these has proved very effective. A new antipsychotic drug clozapine (see above) has a lower risk of extrapyramidal adverse effects.

(iii) The neuroleptic malignant syndrome

The neuroleptic malignant syndrome is a rare but serious idiosyncratic adverse reaction of unknown cause, in which there is usually a sudden onset of fever, akinesia, rigidity, reduced consciousness, and autonomic disturbances, including tachycardia and hypertension. It can be fatal and demands emergency treatment by active cooling and i.v. dantrolene (see p. 593).

32 The relief of pain

Co-author: H. J. McQuay

In this chapter we shall consider the symptomatic treatment of pain, remembering that the treatment of pain should also take account of the cause of the pain (see below).

Pain is a subjective symptom which is affected by a variety of psychological factors. Some patients complain of pain when seemingly negligibly painful stimuli are present; this is known as a low pain threshold. Others do not complain in the face of apparently severely painful stimuli; this is known as a high pain threshold. Even an individual may appreciate the intensity of pain differently at different times, and factors such as anxiety, depression, boredom, or distraction can influence the way in which we perceive pain. It is well known, for example, that men injured in war may not feel the pain of their injuries until long after they have been sustained.

Pain can be reduced in intensity by simple reassurance, by hypnosis, by trance-like meditative states, and by acupuncture. It can also be alleviated by the administration of inactive material: the placebo response, which occurs in about one-third of patients with pain (see Chapter 14). These phenomena have been ascribed to functions of the endogenous opioid peptides, the endorphins and enkephalins, in the brain and spinal cord, but the role of these substances in the physiological control of the mechanisms in the nervous system which process pain sensations has yet to be fully defined. However, in practical terms these observations emphasize that management of the whole patient, rather than the uncritical prescription of analgesics alone, is of great importance in the treatment of pain.

32.1 Anatomical and neuropharmacological mechanisms underlying pain sensation

The chain of central nervous mechanisms which underlie pain sensation is illustrated in Fig. 32.1. The sequence is as follows:

1. Noxious stimuli are detected by receptors in pain-sensitive tissues.

2. The signal generated by these receptors is transferred by sensory nerves, through the dorsal root ganglia, to the dorsal horn of the spinal cord.

3. The signal received through the peripheral sensory mechanisms is processed by the spinal cord segment and transferred via ascending spinal cord pathways to various parts of the brain.

4. The signals received in the thalamic nuclei, periventricular grey matter, and brain-stem reticular formation are processed and passed on to the sensory cortex, giving one the sensation of pain.

5. Signals received in several sites, but particularly in the reticular formation and medulla, descend, through polysynaptic pathways, to the dorsal horn of the spinal cord, where they may either facilitate or inhibit activity.

Although the precise functions of some of the central nervous system relays are not understood, the relevant neuropharmacology is becoming clearer. Opiate receptors and opioid peptides,

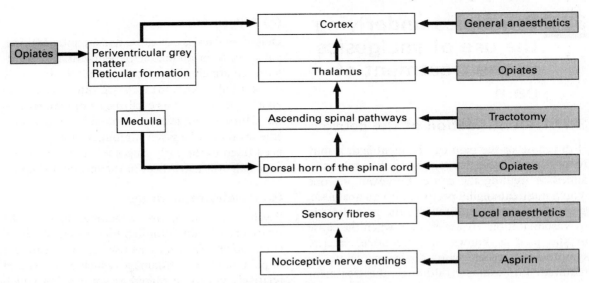

■ **Fig. 32.1** Nervous pathways mediating pain and the sites of action of analgesics.

particularly the enkephalins, are found in the dorsal horn of the spinal cord, in the periventricular grey matter, and in the thalamus. The opioid peptides probably function as neurotransmitters in these areas. Substance P is highly concentrated in the dorsal horn of the spinal cord, where it might function as a neurotransmitter for the relay of nervous impulses. 5-hydroxytryptamine is the neurotransmitter of the system which originates in the medulla and descends to the dorsal horn, where it probably modulates sensory inputs from the periphery.

32.2 Mechanisms of action of analgesics

Against this background the actions of the analgesics can be at least partly understood. Their sites of action are illustrated in Fig. 32.1.

Analgesics are of two broad types, opioid and non-opioid. The non-opioid analgesics include drugs such as aspirin and related salicylates and paracetamol. The opioid analgesics are in turn of two types, the non-synthetic or semi-synthetic compounds related to morphine and the synthetic opioids which are not related to morphine. Opioid analgesics used to be referred to as narcotic analgesics.

Non-opioid analgesics are thought to act peripherally, but there may be central components to their actions. Aspirin is a potent inhibitor of cyclo-oxygenase (prostaglandin synthetase) and it thus inhibits the formation of the prostaglandins. Through this mechanism it produces at least its anti-inflammatory action, and even if inflammation is not primarily involved in the syndrome of pain, the inhibition of prostaglandin synthesis is thought to remove the effect of prostaglandins in lowering the threshold at which pain nerve-endings fire, i.e. it makes them less sensitive to painful stimuli.

The analgesic action of paracetamol is not so easy to explain. It is a poor inhibitor of peripheral prostaglandin synthesis, but it has been suggested that it may inhibit brain prostaglandin synthetase activity and somehow produce an analgesic effect centrally. However, the matter is not settled.

The opioid analgesics all act as complete or partial agonists at opioid receptors, of which there are several types, in the brain and spinal cord and in the periphery (for example in the gut). The three subtypes of opioid receptor which are involved in analgesia are the μ, δ, and κ receptors. Presumably the opioid analgesics mimic the actions of the endogenous opioid peptides, albeit in great excess, and thereby inhibit both the spinal and central processing of pain sensation.

32.3 Principles underlying the use of analgesics in the treatment of pain

32.3.1 Identification of the cause

If the cause of the pain can be identified, it may be possible to treat the pain by specific measures aimed at treating the cause. For example, one would not treat angina pectoris with an analgesic, since glyceryl trinitrate relieves the pain directly by vasodilatation. However, even when the cause of the pain is known and treatable, interim symptomatic relief with analgesics may be required. For example, although the treatment of acute peritonitis involves surgery and antibiotic therapy, opioid analgesics are used to relieve the pain. In the discussion that follows we shall deal only with the symptomatic relief of pain. ∎

32.3.2 The need for adequate dosages of analgesics

When treating pain it is important to give effective dosages of analgesics. Ideally treatment should be given often enough to provide continuous control of pain. In the context of chronic pain this means that one does not control continuing severe pain on the basis of giving doses of analgesics only when the pain makes the patient ask for analgesia, allowing the pain to recur before giving further treatment. Instead, doses of analgesics in such cases should be given in anticipation of pain, based on careful observation of the pattern of symptoms in the individual patient. When there is acute pain there is little time to titrate the dose against the patient's response. This means that one should be prepared to increase the dose quite quickly until the pain is under control.

32.3.3 The use of adjunctive therapy

There are several circumstances in which drugs other than analgesics may be helpful as adjunctive therapy.

(a) Antiemetics

Opioid analgesics can cause nausea and vomiting, particularly in ambulant patients, and in short-term treatment (for example after an acute myocardial infarction) they are often given with an antiemetic, such as cyclizine or prochlorperazine. During long-term oral opioid therapy antiemetics should be given if required. Few patients need them in the early stages of cancer pain, but over half will need them in the terminal stages.

(b) Psychotropic drugs

Psychotropic drugs are sometimes used in the treatment of pain, although their mode of action is unknown. They may be used in the treatment of pain due to nerve damage, which may respond relatively poorly to opioid analgesics, but which may respond to anticonvulsants and tricyclic antidepressants. For example, tricyclic antidepressants are used in postherpetic neuralgia and anticonvulsants in trigeminal neuralgia and diabetic neuropathy. They are also used as adjunctive therapy with opioid analgesics in the management of chronic pain, when tricyclic antidepressants are often used. If anxiety is an important component of pain a benzodiazepine may be of value. Benzodiazepines, chloral hydrate derivatives, or tricyclic antidepressants may also be useful if insomnia is associated with pain.

(c) Laxatives

Laxatives are often necessary to relieve constipation during long-term treatment with opioid analgesics.

32.3.4 Differences in the analgesic and anti-inflammatory properties of analgesic drugs

It is important to note that non-steroidal anti-inflammatory drugs and drugs used as analgesics vary in their analgesic and anti-inflammatory activities, as shown in Table 32.1. Drugs which have both analgesic and anti-inflammatory properties are specifically useful in the treatment of rheumatic and other arthropathies (see Chapter 29) and in the treatment of painful bony metastases.

■ **Table 32.1** Analgesic and anti-inflammatory properties of some commonly used analgesics and non-steroidal anti-inflammatory drugs

	Analgesic activity	Anti-inflammatory activity
Aspirin	+	+
Paracetamol	+	−
Ibuprofen	+	+
Indomethacin	+	+ +
Phenylbutazone	+	+ +
Mefenamic acid	+	+
Flufenamic acid	−	+

■ **Table 32.2** Drugs used in the symptomatic treatment of pain

1. *Non-opioid analgesics (for mild to moderate pain)*
   Aspirin (p. 677)
   Paracetamol (p. 657)
   Some non-steroidal anti-inflammatory drugs (see Table 32.1)

2. *Combinations of non-opioid and opioid analgesics (for mild to moderate pain)*
   Co-codaprin (aspirin + codeine)
   Co-codamol (paracetamol + codeine)
   Co-proxamol (paracetamol + dextropropoxyphene)
   Co-dydramol (paracetamol + dihydrocodeine)

3. *Opioid and other narcotic analgesics* (p. 641)
   For mild to moderate pain
      Codeine
      Dextropropoxyphene
      Dihydrocodeine
      Buprenorphine
   For severe pain
      Morphine
      Diamorphine
      Buprenorphine
      Pethidine
      Dextromoramide
      Dipipanone
      Methadone

32.4 The practical use of analgesics

The various analgesics we shall discuss are listed in Table 32.2. Some examples of the conditions in which they may be used are listed in Table 32.3, and some pain syndromes which have specific forms of treatment are listed in Table 32.4.

32.4.1 Non-opioid analgesics for mild to moderate pain

Non-opioid analgesics are chiefly indicated for the treatment of simple headaches, somatic pain in the musculoskeletal tissues, and other mild to moderate non-visceral types of pain.

Aspirin is the analgesic of choice for musculo-skeletal pain and simple headache. It is particularly effective if there is also an inflammatory element. The main problem with aspirin is gastric irritation, which at its mildest may result in dyspepsia and at its most severe may cause peptic ulceration and symptomatic gastrointestinal bleeding and perforation (see p. 678). Dyspepsia due to aspirin may be lessened by taking it with food and by using soluble or buffered formulations. These formulations are particularly useful for the treatment of acute pain, since they are relatively quickly absorbed. For chronic pain one may use formulations such as microencapsulated or enteric-coated aspirin, or other types of salicylate which cause less gastrointestinal irritation (for example benorylate or salsalate, see p. 677).

Paracetamol is an alternative to aspirin. It should be used instead of aspirin in the treatment of pain in patients with an increased tendency to gastric irritation, which it does not cause, in patients who are sensitive to aspirin (see p. 111), in patients taking warfarin (see p. 136), and in children under 12 years of age, in whom aspirin is contra-indicated because of the small risk that it may cause Reye's syndrome. However, paracetamol has no anti-inflammatory activity and is not a substitute for aspirin in circumstances in which an anti-inflammatory action is required.

32.4.2 Opioid analgesics for mild pain

Dextropropoxyphene and codeine are often used in combination with non-opioid analgesics in the

■ **Table 32.3** Examples of appropriate analgesics for some clinical problems

Condition	Analgesic
Simple headache	Aspirin or paracetamol
Sprained ankle	Aspirin
Pain after dental extraction	Co-codaprin, co-proxamol, or NSAID
Mild sciatic pain	Co-codaprin or co-proxamol
Severe sciatic pain	Dihydrocodeine or buprenorphine
Moderately severe postoperative pain (for example orthopaedic)	Dihydrocodeine or buprenorphine + NSAID
Severe postoperative or traumatic pain	Morphine, diamorphine, or buprenorphine + NSAID
Severe intractable pain of malignancy	Morphine, diamorphine, dipipanone, dextromoramide, etc + NSAID (see text)
Acute myocardial infarction	Morphine or diamorphine
Acute abdominal pain	Pethidine or buprenorphine
Pain of labour	Pethidine or spinal opiates

NSAID = non-steroidal anti-inflammatory drug.

■ **Table 32.4** Some pain syndromes with specific analgesic treatments

Condition	Treatment
Dysmenorrhoea	Mefenamic acid
Bone pain from metastatic malignancy	Opioid analgesics + NSAID
Bone pain from metastatic prostatic carcinoma	Stilboestrol + analgesics or buserelin/gonadorelin (see p. 361)
Trigeminal neuralgia	Carbamazepine
Diabetic neuropathy	Carbamazepine
Lightning pains of tabes dorsalis	Carbamazepine
Migraine (p. 436)	Acute: ergotamine aspirin + metoclopramide paracetamol + metoclopramide sumatriptan Prophylaxis: pizotifen
Giant cell arteritis and polymyalgia rheumatica	Corticosteroids
Postherpetic neuralgia	Amitriptyline

NSAID = non-steroidal anti-inflammatory drug.

treatment of mild pain, increasing analgesia by invoking different mechanisms. They may also have a slight euphoriant action, which potentiates the overall analgesic effect. These opioid analgesics should therefore not be prescribed for long periods of time for trivial reasons, since they carry a slight potential for abuse and also cause constipation.

32.4.3 Opioid analgesics for the treatment of moderate pain

Codeine, dihydrocodeine, and dextropropoxyphene can be useful in patients with moderate to severe visceral pain. However, in high dosages codeine and dihydrocodeine cause constipation, sedation, dizziness, and (especially in old people) confusion. Oral morphine or sublingual buprenorphine are often preferred if increases in dosage requirements are predictable.

32.4.4 Opioid analgesics for the treatment of severe pain

Potent opioid analgesics are particularly indicated for the relief of visceral pain, postoperative pain, severe pain in trauma, and the pain of advanced malignant disease. Morphine and diamorphine have the additional very useful actions of relieving anxiety, producing drowsiness, and allowing sleep. Because they also cause peripheral vasodilatation they are the opioids of choice in the treatment of the pain of acute myocardial infarction.

For the relief of pain in labour pethidine is generally chosen if only short-term relief is required, since it has a short duration of action and therefore causes less respiratory depression in the newborn than other potent opioid analgesics. Epidural anaesthesia is preferred for more long-term relief. Pethidine is also sometimes preferred to morphine in the treatment of biliary and ureteric colic, since it is thought to cause less smooth muscle contraction.

Although there are quantitative differences among the opioid analgesics they all have the potential to produce similar adverse effects, such as respiratory depression, suppression of the cough reflex, nausea and vomiting, constipation, and tolerance and dependence.

Beware of prescribing opioid analgesics for any of the following:

(1) patients with impaired liver function (see p. 109);

(2) patients with increased intracranial pressure, since the level of consciousness and the diameter and reactivity of the pupils in such cases are important guides to the aetiology and prognosis;

(3) patients with reduced respiratory function;

(4) patients with hypotension;

(5) patients with impaired renal function: this is important for opioid analgesics with pharmacologically active metabolites which are excreted via the kidneys, including pethidine (toxic metabolite norpethidine) and morphine (active metabolite morphine-6-glucuronide).

It is important to appreciate that the respiratory depression which opioid analgesics may cause is counterbalanced by pain. Thus, these drugs will produce respiratory depression more readily in patients without pain. If one carefully titrates the dose against the pain, one can achieve effective analgesia with little effect on respiratory function.

Details of the formulations available, dosages, routes of administration, and so on, are given in the Pharmacopoeia (see p. 641), but some points are worthy of emphasis.

For short-term treatment of pain morphine and diamorphine are given parenterally. The choices of parenteral routes are subcutaneous (not generally favoured because of variable absorption), intramuscular (usually the preferred route), and intravenous (usually reserved for very severe acute pain or in acute left ventricular failure with pulmonary oedema). Nowadays it is also common to treat some forms of postoperative pain by giving opiates intrathecally or extradurally, either as a bolus or by continuous administration.

For more chronic pain oral formulations are available, for example as elixirs, particularly in combination with antiemetics, such as chlorpromazine (see the Pharmacopoeia). When patients with chronic pain can no longer take oral therapy subcutaneous infusions may be used. In such cases diamorphine is often used, because it is very soluble and can be given in large doses in relatively small volumes compared with morphine.

The usual dose of morphine i.m. is 10 mg. It takes effect within 15–30 min, reaching a maximum in 1–1.5 h, and lasting 3–6 h. The effective dose when given orally, whether as an elixir or as controlled-release tablets, is unpredictable, and usually a larger dose is needed than by the parenteral route, because of first-pass metabolism. If one uses the controlled-release formulation one should first determine the individual patient's daily dosage requirement using elixir and then substitute the controlled-release tablets, giving half the daily requirement in 12-hourly doses. This is because the time to steady state (see p. 23) will depend on the rate-limiting half-time, which in this case is the half-time of release of morphine from the controlled-release formulation. Since this is very long by comparison with the desired onset of action, treatment from the start with a controlled-release formulation will lead to a long delay in the onset of action and difficulty in titrating the dosage to the needs of the patient.

Dosages of diamorphine by any route are about half of those of morphine.

Pethidine is a poor choice for long-term analgesia, because of its unpredictable systemic availability after oral administration, its short duration of action, and its toxic metabolite, norpethidine.

Dextromoramide, dipipanone, and methadone are generally used in the long-term management of intractable pain, as alternatives to morphine or diamorphine (for example in the pain associated with malignant disease). They have similar adverse effects to morphine and diamorphine, but occasional patients find that they are as effective or more effective and have fewer adverse effects.

Buprenorphine is a selective partial agonist at opioid μ receptors. Since it is a partial agonist, it has a low potential for dependence. It has a duration of action of 6–8 h and can be given both parenterally (i.v. and i.m.) and sublingually, for both acute and chronic pain. The sublingual route obviates its first-pass metabolism by the liver and it is especially useful in treating transient, moderate to severe visceral pain. Note that naloxone (see p. 641) is not very effective as an antagonist of the effects of buprenorphine, because buprenorphine dissociates slowly from the opioid receptors.

32.5 The treatment of intractable pain in terminal malignant disease

Analgesia is only one factor in the treatment of the pain and distress of advanced, metastatic, and terminal malignant disease, the management of which has become a specialty of its own in recent years.

In the treatment of pain in these patients there are certain important principles to be observed, similar to the general principles outlined above.

1. Analgesic therapy must be carefully titrated to suit the needs of the individual.
2. Pain should be relieved quickly and effectively by the administration of adequate doses of analgesics given sufficiently frequently.
3. One should not withhold analgesics simply because of a concern that dependence may occur. When effective pain relief is the chief goal dependence and tolerance are of minimal concern.

The treatment of pain in terminal malignancy can begin with simple non-opioid analgesics, and these may be effective when combined with other methods of general management. If and when the pain becomes worse, an oral opioid analgesic will be indicated; some use the synthetic opioids, such as oral dipipanone, dextromoramide, or methadone, but most prefer morphine.

Whichever analgesic is chosen the starting dose should be at the lower end of the dosage range (for example 10 mg of morphine in a conventional formulation four-hourly), increasing the dose every 24 h until the pain is controlled. If the pain is very severe doses may be increased more often. For morphine the steps in dose should be 10, 20, 30, 45, 60, 90, 120, and 150 mg. As soon as the pain is controlled the effective dose should be repeated at the usual dosage interval (for example four-hourly for morphine), or more frequently if the patient's pain is recurring before the next dose is due. When the daily requirements have been established one can switch to twice-daily dosage of a slow-release formulation.

Parenteral analgesics should be necessary only for the patient who cannot swallow or who is vomiting.

Phenothiazines should be used to prevent nausea and vomiting due to opiate analgesics (see the Pharmacopoeia for lists of some available elixir formulations of opioid analgesics with chlorpromazine).

33 General anaesthesia and local anaesthetics

Co-author: J. W. Sear

Anaesthetists are practical clinical pharmacologists. Through the skilled use of drugs the patient is tranquillized and prepared for operation, quickly and pleasantly rendered unconscious and unfeeling, and kept so at a finely tuned level throughout the operation. During this time muscle relaxants may be used to facilitate surgery, the patient's airways are carefully kept patent, and meticulous attention is paid to oxygenation and the preservation of normal blood gases and acid-base balance. Cardiovascular function and blood pressure are monitored and kept within well-defined acceptable limits.

All of this requires careful handling of the drugs used in anaesthetic practice. Any untoward physiological disturbance during the operation has to be dealt with, often with drugs. After the operation the sooner patients' normal functions are restored the better. They should be independently breathing normally (i.e. respiratory depression and neuromuscular blockade should have been fully reversed), with a stable circulation and normal consciousness, and without post-operative pain (requiring the judicious use of post-operative analgesics).

It is a tribute to the skills of anaesthetists in using drugs and maintaining physiological functions that serious adverse events are so infrequent during anaesthesia.

Here we shall briefly examine the clinical pharmacology of the drugs used in anaesthesia and some of the principles of their use. We shall not deal with precise details of anaesthetic practice. As for mechanisms of action we shall deal only with the muscle relaxants. The actions of opioid and other analgesics, benzodiazepines, and anticholinergic drugs are discussed elsewhere, and the mechanisms of action of the intravenous hypnotics and volatile anaesthetics is still obscure.

The aim of anaesthesia is to depress the functions of the central nervous system whilst maintaining the functions of other vital body organs. The usual requirements during and after general anaesthesia are:

(1) unconsciousness;

(2) analgesia;

(3) muscle relaxation;

(4) the maintenance of physiological stability and the suppression of visceral reflexes.

There is no one anaesthetic agent which will achieve all of these effects when given in normal dosage. Anaesthesia therefore involves the use of combinations of different types of drugs.

There are several distinct stages in the anaesthetic process:

(1) premedication;

(2) induction of anaesthesia;

(3) initiation and maintenance of muscle relaxation;

(4) maintenance of anaesthesia;

(5) analgesia, as part of the premedication, during the operation, and after the operation;

(6) other drug therapy, for example to reverse neuromuscular blockade, to prevent or treat vomiting, and to reverse the residual effects of opioids and benzodiazepines.

The list of drugs used is given in Table 33.1.

■ **Table 33.1**   Drugs used in anaesthesia

---

1. *Premedication*
   (a) *Sedatives and analgesics*
      Narcotic analgesics, for example morphine, pethidine (p. 641)
      Benzodiazepines (p. 564)
         Diazepam
         Lorazepam
         Midazolam
         Temazepam
   (b) *Anticholinergic drugs* (p. 538)
      Atropine
      Glycopyrrolate
      Hyoscine
   (c) *Major tranquillizers*
      Chlorpromazine
      Promethazine

2. *Intravenous anaesthetics (induction and maintenance)*
   Thiopentone
   Diazepam
   Methohexitone
   Midazolam
   Propofol
   Ketamine

3. *Inhalational anaesthetics (for maintenance anaesthesia and for induction in children)*
   Nitrous oxide
   Halothane
   Enflurane
   Isoflurane
   Diethylether

4. *Muscle relaxants*
   (a) *Non-depolarizing muscle relaxants* (p. 647)
      Atracurium
      Vecuronium
      Pancuronium
      Tubocurarine
      Alcuronium
      Gallamine
   (b) *Depolarizing muscle relaxants*
      Suxamethonium (p. 647)

5. *Neuroleptic and narcotic analgesic drugs*
   Droperidol (p. 645)
   Fentanyl and alfentanil
   Phenoperidone
   Morphine (p. 641)

6. *Drugs used during the reversal of anaesthesia*
   Naloxone (p. 641)
   Neostigmine, pyridostigmine, physostigmine, edrophonium (p. 539)
   Flumazenil

33.1 Premedication

The aims of premedication are:

(1) to reduce anxiety;

(2) to reduce salivary secretions;

(3) to suppress autonomic reflexes (for example cardiac arrhythmias);

(4) to cause amnesia;

(5) to provide adjuvants for the maintenance of anaesthesia.

Although drugs are used to produce these effects, the patient's anxiety may be allayed to some extent by careful and sympathetic explanation of what anaesthesia and surgery entail.

A commonly used premedication is the combination of an opioid analgesic with an antimuscarinic drug. The opioid is usually morphine, which in addition to relieving anxiety provides some intraoperative analgesia. Atropine or hyoscine (scopolamine) are used to dry up secretions and to suppress the parasympathetic overactivity caused by suxamethonium and the operative procedures.

Other forms of premedication which may be used, depending on the operative procedure are:

(1) benzodiazepines (for example diazepam, midazolam, lorazepam, temazepam) (note that benzodiazepines provide no analgesia);

(2) droperidol (a neuroleptic drug) with fentanyl (an opioid analgesic), both given i.v., providing swift sedation with analgesia (this combination is called 'neuroleptanalgesia');

(3) phenothiazines (for example trimeprazine, which may be used as a premedication in children).

33.2 Induction of anaesthesia

Thiopentone i.v. is the most commonly used inducing agent for major surgery, acting within 10–30 s. Other options are mentioned in the list of drugs. Suxamethonium i.v. is usually used immediately after thiopentone and before tracheal intubation, if that is to be performed, to provide muscle relaxation of short duration.

33.3 Muscle relaxants

Muscle relaxants are of two types (Table 33.1), the non-depolarizing or competitive blocking agents (of which d-tubocurarine is the prototype) and the depolarizing agent suxamethonium.

Non-depolarizing competitive blocking agents compete with and antagonize the actions of acetylcholine at the muscle motor end-plate. They can themselves be antagonized by acetylcholinesterase inhibitors (for example neostigmine, pyridostigmine, edrophonium), which prevent the metabolism of acetylcholine and cause it to build up at the motor end-plate, thereby overcoming the competitive block.

The depolarizing agent suxamethonium, which is similar in structure to acetylcholine, causes depolarization of the motor end-plate and prevents the response to acetylcholine. Its effects are therefore not reversed by neostigmine, but its action is in any case usually of very short duration. Suxamethonium is used for short periods of muscle relaxation, for example during electroconvulsive shock therapy, bronchoscopy, or orthopaedic manipulations. It is also used at the start of an operation if a rapid sequence of induction and intubation is required, for example to reduce the risk of vomiting and aspiration. However, its adverse effects limit its use when rapid relaxation is not important, and if long periods of muscle relaxation are required, for example during abdominal surgery, non-depolarizing drugs are generally used from the start of anaesthesia.

The non-depolarizing drugs are highly charged and do not pass across cell membranes easily. The speed of onset of neuromuscular blockade after their i.v. administration is therefore determined by the rate of blood flow through the muscle.

Ventilation is necessary after the patient has been paralysed with neuromuscular blocking drugs, and one of the main problems with these drugs is prolonged apnoea, requiring maintenance of assisted ventilation. Prolonged apnoea after non-depolarizing relaxants may be caused by:

(1) metabolic acidosis;

(2) myasthenia gravis;

(3) potassium depletion;

(4) hyponatraemia;

(5) drugs (for example quinidine and the aminoglycoside antibiotics);

(6) decreased elimination (for example because of renal impairment).

Prolonged apnoea after depolarizing drugs may be due to:

(1) deficiency of plasma pseudocholinesterase, either congenital (see Chapter 8) or acquired (for example in liver disease and during pregnancy);

(2) malnutrition;

(3) drugs (for example methotrexate);

(4) 'dual block' (the development of a nondepolarizing block following the primary depolarizing block, usually due to repeated doses of suxamethonium and often precipitated by acid/base and electrolyte disturbances, such as potassium depletion).

33.4 Maintenance of anaesthesia

Induction and initial muscle relaxation may be followed by maintenance anaesthesia and muscle relaxation appropriate to the type of surgical procedure being undertaken. This might involve the administration of a mixture of nitrous oxide and oxygen, with or without a volatile agent, supplemented when necessary by the i.v. administration of an opioid analgesic such as fentanyl, or occasionally by additional doses of an i.v. anaesthetic drug. Muscle relaxation during maintenance anaesthesia of appreciable duration is provided by non-depolarizing muscle relaxants, the choice of which depends on their other (nonrelaxant) properties and their routes of elimination.

It is important to note that the volatile agents halothane, enflurane, and isoflurane are potent inhalational anaesthetics but have no analgesic properties, whereas nitrous oxide is a potent analgesic but a poor anaesthetic. Volatile agents are therefore used in combination with nitrous oxide in order to provide balanced anaesthesia and analgesia.

The above general routine is subject to great variation depending upon the age and medical condition of the patient, the type of operation and surgical technique, the habits and experience of the anaesthetist, and the anaesthetic technology available.

33.4.1 Intravenous anaesthetic agents

Some important pharmacokinetic characteristics of the agents used intravenously in anaesthesia are given in Table 33.2.

(a) Thiopentone

The barbiturate thiopentone is the most commonly used i.v. anaesthetic. It may be used as the sole anaesthetic agent for short and minor operations, and for electroconvulsive therapy. The solution for injection is alkaline and can produce tissue necrosis if injected extravascularly and arterial spasm if injected into an artery.

The onset and duration of action of thiopentone illustrate some important clinical pharmacology. An effective hypnotic dose (up to 5 mg/kg) produces loss of consciousness within the time it takes to travel from the site of injection to the brain (i.e. less than 30 s). This is because the drug is highly lipid soluble and enters the brain very readily. This fast induction of anaesthesia occurs while plasma concentrations are at a peak after injection. The drug then starts to redistribute to other body tissues and the plasma concentration starts to fall as the drug is distributed into muscle and fat. It is mainly the fall in plasma concentration produced by this redistribution phase (with a half-life of about 2.5 min) which is responsible for the short duration of anaesthesia after an initial injection.

However, if large or repeated doses of thiopentone are given, it enters fat depots and because hepatic metabolism is relatively slow (half-time 9–12 h) a distribution equilibrium is set up between blood, fat (and other tissues), and brain, and this can lead to prolonged anaesthesia and unconsciousness, which is a serious hazard postoperatively. This cumulative effect must be

■ **Table 33.2** The pharmacokinetics of some important intravenous drugs used in anaesthesia

Drug	Half-time (h)	Volume of distribution (L)	Clearance (mL/min)
Thiopentone	5–12	120–200	200–350
Methohexitone	2–5	60–80	700–900
Propofol	1–3	1000–1700	1000–1800
Midazolam	2–4	70–130	300–550
Ketamine	2–3	200–250	1250–1400
Etomidate	1–4	140–300	800–1700
Fentanyl	3–4	200–300	900–1000
Alfentanil	1–2	40–70	200–400

allowed for when calculating dosages for administration by intermittent injection or by infusion. This is one reason why maintenance anaesthesia with an inhalational anaesthetic is generally preferred.

Adverse effects of thiopentone include laryngeal spasm, respiratory depression, and hypotension due to vasodilatation and depressed myocardial function.

Thiopentone should be used with caution and in reduced doses in patients with renal impairment, marked congestive cardiac failure, and acute intestinal obstruction, and in gravely ill patients with debilitation or circulatory shock. In states of circulatory shock, with peripheral circulatory failure and hypovolaemia, the speed and effectiveness of the distribution phase may be reduced, and prolonged high blood concentrations may cause prolonged and deep anaesthesia, unexpectedly severe depression of all cerebral functions, and depression of cardiac function (with hypotension and a fall in cardiac output).

Contra-indications to thiopentone include a history of thiopentone sensitivity and, because it is a barbiturate, porphyria (see Chapter 8). It is also contra-indicated in patients with respiratory obstruction or inflammation of the oropharyngeal cavity with accompanying oedema and trismus.

(b) Methohexitone

Methohexitone, another barbiturate, is more potent than thiopentone and it produces a shorter duration of anaesthesia. Recovery from its anaes-thetic effects depends on its redistribution from the brain to other tissues, as with thiopentone. However, its hepatic metabolism is faster than with thiopentone (half-time 100–200 min) and the risk of accumulation during continued administration is therefore less.

Because of its short duration of action, methohexitone is used for out-patient and dental procedures. Its adverse effects include pain and thrombophlebitis after intravenous injection and exaggerated involuntary movements (especially in unpremedicated patients and patients with epilepsy). Like thiopentone it is contra-indicated in porphyria.

(c) Etomidate

Etomidate is an imidazole with a short duration of action, because of rapid metabolism by esterases in the liver and plasma. Repeated administration does not lead to accumulation, in contrast to thiopentone (see above).

Etomidate has a number of important disadvantages. It causes pain on injection (which may be reduced by pretreatment with an i.v. opioid analgesic, such as fentanyl or alfentanil), involuntary myoclonic movements, and reversible inhibition of steroidogenesis (a dose-dependent effect, which is not a major problem with single doses or infrequent intermittent administration).

Despite these disadvantages, etomidate is of value in some circumstances. It causes only minimal cardiorespiratory changes during induction of anaesthesia and may therefore be used in patients with cardiovascular disease. It also has the advantage of not releasing histamine, in contrast to the barbiturates, such as thiopentone and methohexitone, and opioids, such as morphine; it may therefore be used in patients with atopy.

(d) Ketamine

Ketamine is a phencyclidine derivative and is the only true hypnotic agent which also has analgesic effects. In contrast to other agents it increases sympathetic nervous system activity, and this is useful for the rapid induction of anaesthesia in patients who require a high degree of sympathetic activity to maintain cardiovascular function (for example in the presence of pericardial tamponade and hypotension).

Ketamine is not as rapidly effective as the agents discussed above, and recovery from its effects may be complicated by important adverse effects, including hallucinations, which may be minimized by premedication with a benzodiazepine.

Ketamine may be used in poor-risk surgical patients (for example those with poor myocardial function or hypovolaemia), for repeated anaesthesia in patients with burns (for debridement of wounds, painful dressings, and skin grafting), and in short diagnostic or surgical procedures, including cardiac catheterization. Since ketamine may also be given intramuscularly it is sometimes used in children, in patients with poor venous access, and in patients with multiple injuries at the site of an accident.

Ketamine is metabolized in the liver and at least one of its metabolites (norketamine) is active.

(e) Propofol

Propofol is a phenol which is water-insoluble and is formulated as an emulsion. It has a rapid onset of action and since it has a high rate of hepatic clearance recovery from its effects is also rapid. This makes it useful in day-care anaesthesia.

Propofol causes cardiovascular and respiratory depression comparable with thiopentone when it is used for induction of anaesthesia, but these effects may be attenuated if induction is achieved by a continuous intravenous infusion. It commonly causes pain on injection (especially when small veins are used), apnoea, coughing and hiccuping, and involuntary movements.

However, it does not commonly cause postoperative nausea, vomiting, and headache. Because of its cardiovascular effects it should be used with care in patients with cardiac disease or hypovolaemia. It may cause bradycardia and hypotension, particularly if used in combination with fentanyl or alfentanil.

(f) Midazolam

Midazolam is a benzodiazepine which causes sedation, amnesia, and sleep, but not anaesthesia. Unlike diazepam it is water-soluble, is not converted to active metabolites, and is short-acting. However, induction with midazolam is not as rapid as with the barbiturates, and may be accompanied by unexpected ventilatory and cardiovascular depression. Its other unwanted effects include significant respiratory depression in patients with chronic obstructive lung disease, and hypotension associated with hypovolaemia.

33.4.2 Inhalational anaesthetic agents

The depth of anaesthesia produced by these agents is determined by their partial pressure in cerebral arterial blood, which in turn determines their diffusion into and pressure within brain tissue. The partial pressure of the anaesthetic agent in arterial blood is determined by the following factors:

(a) The partial pressure of the agent in alveolar gas

The partial pressure of the agent in alveolar gas depends on its concentration in the inspired air, alveolar ventilation (both of which are controlled by the anaesthetist), and the rate of diffusion of the agent from the alveolar gas into the blood. The rate of diffusion depends on the partial pressure gradient of the agent between alveolar gas and mixed venous blood (which changes as the duration of administration proceeds), pulmonary blood flow (which carries the agent in the blood away from the point of diffusion), and the solubility of the anaesthetic in the blood (see below). The alveolar membrane itself provides no appreciable barrier to diffusion.

(b) The solubility of the anaesthetic agent in the blood

The solubility of an anaesthetic agent in the blood is expressed as the blood/gas partition coefficient. This is the ratio of the concentration in the blood to the concentration in a gas phase across a diffusing membrane when the partial pressures in both phases are equal, i.e. at equilibrium. The more soluble the agent in the blood the higher the partition coefficient. Some blood/gas coefficients are shown in Table 33.3.

If an anaesthetic agent is highly soluble in the blood, more of it must be dissolved in the blood in order to raise its partial pressure there to levels which will produce anaesthesia. Furthermore, in these circumstances more of the agent is removed from the alveolar gas phase, thus reducing the diffusion gradient. In contrast, when the agent is poorly soluble the partial pressure in the blood increases more quickly, and anaesthesia is more rapid.

The potency of anaesthetic gases is expressed as the minimum alveolar concentration (MAC), which is defined as the minimum concentration of gas in the lungs which will produce a state of anaesthesia in 50 per cent of patients. The values of MAC for some inhalational anaesthetics are given in Table 33.3.

(a) Nitrous oxide

Nitrous oxide is a potent analgesic but a weak anaesthetic with a high MAC (see Table 33.3), because of which it cannot be used on its own for anaesthesia. It is therefore used as a background anaesthetic together with oxygen 30–35 per cent and a volatile anaesthetic (for example halothane, enflurane, or isoflurane) to maintain anaesthesia. Its use in combination with the other volatile anaesthetics reduces the magnitude of the increase in arterial carbon dioxide tension which occurs when the other volatile agents are used alone.

Nitrous oxide/oxygen mixture (50/50, Entonox®) is useful for rapid analgesia in sub-anaesthetic doses, and is used for this purpose in obstetric analgesia and for procedures which require short periods of analgesia (for example when dressing burns or during orthopaedic manipulations).

Nitrous oxide is generally non-toxic, but hypoxia must be avoided. It may potentiate respiratory depression due to opioid analgesics.

Bone-marrow depression has occurred with prolonged administration of nitrous oxide (for example during controlled ventilation in the treatment of tetanus). Because nitrous oxide quickly diffuses into air-containing spaces, it may increase the volume of gas in dilated loops of bowel, increase the volume of a pneumothorax, or cause increased pressure in the paranasal sinuses and the middle ear.

(b) Halothane

Halothane is a fluorinated hydrocarbon, a colourless, non-inflammable, volatile liquid anaesthetic, the vapour of which is pleasant to inhale and non-irritating, and with which there is a relatively low incidence of post-operative nausea and vomiting. It is a potent anaesthetic with a low MAC (Table 33.3) and is rapid in its action. However, in low concentrations it is a poor analgesic. Recovery from its anaesthetic effects is rapid. It

■ **Table 33.3** Blood/gas coefficients, O_2/gas coefficients, and minimum alveolar concentrations (MACs) for some commonly used inhalational anaesthetics

Anaesthetic	Blood/gas coefficient	O_2/gas coefficient	MAC
Nitrous oxide	0.47 (very insoluble)	1.4	105
Halothane	2.3	224	0.77
Isoflurane	1.4	91	1.15
Enflurane	1.9	96	1.68
Diethyl ether	12.10 (very soluble)	65	1.92

is used in the maintenance of anaesthesia. Although most of it is eliminated by expiration some is metabolized in the liver and its metabolites, which may be toxic, are cleared slowly.

Halothane itself produces some degree of muscle relaxation, although insufficient for major abdominal surgery, when muscle relaxants should be used. It potentiates the actions of the non-depolarizing muscle relaxants, such as d-tubocurarine, both on the motor end-plate and at autonomic ganglia, and the latter may result in hypotension. Other non-depolarizing muscle relaxants (gallamine and pancuronium) have no ganglion-blocking effects and so do not produce hypotension when used with halothane or other volatile anaesthetics.

Halothane has important effects on the cardiovascular system. It causes a dose-dependent fall in blood pressure, due to depressed myocardial contractility (producing a fall in cardiac output), and disordered baroreceptor function. Halothane also makes the heart more sensitive to the arrhythmogenic effects of endogenous and exogenous adrenaline and other catecholamines and predisposes to ventricular arrhythmias (extra beats, tachycardia, and occasionally fibrillation); hypercapnia worsens these arrhythmogenic effects.

Halothane is a respiratory depressant, and the tendency to hypoventilation must be corrected by assisted ventilation. However, it is a suitable agent for patients with asthma, chronic bronchitis, and emphysema, since it causes bronchodilatation, does not stimulate the production of secretions, and does not irritate the bronchi, pharynx, or larynx.

The main adverse effect of halothane, apart from problems arising during anaesthesia, has been liver damage. Its use is associated with a very small risk of hepatitis, the severity of which can range from acute massive necrosis of the liver, which is very rare, to disturbances of liver function with or without jaundice. The risk of liver damage is increased in the middle-aged, in obese people, and by repeated exposure (particularly when the last exposure was within six weeks). The hepatitis may be a hypersensitivity reaction, perhaps due to an interaction of a metabolite (a hapten) with a protein, or to direct toxicity of halothane metabolites.

The precise incidence of halothane-induced hepatitis is still not known, but it is now widely accepted that repeated exposure should be avoided unless there are good indications. These include the induction and maintenance of anaesthesia in patients with chronic obstructive lung disease and in children and others who are afraid of needles, and the relief of life-threatening bronchoconstriction and hypoxia in patients with acute severe asthma.

Other adverse effects of halothane include inhibition of the hypoxic pulmonary vasoconstrictor reflex, increased intracranial pressure, reduced hepatic blood flow, and malignant hyperpyrexia (see p. 101).

(c) Enflurane

Unlike halothane, enflurane is a fluorinated ether. It is a geometrical isomer of isoflurane (see below).

The effects of enflurane on the cardiovascular and respiratory systems are qualitatively similar to those of halothane. Both reduce myocardial contractility equally, and while both also depress the ventilatory response to hypoxia and hypercapnia, enflurane does this with greater potency than halothane.

Enflurane is unique amongst the currently available volatile anaesthetics in causing central nervous system excitation, and this is associated with a risk of seizures, particularly in the presence of hypercapnia.

Enflurane has been reported to have caused hepatitis, and there is evidence suggesting cross-reactivity between antibodies in the sera of patients with halothane-related hepatotoxicity and antigens produced by the metabolism of enflurane.

Enflurane causes uterine relaxation and increases the risk of uterine haemorrhage. It shares this effect with halothane and isoflurane, but the effect of enflurane is greatest. Its other adverse effects include inhibition of the hypoxic pulmonary vasoconstrictor reflex, increased intracranial pressure, and malignant hyperpyrexia (see p. 101).

Enflurane is metabolized in the liver to free inorganic fluoride ions. These are nephrotoxic in blood concentrations over 50 μmol/L, which can occur during effective anaesthesia in obese patients who are also receiving enzyme inducers (see Chapter 10), in cases of prolonged anaesthesia, and in patients with pre-existing renal impairment. This nephrotoxicity results in polyuria and an impairment of renal concentrating ability.

Enflurane potentiates the effects of the non-depolarizing muscle relaxants.

(d) Isoflurane

Isoflurane is a fluorinated ether, a geometric isomer of enflurane. It has all the favourable properties of halothane and enflurane, in addition to which it has a faster onset of action and wears off more quickly. It is metabolized to a smaller extent than enflurane and halothane, and the risks of renal and hepatic damage are therefore less than with the other volatile agents (see above). Although it reduces systemic vascular resistance, it has little effect on cardiac contractility, and so cardiac output is maintained and the heart rate increases, maintaining the blood pressure. However, hypotension may occur in patients with reduced sympathetic reserve, for example patients taking β-adrenoceptor antagonists.

Isoflurane has some important individual properties. It is an anticonvulsant, it protects the brain against the effects of ischaemia, it reduces the extent to which the heart is sensitized to catecholamines during general anaesthesia, and it is less arrhythmogenic than the other volatile anaesthetics. Because of these characteristics isoflurane is now the most commonly used of the volatile anaesthetics.

The adverse effects of isoflurane include inhibition of the hypoxic pulmonary vasoconstrictor reflex and malignant hyperpyrexia (see p. 101).

33.5 Postoperative medication

Recovery from anaesthesia involves a reversal of the effects described for its production. When a patient is ventilated with a gas which contains no anaesthetic the partial pressure of the agent in the arterial blood falls quickly, the partial pressure in the brain follows suit, and consciousness quickly returns. Anaesthetic agents persist for longer in muscle and fat because of a relatively poorer blood supply.

The analgesia and anaesthesia provided by inhalational anaesthetics quickly reverse as the anaesthetic agent is cleared from the brain. However, analgesia and respiratory depression from opioid analgesics given during anaesthesia may persist into the post-operative phase. Post-operative analgesia may be desirable, but respiratory depression is not. Naloxone, an opioid antagonist, is used to reverse opioid-induced respiratory depression, but careful dosage is required to avoid reversal of analgesia. Post-operative analgesia is usually provided by opioid analgesics.

Non-depolarizing neuromuscular block persisting after the operation is reversed by giving neostigmine i.v., and this may need to be repeated. The muscarinic effects of neostigmine are prevented by the concurrent administration of atropine.

The residual effects of benzodiazepines can be reversed by the specific competitive antagonist flumazenil (200 micrograms i.v. over 15 s followed, if necessary, by further doses of 100 micrograms at 1 min intervals up to a total of 1 mg). However, flumazenil has a very short duration of action (half-time about 1 h), because it is rapidly cleared from the body by hepatic metabolism. Thus, the sedative effects of the benzodiazepine may return a few hours after flumazenil has been given, even when a short-acting benzodiazepine (for example midazolam, half-time 2–4 h) has been used. Flumazenil should not be given to patients with a history of panic attacks, in whom it can cause acute anxiety. Other adverse effects are unusual unless too high a dose is given, when transient dizziness, anxiety, and facial flushing may occur.

Nausea and vomiting are very common after operations and there is no satisfactory method of treatment. This is discussed in Chapter 25 (p. 323).

33.6 Local anaesthetics

Local anaesthetics (listed in Table 33.4) produce a transient reversible blockade of nerve function. They do this by blocking sodium channels in the axonal membrane and thus inhibiting sodium

■ **Table 33.4** Some commonly used local anaesthetics, their maximum doses, and their adverse effects

Local anaesthetic	Maximum doses (mg)		Important adverse effects*
	Alone	With adrenaline	
Amethocaine	100	–	Cardiac depression, asystole, ventricular fibrillation
Bupivacaine†‡	175	250	Cardiotoxicity, drowsiness, convulsions
Cocaine	200	–	Sympathetic stimulation, excitement, restlessness, headache, vomiting, myocardial depression, cardiac arrhythmias
Lignocaine†‡	30	50	Convulsions, psychotic reactions
Mepivacaine†	350	500	Cardiotoxicity
Prilocaine†¶	400	600	Methaemoglobinaemia
Procaine	500	700	CNS toxicity

*All local anaesthetics may cause hypersensitivity reactions (see text).
†These drugs may cause malignant hyperpyrexia.
‡Formulated with and without adrenaline.
¶Formulated with and without felypressin.

conductance; this in turn reduces the rate and degree of depolarization of the nerve cell and prevents propagation of the action potential.

Local anaesthetics penetrate through the epineurium and nerve cell membrane to their site of action in their unionized form, but their effect on sodium conductance is via the ionized form. It is therefore important that the pK_a of local anaesthetics is close to the physiological pH of the tissues, which means that there will be approximately equal amounts of both forms available. The other pharmacological actions of the local anaesthetics may arise through inhibition of the binding of calcium ions to phosphatidyl serine.

Small lightly-myelinated fibres and unmyelinated fibres are blocked first by local anaesthetics and large heavily-myelinated fibres last. The order of loss of nerve function proceeds through pain, temperature, touch, proprioception, and finally skeletal muscle power.

The lipid solubility of a local anaesthetic is the primary determinant of its potency, while its duration of action depends on the rate at which it diffuses from its site of action and its subsequent rate of elimination from the body. For example, procaine and chloroprocaine are very lipid soluble and therefore very potent; however, they are rapidly metabolized by plasma esterases

and therefore have short durations of action. In contrast, tetracaine and bupivacaine are poorly soluble and therefore of low potency; however, they are slowly eliminated and therefore have long durations of action. Intermediate in potency and duration of action between these two groups are lignocaine, mepivacaine, and prilocaine.

The duration of action of a local anaesthetic may be prolonged by using a local vasoconstrictor to slow the rate at which the anaesthetic diffuses from its site action (see below).

The procedures used in applying local anaesthetics to nervous tissues in appropriate concentrations without producing systemic toxicity are the province of surgical and anaesthetics texts, and we shall not consider them here. However, we shall consider some aspects of the use of lignocaine as a local anaesthetic and the adverse effects of all the local anaesthetics.

Lignocaine is a weak base with a pK_a of 7.86. It is formulated in aqueous solution as the soluble hydrochloride salt, and the different types of formulations available for local anaesthesia are listed in Table 33.5.

The onset of action of lignocaine is rapid (within a few minutes). It has a intermediate duration of action, and this can be prolonged by the addition of a local vasoconstrictor. For example, its duration of action when it is injected

■ **Table 33.5** Formulations of lignocaine for use as a local anaesthetic

1. *Lignocaine hydrochloride injection*
   0.5, 1.0, and 2.0 per cent
   1.5 per cent for epidural injection

2. *Lignocaine*   *plus*   *Adrenaline*
   0.5 per cent (5 mg/mL)   1:200 000 (5 micrograms/mL)
   1.0 per cent (10 mg/mL)   1:200 000 (5 micrograms/mL)
   2.0 per cent (20 mg/mL)   1:200 000 (5 micrograms/mL)

3. *Formulations for surface anaesthesia*
   Eutectic cream (lignocaine 2.5 per cent + prilocaine 2.5 per cent)
   Gel (2 per cent)
   Ointment (5 per cent)
   Liquid spray (4 and 10 per cent)

alone in a 1 per cent solution is about 1 h, but when adrenaline is added the duration of action may be prolonged to 1.5–2.0 h. The adverse effects of all the local anaesthetics are similar, and the main effects are on the central nervous system, the cardiovascular system, and the neuromuscular junction.

(a) Central nervous system

Most local anaesthetics readily cross the blood–brain barrier. In the brain they initially cause excitation and then in higher concentrations depression. Plasma lignocaine concentrations correlate well with the associated central nervous system toxicity (see the Pharmacopoeia).

(b) Cardiovascular system

In pharmacological concentrations local anaesthetics cause arterial dilatation and myocardial depression. In toxic concentrations these effects may result in cardiac failure and circulatory collapse. In addition they may depress myocardial conduction pathways and cause cardiac arrhythmias and cardiac arrest. Some of the local anaesthetics (for example procaine) may cause cardiac arrhythmias by a quinidine-like effect on the heart (see p. 671).

(c) Neuromuscular junction

In addition to their effects on sensory fibres, local anaesthetics also affect transmission at the neuromuscular junction and may potentiate the effects of depolarizing and non-depolarizing neuromuscular blocking drugs.

Toxicity can occur if large amounts of local anaesthetics are injected into the tissues or if a normally non-toxic dose is accidentally injected intravenously. In adults toxic effects of lignocaine are unlikely at total doses below 200 mg (i.e. 20 mL of a 1 per cent solution) when no vasoconstrictor is used and 500 mg (i.e. 50 mL of a 1 per cent solution) with solutions which contain a vasoconstrictor (see below). The safe doses of other local anaesthetics and their adverse effects are shown in Table 33.4.

In addition to dose-related effects allergic reactions occasionally occur, with bronchospasm, urticaria, and angio-oedema. These reactions are more common with esterified local anaesthetics (amethocaine, cocaine, and procaine). The local application of amethocaine and benzocaine may cause a local allergic reaction on the skin or mucous membranes, and these local anaesthetics are not commonly used, being reserved for use in ophthalmology (amethocaine) and for oropharyngeal anaesthesia (benzocaine).

The risk of adverse reactions to local anaesthetics can be minimized by using the lowest possible doses, particularly when using combination formulations with adrenaline or felypressin (a vasopressin analogue with vasoconstrictor properties). These vasoconstrictors are added to reduce local blood flow and therefore to prolong anaesthesia, but they have certain dangers.

1. They may cause local ischaemia.
2. Adrenaline may cause systemic toxicity, and the total dose should not exceed 500 micrograms. If more than 50 mL of a local anaesthetic solution is to be used the concentration of adrenaline should be no more than 1:200 000.

3. The effects of adrenaline may be potentiated by tricyclic antidepressants. This is potentially a very important interaction in dental practice. Solutions which contain felypressin should be safer in such patients.

34 Drug dependence and abuse

Co-author: P. J. Robson

Drug dependence, misuse, and abuse pose serious threats to the well-being of society and are responsible for much illness and death among addicts. Although most illicit drug misusers are young people, misuse of benzodiazepines, barbiturates, alcohol, and tobacco tends to occur among older people.

The important classes of chemical agents most commonly subject to abuse are listed below:

(1) opiates (and other narcotic analgesics);

(2) CNS stimulants: amphetamine and related drugs (including methylene dioxymethamphetamine (MDMA, 'ecstasy')), and cocaine;

(3) cannabis;

(4) lysergic acid diethylamide (LSD) and other psychedelic drugs;

(5) alcohol;

(6) benzodiazepines;

(7) barbiturates;

(8) tobacco (nicotine);

(9) volatile substances: toluene in glue and butane.

Terminology in this area is difficult. 'Addiction', 'habituation', and 'compulsive drug abuse' are confusing terms, while 'drug misuse' and 'drug abuse' are terms which spring from cultural perceptions and which represent value judgements.

Two useful independent concepts should be defined: 'drug dependence' and 'problem drug use'.

Drug dependence is characterized by a preoccupation with a drug, to the detriment of other interests or responsibilities, and by a compulsion to take it without concern for the consequences. It may be primarily physical, when an individual requires continued administration of the drug to prevent physical withdrawal symptoms, or psychological, when either a search for pleasure or euphoria or a need to escape unpleasant mood states or the harsh realities of life are the primary drives. A person who is dependent on a drug in this way can be described as an addict.

Problem drug use occurs when continuing consumption of the drug becomes associated with physical, psychological, social, or legal harm.

34.1 Factors which predispose to drug dependence

To become a regular drug user an individual has to make two distinct decisions: to try the drug for the first time, and having tried it to repeat and continue the experience.

The reasons for initial use generally fall into one of four categories: recreational (the large majority), therapeutic (for example opiates for chronic pain, benzodiazepines for insomnia or anxiety), instrumental (for example caffeine or amphetamine to counter fatigue), or cultural (for example cannabis smoking).

Assuming that the drug is available and that the user has some peer group approval, recreational use requires a susceptible individual. Although the idea of an 'addictive personality' is now given little credence, certain personality traits (for example sensation seeking, nonconformity, autonomy, and an ability to tolerate deviance in others) make experimentation with drugs more likely. Continued use then depends on positive and/or negative reinforcement: the ability of the drug to provide pleasure and perhaps enhance performance, or to take away pain or dysphoria. The effects of any drug, both physical and psychological (see Table 34.1), are shaped by the expectations of the user and the setting in which the drug is taken.

34.1.1 Psychological factors

The psychological factors which predispose to drug dependence are discussed in textbooks of psychiatry and a discussion of them here is beyond the scope of this book. There are no sure predictive tests to indicate who may or may not experiment with drugs or become dependent on them.

34.1.2 Neurochemical and neuropharmacological factors

Neurochemical and neuropharmacological factors may operate in the initiation of drug abuse and certainly operate in drug dependence. Presumably there is some pattern of neuronal function, either at the level of the integration of neuronal systems or at a biochemical/pharmacological level, which render an individual more or less likely to react to a drug in such a way as to lead that individual to want to repeat the experience. This biological substrate will then be one of the factors which will continue to predispose the individual to further repetitions. Repeated exposure then leads to pharmacological adaptive changes in the brain, causing physical dependence. When this state is reached the adaptive changes which occur are such that in the absence of the drug neuronal patterns of activity are unveiled and activated, causing a withdrawal syndrome.

There are various hypotheses about the pharmacological causes of dependence on opiates, alcohol, benzodiazepines, and barbiturates. In opiate dependence it is proposed that the exogenous opiate (for example morphine) acts on endogenous opioid (enkephalin) receptors, either turning off endogenous opioid synthesis or reducing its function in some way, such that when the exogenous opiate is withdrawn endogenous opioid function is inadequate. Through a series of events, which probably involves the activation of central noradrenergic systems, the withdrawal syndrome is initiated. Clonidine, an α_2-adrenoceptor agonist, which can inhibit the activity of central noradrenergic systems, can suppress the withdrawal syndrome in some addicts.

In dependence on alcohol, benzodiazepines, and barbiturates attention is currently being focused on the function of the neurotransmitter GABA (γ-aminobutyric acid). It has been proposed that in their different ways alcohol, benzodiazepines, and barbiturates all lead to an increase in the functional activity of GABA receptors in certain areas of the brain, resulting in a reduction in the activity of endogenous GABA. Withdrawal results in the typical withdrawal syndromes due to these drugs because of a loss of GABA-mediated inhibitory influences in the brain. All of these syndromes have some features in common, including anxiety, insomnia, fits, and tremor, although the severity and quality differ in each case.

Similar mechanisms have been proposed for dependence on other substances. Amphetamine dependence may be due to adaptive changes in dopamine or noradrenaline function, occurring as a result of the increase in the release of these neurotransmitters which amphetamine causes. Cocaine dependence may result from changes brought about by inhibition of noradrenaline reuptake, and dependence on LSD may relate to the function of 5-hydroxytryptamine. The pharmacological mechanisms whereby cannabis and nicotine bring about dependence are still a mystery.

In recent years considerable effort has been expended in seeking the neurobiological basis of positive reinforcement, which might underlie psychological dependence as a phenomenon separate from physical dependence. The existence of a 'pleasure pathway' located in dopamine-containing cells of the ventral-tegmental area and the substantia nigra has been proposed. This work raises the possibility of pharmacological approaches to the problem of persistent intense craving.

34.2 Opiates

Opiate dependence is a world-wide public health menace associated with a great deal of criminal activity. For example, in the UK there are currently estimated to be between 100 000 and 150 000 opiate injectors. Heroin (diamorphine) is the most frequently abused opiate. First experiences may occur through smoking, with subsequent graduation to administration subcutaneously and then intravenously. On first use there is often nausea, vomiting, and anxiety, but these symptoms disappear with subsequent use and euphoria becomes predominant. As tolerance develops the addict uses the i.v. route with increasing doses to try to produce the euphoria (the 'high') which results from rapidly increased concentrations of the drug in the blood. Tolerance to constipation and pupillary constriction does not occur to any great extent. Eventually the addict becomes most concerned with combating withdrawal symptoms and must have a regular supply of the drug to avoid these.

Withdrawal symptoms begin at about 8 h after the last dose and reach a peak at about 36–72 h. After methadone the onset of withdrawal symptoms is delayed for 24–48 h and peaks at 3–4 d. Symptoms occur in the following order.

1. Psychological symptoms: anxiety, depression, restlessness, irritability, drug craving.
2. Lacrimation, rhinorrhoea, yawning, and sweating.
3. Restless sleep, after which the above symptoms are accompanied by sneezing, anorexia, nausea, vomiting, abdominal cramps, diarrhoea, bone pain, muscle pain, tremor, weakness, chills and goose-flesh ('cold turkey'), and insomnia. Hypotension, cardiovascular collapse, and convulsions occur rarely.

These symptoms gradually fade over about 5–10 d, during which time general malaise and abdominal cramps persist. This phase may continue for up to 6 weeks if the addict was previously taking methadone.

34.2.1 Medical complications of opiate dependence

The medical complications of opiate dependence are due to effects of the drugs themselves and of the toxic materials and adulterants which may be used as bulking agents and injected with them.

(a) Acute heroin reactions

Some acute reactions are due to overdose and some may be due to adulterants, such as quinine, or to allergic reactions. These reactions tend to present as hypoxia with cyanosis, pulmonary oedema, respiratory depression, and reduced levels of consciousness progressing to coma. Fever and leucocytosis may also occur. Treatment consists of establishing a good airway, maintaining adequate oxygenation (through an endotracheal tube if necessary), giving i.v. glucose and thiamine, and the cautious administration of naloxone i.v. in doses which will lighten consciousness if an opiate is primarily responsible. It is important to remember that the half-time of naloxone is much shorter than that of most opiates, that its effects must be carefully monitored, and that repeated doses may be necessary. Tracheal and bronchial suction, treatment of acute allergic reactions (with corticosteroids and antihistamines), and antibiotic therapy of infection may also be necessary.

(b) Infections

i. HIV and other sexually-transmitted diseases

The risk of HIV infection is high in addicts, because of transmission via shared needles. Other sexually transmitted diseases are also common, particularly in women, because of prostitution or lack of self-care.

ii. Other infections

Infections due to repeated septic injections in opiate addicts may involve any of several organs, and include skin infections, endocarditis, osteomyelitis, hepatitis B, pneumonia and lung abscess, and septicaemia.

(c) Neurological complications

As well as infection, transverse myelitis, peripheral neuropathy, and myopathy can all occur.

(d) Cardiovascular and pulmonary complications

As well as infection, cardiac arrhythmias, emboli, and pulmonary aspiration and collapse can all occur.

(e) Pregnancy

Dependent mothers may give birth to dependent babies, who may suffer from a withdrawal syndrome at birth.

34.2.2 The treatment of opiate dependence

The treatment of opiate dependence is difficult and in the short term not very successful, although after 10 years about 50 per cent of those in whom treatment has been tried will be abstinent. In the UK there are drug dependency units at which addicts can receive controlled amounts of drugs

■ Table 34.1 Some effects of drugs of misuse

Drug(s)	Physical effects	Psychological effects
Opiates		
Acute	Drowsiness, ataxia, miosis, respiratory depression, histamine release	Confusion
Chronic	Tolerance, hormonal effects, constipation	Constant preoccupation
Withdrawal	Yawning, running eyes and nose, tremor, sweating, mydriasis, restlessness, sleeplessness, gastrointestinal disturbances, muscle/bone aches, tachycardia, hypertension	Anxiety, irritation, extreme craving
Stimulants		
Acute	Overactivity, insomnia, sweating, diarrhoea, arrhythmias, fever, changes in blood pressure, convulsions, coma	Binges/crashes, panic, irritability, delusions, hallucinations
Chronic	Tolerance, microvascular damage, dopamine neuronal damage and receptor supersensitivity	Depression, extreme preoccupation, chronic psychosis
Withdrawal	Deep sleep, lethargy	Depression, anhedonia, reduced motivation, extreme craving
Barbiturates		
Acute	Drowsiness, ataxia, nystagmus, slurred speech, respiratory depression, hypotension, coma	Confusion, depression, emotional instability, amnesia
Chronic	*As acute*; selective tolerance, drug interactions (see p. 127)	Aggression, psychosis, paranoid ideas
Withdrawal	Insomnia, nausea, vomiting mydriasis, hypotension, tremor, hyper-reflexia, convulsions	Anxiety, irritability, emotional instability, psychosis
Benzodiazepines		
Acute	Drowsiness, ataxia, vertigo, slurred speech, respiratory depression (massive doses only)	Confusion, amnesia, rebound anxiety
Chronic	Neuroradiological changes	Cognitive impairment, reduced ability to cope
Withdrawal	Increased sensory perception, insomnia, vertigo, cramps, gastrointestinal disturbances, convulsions	Mild to moderate craving, emotional instability, anxiety
Cannabis		
Acute	Tachycardia, hypotension, yawning, red eyes, diuresis, mydriasis, carbohydrate hunger	Thought disorder, panic, paranoid ideas, psychosis (rare)
Chronic	Bronchitis, ?immune suppression, ?reduced fertility	Anxiety, possible psychosis, ?reduced motivation
Withdrawal	Probably none	Mild/moderate craving

Drug(s)	Physical effects	Psychological effects
Hallucinogens		
Acute	Paraesthesiae, tremor, sympathetic and parasympathetic stimulation, leucocytosis	Hallucinations, panic, anger, delusions, impulsive behaviour
Chronic	?Teratogenicity, ?carcinogenicity	Mood lability, psychosis, compulsive use, suicidal impulses
Withdrawal	None	Moderate craving, flashbacks
Solvents		
Acute	Ataxia, slurred speech, arrhythmias, convulsions, coma	Psychosis, aggression, poor judgement, feelings of omnipotence
Chronic	Hepatic or renal damage, bone-marrow suppression, neuropathy, encephalopathy, 'glue-sniffer's rash'	*As acute*
Withdrawal	None	Moderate craving
Methylene dioxymethamphetamine (MDMA, 'ecstasy')		
Acute	Cardiorespiratory collapse because of impurities (rare)	Hallucinations (rare)
Chronic	?Brain damage (ill-defined), ?immune suppression	Fatigue, depression, binges
Withdrawal	None	Flashbacks

and social and psychiatric help. Gradual dosage reduction may be possible and may be helped by the substitution of methadone, a narcotic analgesic, which is an agonist at μ opioid receptors and which can be given orally. Methadone has a prolonged action and in appropriate once-daily dosages can remove the craving for opiates. In some addicts it may become possible after a time to withdraw the methadone gradually.

Every prescriber has a responsibility to avoid worsening dependency or feeding the illicit market, but must balance this against a duty to respond humanely to those who want to break contact with their illicit suppliers as a first step towards a more stable and productive lifestyle. Whilst there are undoubtedly addicts whose main ambition is to gull unwary doctors, there are many others who regard doctors as practical sources of help in attempting to regain some control over their lives.

In the UK drugs of dependence are subject to the requirements of the *Misuse of Drugs Act* of 1971 and of the *Regulations* of 1985, which are described in the *British National Formulary*, as is the procedure for notifying the Chief Medical Officer of Health, through the Home Office

Department, about new addicts. Information from the Home Office Addicts Index, a confidential index maintained by the Chief Medical Officer, can be obtained by ringing the number listed in the *British National Formulary*. Medical practitioners in the UK are now being asked to notify drug misusers to Local Regional Drug Misuse Data Bases. In the UK only practitioners who hold a special licence from the Home Office may prescribe heroin, cocaine, or dipipanone for addicts in relation to their addiction needs. Other practitioners must refer addicts to Drug Addiction Treatment Centres, but they may prescribe these drugs for pain relief in any patient (including an addict).

Further details on the management of drug misuse can be found in *Drug misuse and dependence: guidelines on clinical management*. HMSO, 1991.

34.3 Cocaine and amphetamines

It is estimated that up to 30 million people have used cocaine in the recent epidemic in the USA.

In the UK the use of amphetamines is far more prevalent than the use of cocaine, and appetite suppressants, such as diethylpropion and phentermine, frequently find their way on to the illicit market.

The clinical effects of cocaine (also known as 'coke' or 'snow' and in one particular form as 'crack') and those of amphetamine (also known as 'speed') are not dissimilar, although they have different durations of action, by which those with experience may distinguish them. Their effects include euphoria, increased drive, increased confidence, increased sociability, loquacity, and increased physical and mental capacities. There may also be a reduced need for food, rest, and sleep.

Cocaine may be sniffed, injected intravenously, or smoked as the free base or as 'crack'. Amphetamines are often taken orally, but are also commonly injected. The pattern of usage of these drugs often takes the form of binges of escalating doses terminating in a 'crash', characterized by exhausted sleep followed by depressed mood, which fuels the initiation of the next binge.

Although it was thought that tolerance did not occur to cocaine, it is now clear that some users tolerate very large doses of 'crack', which would be toxic to a naïve user. However, it is less clear whether tolerance occurs to its euphoriant and reinforcing effects. Tolerance does occur to the peripheral and central effects of amphetamines. There is no cross-tolerance between cocaine and amphetamines. The use of prolonged and high dosages may lead to a cocaine- or amphetamine-induced psychosis, not dissimilar from acute paranoid schizophrenia. There are no major physiological withdrawal phenomena from cocaine or amphetamines, but troublesome dysphoria and craving may persist for months or even years.

34.4 Cannabis

Cannabis sativa, the hemp plant, yields marijuana and hashish. The active chemicals in the plant are δ-9-tetrahydrocannabinol (δ-9-THC), δ-8-THC, and numerous other cannabinols.

Marijuana is the dried mixture of crushed leaves and stalks of the plant. The flowering tops of the plant secrete the resin which when compressed forms hashish (or 'hash'), which is more potent than marijuana. These cannabis preparations are also known under a variety of other names, including 'ganja', 'bhang', 'grass', 'pot', and 'kef'. Marijuana is smoked in home-made cigarettes ('joints'), hashish in small pipes. An average 'joint' contains 300–500 mg of herbal material, of which 1–2 per cent is active. The maximal possible absorption is 50 per cent, so that a sophisticated smoker can expect to obtain an average of 2.5 mg of THC per cigarette. Novices or purchasers of heavily adulterated material may absorb little or no active substance, but may on the other hand be exposed to active adulterants, such as opiates. This variability makes self-reporting of consumption highly unreliable and makes much existing research uninterpretable.

Cannabis is used widely throughout the world: in one study 60 per cent of North Americans between the ages of 18 and 25 years said they had used it, and 28 per cent said they were current users. In the UK 3–4 million people have used cannabis, and there are an estimated 1 million current users. There is an increasing debate about the possible merits and demerits of making cannabis more readily available by decriminalizing it, i.e. making it available under license (rather than legalizing it, which would imply unrestricted availability). The crux of the debate is the balance between the secondary harm to the individual and society from the effects of prohibition on the one hand and the primary risks associated with the consumption of the drug on the other. Currently it is thought that the latter outweighs the former, and there is little prospect of a change in the law in the UK.

Cannabis has physical and mental effects which begin within minutes of starting to smoke it. The physical effects include an increase in heart rate, peripheral vasodilatation, conjunctival suffusion, bronchodilatation, dryness of the mouth, and in large doses tremor, ataxia, nystagmus, nausea, and vomiting. The mental effects vary from person to person, depending on such variables as personality, mood, surroundings, expectations, and previous cannabis experience. Generally there is a feeling of well-being, accompanied by feelings of enhanced sensory perception. There may be drowsiness or hyperactivity. Ideas flow rapidly and may be disconnected. Time seems to pass slowly. Motor performance may be altered, as it may be by any sedative drug, and driving skills may be impaired.

There may be mild tolerance and a mild withdrawal syndrome, rather like a mild benzodiazepine withdrawal syndrome. Physical dependence does not seem to be a big problem.

Heavy use of marijuana is associated with social apathy, but this often precedes drug use and may not be an adverse effect. Adverse psychological effects include occasional cases of depression, anxiety, acute panic reactions, and paranoid ideas. Single large doses may cause an acute toxic psychosis with confusion and hallucinations. There is controversy as to whether marijuana can produce a prolonged psychosis.

34.5 LSD and other psychedelic drugs

The psychedelic drugs include the ergotamine analogue lysergic acid diethylamide (LSD, also called 'acid'), psilocybin, psilocin, dimethyltryptamine, diethyltryptamine, mescaline, and some molecular analogues of amphetamine.

The effects of LSD usually occur at a dose of 200 micrograms, but may be seen at doses down to 20 micrograms. Within 20 min autonomic effects are apparent, including mydriasis, hyperthermia, tachycardia, increased blood pressure, piloerection, and sometimes nausea. Mental effects occur within 1–2 h and their nature and intensity depend on the environment and the state of mind of the individual. They include heightened perception (particularly of colours), the fusion of after-images with true images, melting visual perceptions, an increased sense of clarity, increased awareness, the impression that one's thoughts are of great importance (although they are generally mundane or trivial), a sensation that time is passing slowly, and impressions of distorted body images. Mood varies, and there can be euphoria or dysphoria, calmness or anxiety, elation or depression, sociability or paranoia. 'Bad trips' with acute panic reactions sometimes occur and can lead to suicide.

Tolerance to LSD develops quickly, but physical dependence does not occur and psychological dependence is unusual. During long-term use a curious phenomenon known as 'flashback' is sometimes experienced. This is the recurrence of some effects of the drug, usually brief visual experiences, which may be worrying or unpleasant, at a time when the individual is drug-free. Persistent psychosis is a rare complication of LSD dependence.

Both acute intoxication with LSD and flashback can be treated with dopamine receptor antagonists, such as chlorpromazine.

34.6 Alcohol

The morbidity and mortality associated with alcohol abuse pose considerable public health problems. There are three main medical and psychiatric problems:

(1) acute alcohol intoxication (see the Pharmacopoeia p. 546);

(2) chronic alcoholism (with its attendant physical effects, for example cirrhosis);

(3) Alcohol withdrawal reactions (delirium tremens).

Drug therapy plays little part in the first two of these, except for aversion therapy with disulfiram, but does have a place in the management of delirium tremens.

Delirium tremens is an acute withdrawal reaction which is important to recognize, because it has a high rate of mortality. It can occur in a chronic alcoholic who simply cannot get a drink, but in general medical practice it is more common in a chronic alcoholic admitted to hospital with an intercurrent illness, such as trauma, pneumonia, stroke, or myocardial infarction. It also occurs in patients with alcoholic cirrhosis admitted to hospital with gastrointestinal bleeding.

The symptoms of delirium tremens come on within a few hours after the last drink and mount over the next 2–3 days. At first there is anxiety, agitation, tremulousness, and tachycardia. These are later accompanied by confusion, severe agitation, and hallucinations (often visual). The patient is tremulous, sweating, and tachypnoeic, and may be pyrexial. The blood pressure may be high, low, or normal. Nausea and vomiting are common. Seizures may occur and are serious.

The drug management of delirium tremens includes the maintenance of fluid and electrolyte balance, the administration of vitamins (particularly thiamine to prevent Wernicke's encephalopathy), a high carbohydrate and high calorie diet, and the use of sedating drugs. Choices for the drug treatment of the delirium are from among the benzodiazepines, the barbiturates, and chlormethiazole. Besides the delirium another important consideration is the prevention of seizures, and in those with a previous history of convulsions during alcohol withdrawal phenytoin may be indicated. Most physicians treating alcohol withdrawal states now use chlormethiazole, diazepam, or chlordiazepoxide.

Chlormethiazole can be given as an i.v. infusion of a 0.8 per cent solution, 40–100 mL (320–800 mg) over 5–10 min, to produce drowsiness and to remove restlessness and agitation. The subsequent infusion rate is adjusted according to the response. Oral chlormethiazole can be substituted for the infusion in dosages of three capsules 6-hourly for 2 d, two capsules 6-hourly for 3 d, and then one capsule 6-hourly for 4 d (one capsule = 192 mg of chlormethiazole).

Chlormethiazole has itself a tendency to produce dependency in alcoholic patients and because of this hazard it should not be given for longer than necessary. In patients with alcoholic cirrhosis its first-pass metabolism is impaired and oral dosages should be reduced because of the risk of hepatic encephalopathy; i.v. dosages are not affected by this.

Diazepam is given in doses of 10 mg i.v. four-hourly as required. Oral diazepam can be substituted as the critical stage passes.

Chlordiazepoxide is given in doses of 50–100 mg by deep intramuscular injection when the patient is very agitated or confused. This is followed by 50–100 mg orally 6-hourly. Once the patient is stabilized withdrawal can be carried out over a period of 2–3 weeks.

34.7 Benzodiazepines

There are two broad categories of benzodiazepine misuse.

1. Illicit misuse of benzodiazepines which have been obtained other than by prescription.

2. Misuse of benzodiazepines prescribed for therapeutic purposes.

Illicit misuse is not uncommon, and there is quite a large illicit market in benzodiazepines. They may be taken orally, or oral formulations may be liquefied for injection. The risks of this include thrombophlebitis, abscesses, septicaemia, and (in the case of needle sharing) infection with HIV. Generally this type of misuse is associated with the misuse of other drugs.

Those who misuse benzodiazepines which they have received on prescription probably constitute a much larger category and pose a serious problem. If a benzodiazepine is taken for longer than say 6 weeks, dependence may occur. When the drug is withdrawn there may be a withdrawal syndrome of variable intensity. This occurs within 2–3 days after the withdrawal of a short-acting benzodiazepine (for example lorazepam) and within about 7 d in the case of a long-acting benzodiazepine (for example diazepam).

In the patient who has been given a benzodiazepine for anxiety, the withdrawal syndrome consists of rebound anxiety and its physical accompaniments, with other manifestations in severe cases (see below). This causes the patient to ask for a further supply of the drug, thus fuelling dependence. Tolerance to the anxiolytic and euphoriant effects of the benzodiazepines may occur and lead to the need for increased dosages if long-term therapy is embarked upon. In the patient who has been treated for insomnia the withdrawal syndrome consists of rebound insomnia, and similar principles apply.

■ **Table 34.2** Dosages of some benzodiazepines equivalent to 30 mg of diazepam

Benzodiazepine	Dose equivalent to 30 mg of diazepam (mg)
Chlordiazepoxide	90
Lorazepam	15
Nitrazepam	30
Oxazepam	90
Temazepam	60

In severe dependence the withdrawal syndrome consists of the psychological and physical symptoms and signs of anxiety with sweating, insomnia, headache, shaking, nausea, and feelings of disordered perception, such as unreality, abnormal body sensations, and hypersensitivity to stimuli. Psychoses and epilepsy may also occur. Note the resemblance of this syndrome to the syndrome of alcohol withdrawal (delirium tremens). The symptoms of withdrawal may last for 1–2 weeks, but in some cases may continue for weeks or months.

It is difficult to predict how dependent an individual may become, but the benzodiazepine withdrawal syndrome is common, and it is now accepted that benzodiazepines should generally not be prescribed in anxiety for more than 2–4 weeks at a time and only for severe anxiety. They should generally not be used as hypnotics for more than 2 weeks at a time and only for severe insomnia.

In the treatment of benzodiazepine dependence one should try to withdraw the benzodiazepine slowly by gradual reductions in dosage. If the patient who has been taking a short-acting benzodiazepine is unable to do this one would substitute diazepam, which can be given once a day (because of its long half-time, which is attributable to its active metabolite desmethyldiazepam). Then one would start to withdraw the diazepam slowly, in steps of 2 mg every two weeks, until the drug is withdrawn or symptoms return. If the symptoms return one would prescribe the lowest dose at which there were no symptoms and start to withdraw more slowly (for example reducing the daily dose by 1 mg every two weeks). In the extreme case, if more than 30 mg of diazepam equivalents are being taken per day (see Table 34.2), withdrawal should be very slow, over several months to a year. This requires a great deal of support and specialist management.

34.8 Barbiturates

In the UK barbiturate dependence is usually due to illicit drug abuse. Tolerance may be marked and is often associated with i.v. use. Withdrawal symptoms can be severe and resemble delirium tremens.

34.9 Tobacco (nicotine)

The adverse effects of smoking, and particularly of smoking cigarettes, pervade medical practice. Acute and chronic bronchitis, emphysema, bronchogenic carcinoma, some other carcinomas, peripheral arterial disease, coronary artery disease, and peptic ulceration are all associated with the use of cigarettes, and about one-third to a half of all smokers die of a smoking-related disease.

It is hard to pin down exactly what pleasure smoking brings. It is a habit which generally needs working at to establish its pleasure, but once established it can engender both relaxation of the mind and increased drive at different times and in different circumstances.

Withdrawal symptoms include a craving for tobacco, increased appetite, and irritability.

Because it induces hepatic drug-metabolizing enzymes, smoking increases the metabolism of drugs such as caffeine, theophylline, and imipramine. A history of smoking should always be considered as a factor in variable drug response.

Chewing-gum containing nicotine may help those trying to give up smoking. However, the main factor in successfully breaking the tobacco habit is the motivation of the individual. Anti-smoking clinics help people to give up smoking and provide encouragement and reassurance.

34.10 Personal accounts of drug dependence

Several well-known writers have described their own experiences with drugs of abuse. The following may be of interest:

Confessions of an English opium eater, Thomas de Quincy (1822).
Opium. The diary of a cure, Jean Cocteau (1930).
Junkie, William Burroughs (1953; heroin).
The doors of perception, Aldous Huxley (1954; mescalin).
Return trip to nirvana, Arthur Koestler (1961; psilocybin). Reprinted in *Drinkers of infinity* (1968).

35 The management of poisoning

Co-author: D. J. M. Reynolds

The vigour with which one treats a case of poisoning varies from simple observation only to large-scale intensive action to maintain vital body functions. Almost all poisoned patients will survive, if necessary with intensive supportive treatment. Although many patients will be given an emetic and perhaps activated charcoal (see below), only a few patients will need either an antidote specific to the drug they have taken or special treatment to hasten elimination of the poison from the body.

35.1 The immediate management of the acutely ill patient

In Table 35.1 are summarized the various components of the immediate management of the acutely ill patient.

35.1.1 Respiratory function

Respiratory function may be assessed by observing ventilation and more formally by measurements of blood gases, including oxygen saturation. It is important to maintain a clear airway at all times. If the patient is drowsy or unconscious, but breathing spontaneously, it is sufficient to ensure an open airway by keeping the patient semi-prone with the neck extended, by inserting an oral airway, and by sucking out secretions at regular intervals. Unconscious patients should be turned on to the left side. Remove all obstructions from the mouth (including dentures) and suck out any secretions or debris.

If the patient is not maintaining adequate spontaneous respiration, ventilation should be assisted using a face mask and an Ambu bag; if possible, a cuffed endotracheal tube should be inserted as soon as possible and the patient should be moved to a facility in which mechanically assisted ventilation can be carried out.

In determining the need for oxygen the degree of cyanosis is an unreliable guide to the degree of oxygenation. Pulse oximetry, if available, is a simple non-invasive way of measuring the oxygen saturation and it may be used continuously to monitor patients who are deeply unconscious. Arterial blood gas measurement is the best way of measuring the adequacy of gas exchange.

If there is hypoxaemia oxygen should be given according to the following guidelines:

P_AO_2 between 8 and 11 kPa (62 and 85 mmHg) and P_ACO_2 between 5 and 7 kPa (38 and 54 mmHg): give 24 per cent oxygen, increasing to 28 per cent after 30 min if the P_ACO_2 has not risen;

P_AO_2 below 8 kPa or P_ACO_2 above 7 kPa: assisted ventilation will be required.

During oxygen therapy the arterial blood gases should be used as a guide to dosage, since oximetry will give information about oxygen saturation but not about carbon dioxide tension (see p. 301).

In carbon monoxide poisoning carboxyhaemoglobin in the circulation will give a falsely high apparent oxygen saturation, and oximetry cannot be used to monitor progress. The treatment of choice in carbon monoxide poisoning is hyperbaric oxygen, when available, or 100 per cent oxygen.

35.1.2 Cardiovascular function

Measure and monitor the heart rate and blood pressure. There are no hard-and-fast rules, but

▌ **Table 35.1**   A summary of the management of acute poisoning (see text for detailed discussion)

1.	Respiratory function	Check gag reflex
		Remove dentures
		Clear out oropharyngeal
		   obstructions/debris/secretions
		Lay on left side with head down
		Insert oral airway or, if cough reflex lost, an
		   endotracheal tube
		Give oxygen if hypoxic
		Assist respiration if required

2.	Circulatory function	Check heart rate and blood pressure
		If systolic blood pressure below 80 mmHg
		(young patients) or 90 mmHg (old patients):
		   Raise end of trolley/bed
		   If ineffective, give volume expanders
		If fluid overload and oliguria:
		   Give dopamine and/or dobutamine

3.	Renal function	Monitor urine output
4.	Consciousness	Assess level of consciousness (see text)
5.	Temperature	Take temperature rectally If below 36°C reheat slowly Warm all inspired air and i.v. fluids
6.	Convulsions	Treat with diazepam, chlormethiazole, phenytoin, or anaesthesia with assisted ventilation
7.	Cardiac arrhythmias	Treat as required (see text and Chapter 23)

8.	Gastric lavage and
	ipecac-induced emesis
		See Table 35.2 for indications, contra-indications,
		   and risks
		Add non-specific or specific antidotes to lavage fluid
		   or leave in stomach after lavage (see Table 35.3)

9.	Fluid and electrolyte balance	Dehydration: oral fluids usually enough Unconscious patients: use i.v. fluids and insert a central venous pressure line Treat hypokalaemia (see p. 349)
10.	Specific emergency measures	See section 35.2.5
11.	Chest radiography	In drowsy or comatose patients who vomit After endotracheal intubation
12.	Collection of specimens	Gastric aspirate (drugs) Urine (drugs, renal function) Blood (drugs, arterial gases, electrolytes)

in general the minimum acceptable systolic pressure is 80 mmHg if the patient is below 50 years of age, or 90 mmHg over 50 years of age. If there is hypotension raise the end of the trolley or bed about 20 cm. If the blood pressure remains low set up an intravenous infusion and give plasma volume expanders, such as colloid solutions (dextrans, gelatins, or hydroxyethyl starches, see p. 413). If this is done a urinary catheter should be inserted and urinary output should be monitored every hour. However, patients are often in positive fluid balance, or at least not fluid-depleted, and great care must be taken not to cause fluid overload. Sometimes it may be necessary to insert a central venous pressure line, so that fluid requirements can be assessed precisely. If plasma volume expanders do not cause an increase in blood pressure, or if urine output is below 30 mL/min, then inotropic drug therapy is indicated. Some would recommend the use of a β-adrenoceptor agonist, such as dobutamine (2.5–10 micrograms/kg/min by continuous i.v. infusion), but if one's chief concern is renal blood flow then low doses of dopamine (for example 5 micrograms/kg/min) may be sufficient, or may be combined with dobutamine. Higher doses of dopamine (10–20 micrograms/kg/min) also have a β-adrenoceptor agonist effect, but at higher doses both drugs have α-adrenoceptor agonist effects, and may cause peripheral and renal vasoconstriction. Whatever agent is used it is wise not to raise the systolic pressure above 100 mmHg.

35.1.3 Renal function

Renal function may be assessed by measuring plasma urea and creatinine concentrations and should be carefully monitored by measuring urine output, if necessary by catheterization. The use of dopamine to improve renal blood flow, and hence urine flow, is mentioned in the previous section.

35.1.4 Level of consciousness

This will already have been roughly assessed while assessing respiratory and cardiovascular function, but now is the time to assess it more rigorously according to the following scheme, so that progress can be monitored:

Grade 0. Fully conscious.
Grade 1. Drowsy, but responds to commands, or asleep but easily roused.
Grade 2. Unconscious, but responds to standard minimally painful stimuli.
Grade 3. Unconscious, but responds to standard maximally painful stimuli.
Grade 4. Unconscious, and does not respond to any stimuli.

Useful 'standard' stimuli are rubbing the sternum vigorously with the knuckles or pinching the Achilles tendon. Pressure over the supra-orbital fissure should not be used because of the risk of damage to the eye if the hand slips.

The main virtue of this system is that it may be used to provide objective evidence of a change in conscious state over a period of time. In addition gastric lavage should not be carried out without prior endotracheal intubation in patients who have no gag reflex, or who seem likely to aspirate, or who may have seizures. Impairment of consciousness of any grade in patients who have taken salicylates is an important sign and (in the absence of alcohol) suggests serious poisoning.

35.1.5 Temperature

Hypothermia can be a serious problem in unconscious patients who have been exposed to a low ambient temperature. In an unconscious patient measure the temperature rectally with a low-reading clinical thermometer or a thermocouple. Hypothermia (rectal temperature below 36°C) should be treated slowly by keeping the patient in a warm environment and by the use of a 'foil' blanket or gentle rewarming with an electric blanket. All inspired air and infusion solutions should be warmed before administration.

Hyperthermia should be treated by fanning and tepid sponging.

35.1.6 Convulsions

Convulsions may be treated with either diazepam (as Diazemuls®, 10 mg i.v., repeated at 30 min intervals to a total of 30 mg, and followed if required by a continuous infusion at a rate of 100 micrograms/kg/h in saline) or chlormethiazole (40–100 mL of a 0.8 per cent solution given by i.v. infusion over 5–10 min, followed if necessary by a continuous i.v. infusion at a rate depending on the patient's response). If this fails, the treatment advised for status epilepticus (see p. 435) should be used and if possible the patient should be moved to an intensive therapy unit.

35.1.7 Cardiac arrhythmias

Record a 12-lead electrocardiogram and monitor the cardiac rhythm in patients who are deeply unconscious or hypothermic, or who have taken digoxin, antiarrhythmic drugs, β-adrenoceptor antagonists, anticholinergic drugs (for example tricyclic antidepressants), potassium, sympathomimetic drugs, or unknown drugs. If cardiac arrhythmias occur check for and correct electrolyte abnormalities (especially hypokalaemia), hypoxia, and acidosis.

In general it is better to avoid treating tachyarrhythmias if the blood pressure is unaffected and the urine output is maintained. This is because antiarrhythmic drugs often have a negative inotropic effect on the heart and because the potential for complex drug interactions in cases of poisoning is considerable. However, certain arrhythmias do require treatment.

Sustained ventricular tachycardia and ventricular fibrillation should be treated by direct current shock. For digitalis-induced arrhythmias antidigoxin antibody administration, or phenytoin if antibody is not available, is the treatment of choice. Supraventricular arrhythmias generally do not need treatment, unless there is chest pain or evidence of haemodynamic instability. If sinus bradycardia needs to be treated atropine may be used, but a transvenous pacemaker may be required.

35.1.8 Removal of poison from the stomach

If the patient is seen within 4 h of poisoning it is worth attempting to remove tablets or capsules from the stomach by gastric lavage or induced emesis. These procedures may also be of value up to 24 h or longer after poisoning with iron salts or salicylates, which can cause pylorospasm, and up to 8 h after opiates or drugs with anticholinergic effects (for example tricyclic antidepressants), which decrease gastrointestinal motility. The indications, contra-indications, and risks of induced emesis and gastric lavage are listed in Table 35.2.

▮ **Table 35.2** Indications, contra-indications, and risks of gastric lavage and ipecac-induced emesis

	Gastric lavage	**Ipecac-induced emesis**
Indications	Within 4 h of any overdose Within 8 h of anticholinergic drugs (for example tricyclic antidepressants) and opiates Within 12 h of salicylates and iron At any time in unconscious patients	Within 4 h of any overdose Within 8 h of anticholinergic drugs (for example tricyclic antidepressants) and opiates Within 12 h of salicylates and iron To be preferred in children and after digitalis
Contra-indications	Petroleum distillates Corrosive agents	Petroleum distillates Corrosive agents Antiemetics If patient unconscious
Risks	Aspiration (intubate if unconscious) Rupture of oesophageal varices in alcoholics	Aspiration Ipecac toxicity

(a) Induced emesis

This should only be carried out in a patient with a normal gag reflex. In an emergency vomiting may be induced by pharyngeal stimulation with a finger or the back of a spoon. In hospital, syrup of ipecacuanha or paediatric ipecacuanha emetic draught is used in a dose of 15 mL (10 mL in a child under 18 months) with 200 mL of water or fruit juice. It should have an effect within about 30 min, but if not the dose should be repeated. No more than two doses should be given, because of the risk of ipecac toxicity. Ipecac should not be given to a patient who has taken an antiemetic.

(b) Gastric lavage

Before carrying out gastric lavage check that the gag reflex is intact. If it is not, a cuffed endotracheal tube must be inserted before gastric lavage is carried out in order to minimize the risk of aspiration of lavage fluid or gastrointestinal contents, and suction apparatus should be available.

The patient should be laid on the left side, the head below the level of the rest of the body, and a wide-bore tube should be passed via the mouth into the stomach. We use a 150 cm tube with a 7 mm internal diameter and extra perforations in the final 10 cm or so. The usual lavage fluid is warm water, but in young children warm saline should be used. In some cases specific antidotes may be added to the lavage fluid (see Table 35.3) or left in the stomach at the end of lavage. The lavage fluid in volumes of 300 mL is passed, via a large funnel held above the patient, down the tube into the stomach. The funnel is then lowered beneath the level of the patient and the gastric contents are allowed to drain into a bucket or aspirated with a large syringe. This procedure is

■ **Table 35.3** Agents used in decreasing the absorption of ingested poisons

Poison	Additions to lavage fluid (warm water or saline)	Agent(s) to be left in stomach after lavage or to be given orally
Cyanide	Sodium thiosulphate 5%	Sodium thiosulphate 25%, 300 mL
Digitoxin		Colestipol or cholestyramine; activated charcoal
Hydrofluoric acid		Calcium gluconate 10%, 300 mL
Iron	Desferrioxamine (see text)	Desferrioxamine (see text)
Opiates	Potassium permanganate (one tablet BPC in 3.5 L)	Wash all permanganate out of stomach
Oxalic acid (for example in bleach)	Calcium gluconate 1%	Calcium gluconate 1%, 300 mL
Paraquat	Fuller's earth, 150 g/L	Fuller's earth, 150 g/L (see text)
Phenol, cresol, lysol	Castor oil in water, 1:2	Castor oil, 50 mL (or another vegetable oil, such as arachis oil or olive oil)
Phosphorus	Copper sulphate 0.1%	Copper sulphate 0.1%, 50 mL
Sodium hypochlorite (for example in bleach)	Sodium thiosulphate 5%, or milk, or milk of magnesia (magnesium hydroxide 8.5%)	Copper sulphate 0.1%, 100 mL
Various (see text)		Activated charcoal

repeated until the fluid returning from the stomach is clear. Some of the initial return should be kept for chemical analysis if later required.

There is no place for carrying out gastric lavage as a punitive measure in a case of self-poisoning. If a patient is unco-operative force should not be used.

35.1.9 Prevention of further absorption of drug from the gut

There are several agents which may be used to prevent the further absorption of drugs from the gut. Foremost among these is activated charcoal, which may be instilled into the stomach after gastric lavage (5–10 g in 100 mL of water) and which will adsorb various drugs, thereby reducing their absorption. Examples include salicylates, barbiturates, tricyclic antidepressants, dextropropoxyphene, digitalis, and paraffin. Repeated oral doses of activated charcoal may adsorb some drugs which are secreted into the gut via the gastrointestinal epithelium or excreted via the bile, and may thus increase the rate of their excretion. Activated charcoal should not be given together with ipecacuanha, since ipecac may cause the charcoal to be vomited and charcoal renders ipecac ineffective by adsorption. Other agents which may be added to gastric lavage fluid or left in the stomach at the end of lavage are listed in Table 35.3.

35.1.10 Fluid and electrolyte balance

Most patients have either normal fluid and electrolyte balance or slight fluid overload. For those who are fluid depleted (for example because of vomiting), but who are conscious, oral fluids are usually sufficient. In most unconscious patients simple replacement with 5 per cent dextrose and physiological saline (in a ratio of 2:1) is usually sufficient. Central venous pressure monitoring may be required in severely ill patients. Hypokalaemia may be treated with either oral or i.v. potassium chloride.

35.1.11 Specific measures

Some drugs require immediate specific treatment. The most important are cyanide and paraquat,

discussed below. The treatment of paracetamol poisoning should be instituted as soon as possible, without necessarily waiting for the result of the plasma paracetamol concentration measurement, in patients who are seen within 10–12 h after ingestion or even later. Opiate poisoning should be treated as soon as possible with naloxone, and carbon monoxide poisoning with oxygen.

Other specific measures which are not quite so urgent are dealt with under the specific drug headings below.

35.1.12 Chest radiography

A chest X-ray should be taken in any drowsy or comatose patient who has vomited, to rule out aspiration pneumonia, and in any patient who requires endotracheal intubation, to check the position of the endotracheal tube. A chest X-ray is not usually necessary in a fully conscious patient even after induced emesis or gastric lavage.

35.1.13 Collection of specimens

A urine sample and a blood sample (20 mL in two heparinized tubes) taken on admission and a sample of gastric aspirate obtained by lavage should be kept in case later analysis is required in unconscious or severely poisoned patients and in poisoning with any unusual poison (especially new drugs). Always label the containers carefully with the patient's full name, and the date and time of the sample.

In cases of suspected criminal poisoning the accurate identification of samples is crucial. Normal hospital practice in the UK is not sufficient to ensure legally acceptable identification of samples, and samples should be taken in the presence of witnesses and preferably in the presence of a 'scenes of crime' officer from the local police.

Emergency analysis of drugs in the blood is indicated only if the result will affect the management of the case, and is usually restricted to aspirin and paracetamol, each of which is discussed below under its own heading. Measurement of barbiturate concentrations serves principally in making the diagnosis in cases of coma of unknown cause and in identifying the type of barbiturate used (i.e. long-, intermediate-, or short-acting). However, the plasma barbiturate concentration does not reflect prognosis, because of wide interindividual variability, and should not be used as a guide to treatment.

Paraquat may be identified in both gastric aspirate and urine by a simple colorimetric test. This test is useful in excluding the diagnosis and in monitoring progress.

In the majority of uncomplicated cases routine measurements of plasma urea, creatinine, and electrolyte concentrations are not necessary, but they should be made in all ill patients to assess renal function, hepatic function, and state of hydration. In some cases tests should be carried out specific to the effects of the drug (for example blood glucose, arterial blood gases, and prothrombin time for aspirin, and liver function tests for paracetamol).

The indications for various blood tests are summarized in Table 35.4.

35.2 The detailed management of poisoning

There are six components to the management of self-poisoning.

1. Emergency and general supportive measures.
2. Removal of poison from the gut.
3. Prevention of further drug absorption.
4. Hastening of drug elimination from the body.
5. Measures specific to the drug.
6. Psychiatric assessment (not discussed here).

35.2.1 Emergency and general supportive measures

These have been discussed above under the headings of respiratory function, cardiovascular function, renal function, temperature, convulsions, cardiac arrhythmias, and fluid and electrolyte balance.

35.2.2 Removal of poison from the gut

Induced emesis and gastric lavage are discussed in section 35.1.8.

35.2.3 Prevention of further drug absorption

The use of activated charcoal and other measures intended to prevent the further absorption of ingested drug from the gastrointestinal tract is discussed in section 35.1.9. Drugs which should be used to limit the absorption of specific poisons are listed in Table 35.2.

35.2.4 Hastening of drug elimination from the body

(a) Diuresis in acid or alkaline urine

Certain lipophilic ionizable drugs are subject to extensive pH-dependent passive reabsorption by

■ **Table 35.4** Indications for laboratory tests in self-poisoning

Test	Indication
Plasma drug concentration	Aspirin, paracetamol (barbiturates, iron, lithium)
Urine drug concentration	Paraquat
Arterial blood gases	Coma, aspirin, unexplained hyperventilation, hypoxia (for example due to carbon monoxide poisoning)
Plasma electrolytes (especially potassium)	Severe aspirin poisoning, digoxin, potassium, insulin, sulphonylureas, sympathomimetics
Blood glucose	Unexplained coma, alcohol, hypoglycaemic drugs, aspirin
Prothrombin time	Aspirin, paracetamol (not urgent)
Liver function tests	Paracetamol (not urgent)

the renal tubules and have clearance rates close to the normal rate of urine flow (1–2 mL/min). The clearance rates of such drugs can be increased by altering the pH of the urine and to a lesser extent by increasing the urine flow rate. Examples of drugs affected in this way are salicylates and lithium (clearance enhanced in an alkaline urine) and amphetamine (clearance enhanced in an acid urine). A useful regimen for salicylates is discussed below.

(b) Dialysis

Removal of drugs by dialysis procedures is reserved for severe cases of poisoning. It is useful only for drugs which are not widely distributed to the body tissues and which are not highly bound by plasma proteins. It may be of value in serious poisoning with salicylates, barbiturates, chloral hydrate and its derivatives, iron, and lithium, among others.

(c) Charcoal haemoperfusion

Because charcoal adsorbs many drugs, charcoal haemoperfusion (i.e. passing the blood from the body through a charcoal column and returning it to the body) can be used to remove a drug from the circulation. It is of value even when there is high plasma protein binding, but wide distribution of the drug to the tissues limits its usefulness. The problems of thrombocytopenia, leucopenia, febrile reactions, and charcoal emboli encountered with early forms of charcoal columns have been diminished by the more modern types. If available, charcoal haemoperfusion may be of value in serious poisoning with salicylates, barbiturates, glutethimide, meprobamate, methaqualone, theophylline, and derivatives of chloral hydrate. Despite its widespread use in the treatment of paraquat poisoning there is no evidence that it is effective.

(d) Oral activated charcoal

Some drugs are eliminated from the body by being excreted into the gut either via the bile or by secretion via the intestinal epithelium. However, these drugs may also be reabsorbed from the gut. It is therefore possible to increase their rates of excretion by the repeated oral administration of activated charcoal. Examples of drugs whose clearance rates may be increased in this way are phenobarbitone, carbamazepine, phenytoin, dapsone, and the tricyclic antidepressants.

35.2.5 Measures to be taken in specific cases of poisoning

In Table 35.6 at the end of this chapter are listed the compounds which can be used in the specific treatment of cases of poisoning, and some aspects of their uses are also summarized. The following merit extra discussion.

(a) Salicylates

The clinical features of salicylate poisoning are tinnitus, deafness, hyperventilation, hyperpyrexia with sweating and dehydration, and epigastric pain and vomiting. Patients are generally fully conscious, and any impairment of consciousness is a sign of serious poisoning or of poisoning with other agents (for example alcohol). There may be hypoglycaemia. Bleeding may occur, with a reduction in prothrombin time due to a warfarin-like effect on vitamin K reductases.

Salicylates directly stimulate the respiratory centre, causing a respiratory alkalosis due to hyperventilation. In addition there is a metabolic acidosis, because salicylic acid uncouples oxidative phosphorylation. In adults the respiratory alkalosis is usually the major feature, but in children the metabolic acidosis tends to predominate and poisoning in children is more serious at any plasma salicylate concentration than in adults.

The plasma salicylate concentration may be measured as a guide to therapy, but because salicylate is highly protein-bound the total (protein-bound and unbound) plasma concentration is not a good guide to the severity of poisoning, and should always be interpreted with the patient's clinical state in mind. The arterial blood gases give a better indication of the severity of poisoning.

Gastric lavage should always be carried out, even if the patient presents many hours after ingestion. If the plasma salicylate concentration is above 3.0 mmol/L in adults or 1.8 mmol/L in children and the patient has obvious signs and symptoms of toxicity, then alkaline diuresis should be begun. The following i.v. regimen is considered safe:

Physiological saline (500 mL), 5 per cent dextrose (1 L), and 1.26 per cent sodium bicarbonate (500 mL) are infused concurrently over 3 h and thereafter at 1 L per hour until clinical improvement occurs. Potassium chloride should be added at a rate of 20 mmol/h. In children the infusion rate of this solution should be 30 mL/kg/h. Plasma electrolyte measurements should be made every 2–4 h. Because alkalinization of the urine is more important than the diuresis an alternative is sodium bicarbonate alone (1500 mL of a 1.26 per cent solution over 4 h). The pH of the urine should be monitored to ensure that alkalinization is adequate, which means keeping the urinary pH above 8.

It is important to avoid fluid overload in patients receiving this regimen and frusemide may be added to ensure this. Urinary output should be carefully monitored and a central venous line may be necessary in elderly patients who are frail or who have heart disease. Forced diuresis should not be carried out in patients with circulatory failure, renal failure, or pre-existing fluid overload, and in those cases bicarbonate alone can be used with careful monitoring of fluid balance. Peritoneal dialysis or haemodialysis are more satisfactory alternatives.

Hypoglycaemia is usually reversed by the dextrose in the infusion solution. If the prothrombin time is prolonged vitamin K should be given (10 mg of phytomenadione slowly i.v.) or fresh frozen plasma if bleeding is a problem.

In drowsy or unconscious patients acidosis should be corrected with i.v. sodium bicarbonate before starting other treatment. In such patients peritoneal dialysis or haemodialysis are to be preferred to alkaline diuresis.

(b) Paracetamol

Paracetamol poisoning is an acute medical emergency and there must be no delay in treating it. There is usually little in the way of acute symptoms, apart from nausea and vomiting. However, in severe poisoning (more than 10 g) there are several delayed effects. The most important of these is liver damage, the cause of which can be understood by considering the metabolism of paracetamol, illustrated in Fig. 35.1. In usual analgesic doses paracetamol is metabolized about 85 per cent by conjugation with glucuronide and sulphate and about 10 per cent by conjugation with glutathione. In overdose the glucuronide and sulphate pathways are saturated and the excess paracetamol is metabolized by conjugation

with glutathione. However, hepatic glutathione is rapidly depleted, and an intermediate hydroxylamine metabolite accumulates and binds irreversibly to liver proteins, causing damage. Compounds with sulphydryl (SH) groups, which conjugate the toxic hydroxylamine metabolite, can therefore prevent liver damage, but only if they are given before enough of the metabolite is formed and has had enough time to damage the liver. The most useful SH donor is *N*-acetylcysteine.

The signs of serious paracetamol toxicity occur late (about 48–72 h after ingestion), but careful studies in poisoned patients have led to the development of guidelines for early treatment, based on the plasma paracetamol concentration and the time since ingestion, which allow one to decide whether or not to institute treatment. The guidelines are illustrated in Fig. 35.2, which consists of a graph of plasma paracetamol concentrations versus time. The vertical axis is in logarithmic scale and shows plasma paracetamol concentrations from 0.3 to 1.2 mmol/L. The horizontal axis is in linear scale and shows the time after ingestion from 4 to 12 h. A line is drawn between two points representing concentrations of 1.2 and 0.3 mmol/L at 4 h and 12 h respectively.

This graph is used as follows. Measure the plasma paracetamol concentration at the time of admission, if between 4 and 12 h after ingestion. Plot the value of the patient's plasma paracetamol concentration against the time after ingestion. If the point falls on or above the line treatment is indicated. If the point falls below the line treatment is not indicated.

In patients who present within 4 h of ingestion, the plasma paracetamol concentration is unreliable, because absorption will still be continuing. If the patient has taken more than 10 g start treatment and measure the plasma paracetamol concentration at 4 h (treatment does not alter the concentration). Treatment can then be stopped if the point falls below the line.

The above advice applies to patients who present up to 12–15 h after ingestion. Recently it has been advised that any patient who presents after 12–15 h, and certainly up to 36 h, may benefit from treatment with *N*-acetylcysteine.

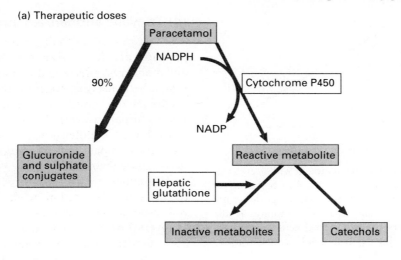

(a) Therapeutic doses

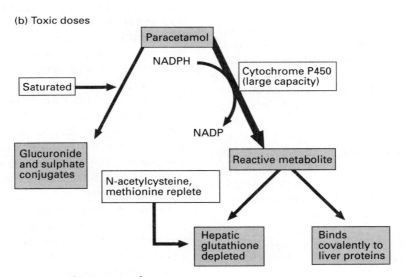

(b) Toxic doses

■ **Fig. 35.1** The metabolism of paracetamol.

In patients who have been taking drugs which induce hepatic drug-metabolizing enzymes (for example phenobarbitone, phenytoin, carbamazepine, rifampicin, griseofulvin) the toxic effects of paracetamol may be enhanced. The effects are also enhanced in chronic alcoholism, perhaps because of depletion of hepatic glutathione. There is no good guidance as to when treatment should or should not be given in such cases, and it is probably wise at present to treat all such patients if they present within 36 h of ingestion.

Treatment should be with intravenous *N*-acetylcysteine as follows:

(1) 150 mg/kg i.v. over 15 min;

(2) 50 mg/kg i.v. in 500 mL of 5 per cent dextrose over 4 h;

(3) 100 mg/kg i.v. in 1 L of 5 per cent dextrose over 16 h.

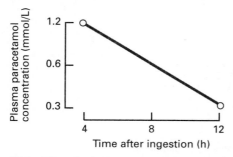

∎ **Fig. 35.2** The criteria for treatment with acetylcysteine after poisoning with paracetamol to prevent liver damage. Plot the value of the plasma paracetamol concentration against the time of sampling. If the plotted point lies above the line treatment is indicated. The conversion for paracetamol concentrations from mmol/L to µg/mL is 1.2 mmol/L ≈ 180 µg/mL.

Methionine is sometimes used as an alternative to i.v. acetylcysteine, but it is given orally and is therefore less reliable and its usefulness may be limited by vomiting. Some proprietary formulations of paracetamol now also contain methionine in amounts sufficient to provide immediate treatment in cases of poisoning.

In any patient who has required treatment with acetylcysteine or methionine liver enzymes and the prothrombin time (INR) should be monitored. Such patients should be kept in hospital for at least 48 h for observation, since the chances of moderate to severe liver damage are high if the liver enzymes continue to rise or the INR rises above 2 at 24 h. Generally the maximum rises in AsT and INR occur at 72–96 h after ingestion.

If there is evidence of severe liver damage and the prospect of hepatic encephalopathy, one should begin intensive management of liver failure (see p. 340). If transfer to a specialist unit is contemplated it should be done before intensive management is required, if possible. If intensive therapy fails to halt the progression of liver damage, liver transplant may be considered.

In patients who have taken paracetamol as co-proxamol remember also to treat dextropropoxyphene poisoning with naloxone (see below).

Remember also that many over-the-counter medicines contain paracetamol.

(c) Tricyclic antidepressants

The features of poisoning with tricyclic antidepressants are due to their peripheral and central anticholinergic effects and to the potentiation of sympathetic nervous system activity. The clinical results are dry mouth, dilated pupils and blurred vision, urinary retention, tachyarrhythmias and heart block, hypotension, impairment of consciousness, impairment of respiration, hallucinations, and convulsions.

The majority (over 80 per cent) of patients require only observation, while most of the rest will respond to simple supportive measures, such as reversal of hypoxia with oxygen and of lactic acidosis with sodium bicarbonate.

The risk of seizures or cardiac arrhythmias can be judged from the duration of the QRS complex on the ECG. If the QRS complex is shorter than 0.10 s there is no risk, if it is between 0.10 and 0.16 s there is a risk of seizures, and if it is greater than 0.16 s there is a risk of both seizures and cardiac arrhythmias. If there are life-threatening ventricular tachyarrhythmias, a β-blocker, lignocaine, or phenytoin may be tried. If there is impaired cardiac function as a result of an arrhythmia DC cardioversion may be required. Bradycardia and heart block should be treated by a transvenous pacemaker. Respiratory depression may require assisted ventilation. Convulsions should be treated with diazepam or chlormethiazole.

Physostigmine has been used to treat the severe adverse effects of poisoning with tricyclic antidepressants, but it is not recommended, since it has a short duration of action and can itself cause serious adverse effects.

(d) Barbiturates

Barbiturate poisoning presents with the signs and symptoms of central nervous system depression, including any degree of impairment of consciousness from drowsiness to coma, restlessness, delirium, hallucinations, convulsions, and respiratory depression. Other effects include hypotension and shock, sometimes causing renal failure, hypothermia, and the characteristic but non-specific skin blisters, which may also be seen in poisoning with other compounds, including tricyclic antidepressants and carbon monoxide.

The effects of poisoning may last several days with the long-acting barbiturates, such as phenobarbitone and pentobarbitone.

Gastric lavage and supportive measures are indicated. Repeated oral doses of activated charcoal increase the rate of barbiturate elimination. In seriously ill patients haemodialysis or charcoal haemoperfusion may be required if deterioration occurs despite intensive support.

(e) Paraquat

This is a serious and often fatal poisoning with a herbicide used in various proprietary weedkillers (for example Weedol®, Gramoxone®, Pathclear®). Fatalities are much less common after the ingestion of granular (domestic) forms of paraquat than after liquid (commercial) forms, which can be fatal in ingested volumes of 10 mL. Most paraquat formulations now contain an emetic and are brightly coloured and malodorous.

Paraquat irritates the skin and mucous membranes, producing burning sensations in the mouth and abdomen, followed by local ulceration in the oropharynx and oesophagus and nausea and vomiting. However, the major effect takes some days to develop: pulmonary oedema secondary to alveolitis and bronchiolitis, due to the effects of a toxic superoxide. It usually results in fatal respiratory failure or renal failure. Treatment in suspected cases should therefore be started immediately and withdrawn if urine testing fails to show the presence of paraquat.

The poison should be vigorously washed away from the skin and eyes and antibiotic drops should be applied to the eyes if affected. In an emergency vomiting should be induced by pharyngeal stimulation. Gastric lavage must be carried out as soon as possible, preferably with a 15 per cent solution (i.e. 150 g/L) of fuller's earth, which adsorbs paraquat. After lavage 1 L of a suspension of 150 g of fuller's earth, with 200 mL of a 20 per cent solution of mannitol as a purgative, should be left in the stomach. This treatment should then be repeated as often as the patient can tolerate it, say half-hourly, until fuller's earth appears in the stools. During this time a nasogastric tube should be kept in position so that the fuller's earth and mannitol can be given directly into the stomach. Fuller's earth 100 g will irreversibly bind 5 g of paraquat. Bentonite 7 g may be used instead of fuller's earth, but it is less effective. In addition alkaline diuresis, as for salicylate poisoning, should be carried out.

(f) Cyanide

Cyanide poisoning (by ingestion or inhalation) is a medical emergency, requiring rapid treatment. If cyanide has been swallowed, gastric lavage should be performed with 5 per cent sodium thiosulphate, 300 mL of 25 per cent sodium thiosulphate should be left in the stomach. Dicobalt edetate (dicobalt EDTA) should be given i.v. as soon as possible in all cases of poisoning in a dose of 600 mg in 40 mL over 1 min. If recovery does not occur within a minute or two another 300 mg of dicobalt edetate should be given. Oxygen (100 per cent) should also be given and acidosis should be corrected with sodium bicarbonate.

(g) Carbon monoxide

Despite the replacement of coal gas by North Sea gas, carbon monoxide poisoning is still the commonest cause of death from self-poisoning in the UK, due to poisoning with car exhaust fumes. In the home, incomplete combustion of methane in North Sea gas (for example in a faulty gas fire) causes the formation of carbon monoxide, which may accumulate in poorly ventilated surroundings, and this is responsible for a large number of accidental deaths each year.

Carbon monoxide poisoning can cause nausea and vomiting, headache, confusion, loss of consciousness, hemiplegia, monoplegia, cerebral oedema, and cardiac arrhythmias. Even if recovery is complete there may be long-term neuropsychiatric damage.

Treatment is by removal from the source of the gas, and by the early administration of oxygen. Carbon monoxide has a higher affinity for haemoglobin than oxygen and forms carboxyhaemoglobin, which has a half-time of about 4 h. This is reduced to 1 h if the patient is breathing 100 per cent oxygen and to 0.5 h if hyperbaric oxygen is given. Since most centres do not have ready access to hyperbaric oxygen, it should be reserved for those who are unconscious or severely acidotic, or who have signs of cardiac or neurological damage. In severe cases when hyperbaric oxygen is not available intubation and mechanical ventilation should be considered. Treat cerebral oedema with mannitol (500 mL of a 20 per cent solution) and cardiac arrhythmias as required.

(h) Narcotic analgesics

The opioid receptor antagonist naloxone rapidly reverses the effects of both opiate analgesics and other narcotic analgesics (for example pethidine, pentazocine, dextropropoxyphene). It is given in a dose of 0.4 mg i.v. initially, repeated every 2–3 min if required. A total dose of 1.2 mg is usually sufficient. In buprenorphine poisoning naloxone produces only partial reversal and in severe cases ventilation may be required. Naloxone is eliminated from the body with a half-time of about 1 h, i.e. faster than the narcotic analgesics, and its effects may therefore wear off. One must therefore be prepared to administer another dose if required, and patients may need to be persuaded to stay in hospital in case this should be necessary.

Great care should be taken in reversing opiate-induced coma in opiate addicts, because of the risk of inducing an acute withdrawal syndrome (see p. 479).

(i) Organophosphorus insecticides

These compounds are irreversible inhibitors of acetylcholinesterase. They are very toxic and since they are absorbed through the skin, rubber gloves should be worn when in contact with the patient or the patient's clothes. Intensive respiratory support is required, and when cyanosis has been reversed atropine should be given, 2 mg i.v. every 10 min until the skin is dry and there is a sinus tachycardia, or other evidence of full atropinization. A cholinesterase reactivator should also be given, such as pralidoxime 30 mg/kg i.v. at a rate of no more than 500 mg/min, and repeated after 30 min. Cholinesterase reactivators are not widely stocked by hospitals, but are available at certain UK centres whose names are held by the poisons information centres. Convulsions should be treated with diazepam or chlormethiazole.

(j) Digitalis

In this instance ipecac-induced emesis is preferable to gastric lavage, since there may be an increased risk of cardiac asystole during lavage. If a large dose has been taken (for example more than 5 mg of digoxin) a transvenous pacemaker should be inserted as soon as possible, even in the absence of arrhythmias or heart block, since its insertion

at a later time when it is seen to be needed is more likely to cause arrhythmias than early on. Oral activated charcoal may help reduce the absorption of digitalis drugs, and an anion exchange resin, such as cholestyramine or colestipol, is also effective in reducing digitoxin absorption.

Definitive treatment of severe digitalis toxicity is with the Fab fragments of antidigoxin antibody, which are effective in reversing the effects of not only digoxin, but also of other digitalis drugs, including digitoxin and lanatoside C. The ways to calculate the appropriate doses are shown in Table 35.5. Abnormalities of potassium balance may also require specific therapy. After successful reversal of digitalis intoxication with antidigoxin antibody it may be necessary to treat heart failure or atrial fibrillation if the therapeutic effects of digitalis have been lost.

If antidigoxin antibody is not available or if cardiac arrhythmias and heart block occur before it can be given or takes effect, they should be treated as described in Chapter 24 (p. 285).

■ **Table 35.5** Calculations of the appropriate doses of Fab fragments of antidigoxin antibody in cases of digitalis intoxication or overdose

1. *Digoxin*
   (a) When the dose of tablets is known:
       Dose in mg × 40
   (b) When the plasma concentration is known:
       Concentration in ng/mL ×
           lean body weight × 0.34
       or
       Concentration in nmol/L ×
           lean body weight × 0.26

2. *Digitoxin*
   (a) When the dose is known:
       Dose in mg × 60
   (b) When the plasma concentration is known:
       Concentration in ng/mL ×
           lean body weight × 0.034
       or
       Concentration in nmol/L ×
           lean body weight × 0.026

Example: Plasma digoxin concentration 24 ng/mL in a patient with estimated lean body weight 75 kg. Give 24 × 75 × 0.34 = 612 mg.

(k) Benzodiazepines

In the vast majority of cases only supportive measures are required in cases of benzodiazepine poisoning. Recently flumazenil, a benzodiazepine antagonist, has been introduced for the reversal of the central sedative effects of benzodiazepines after anaesthesia and in intensive care units. It is not indicated for the reversal of coma or sedation associated with uncomplicated benzodiazepine overdose, but it may be kept in mind in complicated cases in which respiratory depression and hypotension occur or in a patient who is old or has worrying underlying disease, such as chronic obstructive lung disease. In patients who have been taking benzodiazepines for more than a few weeks one should bear in mind the risk of an acute benzodiazepine withdrawal syndrome, which may cause fits and cardiac arrhythmias. Flumazenil should not be given to patients who have taken a tricyclic antidepressant, because of the risk of convulsions and cardiac arrhythmias.

(l) Notes on some other important poisonings (see also Table 35.5)

1. Major tranquillizers

This includes phenothiazines, such as chlorpromazine, butyrophenones, such as haloperidol, and thioxanthenes, such as flupenthixol. Intensive supportive measures may be required. Dyskinesias should be treated with benztropine (2 mg i.v.) or procyclidine (5 mg i.v.), and convulsions with diazepam or chlormethiazole.

2. Monoamine oxidase inhibitors

Dopamine or dobutamine should not be used for treating shock, since their metabolism is inhibited by MAO inhibitors. Instead use hydrocortisone, 100 mg i.v. six-hourly. For hyperthermia use a fan and tepid sponging or chlorpromazine (100 mg i.m.). Chlorpromazine is also useful for treating the cerebral stimulatory effects of MAO inhibitors.

3. Lithium

Lithium excretion is hastened by alkalinization of the urine, but very careful plasma electrolyte monitoring must be carried out. Diuretics should not be used, since they inhibit the renal excretion of lithium. In severe cases dialysis or charcoal haemoperfusion may be required.

4. Iron

Gastric lavage should be carried out with a solution of desferrioxamine, 2 g/L, and 10 g of desferrioxamine should be left in the stomach at the end. Desferrioxamine should also be given as soon as possible both i.m. and i.v. The doses are: i.m. 2 g (1 g in a child) repeated after 12 h; i.v. 15 mg/kg/h to a maximum of 80 mg/kg/d. If there is oliguria start dialysis immediately. Rarely i.v. desferrioxamine may cause acute anaphylaxis or reversible hypotension.

5. Methanol

Give ethyl alcohol 1 mg/kg of a 50 per cent solution orally immediately, followed by an i.v. infusion of 5 per cent ethyl alcohol in 5 per cent dextrose at a rate of 5–10 mL/h, aiming for a minimum blood ethanol concentration of 22 mmol/L (100 mg/dL). Increase the dose by 8 mL/h during dialysis. Treat acidosis with sodium bicarbonate. In severe cases haemodialysis or peritoneal dialysis is necessary, for example if the blood methanol concentration is over 16 mmol/L (500 mg/L) or if there are neurological or ophthalmic complications or severe acidosis.

35.3 Sources of information

For the names of some textbooks describing the presentation and management of acute poisoning see the bibliography (Chapter 20). For information on individual drugs in the UK a poisons information centre should be contacted. The telephone numbers of these centres are listed in *The British National Formulary*.

For specific advice on paraquat poisoning one of the many paraquat treatment centres should be contacted (see *Br. Med. J.* (1979). **ii**, 619).

35.4 Agents used in the treatment of poisoning

In Table 35.6 are shown the various therapeutic agents which may be used in the treatment of poisoning, arranged alphabetically in order of agent. There is also a cross-index to the table, arranged alphabetically in order of the poisons to be treated.

■ **Table 35.6** Agents used in the treatment of self-poisoning

Agent	Used in poisoning by	Mode of action	Dosage	Comments
N-acetylcysteine	Paracetamol	Sulphydryl compound: prevents hepatic necrosis by assisting conjugation of toxic hydroxylamine metabolites of paracetamol	See text (p.494)	May cause anaphylactoid reactions
Acids, dilute acetic acid 1% w/v, lemon juice, vinegar 1:4	Caustic alkalis (for example ammonia, potassium or sodium hydroxide)	Neutralizing effect	Oral: 100–200 mL, or as much as can be tolerated	
Alcohol (ethanol, ethyl alcohol) (p. 546)	Methyl alcohol, ethylene glycol (and other glycols)	Competes with methyl alcohol for metabolism by hepatic enzyme alcohol dehydrogenase, preventing formation of toxic formic acid and formates; prevents breakdown of glycols into toxic oxalic acid and oxalates	See text	
Ascorbic acid	As an alternative to methylene blue (but less effective)	See methylene blue	I.v.: 1 g slowly Oral: 200 mg t.d.s.	
Atropine sulphate (p. 538)	1. Organophosphorus insecticides, for example malathion, parathion, and other acetylcholinesterase inhibitors, including carbamates 2. Neostigmine and other parasympathomimetics	Competes with acetylcholine at parasympathetic nerve endings; no effect at neuromuscular sites	1. Mild cases: i.m., s.c.: initially 0.6–1.2 mg. Severe cases: i.v.: 0.25–2 mg repeated at 15–30 min intervals to maintain atropinization 2. I.m., s.c.: 0.6–1.2 mg to control muscarinic effects (may be given i.v. in severe cases)	
Benztropine (p. 538)	Butyrophenones Phenothiazines Reserpine	Cholinoceptor antagonist for control of the extrapyramidal effects of these drugs	I.v.: 1–2 mg will give rapid relief of symptoms; the dose may be repeated	

Agent	Poisoning	Mechanism	Dose/route	Notes
Calcium gluconate	1. Hydrofluoric acid	Binds fluoride ion in a less soluble complex	Oral: after ingestion, 30 g well diluted. Eye-drops: 10% sterile solution, a few drops. Topical: applied to affected skin repeatedly (for example in dressings) after pain subsides. I.v.: for convulsions 10 ml of a 10% solution, repeat if necessary	Give by slow i.v. injection; high blood concentrations of calcium ions may depress cardiac function. Solution irritant, take care during i.v. injection
	2. Lead	Relieves pain of colic after acute poisoning	I.v.: 10–20 mL of a 10% solution	
	3. Oxalic acid	Prevents tetany	Oral: after ingestion 100 mL of a 1% solution	
Chlormethiazole (p. 579)	Agents causing convulsions	Anticonvulsant	See text	
Chlorpromazine (p. 645)	LSD, amphetamines, MAO inhibitors	Tranquillizer; reduces hyperpyrexia	I.m.: 100–200 mg	Contra-indicated in comatose patients
Desferrioxamine mesylate	Iron	Iron chelator (100 mg chelates approximately 8.5 mg of iron)	Oral, i.m., and i.v.: See text	Rapid i.v. injection may cause allergic reaction; local pain may occur with i.m. injection
Dextrose	Hypoglycaemic drugs	Maintains blood glucose	Oral, i.v.: as required	
Diazepam (p. 564)	Agents causing convulsions	Anticonvulsant	See text	
Dicobalt edetate	Cyanide	Forms stable complex with cyanides	I.v.: 300 mg (20 mL) over 1 min; may be repeated if the response is inadequate	If no improvement give nitrite/thiosulphate therapy
Dimercaprol (British anti-Lewisite, BAL)	Arsenic, mercury, antimony, bismuth, heavy metals, gold, thallium, lead (combined with sodium calcium edetate for encephalitis), nickel	Chelator; combines with metals which inhibit the pyruvate oxidase system by competing with sulphydryl groups in proteins; dimercaprol has a higher affinity for the metals than the proteins do	4 mg/kg i.m. every 4 h for 2 d, followed by 3 mg/kg b.d. for up to 8 d if required	High doses produce adverse effects in 50% of patients (nausea, vomiting, headache, burning sensation of lips, mouth, throat, and eyes, salivation, lachrymation, hypertension, muscle spasm, tachycardia); these are at a maximum 20 min after injection and subside in 2 h; there may be pain at the site of injection; do not use in patients with impaired liver function; contra-indicated in cadmium and iron poisoning

Agent	Used in poisoning by	Mode of action	Dosage	Comments
Flumazenil	Benzodiazepines	Antagonist at benzodiazepine receptors	See p. 473	Rarely needed because of the safety of benzodiazepine poisoning; risks of convulsions and cardiac arrhythmias in patients who have taken a tricyclic antidepressant or long-term benzodiazepines; in UK licensed only for use in ITUs
Fuller's earth suspension (150 g/L)	Paraquat, diquat, and other bipyridylium compounds	Adsorption of poison in the gastrointestinal tract, preventing absorption	See text	
Glucagon	1. Hypoglycaemic drugs	1. Increases hepatic glycogen mobilization to increase plasma glucose	1. I.m., s.c., or i.v.: 0.5–2 mg; may be repeated once or twice if there is no response	1. Response takes 5–20 min, so i.v. dextrose is the treatment of choice
	2. β-adrenoceptor antagonists	2. Stimulates adenyl cyclase activity	2. I.v.: 2 mg, repeated according to response (i.v. up to 40 mg over 12 h has been used)	2. The diluent of glucagon may contain phenol 0.2%, which may cause toxic effects if repeated doses are necessary
Methylene blue (ascorbic acid is an alternative, but is less effective)	Chlorates, phenacetin, glyceryl trinitrate, phenazone, nitrobenzene, toluidine, nitric acid, nitrites, dinitrophenol, aniline derivatives	For methaemoglobinaemia: hastens the conversion of methaemoglobin to haemoglobin	I.v.: 10 mL of a 1% solution repeated as required (1–4 mg/kg body weight)	Take care to avoid extravasation
Naloxone hydrochloride (p. 641)	Narcotic analgesics	Opioid antagonist; counteracts respiratory depression	I.v.: initially 0.4–1.2 mg, repeated once or twice at 2–3 min intervals	Pure antagonist; does not cause respiratory depression (cf nalorphine); may cause cardiac arrhythmias in opiate addicts
D-penicillamine (p. 657)	1. Lead: chronic poisoning or in the control of plumbism after acute overdose (NOT for tetra-ethyl lead poisoning) 2. Gold: if adverse reaction to dimercaprol treatment	Chelating agent, aids elimination of the metallic ion	Oral: 1–4 mg daily in divided doses. Children: 5 years 150 mg b.d.; 6–12 years 300 mg b.d.	Allergic reactions; patients sensitive to penicillin may react to penicillamine

Phentolamine mesylate (p. 542)	Amphetamine and sympathomimetic agents, such as ephedrine. Clonidine. Hypertensive crises in patients taking MAO inhibitors	α-adrenoceptor antagonist	I.v.: 5–10 mg, repeated as necessary	
Physostigmine (p. 539)	1. Anticholinergic drugs, such as atropine, hyoscine, propantheline 2. Tricyclic antidepressants (but see text)	Acetylcholinesterase inhibitor; reverses both peripheral and central effects 2. See text	1. i.v., i.m., s.c.: 1–2 mg every 1–2 h or as required	
Procyclidine (p. 538)	Butyrophenones Phenothiazines Reserpine	Cholinoceptor antagonist for control of the extrapyramidal effects of these drugs	I.v.: 5–10 mg will give rapid relief of symptoms; the dose may be repeated after 20 min	
Salbutamol (p. 541)	β-adrenoceptor antagonists	Selective β_2-agonist; relieves β-blocker-induced bronchoconstriction	Inhalation: 1–2 mg/h via nebulizer	
Sodium calcium edetate	Lead (acute and chronic). More effective if used in combination with dimercaprol	Exchanges calcium ions for lead ions in the blood and forms a stable, non-ionizable, water-soluble lead compound, which is readily excreted unchanged in the urine	I.v.: 40 mg/kg/day in two divided doses for 3–5 days; combined with dimercaprol Note: if there is encephalopathy and increased intracranial pressure the dose may be given i.m. to avoid giving excess fluid	Nausea, diarrhoea, and abdominal pains often occur during i.v. injection, as can a burning sensation at the site of injection. Thrombophlebitis can occur if the concentrated solution is injected quickly. Nephrotoxicity can cause albuminuria, casts and cells in the urine, oliguria, and renal failure
Sodium nitrite	Cyanide	Converts haemoglobin to methaemoglobin, which competes with cytochrome oxidase for cyanide, forming cyanhaemoglobin	See text	Used with sodium thiosulphate. Dicobalt edetate is the usual first-line therapy for cyanide poisoning
Sodium thiosulphate	Cyanide	Hastens conversion of cyanmethaemoglobin to thiocyanate by the action of tissue rhodanase	See text	Used with sodium nitrite

Poisoning by	Agent(s) used (Table 35.6)	Poisoning by	Agent(s) used (Table 35.6)
Acetylcholinesterase inhibitors	Atropine	Iron	Desferrioxamine
Alkalis, caustic	Acids	Lead	Calcium gluconate, dimercaprol, penicillamine, sodium calcium edetate
Ammonia	Acids	LSD	Chlorpromazine
Amphetamines	Chlorpromazine, phentolamine	Malathion	Atropine
Analgesics, narcotic	Naloxone	Mercury	Dimercaprol
Aniline derivatives	Ascorbic acid, methylene blue	Methyl alcohol (methanol)	Alcohol (ethanol)
Anticholinergic drugs	Physostigmine	Monoamine oxidase inhibitors	Chlorpromazine
Antidepressants, tricyclic	Physostigmine	Monoamine oxidase inhibitors ('cheese reaction')	Phentolamine
Arsenic	Dimercaprol	Narcotic analgesics	Naloxone
Atropine	Physostigmine	Neostigmine	Atropine
β-adrenoceptor antagonists	Glucagon, salbutamol	Nickel	Dimercaprol
Benzodiazepines	Flumazenil	Nitric acid	Ascorbic acid, methylene blue
Bipyridylium compounds	Fuller's earth	Nitrites	Ascorbic acid, methylene blue
Bismuth	Dimercaprol	Nitrobenzene	Ascorbic acid, methylene blue
Butyrophenones	Benztropine, procyclidine	Organophosphorus insecticides	Atropine
Carbamates	Atropine	Oxalic acid	Calcium gluconate
Caustic alkalis	Acids	Paracetamol	Acetylcysteine
Chlorates	Ascorbic acid, methylene blue	Paraquat	Fuller's earth
Clonidine	Phentolamine	Parasympathomimetic agents	Atropine
Convulsive agents	Chlormethiazole, diazepam	Parathion	Atropine
Cyanide	Dicobalt edetate; sodium nitrite + sodium thiosulphate	Phenacetin	Ascorbic acid, methylene blue
Dinitrophenol	Ascorbic acid, methylene blue	Phenazone	Ascorbic acid, methylene blue
Diquat	Fuller's earth	Phenothiazines	Benztropine, procyclidine
Ephedrine	Phentolamine	Potassium hydroxide	Acids
Ethylene glycol	Alcohol (ethanol)	Propantheline	Physostigmine
Glyceryl trinitrate	Ascorbic acid, methylene blue	Reserpine	Benztropine, procyclidine
Glycols	Alcohol (ethanol)	Sodium hydroxide	Acids
Gold	Dimercaprol, penicillamine	Sympathomimetic agents	Phentolamine
Hydrofluoric acid	Calcium gluconate	Thallium	Dimercaprol
Hyoscine	Physostigmine	Toluidine	Ascorbic acid, methylene blue
Hypoglycaemic drugs	Dextrose, glucagon	Tricyclic antidepressants	Physostigmine
Insecticides, organophosphorus	Atropine		

Cross-index for Table 35.6

36 The principles of cancer chemotherapy

Co-author: J. Carmichael

Cancers kill 20 per cent of people. Although certain cancers can be cured by local treatments, such as surgery and radiotherapy, many are incurable because of systemic spread. The management of disseminated tumours is complex, and often involves several different types of therapy, even with tumours which are sensitive to cytotoxic drugs. The use of drugs in the management of malignant disease requires much experience and skill. However, although such treatment is carried out in specialist units the general continuing care of these patients is part of the responsibility of every surgeon, physician, and general practitioner. A knowledge of the principles of cancer chemotherapy is therefore of importance.

The first point to note is that drug therapy is only part of the treatment of the patient with malignant disease. The general management of the patient and family, the control of symptoms such as pain, the treatment of complications such as obstruction of urinary flow in carcinoma of the prostate, and the place of surgery and radiotherapy in overall management are all of vital importance. Because the toxic:therapeutic ratios of cytotoxic drugs are generally low, and because cytotoxic drug toxicity can be symptomatically very distressing and occasionally fatal, the judgement as to when such treatment should be used is based on several important variables. These include the known efficacy of chemotherapy in similar cases, and the mental and physical condition and social circumstances of the individual patient. The mixture of skills required in each case varies, and the integration and organization of chemotherapeutic, surgical, and radiotherapeutic, programmes have in recent years led to the establishment of the specialties of medical, surgical, and radiation oncology.

Although the five-year survival rates for the major solid neoplasms (for example colon, rectum, lung, breast, uterus) have not increased dramatically since the 1940s, there have been startling successes in some neoplastic conditions, such as tumours of the haemopoietic system and germ cell malignancies.

36.1 Tumour responsiveness to chemotherapy

Tumour responsiveness to chemotherapy can be classified into three categories: tumours which are highly chemosensitive, moderately chemosensitive, and chemoresistant (Table 36.1).

36.1.1 Chemosensitive tumours

Chemosensitive tumours have a high complete response rate to chemotherapy. They are generally sensitive to several drugs, and combination chemotherapy is to be preferred to single agent therapy. Chemotherapy should be considered in all such cases and many patients with certain tumour types will be cured.

36.1.2 Moderately chemosensitive tumours

Moderately chemosensitive tumours have a low complete response rate to chemotherapy (about 10 per cent) but a high partial response rate (about 50 per cent). Combination chemotherapy is mar-

▌ **Table 36.1** Examples of tumour responsiveness to cancer chemotherapy

	Tumour	Treatment
1. *Chemosensitive*	Hodgkin's lymphoma	Combination chemotherapy, radiotherapy (pp. 405, 515)
	Non-Hodgkin's lymphoma	Combination chemotherapy, radiotherapy (p. 406)
	Acute leukaemias	Combination chemotherapy (pp. 406, 514)
	Choriocarcinoma	Methotrexate, actinomycin
	Testicular carcinoma (seminoma/teratoma)	Surgery, radiotherapy, chemotherapy (p. 515)
	Wilms' tumour (children)	Surgery, radiotherapy, chemotherapy
	Burkitt's lymphoma	Cyclophosphamide
	Rhabdomyosarcoma	Surgery, radiotherapy, chemotherapy
	Retinoblastoma	Radiotherapy, cyclophosphamide
	Acute adult leukaemias	Combination chemotherapy (p. 406) + surgery/radiotherapy
2. *Moderately chemosensitive*	Breast carcinoma	Surgery, radiotherapy, chemotherapy
	Multiple myeloma	Combination chemotherapy (p. 407)
	Bladder carcinoma	Combination chemotherapy (local and systemic)
	Carcinoma of prostate	Hormonal therapies (p. 361)
	Ovarian carcinoma	Combination chemotherapy, surgery
	Oat cell bronchogenic carcinoma	Combination chemotherapy
	Endometrial carcinoma	Hormonal and cytotoxic chemotherapy, surgery
	Head and neck cancers	Chemotherapy + surgery/radiotherapy
	Gastric carcinoma	Surgery, combination chemotherapy
3. *Chemoresistant*	Pancreatic islet cell carcinoma	Surgery, combination chemotherapy
	Adrenocortical carcinoma	Combination chemotherapy
	Squamous cell bronchial carcinoma	Surgery and radiotherapy ± chemotherapy
	Colorectal carcinoma	(Surgery can be effective)
	Malignant melanoma	Surgery
	Pancreatic adenocarcinoma	Surgery
	Gliomas	Surgery
	Hypernephroma	Surgery, chemotherapy, immunotherapy

ginally more effective than single agent treatment. Chemotherapy may be used at some stage of the disease in such cases, but would not be first-line treatment. Chemotherapy is often useful as an adjuvant to surgery and radiotherapy.

36.1.3 Chemoresistant tumours

Chemoresistant tumours have response rates in the region of 20 per cent and complete responses are rare, although for certain tumour types chemotherapy has an adjuvant role. Combination chemotherapy is rarely more effective than treatment with a single drug. In such cases new drugs may be used as single first-line agents, in the hope of obtaining some response. This also provides information on such drugs for future use. Cytotoxic drugs may also be used in such cases to alleviate symptoms when local measures have failed.

36.2 The actions of chemotherapeutic drugs relevant to their clinical uses

Some of the drugs used in cancer chemotherapy are listed in Table 36.2 and their modes of action are summarized in the Pharmacopoeia. However, there are certain points to emphasize in relation to their use in cancer chemotherapy.

36.2.1 Mechanisms of action

There are several different mechanisms by which cytotoxic drugs interfere with cell growth and division. Their different sites of action in regard to the molecular biochemistry of the cell are illustrated in Fig. 36.1. The fact that cytotoxic drugs differ in their mechanisms of action gives the opportunity for producing cumulative biochemical lesions in the cell during therapy, by using combinations of drugs with different mechanisms of action.

■ **Table 36.2** Some drugs used in cancer chemotherapy

1. *Alkykating agents*
   Busulphan (p. 566)
   Carmustine
   Chlorambucil (p. 573)
   Cyclophosphamide (p. 590)
   Estramustine
   Ifosfamide
   Lomustine
   Melphalan (p. 631)
   Mustine (p. 640)
   Thiotepa
   Treosulfan

2. *Antimetabolites*
   Cytarabine (p. 592)
   Deoxycoformycin
   Fluorouracil (p. 607)
   Mercaptopurine (p. 561)
   Methotrexate (p. 632)
   Thioguanine

3. *Cytotoxic antibiotics*
   Actinomycin (p. 540)
   Bleomycin (p. 565)
   Doxorubicin (p. 601)
   Epirubicin
   Mitomycin
   Mitozantrone

4. *Hormones and hormone antagonists*
   Anti-oestrogens
     Tamoxifen (p. 692)
     Toremifene

   Anti-androgens
     Cyproterone
   Glucocorticoids (p. 584)
   Oestrogens, for example stilboestrol (p. 678)
   Progestogens, for example
     medroxyprogesterone (p. 678)
   LHRH agonists
     Buserelin
     Goserelin
   Aromatase inhibitors
     Aminoglutethimide

5. *Vinca alkaloids* (p. 704)
   Vinblastine
   Vincristine
   Vindesine

6. *Epipodophyllotoxins*
   Etoposide (VP 16)
   Tenoposide (VM 26)

7. *Immunotherapies*
   Interferons (α, β, γ)
   Interleukin 2
   Tumour necrosis factor

8. *Others*
   Amsacrine
   Carboplatin
   Cisplatin (p. 583)
   Dacarbazine
   Hydroxyurea
   Procarbazine
   Razoxane

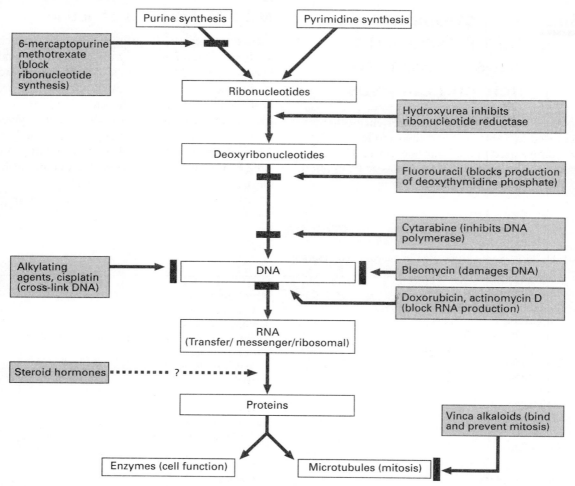

■ **Fig. 36.1** Cellular biochemistry and the sites and mechanisms of action of cytotoxic drugs.

36.2.2 The effects of cytotoxic drugs on different phases of the cell cycle

All cells which synthesize DNA go through a regular cycle which has several different phases (illustrated in Fig. 36.2).

(i) G_1 phase

The G_1 phase is a resting phase, the duration of which is a major factor determining the duration of the cell cycle time. It occurs after cell division (mitosis) is complete. During G_1 there is no DNA synthesis, but RNA and protein synthesis occur normally and the cells subsequently go into S phase. However, after mitosis cells may go into a different kind of resting phase, G_0, in which they are out of the cycle but are still capable of proliferating.

(ii) S phase

The S phase is a phase of DNA synthesis which occurs after G_1, and is preceded by an increase in the rate of RNA synthesis. This results in a doubling of the DNA content of the cell and the production of sister chromatids.

(iii) G_2 phase

G_2 is another resting phase, which occurs immediately after the S phase. DNA synthesis once more stops while RNA and protein synthesis continue.

(iv) M phase (mitosis)

During mitosis there is a reduction in the rate of RNA and protein synthesis. At this point the chromosomes condense and the sister chromatids separate, the cell divides, and the resting phases occur again.

Different cytotoxic drugs may act at different phases of the cell cycle, as illustrated in Fig. 36.2. Certain principles follow from these observations.

(a) The effect of the growth fraction on the response to chemotherapy

The growth fraction is the proportion of cells that are in cycle at any time. It is an important factor in the response of a tumour to chemotherapy, since tumours with a high growth factor are generally more sensitive to chemotherapy. Conversely, cells in G_0 are resistant to cytotoxic drugs.

(b) The effect of the speed of cell cycle on the response to chemotherapy

The faster the cell cycle proceeds the more likely it is that treatment with cytotoxic drugs will 'catch' the cell in a sensitive phase. Unfortunately, in general the faster the cell cycles the more malignant is the condition. As a corollary of this, normal cells with fast cycles, for example bone-marrow, gastrointestinal epithelium, lymphoid tissue, and skin, suffer most from cytotoxic therapy. Cytotoxic drugs are therefore usually given in cycles of treatment at intervals of 3–4 weeks, rather than continuously, since this allows recovery of susceptible tissues, such as the bone-marrow.

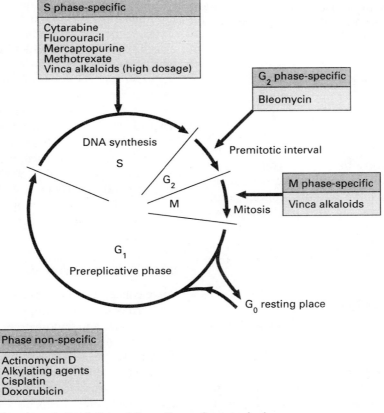

■ **Fig. 36.2** The cell cycle and the timing of the actions of cytotoxic drugs.

(c) Synchrony of the cell cycle in the cells in a tumour

Theoretically if more tumour cells are synchronized in a sensitive phase of the cycle there will be a greater chance that the tumour will respond to a pulse of cytotoxic drug therapy. The fewer cells there are in a sensitive phase the less effective drug treatment will be and the more necessary prolonged therapy will be, with a consequent increase in toxicity. Sometimes an attempt is made to recruit cells into cycle, for example, the recruitment of breast cancer cells with oestrogens, although the efficacy of this approach is unproven.

Alternatively, cytotoxic drugs can be used to arrest cells at different points of the cycle, thus modifying the effects of other treatments. For instance, cells can be brought into synchrony with a mitotic spindle poison, such as a vinca alkaloid, which might arrest cells in their cycle, after which they could be treated with an inhibitor of DNA synthesis, say cytarabine, as they are progressing through S phase. Whether such a combination works in this way in practice is difficult to prove, but it does work in experimental mouse leukaemias.

(d) The effects of tumour size on treatment

Large tumours are relatively unresponsive to cytotoxic drugs, for two reasons. Firstly, many cells tend to be in G_0, the resting phase in which cells are unresponsive to drugs. Secondly, penetration of drugs through a rather poor vasculature is insufficient to achieve cytotoxic concentrations for long enough without also producing severe systemic toxicity. It is better, if possible, to remove large tumour bulk and to treat remaining small tumour masses with chemotherapy, except in highly chemosensitive tumours.

(e) Kinetics of cell kill

Because cytotoxic drugs are generally more effective in particular phases of the cell cycle, they kill a proportion of all cells of a type during each course of treatment, rather than a fixed number of cells. Furthermore, since many human tumours are heterogeneous in their cell populations there may be great variability in the responses of individual cell types. It is therefore difficult to kill off every tumour cell, although if cure is the aim this is essential. Because of this proportionality of cell kill, chemotherapy can often reduce tumour mass sufficiently to result in clinical remission, often quite easily, but without eradicating the tumour, as with small cell lung cancer. Remember that the faster the cells divide, the more easily they are killed by cytotoxic drugs and the faster the onset of clinical remission. Unfortunately, if the tumour cells are not completely eradicated, rapidly-dividing cells also produce clinical relapse quickly, for example in acute myeloid leukaemia or small cell lung cancer.

(f) Resistance of cancer cells to cytotoxic drugs

As noted above there are differences in the responsiveness of some cancer cells to drugs. Many biochemical mechanisms are involved in this resistance, including differences in drug metabolizing enzymes, detoxification mechanisms, and DNA repair. In recent years a specific form of multiple drug resistance has been identified which seems to be important in many solid tumours. This mechanism is mediated by a P-glycoprotein, which pumps cytotoxic drugs out of cells before they can act. This pump can be inhibited, by mechanisms which are not completely understood, by a variety of structurally unrelated drugs, including nifedipine, verapamil, cyclosporin, and tamoxifen. These drugs have been used in combination with chemotherapy in order to block this glycoprotein and reverse this type of drug resistance.. There have been encouraging results with this approach in blood cancers, but resistance in solid tumours has proved more difficult to overcome.

36.2.2 Hormonal drugs

Some cancers can be considered to be dependent on hormones, for example breast cancer, prostatic cancer, and endometrial cancer. Hormones and hormone antagonists can therefore be used in their treatment.

In breast cancer there are now many hormonal treatments available, including the oestrogen antagonist tamoxifen, the progestogen medroxyprogesterone, the LHRH agonist goserelin, and the aromatase inhibitor aminoglutethimide. All of these produce response rates of around 30 per cent in advanced breast cancer and the likelihood of response increases with the patient's age.

Oestrogens were used in the past to treat prostatic cancer, but they have been abandoned because of their adverse effects. It is common nowadays to use an LHRH agonist, such as goserelin. Early tumour flare-ups can occur with goserelin and can be prevented with an anti-androgen, such as cyproterone acetate.

36.2.3 Immunological agents

There has been great interest recently in the use of immunological agents in the treatment of cancers, starting with the interferons. Interferons are effective in hairy cell leukaemia and in low-grade lymphomas, and they may enhance the effectiveness of certain cytotoxic drugs when used in combination.

The cytokine interleukin 2 has recently been used in the treatment of renal cancer, with response rates of 20–30 per cent with interleukin 2 alone and slightly better results in combination with LAK (lymphokine-activated killer) cells.

36.3 Clinical evaluation of tumours before and after treatment

Because of the serious toxicity of cancer chemotherapy it is vital that patients be properly assessed before treatment in order to evaluate their likely response and progress. Careful histopathology and clinical staging by radiological techniques, such as scanning by computerized tomography (CT) and magnetic resonance imaging (MRI), lymphangiography, and surgical exploration, are essential. These procedures are particularly important in curable cancers, such as Hodgkin's lymphoma, in which the choice of treatment depends on the stage of the disease (see p. 405).

In some cases there may be tumour markers detectable in the serum the measurement of which may be used to assess tumour burden, the response to treatment, or recurrence. For example, α-fetoprotein and human chorionic gonadotropin in teratomas, myeloma proteins, α-fetoprotein in hepatocellular carcinoma, ectopic hormones in oat cell carcinoma of bronchus, carcinoembryonic antigen in colorectal carcinoma, prostate-specific antigen in prostatic carcinoma, and CA 125 in ovarian carcinoma.

During therapy tumour responsiveness should be evaluated regularly to give guidance on the advisability of further courses of chemotherapy. Nearly every tumour that is chemosensitive will respond within two courses of chemotherapy (i.e. within about 6 weeks). When staging of the disease has been carried out it should be repeated after three courses. If there has been a good response chemotherapy can be continued with confidence. If the response has been poor other drugs or strategies may have to be considered.

36.4 Combination chemotherapy

Combinations of chemotherapeutic agents are particularly effective in chemosensitive tumours. They are used because:

1. Human malignancies tend to be resistant to one agent; this may or may not be due to cell heterogeneity.
2. Cell resistance is often acquired during treatment with a single agent, one possible reason being the proliferation of mutant cells with biochemical properties which confer resistance to particular agents.
3. Multiple sites of attack on tumour cells are possible with drugs which have different toxic effects on normal cells. Thus, greater overall efficacy of treatment can be achieved without unacceptable toxicity. For instance, vincristine and prednisolone do not have great marrow toxicity and can be combined successfully with doxorubicin in the treatment of acute lymphoblastic leukaemia.

36.5 Regimens for cancer chemotherapy

The main aim of any regimen used in the treatment of cancer is to try to get enough drug to the tumour cells for long enough to achieve a reasonable kill, while at the same time avoiding unacceptable toxicity. Most regimens are based on intermittent administration of drugs, with intervals of a few weeks between courses; this allows time for recovery of normal bone-marrow and immune functions between courses. However, sometimes continuous treatment is more appropriate, for example in the maintenance treatment of chronic lymphocytic leukaemia with chlorambucil, the use of hormones and hormone antagonists in the treatment of carcinoma of the prostate and breast, and the maintenance treatment of chronic myeloid leukaemia with busulphan.

Sometimes special action must be taken to get at cells in sites not easily accessible to drugs given systemically, for example, pleural, pericardial, or peritoneal malignant effusions and CNS spread. The instillation of cytotoxic drugs, such as bleomycin or thiotepa, into malignant effusions can be palliative, reducing the size of the effusion. Large effusions can also cause problems by altering the clearances of cytotoxic drugs, such as methotrexate, and this can result in serious toxicity.

CNS spread is a problem with leukaemias and some solid tumours, since the penetration of many cytotoxic drugs into the brain is poor. Intrathecal methotrexate and radiotherapy to the cranium are now routinely used with great success in preventing CNS involvement in acute lymphoblastic leukaemia in children.

36.6 Adverse effects of drugs used in cancer chemotherapy

The main problem limiting the use of cytotoxic drugs is the occurrence of adverse effects. Although these are listed under the individual agents in the Pharmacopoeia, many are common to most cytotoxic drugs.

36.6.1 Nausea and vomiting

Nausea and vomiting are most common during high-dose pulse therapy. The worst offenders are the mustines, cisplatin, and doxorubicin, but nausea and vomiting can be caused by many cytotoxic drugs and can be a major factor in a patient's tolerance of cancer chemotherapy.

The prevention and treatment of cytotoxic drug-induced nausea and vomiting are not yet satisfactory. Various antiemetics, such as the phenothiazine prochlorperazine and other dopamine receptor antagonists such as domperidone and metoclopramide, are often used. Recently specific antagonists at 5-HT$_3$ receptors, such as ondansetron, have been introduced for this purpose and are very effective.

Cytotoxic drugs are often given at night, so that sedation and sleep can add to the antiemetic effect. Whenever possible antiemetics should be given 24 h before starting chemotherapy so that they may have time to take effect. They should also be taken continuously in order to prevent symptoms rather than simply to alleviate them when they occur. For drugs which are moderately emetic, different types of antiemetics should be given in combination. They may have to be given parenterally if vomiting has already started.

36.6.2 Bone-marrow toxicity

Bone-marrow suppression is relatively common with intensive combination chemotherapy. It can affect the production of any or all of the formed elements of the blood, resulting in anaemia, leucopenia (neutropenia and lymphocytopenia), and thrombocytopenia.

Neutropenia and lymphocytopenia are associated with an increased risk of infections, including bacterial infections, viral infections, and candidiasis. Unusual infections can occur, including infection with *Pneumocystis carinii* and cytomegalovirus, especially if there is protracted immunosuppression. Sepsis due to neutropenia can be rapidly fatal, and infections or febrile illnesses should be treated seriously in all patients taking chemotherapy (see p. 410).

Thrombocytopenia can lead to haemorrhagic complications. Anaemia, common as part of the disease, is worsened by impaired red cell production.

It is customary to delay drug administration or reduce the dosages of cytotoxic drugs when there is bone-marrow toxicity (i.e. a white cell count below $3 \times 10^9/L$ and/or a platelet count below $100 \times 10^9/L$), unless there is evidence of bone-marrow infiltration or when a greater risk is acceptable in the case of a readily curable tumour, particularly if good supportive care can be offered.

The adverse effects of high-dose methotrexate on the bone-marrow can be reversed by the use of folinic acid, whose synthesis it blocks. Of course, the cytotoxic action of methotrexate would be nullified by this, so the procedure is to give a high dose of methotrexate over a short period, to wait for a few hours for the methotrexate to affect a reasonable number of cancer cells going through S phase, then to give folinic acid, thus protecting the bone-marrow. A regimen of this kind is described in the Pharmacopoeia (p. 632). Alternatively folinic acid can be used in combination with 5-fluorouracil, because it stabilizes the 5-dUMP/thymidylate synthase complex, thus enhancing the effect of the fluorouracil, for example in colorectal carcinoma.

36.6.3 Gastrointestinal toxicity

Stomatitis and oral ulceration are common. Superinfection with *Candida albicans* may occur, causing oral candidiasis (moniliasis or thrush). Intestinal ulceration and mucosal shedding may be associated with diarrhoea and intestinal infections can occur.

36.6.4 Alopecia

Hair falls out during treatment with many cytotoxic drugs because of effects on the hair follicle. However, it usually regrows when therapy is over. Certain drugs cause marked hair loss (for example the anthracyclines) while others have little effect (for example chlorambucil).

36.6.5 Gonadal effects

In women menstrual irregularities and amenorrhoea are common and occasionally infertility may occur, especially in women over 35 years of age. In men impaired spermatogenesis is common and sterility may occur; banking of sperm may help. These effects are more common with the alkylating agents.

36.6.6 Hyperuricaemia

If a tumour is responsive to chemotherapy cell breakdown may cause the release of large amounts of purines, which will be metabolized to uric acid, excess production of which can lead to gout and renal damage. When tumours are very sensitive allopurinol may be given to prevent the conversion of hypoxanthine and xanthine to uric acid. If possible, allopurinol therapy should be started a day or two in advance of cytotoxic drugs in order to allow the allopurinol to reach its full effect. However, beware of drug interactions. Allopurinol inhibits the metabolism of 6-mercaptopurine and azathioprine and thus enhances their toxicity; it may also enhance the bone-marrow toxicity of cyclophosphamide (see the Pharmacopoeia, p. 551).

36.6.7 Mutagenesis and carcinogenesis

Cytotoxic drugs may cause mutagenic changes in body cells. This is particularly true of alkylating agents and the vinca alkaloids. Because of this mutagenic potential it is recommended that 6 months should elapse after treatment before attempts at conception are made. It is also important to emphasize that staff who are involved in the use of these drugs should protect themselves from direct exposure. Pregnant women should not handle these drugs at all.

Cytotoxic therapy is associated with an increased risk of other malignant tumours. Whether this is because of the induction of mutations or because of immunosuppression is unknown. This risk must be weighed against the efficacy of treatment. There is an increased risk of myelomonocytic leukaemia, with a peak incidence at 5 years. Later there is also an increased incidence of solid tumours, although the risk is relatively low.

These adverse effects may occur with any cytotoxic drug, although they are of variable importance with different drugs. In addition there are some adverse effects which are specific to individual drugs. Some of these are listed in Table 36.3.

One particular adverse effect of cyclophosphamide and ifosfamide is preventable, namely

■ **Table 36.3** Specific adverse effects of individual cytotoxic drugs

Drug	Adverse effect
Bleomycin	Pulmonary fibrosis, skin pigmentation
Busulphan	Pulmonary fibrosis
Cisplatin	Renal toxicity, ototoxicity, peripheral neuropathy
Cyclophosphamide	Haemorrhagic cystitis, inappropriate ADH secretion
Doxorubicin	Cardiac arrhythmias, cardiomyopathy
Fluorouracil	Skin pigmentation, mucositis
Methotrexate	Hepatic damage (chronic treatment), pulmonary fibrosis
Vincristine	Peripheral neuropathy, autonomic neuropathy

haemorrhagic cystitis. This is due to the formation of a toxic metabolite, acrolein, which can be inactivated in the urinary tract by a substance called mesna, which binds acrolein via its sulphydryl group. Mesna is given in a dose equivalent to 20 per cent of the dose of the cytotoxic drug at the time of administration and (because mesna has a faster rate of clearance) again 4 and 8 h later. Sometimes a larger dose may be necessary.

36.6.8 The effects of disease on the disposition of cytotoxic drugs

Many cytotoxic drugs are extensively metabolized in the liver via the cytochrome P450 mixed function oxidase system, and dosages of cytotoxic drugs may therefore have to be reduced in patients with liver disease. This is particularly so for the anthracyclines, such as doxorubicin, and the vinca alkaloids.

Renal clearance is important for other drugs, including carboplatin and methotrexate.

36.6.9 Drug interactions

Specific interactions of cytotoxic drugs with other drugs are described in the relevant entries in the Pharmacopoeia. It should also be noted that there is a theoretical risk of using live vaccines (see p. 248) in patients taking cytotoxic drugs, since their immune responses may be reduced. This may result in an exaggerated local reaction to the vaccine or even severe systemic infection. This has been reported, for example, after smallpox vaccination in patients taking methotrexate.

36.7 The practical use of cytotoxic drugs

The following three examples of chemotherapeutic regimens will give an idea of the practicalities involved. Note that many of the dosages are expressed in mg per square metre of body surface area. This is because animal experiments have shown a closer relationship between dose and effect when dose is corrected for body surface area rather than body weight. As a rough guide the surface area of a 70 kg man is generally taken to be about 1.7 m^2.

36.7.1 Acute lymphoblastic leukaemia in children

(a) Induction therapy (to induce a remission)

Vincristine 1.5 mg/m^2 i.v. weekly for 4–6 weeks.
Prednisolone 40 mg/m^2 orally daily for 4–6 weeks. The response is monitored by peripheral blood count and bone-marrow aspiration.

(b) CNS prophylaxis

Cranial irradiation and/or intrathecal methotrexate are used. There is some concern about the toxicity to the brain of combined cranial irradiation and intrathecal methotrexate, and in some cases intrathecal methotrexate alone is used.

(c) Maintenance therapy (to maintain a remission)

Mercaptopurine 50 mg/m^2 orally once daily.
Methotrexate 20 mg/m^2 orally once weekly.

Depending on the severity of the leukaemia this may be backed up by a single dose of vincristine i.v. once a month and prednisolone orally for 5 days a month. Other cytotoxic drugs may be added to maintenance therapy if required, but on a monthly basis. Maintenance therapy should be continued for 2–3 years. Children who remain in remission for 4 years after completing 2–3 years of treatment have a very good chance of a cure.

36.7.2 Testicular carcinomas

The treatment of testicular carcinomas (seminomas and teratomas) consists of surgical removal of the testis. The disease is staged according to the extent of spread and radiotherapy or chemotherapy may then be used.

(a) Seminoma

For seminoma radiotherapy is often used after surgery, unless there is bulky lymph node disease or metastases, when chemotherapy can be given.

(b) Teratoma

For testicular teratoma chemotherapy is used after surgery if there is evidence of residual disease or if the concentrations of tumour markers remain increased. Chemotherapy is given as follows:

cisplatin 20 mg/m^2 i.v. daily for 5 d every 3 weeks for four courses;
etoposide 120 mg/m^2 i.v. on days 1, 3, and 5 every 3 weeks;
bleomycin 30 mg i.v. on days 2, 9, and 16 of each course of cisplatin.

After four courses of chemotherapy the disease should be restaged; residual tumour should be removed surgically and further chemotherapy given if appropriate.

36.7.3 Hodgkin's lymphoma

In the literature on cancer chemotherapy one is frequently confronted with acronyms for combination cytotoxic drug therapy, each letter standing for either the approved name or a proprietary name of the drug. One such example is the 'MOPP' regimen for Hodgkin's lymphoma:

M = mustine (6 mg/m^2 i.v. on days 1 and 8);
O = vincristine (Oncovin®) (1.5 mg/m^2 i.v. on days 1 and 8);
P = procarbazine (100 mg/m^2 orally daily on days 1–14);
P = prednisolone (40 mg orally daily on days 1–14).

This treatment is repeated every 4 weeks for a minimum of six treatments. Combination therapy in Hodgkin's lymphoma is currently recommended for the more severe forms (some classes of stage III and all classes of stage IV) (see p. 405).

It will be seen from the demands of these regimens on the patients, the occurrence of adverse effects, the need for careful monitoring of haematological and biochemical functions, and the medical care necessary to cope with infection, that cancer chemotherapy must be carried out by teams experienced in it and equipped to do it properly.

36.7.4 Individualizing therapy

We have given some sample recipes for different tumours. However, it is important in cancer chemotherapy, as in other areas of drug therapy, to individualize treatment wherever possible, rather than blindly following a preset regimen. This can be done in several ways.

Firstly, the nature of the tumour will determine the best drugs to use, and whether or not combinations are likely to be helpful. Secondly, by repeated assessments of clinical progress, as mentioned above, it is possible to decide whether or not to continue with aggressive therapy. Thirdly, the continual monitoring of bone-marrow function both before and during therapy will allow one to pursue more vigorous therapy in those who have no marrow toxicity; conversely, impaired marrow function directs one to reduce the intensity of one's regimen. Finally, the careful use of drugs which can modify the adverse effects of chemotherapy, for example effective antiemetics and bone-marrow growth factors (see pp. 411–12), will improve the therapeutic:toxic ratio of chemotherapy.

37 Immunosuppression and the drug therapy of allergies, connective tissue disorders, and primary immunodeficiencies

Co-author: G. P. Spickett

37.1 Immune disease: pathogenesis and mechanisms of action of drugs

Although the precise details of the mechanisms of action of the drugs which are used in the treatment of allergic and immune diseases have not been fully worked out, sufficient is known to fit the drugs into a scheme which depends on an understanding of the four different types of immune reaction. The drugs used are listed in Table 37.1.

37.1.1 Type I reactions: immediate hypersensitivity

Type I allergic reactions are those in which exposure to an antigen in a predisposed individual leads to the production of IgE antibodies which bind to the cell surfaces of mast cells and basophil polymorphonuclear leucocytes. A subsequent exposure of the individual to the antigen leads to an antigen–antibody reaction at the cell surface and the activation of a system which leads to the release of inflammatory mediators from the cell. These mediators include histamine, leukotrienes, 5-hydroxytryptamine, and kinins. These substances together cause vasodilatation, increased capillary permeability, and oedema in the various tissues which they affect.

The clinical manifestations of the effects of these inflammatory mediators depend on the organs affected. Their effects in the skin cause itching and urticaria, in the nasal mucosa and eyes acute allergic rhinitis and conjunctivitis (hay fever), and in the bronchial mucosa extrinsic allergic asthma. In the syndrome called angio-oedema the effects of inflammatory mediators on the skin and airways result in oedematous facial swelling with urticaria and erythema of the face

■ **Table 37.1** Drugs used in the treatment of allergic disorders and in immune suppression

1. *Allergic disorders*
   Antihistamines (p. 559)
   Adrenaline (p. 541)
   Glucocorticoids (p. 584)
   Sodium cromoglycate and nedocromil (p. 590)

2. *Immune suppression*
   Glucocorticoids
   Cytotoxic drugs
     Azathioprine (p. 561)
     Methotrexate (p. 632)
     Cyclophosphamide (p. 590)
   Cyclosporin (p. 591)

3. *Immunotherapy*
   Antilymphocyte globulin
   Antithymocyte globulin
   Monoclonal antibodies (OKT3)
   Intravenous immunoglobulin (p. 616)

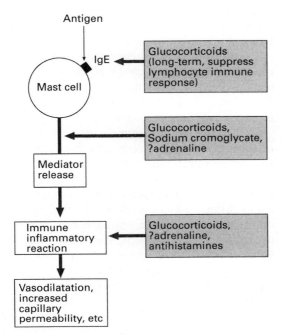

■ **Fig. 37.1** The pathophysiology of immediate hypersensitivity reactions and the sites of action of drugs used in their treatment.

and neck, laryngeal oedema which threatens the airways, and sometimes bronchoconstriction. In the most severe form of allergic reaction, acute anaphylaxis, there is massive release of mediators from cells in many tissues.

The actions of drugs which are used to treat acute immediate hypersensitivity reactions are illustrated in Fig. 37.1. In addition to these drugs, danazol is used to treat the special case of hereditary angio-oedema (discussed separately below).

(a) Histamine (H₁) receptor antagonists

The histamine (H_1) receptor antagonists block the action of histamine at H_1 receptors.

(b) Adrenaline

Adrenaline is used as immediate treatment in life-threatening acute angio-oedema and anaphylactic shock. Exactly how it works is not known, but it is thought to inhibit the mechanisms of release of inflammatory mediators and to decrease capillary permeability. Furthermore, since it is an

adrenoceptor agonist, it relaxes bronchial smooth muscle.

(c) Glucocortiocoids

Glucocorticoids (for example hydrocortisone or prednisolone) have multiple pharmacological effects which interfere with immune reactions. They inhibit the release of inflammatory mediators and suppress the components of the inflammatory reaction, including vasodilatation, increased capillary permeability, and tissue oedema. Glucocorticoids inhibit the release of arachidonic acid from cell membrane phospholipids and so interfere with the synthesis of prostaglandins and leukotrienes.

These effects of glucocorticoids on mediator release and the inflammatory response take some time to come on, even in the high doses which it has become fashionable to use in recent years. So although glucocorticoids should be given as soon as possible in a severe allergic crisis (for example angio-oedema with laryngeal oedema, anaphylactic shock), adrenaline and antihistamines, which have immediate effects, should be used first.

In the longer term glucocorticoids suppress the immune function of lymphocytes and interfere with both humoral- and cell-mediated immune reactions (see below).

37.1.2 Type II reactions: membrane reactive immunity

In Type II reactions an antigen on the surface of a cell combines with antibody, this antigen–antibody complex fixes complement, and damage to the cell membrane results in cell lysis.

Examples of type II reactions are autoimmune thrombocytopenia, autoimmune haemolytic anaemia, and haemolytic anaemia of the newborn (rhesus incompatibility). This type of reaction is also involved in the autoimmune haemolytic anaemia occasionally produced by α-methyldopa. The antibodies in this case are directed against altered components of the rhesus complex. Although a direct Coombs' antibody test may be positive in as many as 5–10 per cent of patients taking methyldopa for longer than a few months, the occurrence of frank haemolysis is rare. The antibody disappears on withdrawal of the drug.

Glucocorticoids and intravenous immuno-globulin have been used to treat type II allergic reactions. Glucocorticoids are used to suppress lymphocyte function and immunoglobulin production in autoimmune haemolytic anaemia. Intravenous immunoglobulin is effective in high doses in treating autoimmune thrombocytopenia and less so in autoimmune haemolytic anaemia. Its mechanism of action is unknown but involves suppression of antibody production and inhibition of the phagocytic function of the reticulo-endothelial system.

37.1.3 Type III reactions: immune complex disease

Immune complex disease is caused by the deposition of antigen–antibody complexes in the capillary beds of tissues, resulting in activation of the complement system and local inflammatory injury. Immune complex damage can produce at least part of the pathological picture of serum sickness, glomerulonephritis, rheumatoid arthritis, and infective endocarditis. Serum sickness may occur as an immune response to drugs such as penicillin, streptomycin, and sulphonamides.

Glucocorticoids suppress the inflammatory response and reduce lymphocyte function and immunoglobulin production in immune complex disease.

37.1.4 Type IV reactions: cell-mediated immune reactions

In type IV reactions the antigen stimulates T lymphocytes to produce lymphokines. Antibody is not involved. Lymphokines cause the tissue changes associated with cell-mediated hypersensitivity in several ways. Some lymphokines affect macrophage function and cause macrophages to accumulate at the site of the reaction; others have chemotactic properties for polymorphonuclear leucocytes, while others promote or suppress lymphocyte antibody production. Interferons are lymphokines which are produced by T cells in response to viral infections and inhibit viral replication.

Type IV reactions are most commonly caused by viral and bacterial agents which have a predominantly intracellular site of action, for example *Mycobacterium tuberculosis*, *Brucella*,

Bordetella pertussis, *Treponema pallidum*, and viruses.

Organ transplant rejection and contact dermatitis are examples of type IV reactions, and cell-mediated hypersensitivity is also of importance in a large number of chronic inflammatory diseases, including sarcoidosis.

Cell-mediated hypersensitivity reactions can be suppressed with glucocorticoids or with more specific immunosuppressive agents, such as the cytotoxic immunosuppressants, or cyclosporin. Furthermore, immunosuppresive therapy using combinations of glucocorticoids with one or other of azathioprine, cyclophosphamide, or occasionally chlorambucil, has been tried in a variety of chronic inflammatory conditions, including systemic lupus erythematosus, necrotizing vasculitis, scleroderma, polymyositis, rheumatoid arthritis, regional enteritis (Crohn's disease), ulcerative colitis, chronic active hepatitis, and glomerulonephritis. However, these are disorders for which specialist care is essential for several reasons: immunosuppression is associated with an increased risk of viral, fungal, and bacterial infections; the drugs have direct toxic effects, such as bone-marrow suppression, hair loss, and infertility; and there is an increased risk of cancers, usually of lymphoid origin, with long-term immunosuppressive therapy.

(a) Glucocorticoids

Glucocorticoids suppress the inflammatory reaction by reducing macrophage chemotaxis and phagocytosis. They also alter lymphocyte function in several ways. They produce a lymphopenia, particularly of T lymphocytes, by a redistribution of cells into lymphoid tissue. They interfere with lymphocyte proliferation, activation, and differentiation, and with many different aspects of lymphocyte function involved in the immune response. They are not very effective in suppressing B cell antibody production, and the beneficial effects of corticosteroids in antibody-mediated and immune-complex-mediated diseases is more likely to be due to their anti-inflammatory actions.

(b) Cytotoxic immunosuppressants

The cytotoxic drugs azathioprine, methotrexate, and cyclophosphamide impair lymphocyte proliferation and function.

(i) Azathioprine

Azathioprine is most active on dividing cells, acting through its metabolite 6-mercaptopurine. It inhibits type IV immune reactions and does not interfere so much with normal humoral antibody production, presumably because it is more active against T cells than B cells. Although bone-marrow suppression is always a risk, one can obtain the beneficial effects of azathioprine on lymphocyte proliferation and function with dosages lower than those which usually produce marrow suppression and lower than the equivalent dosages of 6-mercaptopurine used in cancer chemotherapy.

Azathioprine is generally used as a steroid-sparing agent or when corticosteroids have been relatively ineffective in the treatment of some autoimmune diseases which can be life-threatening, such as systemic lupus erythematosus, particularly with nephritis, and chronic active hepatitis, and in some chronic inflammatory diseases, such as Crohn's disease. It is also used in preventing the rejection of transplanted organs, along with cyclosporin (see below).

(ii) Cyclophosphamide

Cyclophosphamide is active against B lymphocytes and impairs humoral immunity to a greater extent than cell-mediated immunity. It is used in minimal-change glomerulonephritis when the disease cannot be adequately controlled with steroids and it is also beneficial in a number of diseases characterized by necrotizing vasculitis, for example Wegener's granulomatosis and polyarteritis nodosa, and in antibody-mediated diseases.

(iii) Methotrexate

Methotrexate is used in the treatment of severe psoriasis and in rheumatoid arthritis (see p. 419). Its mechanism of action in psoriasis is not known, but may be via inhibition of the proliferation of epithelial cells or via immunosuppression, since it also benefits the arthritis associated with psoriasis.

(c) Cyclosporin

Cyclosporin has specific actions on T lymphocytes. It suppresses both the induction and proliferation of T-effector cells and inhibits the production of lymphokines. It is used in the prevention and treatment of rejection of organ transplants and in graft-versus-host disease. It has a wide range of adverse effects, including nephrotoxicity, abnormalities of liver function, gum hypertrophy, transient hirsutism, and lymphomas (particularly with high dosages). However, it has little effect on the myeloid system of the bone-marrow. Nor does it have the wide cytotoxic actions of azathioprine and cyclophosphamide.

(d) Immunotherapy

(i) Antilymphocyte globulin and antithymocyte globulin

Antilymphocyte globulin and antithymocyte globulin are generally prepared by immunizing rabbits with human lymphocytes or thymocytes, followed by purification of the IgG fraction of the antiserum. They are potent immunosuppressive agents which act by destroying T lymphocytes. Because they are foreign proteins adverse reactions, such as serum sickness, may occur. They are used mainly to treat graft rejection, graft-versus-host disease, and aplastic anaemia.

(ii) Monoclonal antibodies

Mouse monoclonal antibodies to human lymphocyte antigens may be used in place of antilymphocyte globulin or antithymocyte globulin and may cause the same sort of adverse reactions. The antibody OKT3, which is directed against T lymphocytes, is used to treat graft rejection. Genetic engineering has led to the production of human types of antibody from these mouse antibodies and to the production of antibodies which are targeted more specifically at effector cells.

(iii) Intravenous immunoglobulin

Intravenous immunoglobulin, derived from pooled human plasma, has been used as an immunomodulating agent in a wide variety of autoimmune conditions. Its mode of action is unclear, but it reduces auto-antibody production and blocks the phagocytic function of the reticuloendothelial system. In high doses it may have other effects on T and B lymphocyte function.

37.2 The use of glucocorticoids as anti-inflammatory, antiallergic, and immunosuppressive agents

Glucocorticoids are used for their pharmacological actions on the processes of inflammation and the immune response in diverse situations, some examples of which are given in Table 37.2.

Despite the potential hazards of their adverse effects, which should never be underestimated, and in spite of the generally circumspect use of glucocorticoids in medicine, the justified indications for their systemic use, particularly in hospital, are numerous and include the following (see also the Pharmacopoeia):

severe allergic reactions (anaphylactic shock, angio-oedema, severe urticaria);
acute severe asthma (status asthmaticus);
complicated sarcoidosis;
connective tissue disorders (for example systemic lupus erythematosus, polyarteritis nodosa, giant cell arteritis, polymyalgia rheumatica, and rheumatoid arthritis in a very few patients);
minimal-change glomerulonephritis associated with the nephrotic syndrome;
ulcerative colitis;
cerebral oedema;
pemphigus;
acute leukaemias and lymphomas (in combination therapy);
autoimmune haemolytic anaemia;
idiopathic thrombocytopenic purpura;
chronic active hepatitis.

It is therefore well to have some general guidelines for the use of corticosteroids.

1. Make sure of the 'state of the art' for steroid therapy in the disease you want to treat, because new assessments of benefit versus risk occur frequently. For example, for many years corticosteroids were used in the treatment of cerebral malaria until their use was shown to be deleterious.

2. If you do decide to treat with steroids, treat with adequate dosages and if no response occurs withdraw gradually. Nothing is worse than to treat a potentially steroid-responsive condition with an inadequate dosage, since the adverse effects may then occur without the therapeutic benefits. Although an adequate dosage must be used initially, once the disorder seems to be under control cut back to the smallest effective dosage necessary. If the particular condition allows (for example acute severe asthma, giant cell arteritis, or an acute flare-up of rheumatoid arthritis) tail off the treatment gradually. In some acute allergic conditions therapy may be required for only a few days.

3. Certain conditions may be aggravated by glucocorticoids and may constitute contraindications to therapy. These should be borne

■ **Table 37.2** Examples of the uses of glucocorticoids as anti-inflammatory or immunosuppressive drugs

	Anti-inflammatory action	Immunosuppressive action
Pneumonitis after aspiration	+ + +	−
Systemic lupus erythematosus	+ + (joints)	+ +
Acute severe asthma	+ + (allergic response)	−(?)
Autoimmune haemolytic anaemia	−	+ +
Prevention of transplant rejection	+ (acute rejection)	+ +

in mind when contemplating therapy with corticosteroids:

(a) a history of peptic ulcer;
(b) diabetes mellitus;
(c) sodium retention (heart failure, oedema; here there is the additional risk of potassium depletion, particularly in patients also taking diuretics);
(d) osteoporosis;
(e) affective disorders;
(f) children (suppression of growth).

4. Get used to certain formulations. For example, hydrocortisone hemisuccinate suffices for most i.v. uses (except when huge doses are given, for example in the treatment of states of shock, when methylprednisolone is usually used). Prednisolone is generally preferred for oral therapy. Dexamethasone is traditionally used in the treatment of cerebral oedema.

5. The commonly used dosages of corticosteroids are listed in the Pharmacopoeia. It is possible to get some perspective on the dosages of prednisolone commonly used by considering that the usual replacement dose of hydrocortisone for patients with bilateral adrenalectomy is 20–30 mg daily, which is equivalent to a dose of prednisolone of 5–7.5 mg daily. Thus, a daily dose of prednisolone of 40 mg is about eight times the normal glucocorticoid output of the adrenal cortex, and will completely suppress ACTH secretion and cause adrenocortical atrophy. At a dosage of prednisolone of 5 mg daily ACTH secretion might not be completely suppressed, while at dosages of 10 mg daily or more Cushingoid adverse effects are frequent.

6. The adverse effects of glucocorticoids are detailed in the Pharmacopoeia. There are two ways of reducing the risk of adverse effects, by appropriate timing of the doses during the day and by alternate-day therapy.

    Appropriate timing – the inhibitory effects of exogenous corticosteroids on endogenous steroid secretion are much less marked when the steroids are taken in the morning than at night. Thus, the risk of adrenal suppression may be reduced by giving all of the dose in the morning or by splitting it between the morning and early afternoon. Of course this does not apply to corticosteroid replacement therapy, when the dose should be divided and taken two-thirds in the morning and one-third at night to mimic the normal pattern of endogenous steroid secretion.

    Alternate-day therapy – alternate-day glucocorticoid therapy may reduce the unwanted catabolic effects of the corticosteroids and lessen the degree of suppression of the hypothalamic–pituitary–adrenal axis. However, since the anti-inflammatory and immunosuppressive effects continue over 48 h these are not necessarily lost. In some patients it may therefore be possible to reduce a dosage of prednisolone of, for example, 60 mg daily to 80 mg on alternate days, a reduction in total daily dosage of 20 mg. However, in some patients, notably those with asthma and rheumatoid arthritis, alternate day therapy is not suitable, because for some reason the therapeutic effect is also lost.

7. Patients must be informed of the dangers of sudden withdrawal of corticosteroids, of the hazards of intercurrent infection, of the necessity for careful medical care, and of the need to inform all doctors, nurses, and dentists attending them that they are taking steroids. Warning cards are available and should be carried by the patient (see Fig. 37.2).

8. Withdrawal of glucocorticoid therapy is a hazardous, difficult and variable business. Any patient who is taking a glucocorticoid and who cannot take oral therapy (for example when vomiting or during a surgical procedure) must be protected by being given an adequate dose of hydrocortisone or methylprednisolone i.m. or i.v.

Withdrawal of glucocorticoids after long-term administration should be undertaken very slowly, because of suppression of ACTH secretion and consequent adrenocortical atrophy. With dosages of prednisolone of 20–30 mg daily for a few months it can take many months for the pituitary–adrenal axis to regain its normal responsiveness (see Fig. 5.4).

When glucocorticoid therapy is withdrawn the dosage should be reduced gradually over a period of weeks or months at a rate which depends on the dosage and previous duration of therapy. If

INSTRUCTIONS

1 DO NOT STOP taking the steroid drug except on medical advice. Always have a supply in reserve.

2 In case of feverish illness, accident, operation (emergency or otherwise), diarrhoea or vomiting the steroid treatment MUST be continued. Your doctor may wish you to have a LARGER DOSE or an INJECTION at such times.

3 If the tablets cause indigestion consult your doctor AT ONCE.

4 Always carry this card while receiving steroid treatment and show it to *any* doctor, dentist, nurse or midwife or anyone else who is giving you treatment.

5 After your treatment has finished you must still tell any doctor, dentist, nurse or midwife or anyone else who is giving you treatment that you have had steroid treatment.

Printed in the UK for HMSO 9/90 8264406 1154m 15474   STC1

I am a patient on–

STEROID
TREATMENT

which must not be stopped abruptly

and in the case of intercurrent illness may have to be increased

full details are available from the hospital or general → practitioners shown overleaf

■ **Fig. 37.2** An example of the kind of warning card which should be carried by patients taking corticosteroid therapy. (Issued by the Department of Health in the UK, and reproduced with the permission of the Controller of Her Majesty's Stationery Office.)

in doubt do not reduce the daily dosage by more than 1 mg every month.

Both during steroid treatment and for some time after steroid withdrawal it is necessary to be on the lookout for signs of a flare-up of the disease process and for the occurrence of major stresses, such as infection, trauma, or surgery, which will cause the need for extra steroid cover because of the relative unresponsiveness of pituitary–adrenal function. It is possible during withdrawal to monitor pituitary function (by measuring plasma concentrations of ACTH) and adrenal function and responsiveness (by measuring plasma concentrations of cortisol both at baseline and in response to exogenously administered ACTH).

37.3 The drug therapy of allergic and auto-immune disorders

37.3.1 Allergic rhinitis (hay fever and perennial rhinitis)

The clinical problems in hay fever and perennial rhinitis are allergic conjunctivitis (runny itchy eyes), allergic rhinitis (continual sneezing and an itchy and runny nose), and asthma.

Avoidance of the allergen and desensitization with specific allergens are alternatives to drug therapy. Avoidance of the allergen is effective, but not always attainable. Desensitization is usually only moderately effective or not effective at all.

(a) Antihistamines

Symptomatic therapy often begins with an antihistamine (an H_1 receptor antagonist). Partly because they do not alter the effects of histamine which has already been released, antihistamines are usually only partly effective. Their main adverse effect is drowsiness, which can be dangerous when driving or operating machinery. Newer antihistamines, such as astemizole and terfenadine, which penetrate the brain less well than earlier drugs, cause less drowsiness and are to be preferred. Astemizole has a slow onset of action and should only be used for treatment of a long-term problem (for example in perennial rhinitis). Examples of prescribing for hay fever would be astemizole 10 mg orally o.d. or terfenadine 60 mg orally b.d. Individuals vary in their responses to antihistamines, particularly in the severity of drowsiness, and if drowsiness is a problem (even with one of the newer drugs) it is worth trying another antihistamine.

(b) Sodium cromoglycate and nedocromil

Sodium cromoglycate can be given as a nasal spray for allergic rhinitis, as eyedrops for allergic conjunctivitis, or as an insufflation for asthma. Nedocromil can also be given as an insufflation (see the treatment of asthma, p. 308). These formulations should be taken at regular intervals 4–6 times during the day, since their use is mainly prophylactic.

(c) β-adrenoceptor agonists

β-Adrenoceptor agonists, such as salbutamol, can be used in inhalers to treat the asthma of hay fever (see the treatment of asthma, p. 308).

(d) Ipratropium

Ipratropium can be used in an inhaler to treat the asthma of hay fever (see the treatment of asthma, p. 308). It is also available in a nasal spray for treating watery rhinorrhoea in perennial rhinitis. In that case it would be applied to the nostrils up to four times a day.

(e) Glucocorticoids

For allergic rhinitis glucocorticoids are formulated as nasal sprays (beclomethasone and flunisolide), nasal aerosols (beclomethasone and budesonide), and nasal drops (betamethasone). For asthma one would use one of the several aerosols available (see the treatment of asthma, p. 309). For allergic conjunctivitis eye drops are available (betamethasone), but they are not generally recommended because of their adverse effects, which include glaucoma.

Oral and i.m. formulations of corticosteroids are also not generally recommended, for the same reason, but in very severe cases of allergic rhinitis, when sleep is disturbed and the patient's critical duties are being interfered with, a short course of prednisolone may be given (for example 30 mg daily, reducing on every other day by 5 mg a day), having first checked carefully for contra-indications (see p. 520).

(f) Nasal decongestants

The nasal decongestants are sympathomimetic agents which act as vasoconstrictors and reduce congestion and oedema of the nasal mucosa. Formulations for local use contain sympathomimetics such as ephedrine and phenylephrine (indirect sympathomimetics which cause the release of noradrenaline) and oxymetazoline and xylometazoline (direct α-agonists). Systemic decongestants, of which 28 formulations of 17 brands are listed in the current edition of the *British National Formulary*, contain mixtures of paracetamol, antihistamines, and the sympathomimetic decongestants.

Although decongestants are widely used they are not recommended. The local decongestants are not generally effective for more than a few days because of tolerance. If tolerance occurs and the drug is withdrawn rebound vasodilatation will occur. The local decongestants can also cause damage to the nasal mucosa and cilia. Although the systemic decongestants do not cause rebound vasodilatation, they can cause drowsiness (because they contain antihistamines) and tachycardia and hypertension (because they contain sympathomimetics). A hypertensive crisis may particularly be precipitated by these drugs in patients taking an MAO inhibitor (see p. 639).

37.3.2 Urticaria and angio-oedema

Local symptomatic relief in urticaria can be obtained with calamine lotion, which is cooling. For the systemic treatment of an acute attack of mild to moderate urticaria due to exposure to an allergen, an antihistamine, such as terfenadine 60 mg orally b.d., may be sufficient until the reaction has run its course. If the urticaria is severe then a short course of oral corticosteroids may be indicated (see below). If there is associated angio-oedema, particularly if laryngeal oedema develops or if there is bronchoconstriction, this should be treated as a serious medical emergency with adrenaline, an antihistamine, and corticosteroids.

Adrenaline 0.5–1 mL of a 1:1000 solution should be given i.m. This can be life-saving if there is laryngeal obstruction. Also give as soon as possible an antihistamine i.m., for example chlorpheniramine 10–20 mg (some authorities recommend this by slow i.v. injection). Follow this up with oral or i.m. chlorpheniramine 4–8 mg four-hourly until all signs have gone. Also give hydrocortisone 200 mg i.v. and follow this up with prednisolone 30 mg orally daily, gradually tailing this off over the following week.

Occasionally urticaria responds poorly to antihistamines and corticosteroids, in which case the combination of H_1 and H_2 receptor antagonists may be helpful.

37.3.3 Hereditary angio-oedema

Hereditary angio-oedema is caused by deficiency of the C_1 esterase inhibitor of the complement cascade. Attacks may be prevented if patients avoid the stimuli which they have identified as precipitating factors, including drugs. In an acute attack purified C_1 esterase inhibitor is the treatment of choice. If it is not available give fresh frozen plasma. Adrenaline, antihistamines, and corticosteroids are relatively ineffective in this condition.

Anabolic steroids have been used to prevent attacks. They may increase C_1 esterase inhibitor concentrations, but even if they do not they may suppress attacks. Danazol, which has less androgenic effects than other anabolic steroids can be used in a dosage of 100–400 mg daily orally; stanozolol may be used as an alternative. The anabolic steroids cause increased weight and in women some androgenic changes, and the benefits must be weighed against these adverse effects.

Antifibrinolytic drugs, such as ε-aminocaproic acid and tranexamic acid, have also been used to try to suppress attacks, on the basis that their action in inhibiting proteolysis might spare the C_1 esterase inhibitor. However, they are not first-line drugs, because of adverse effects such as vascular thrombosis.

Idiopathic angio-oedema not associated with C_1 esterase inhibitor deficiency may respond dramatically to antifibrinolytic drugs, such as tranexamic acid, which act here by interfering with the production of kinins.

37.3.4 Anaphylactic shock

Anaphylactic shock occurs so swiftly and with such severity that controlled clinical studies of treatment have never been possible (nor would

be ethical). What follows are the usual treatment procedures used.

Prevention is, of course, most important. A history of previous allergic reactions to drugs, vaccines, serum, or blood transfusion must be sought from anyone about to undergo treatment with the slightest hazard of this kind (see p. 110). Patients who are predisposed to allergic reactions should wear an alerting bracelet or necklace (for example Medic-Alert®).

If an injection causes an anaphylactic reaction place a tourniquet proximal to the injection site to minimize further absorption. In another limb give adrenaline (0.5–1 mL of a 1/:1000 solution i.m.), first withdrawing the plunger to ensure that the needle is not in a vein. If there is laryngeal and/or epiglottal oedema, intubation or emergency tracheotomy may be required to establish an airway. Bronchospasm may be relieved by the adrenaline, but inhaled or i.v. salbutamol and/or i.v. aminophylline will generally be needed (see the treatment of asthma p. 310). Oxygen may also be necessary.

The hypotension of anaphylactic shock is presumably due to vasodilatation and increased capillary permeability. Adrenaline will help, but rapidly infused fluids (for example sodium chloride 0.9 per cent, i.e. 'normal saline') should be given to correct relative hypovolaemia. If hypotension persists, despite adrenaline and i.v. fluids, give corticosteroids and an antihistamine as described above under angio-oedema. This is one condition in which α-adrenceptor agonists might be of help, for example metaraminol 2–10 mg i.m. or noradrenaline by i.v. infusion of 8–12 micrograms/min. If these drugs are used monitor for arrhythmias and treat appropriately.

37.3.5 The treatment of connective tissue disorders

(a) Systemic lupus erythematosus

The cutaneous and joint manifestations of systemic lupus erythematosus are frequently helped by antimalarial drugs, such as chloroquine (150 mg daily) or hydroxychloroquine (200–400 mg daily in divided doses). If treatment is required for other manifestations, systemic corticosteroids (for example prednisolone

10–60 mg daily) should be used first. The dosage should be the minimum required to control symptoms.

Cyclophosphamide and azathioprine are used when the response to steroids is poor and as steroid-sparing agents. Intravenous methyl-prednisolone and cyclophosphamide may be used in severe disease, especially if there is renal involvement. Photosensitivity requires the use of a sun-blocking cream. Treatment of the so-called lupus anticoagulant (cardiolipin) syndrome is by long-term anticoagulation with warfarin.

(b) Systemic sclerosis

Immunosuppressive treatment is not effective in preventing the progression of systemic sclerosis, but corticosteroids may relieve associated joint symptoms. Penicillamine and colchicine have also been used, with variable results, but their adverse effects are often severe. Treatment is therefore best directed at providing symptomatic relief. Raynaud's phenomenon may be severe and digital gangrene may occur.

Peripheral vasodilators, such as the calcium antagonists (for example nifedipine), may help, although large dosages may be required. Altern-atively, some patients get relief from rubbing glyceryl trinitrate ointment into their fingers. In severe cases an infusion of prostacyclin may give prolonged relief, even though the half-time of circulating prostacyclin is very short.

Oesophageal reflux is common in systemic sclerosis, and standard treatment is used (see p. 325). Bacterial overgrowth in the small bowel may worsen malabsorption and may be treated by long-term oxytetracycline.

(c) Polymyalgia rheumatica

In polymyalgia rheumatica prednisolone 10–15 mg daily for 1–3 months is usually enough to induce a remission, after which the dosage is very gradually reduced over the next 2 years and then stopped, as described in the section on corticosteroid use above. Flare-ups are common when the dosage is reduced, and it is then neces-sary to return to a higher dosage and to begin dosage reduction again.

(d) Polymyositis and dermatomyositis

Initial therapy should be with high dosages of corticosteroids (for example prednisolone 60–80 mg daily), followed by a gradual reduction to a maintenance dosage according to the clinical response and biochemical evidence of muscle damage. If there is a poor response to steroids alone, azathioprine or cyclophosphamide should be used. Methotrexate may also be helpful in resistant cases.

(e) Giant cell arteritis and Wegener's granulomatosis

These conditions should be treated with high-dose corticosteroids (for example prednisolone 60–80 mg daily), together with azathioprine or cyclophosphamide. Corticosteroids alone are less effective in inducing and maintaining a remission. In severe cases steroids may be given intraven-ously to start with. Once a remission is induced the dosage of corticosteroid may be reduced. Therapy needs to be continued for 2–3 years and adverse effects are common.

(f) Kawasaki syndrome

Kawasaki syndrome is a vasculitis which involves the coronary arteries in children. It is treated with high-dose aspirin (up to 100 mg/kg/d for 14 days, depending on toxicity) together with intra-venous immunoglobulin (400 mg/kg/d for 5 days or 2 g/kg as a single dose). This reduces the occurrence of coronary artery aneurysms, but only if it is given early in the disease. Corticosteroids worsen the coronary artery damage and should not be used.

37.4 The management of primary immunodeficiencies

37.4.1 Humoral immune deficiency

Antibody deficiency syndromes require the replacement of the missing antibodies. In the past intramuscular immunoglobulin (25 mg/kg/week) was used, but it is painful and does not prevent infections adequately. Intravenous immunoglob-ulin allows much larger doses to be given less often and is the treatment of choice. The dosage should be tailored to the patient's requirements, but is usually within the range of 200–600 mg/kg every 2–4 weeks. The numerous products which are available are not therapeutically equivalent (see the Pharmacopoeia).

When infections occur antibiotic treatment should be continued for at least 14 days and higher dosages than usual may be required. Infections may be with unusual organisms, such as *Ureaplasma*. Enteric infections may be particularly prolonged, especially giardiasis, and repeated courses of metronidazole or tinidazole may be required.

37.4.2 Cellular immune deficiency

The treatment of choice in cases of cellular immune deficiency is usually bone-marrow transplantation. Opportunistic infections are common (see p. 410). Intravenous immunoglobulin may be required, as in humoral immune deficiency (see above). Patients with chronic granulomatous disease may benefit from regular γ-interferon.

Specialist advice is essential in the management of all primary immunodeficiencies.

37.5 Immunosuppression in tissue and organ transplantation

Immunosuppressive therapy in the prevention of graft rejection and in the the treatment of graft-versus-host disease in bone-marrow, heart/lung, kidney, and liver transplantation is a complex, often changing, and specialist procedure, and different authorities use different methods.

The drugs used in these procedures are cyclosporin, azathioprine, corticosteroids, antilymphocyte globulin, and OKT3 antibody. The details of their use in transplantation must be sought in the specialist literature. Here we shall simply illustrate the principles of their use in relation to kidney transplantation.

Immunosuppression after kidney transplantation begins with a large dose of methylprednisolone (500 mg i.v.) at the time of operation. If renal function is good after the operation, prednisolone, azathioprine, and cyclosporin are given. Cyclosporin is omitted at this stage if renal function is poor, because it is nephrotoxic, and it can be added later when renal function recovers. The use of cyclosporin reduces the dosage requirements of prednisolone and azathioprine (for example from 1.5 mg/kg/d of prednisolone to 1.0 mg/kg/d and from 2 mg/kg/d of azathioprine to 1 mg/kg/d). However, the maintenance dosages of these drugs should be adjusted according to the white cell count and in the case of cyclosporin the whole blood concentration (see p. 93).

Acute transplant rejection can be treated with high doses of methylprednisolone (for example 1 g i.v. daily for 3 days), but in severe cases antilymphocyte globulin or OKT3 antibody may be required. Chronic rejection is more difficult to treat, and interim dialysis and another transplant may be necessary.

In addition to the expected adverse effects of these drugs when used alone, there is also an increased incidence in these patients of lymphomas and skin cancers.

Section IV

Pharmacopoeia

Introduction

In this Pharmacopoeia we have listed those drugs which are most commonly used in clinical practice (a total of about 300 compounds). Each drug is dealt with either on its own (for example allopurinol) or in conjunction with other drugs with which it forms a distinct group (for example the aminoglycoside antibiotics). Each section contains the following information.

1. Structure

This is given in full in the case of a single drug. In the case of a group the general structure is given and the individual differences are listed below or indicated.

2. Mode of action

By this we mean the mechanisms of the effects a drug produces at a relevant level of discrimination, for example physiological, cellular, or molecular (see Chapter 4).

3. Uses

The uses of individual drugs are given. In the case of a group of drugs, individual members of which have different indications, those drugs which are usually prescribed for a particular indication are listed as such (for example see acetylcholinesterase inhibitors).

4. Dosages

The dosages given are those most commonly used. However, one should remember that it may be necessary to go outside the usual range on occasion (see p. 202). For some drugs with complicated dosage regimens larger texts should be consulted. We have generally not taken account of the special formulations (for example enteric-coated or slow-release tablets) and manufacturers' literature (i.e. Data Sheets or package inserts) should be consulted. All dosages relate to adults unless specifically stated. Information on paediatric dosages should be sought elsewhere.

5. Kinetic data

Absorption after oral administration has been designated as 'well absorbed' (usually >70 per cent) or 'poorly absorbed' (usually <50 per cent). In some cases we have given percentage values. Values of $t_{1/2}$ quoted are means culled from published literature and there may be wide individual variations from these means. Extent of metabolism or urinary excretion has generally been approximately graded using terms such as 'mostly metabolized' or 'mainly excreted unchanged'. We have indicated the major route of elimination of pharmacologically active compounds and in some cases given more specific information. Information on the apparent volume of distribution and protein binding of some important drugs is given in Tables 3.2 and 3.3.

6. Important adverse effects

Where we have not given percentage incidence figures we have used terms such as the following: 'common' (usually >5 per cent); 'occasional' (1–5 per cent); 'unusual' or 'rare' (<1 per cent).

Where relevant we have also discussed the interactions of drugs with diseases, since such interactions may lead one to prescribe cautiously in particular circumstances. Occasionally such considerations will dictate a contra-indication.

7. Interactions

Of the numerous reported drug interactions (see Chapter 10) we have tried to list only those of clinical relevance.

Abbreviations

i.v., intravenously;
i.m., intramuscularly;
s.c., subcutaneously;
o.d., once daily;
b.d., twice daily;
t.d.s., three times daily;
q.d.s., four times daily.

Index to drugs listed in the Pharmacopoeia

Acetazolamide

Structure

$$CH_3CONH \underset{N \text{——} N}{\overset{S}{\diagdown}} SO_2NH_2$$

Mode of action

Acetazolamide is an inhibitor of carbonic anhydrase. Inhibition of carbonic anhydrase in the kidney leads to an 80–90 per cent reduction in bicarbonate absorption by the proximal tubule, resulting in a large increase in urine pH and an increase in the excretion of sodium, potassium, and phosphate. In the eye it leads to reduction in the formation of aqueous humour.

Uses

Acetazolamide is a weak diuretic and is never used as such. It inhibits the formation of aqueous fluid in the eye and is used in the treatment of some types of glaucoma. It is also used as a prophylactic agent against mountain sickness.

Dosages

0.25–1 g daily in divided doses orally.

Kinetic data

Rapidly absorbed from the gastrointestinal tract. Plasma $t_{1/2}$ 8 h. Excreted unchanged in the urine.

Important adverse effects

Severe hypokalaemia can occur during the first few weeks of treatment because of a high kaliuresis, but the acidosis which occurs secondary to reduced bicarbonate reabsorption compensates for this and plasma potassium concentrations return to normal. Other adverse effects include paraesthesiae, particularly of the lips, drowsiness, dizziness, headache, flushing, fatigue, and gastrointestinal upsets. Avoid acetazolamide in severe renal impairment and do not use it for chronic congestive closed-angle glaucoma.

Interactions

Aspirin reduces the excretion of acetazolamide. Excretion of the antiarrhythmic drugs flecainide, mexiletine, and quinidine is reduced in an alkaline urine; lithium excretion is increased. Hypokalaemia due to acetazolamide may potentiate the effects of digitalis and alter the actions of antiarrhythmic drugs.

Acetylcholinergic agonists (cholinoceptor agonists)

Structures
General

$$R \text{——} CH \text{——} CH_2N^+(CH_3)_3$$
$$O \text{——} CO \text{——} NH_2$$

Bethanecol: $R = CH_3$; carbachol: $R = H$. Pilocarpine is also a cholinoceptor agonist.

Mode of action

These drugs have direct agonist effects on acetylcholine receptors leading to:
(1) stimulation of the smooth muscle of bowel and bladder and relaxation of their sphincters;

(2) pupillary constriction.

The effects of bethanecol and pilocarpine are chiefly muscarinic. Carbachol has some nicotinic activity in addition.

Uses

Relief of postoperative urinary retention or bowel distension (bethanecol and carbachol).
Treatment of open-angle and closed-angle glaucoma (pilocarpine).
Reversal of pupillary dilatation (pilocarpine).

Dosages

Bethanecol, 5 mg s.c.
Carbachol, 250–500 micrograms s.c.

Pilocarpine, two drops of an 0.5–4 per cent solution to the eyes (t.d.s. for glaucoma, once only for reversal of mydriasis).

Kinetic data

Little is known about the kinetics of bethanecol and carbachol, but neither is metabolized by cholinesterases.

Pilocarpine rapidly enters the aqueous humour after topical application to the eye and cannot be detected 2 h later.

Important adverse effects

Commonly abdominal colic, urinary urgency or bladder pain, pupillary constriction, bradycardia, bronchial constriction, flushing, and sweating. These effects are readily reversed by atropine. Do not give these drugs to patients with asthma (risk of bronchoconstriction), hyperthyroidism (may precipitate atrial fibrillation), ischaemic heart disease (may precipitate angina/infarction), or peptic ulcer (increased gastric acid secretion). Do not

use the i.v. or i.m. routes. Remember that urinary retention in old men is usually due to prostatic obstruction, which will not be relieved by stimulating the bladder.

Pilocarpine may cause blurred vision, myopia, and painful ciliary spasm. Other effects include a stinging sensation, lachrymation, headache, photophobia, and local hypersensitivity reactions. It should not be used in glaucoma due to inflammation.

Interactions

Bethanecol and carbachol should not be given in conjunction with other cholinergic drugs or anticholinesterases, because of the risk of potentiation of effects.

Pilocarpine *inhibits* the miotic action of the anticholinesterases, since it prevents the action of acetylcholine whose concentration they increase; this combination should not be used. Pilocarpine also reverses the mydriatic action of the anticholinergic drugs and can be used to reverse their effects after local application.

Acetylcholinergic antagonists (cholinoceptor antagonists)

Structures

Atropine and hyoscine (scopolamine) are stereoisomers. Atropine is shown here:

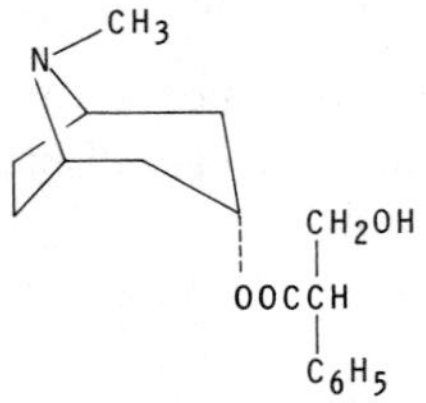

The other drugs discussed here have widely different structures. We give benzhexol hydrochloride as an example:

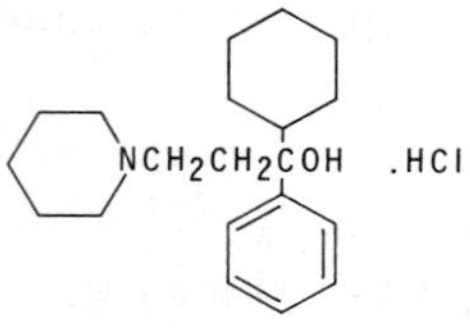

Mode of action

Direct antagonist effect on muscarinic cholinergic receptors leading to:

(1) relaxation of the smooth muscle of bowel and bladder and stimulation of their sphincters;

(2) pupillary dilatation;

(3) decrease in secretions from sweat, bronchial, and other glands;

(4) increased heart rate;

(5) bronchiolar dilatation.

Uses

To decrease glandular secretions preoperatively (atropine, hyoscine).

To dilate pupils (cyclopentolate, tropicamide).

To speed the heart rate in sinus bradycardia (atropine).

To relieve bronchoconstriction in asthma (ipratropium).

To prevent bowel spasm during radiological procedures (hyoscine butyl bromide).

To treat some forms of Parkinson's disease.

To reverse drug-induced Parkinsonism and dystonias (for example procyclidine, benzhexol, benztropine, orphenadrine).

To prevent travel sickness (hyoscine hydrobromide).

Dosages

Atropine: sinus bradycardia, 500 micrograms, i.v.; preoperatively, 600 micrograms i.m.

Hyoscine hydrobromide: travel sickness, 300 micrograms orally 30 min before travel and then six hourly for up to 48 h (maximum 900 micrograms in a day), or one 500 microgram transdermal patch applied a few hours before travel and left in place for up to 72 h; preoperatively, 600 micrograms s.c.

Hyoscine butylbromide: prevention of bowel spasm, 20 mg, i.v. or i.m.

Cyclopentolate: to the eyes, two drops of a 0.5 per cent solution.

Tropicamide: to the eyes, two drops of an 0.1 per cent solution.

Ipratropium: inhalation, one or two puffs (each 20 micrograms) t.d.s.

Procyclidine: orally, 2.5 mg t.d.s. initially, increasing if necessary to 30 mg daily; i.v., 5–10 mg.

Benzhexol: orally, 1 mg o.d. initially, increasing in 2 mg increments every 3–5 d as required up to 15 mg daily; i.v., 2 mg.

Benztropine: orally, 0.5 mg o.d. initially, increasing in 0.5 mg increments every 5–6 d as required to 6 mg daily; i.v., 2 mg.

Kinetic data

Atropine is well absorbed but metabolized during its first passage through the liver. Only about 50 per cent appears unchanged in the urine and parenteral routes are therefore more reliable. $t_{1/2} = 24$ h.

Hyoscine hydrobromide is well absorbed and almost completely metabolized. Its effects last about 2 h.

In the eye the effects of cyclopentolate last up to 24 h, of tropicamide up to 8 h.

Important adverse effects

Unwanted effects are almost unavoidable, especially drying of the mouth, blurred vision, and constipation. In patients with prostatic hypertrophy acute urinary retention may occur. Glaucoma may be precipitated in susceptible individuals. Common central nervous effects include confusion, restlessness, and hallucinations, but hyoscine hydrobromide causes sedation. Tachycardia occurs with all but hyoscine, which may cause bradycardia.

These effects may be reversed with an acetylcholinesterase inhibitor, such as physostigmine.

Tolerance to the action of hyoscine may occur after a single transdermal dose.

Interactions

The anticholinergic effects of other drugs (for example tricyclic antidepressants, disopyramide) may be potentiated.

Acetylcholinesterase inhibitors

Structures

These drugs are quaternary ammonium compounds. Neostigmine is given as an example:

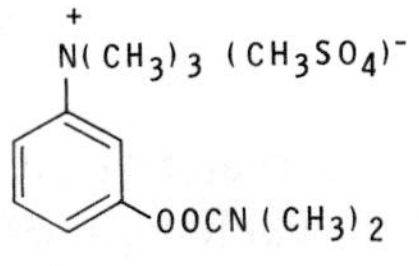

Mode of action

Inhibition of acetylcholinesterase, leading to accumulation of endogenous acetylcholine in cholinergic synapses. This results in:

(1) stimulation of the smooth muscle of bowel and bladder and relaxation of their sphincters;

(2) pupillary constriction;

(3) increased secretion from sweat, salivary, bronchial, and other glands;

(4) depolarization of the motor end-plates of skeletal muscle.

Uses

Myasthenia gravis: diagnosis (edrophonium) and treatment (neostigmine, pyridostigmine).
Reversal of curariform effects (neostigmine).
Glaucoma (physostigmine).
Reversal of pupillary dilatation (physostigmine).
Tricyclic antidepressant overdose (physostigmine, but not usually recommended, see p. 496).

Dosages

Neostigmine: myasthenia gravis. 75–300 mg daily, orally, in divided doses, taken when most needed; reversal of curariform effect of skeletal muscle relaxants 1–2.5 mg.

Physostigmine: glaucoma, 2 drops of an 0.25–0.5 per cent solution once or twice a day to the eyes.

Edrophonium: myasthenia gravis (specific uses, see pp. 440–1), 2 mg, i.v., initially followed by 8 mg if no adverse reaction occurs.

Kinetic data

Absorption after oral administration is generally poor. The half-times and durations of action of these drugs are mostly short. The very short duration of action of edrophonium makes it a useful drug for the diagnosis of myasthenia gravis and the differential diagnosis of myasthenic crisis from overdose of other cholinesterase inhibitors (see p. 439). Physostigmine crosses the blood–brain barrier.

Important adverse effects

Symptoms of excessive cholinergic effects are common, for example abdominal cramps, hypersalivation, sweating, bradycardia (all muscarinic effects) and muscle cramps (nicotinic). The muscarinic effects are reversible by atropine.

Acetylcholinesterase inhibitors should be given cautiously to patients with cardiac disease, for example bradycardia, hypotension, myocardial ischaemia.

Actinomycin D

Structure

Mode of action

Actinomycin D (or dactinomycin) is a cytotoxic antibiotic. It inhibits DNA-dependent RNA synthesis, especially ribosomal RNA, by intercalating between DNA base pairs. It is not specific for any phase of the cell cycle.

Uses

Wilms' tumour of the kidney.
Choriocarcinoma.
A variety of sarcomas.

Dosage

Actinomycin D is given i.v. and usually in combination with other cytotoxic drugs. Dosages vary widely, but a typical dosage regimen (for example in choriocarcinoma) would be 15 micrograms/kg i.v. daily for 5 d over 2–3 weeks.

Kinetic data

Poorly absorbed and therefore given i.v. Excreted mostly in the bile as **unchanged drug and dosages** should therefore be reduced in liver disease. $t_{1/2} = 36$ h.

Important adverse effects

Anorexia, nausea, vomiting, diarrhoea, and stomatitis are common. Bone-marrow suppression is dose-related (see cancer chemotherapy, Chapter 33). Alopecia and skin rashes may occur.

Interaction

For the possible interaction with live vaccines see p. 251.

Adrenoceptor agonists (except dopamine)

Structures

Examples

	R_1	R_2
Adrenaline (epinephrine)	OH	C(OH)HCH₂NHCH₃
Noradenaline (norepinephrine)	OH	C(OH)HCH₂NH₂
Isoprenaline	OH	C(OH)HCH₂NHCH(CH₃)₂
Salbutamol (albuterol)	CH₂OH	C(OH)HCH₂NHC(CH₃)₃
Salmeterol	CH₂	CH(OH)CH₂NH(CH₂)₆ O(CH₂)₄Ph
Dobutamine	OH	(CH₂)₂NHC(CH₃)H(CH₂)₂ C₆H₄OH

Mode of action

Direct agonist effects on α- and β-adrenoceptors with the following relative specificities:

	α	β_1	β_2
Adrenaline	+ +	+ +	+ +
Noradrenaline	+ +	+	+
Isoprenaline	+	+ +	+ +
Salbutamol	0	±	±
Salmeterol	0	±	±
Dobutamine	0	+ +	±

α-adrenoceptor stimulation leads to arteriolar vasoconstriction and pupillary constriction.

β-adrenoceptor stimulation leads to arteriolar vasodilatation (mainly in muscle, i.e. β_2), bronchodilatation (β_2), uterine relaxation (β_2), and cardiac effects (increase in heart rate and contractility, β_1).

The mode of action of adrenaline in glaucoma is not understood.

Uses

To relieve bronchoconstriction in asthma (salbutamol and salmeterol).

To treat allergic reactions, especially anaphylactic shock (adrenaline).

To produce local vasoconstriction and enhance the effects of local anaesthetics (adrenaline).

To prevent and treat premature labour (salbutamol, ritodrine, isoxsuprine).

To treat open angle glaucoma (adrenaline).

To treat myocardial pump failure, for example cardiogenic shock, after cardiopulmonary bypass (dobutamine).

Dosages

Adrenaline: acute allergic reactions, 0.5 ml of a 1:1000 solution i.m.; glaucoma, one drop of a 1 per cent solution o.d. or b.d.

Salbutamol: asthma, orally, 2–4 mg t.d.s.; i.v., 5 micrograms/min, increasing as required up to 20 micrograms/min; inhalation, one puff (100 micrograms) once or twice daily as required, up to q.d.s.; premature labour, 10 micrograms/min i.v., increasing as required up to 45 micrograms/ min.

Salmeterol: asthma, 25–50 micrograms, aerosol inhalation, one to two puffs b.d. (duration of action about 12 h).

Dobutamine: 2.5–10 micrograms/kg/min by continuous i.v. infusion depending on response. Doses should be reduced gradually on withdrawal.

Important adverse effects

Adverse effects are dose-related. They include anxiety, restlessness, tremor, tachycardia, nausea, hypertension, cardiac arrhythmias, and angina.

Adverse effects after aerosol administration are uncommon. However, recently it has been suggested that the β_2-adrenoceptor agonists given by inhalation may increase the death rate from acute severe asthma. The mechanism of this has not been elucidated and it has been especially associated with fenoterol, which is now not recommended.

Kinetic data

	Absorption	Elimination	$T_{1/2}$
Adrenaline	Nil	Metabolized	Minutes
Salbutamol	Good	40% metabolized	4 h
Dobutamine	Nil	Metabolized	Minutes

The long duration of action of salmeterol is attributed to its lipophilic tail (see structure above), which causes it to bind with high affinity to a region of the cell membrane immediately adjacent to the β_2-adrenoceptor, called the exo-receptor.

Adrenoceptor antagonists: non-selective α-blockers

Structures

Phentolamine

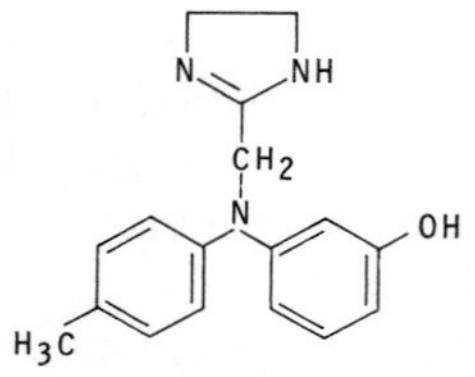

Phenoxybenzamine

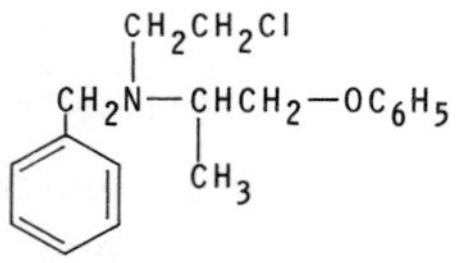

Prazosin, doxazosin, and indoramin, which block α_1-adrenoceptors selectively, are dealt with in a separate monograph.

Mode of action

Direct effect on adrenoceptors, preventing the pharmacological action of released noradrenaline on α_1 (postsynaptic) and/or α_2 (mostly presynaptic) adrenoceptors. The drugs dealt with in this section are not selective for α_1 and α_2 adrenoceptors (cf. prazosin, doxazosin, and indoramin).

Uses

Treatment of hypertension due to:

phaeochromocytoma;
overdose of α-adrenoceptor agonists;
clonidine withdrawal;
amine–MAO inhibitor interactions;
vasospastic states (for example ergotism).

For these conditions i.v. phentolamine would normally be used. In the chronic treatment of phaeochromocytoma oral phenoxybenzamine is used. The value of these drugs in peripheral vascular disease is minimal.

Dosages

Phenoxybenzamine: orally, 10 mg o.d., increasing as required in 10 mg increments at 4-d intervals to a maximum of 60 mg t.d.s.
Phentolamine: i.v., 5–15 mg.

Kinetic data

Little is known about the pathways of elimination of these drugs, but they are probably metabolized in the liver.

Important adverse effects

Common are vasodilatation leading to sinus tachycardia, other arrhythmias, angina pectoris, and orthostatic hypotension. Nasal congestion and failure to ejaculate are common during long-term treatment.

Adrenoceptor antagonists: α_1-blockers

Structures
Prazosin

Doxazosin

Indoramin

Mode of action

These drugs are antagonists at α_1 (postsynaptic) adrenoceptors. They cause peripheral arteriolar vasodilatation, which leads to a fall in blood pressure in hypertension and a decrease in afterload in cardiac failure.

In cardiac failure the blood pressure tends not to fall, because of a concomitant rise in cardiac output; nevertheless, in cardiac failure care should be taken to avoid hypotension. The hypotension is not accompanied by a significant tachycardia, because α_2 (presynaptic) adrenoceptors are not affected, and noradrenaline in the synapse acts upon these receptors to inhibit further noradrenaline release. This contrasts with phenoxybenzamine and phentolamine, which act at both α_1 and α_2 adrenoceptors.

Uses

Hypertension.
Cardiac failure.

Dosages
Prazosin

Since profound hypotension often occurs after the first dose of prazosin, in both hypertension and cardiac failure, the first dose should be small (0.5 mg orally) and should be taken with an evening meal or in bed. Thereafter the initial dosage should be 0.5 mg t.d.s. orally, increasing at intervals of a few days if required to a maximum of 5 mg q.d.s.

Doxazosin

Take the same precautions for the first dose as for prazosin. Initially 1 mg orally daily, increasing after 2–4 weeks to 2 mg daily and later to 4 mg daily if required.

Indoramin

25 mg orally b.d. initially, increasing at 2-weekly intervals by daily dosages of 25–50 mg to a maximum of 100 mg b.d.

Kinetic data

Prazosin and doxazosin are well absorbed and mostly metabolized in the liver. The $t_{1/2}$ of prazosin is 4 h and that of doxazosin 11 h, but the therapeutic effects last for up to about 12 h and 24 h respectively. Dosages should be reduced in renal failure, not because there is accumulation, but because of increased sensitivity.

Indoramin is well absorbed, but almost completely metabolized on its first passage through the liver. The $t_{1/2}$ is 5 h. It is not clear how active the metabolites are by comparison with indoramin itself.

Important adverse effects
Prazosin and doxazosin

Dizziness and loss of consciousness may occur after the first dose, because of profound hypotension (see above). This effect is especially marked in patients taking diuretics or α-adrenoceptor antagonists. Other common effects include dry mouth, headache, postural dizziness, and tachycardia.

Indoramin

The most common adverse effect of indoramin is sedation, which is dose-related. Postural hypotension occurs occasionally, particularly at high dosages. Other occasional adverse effects include failure of ejaculation, depression, dizziness, dry mouth, and nasal congestion.

Interactions

The therapeutic effects of these drugs are enhanced by other antihypertensive drugs, such as diuretics and β-adrenoceptor antagonists.

Indoramin should not be used in combination with MAO inhibitors.

Adrenoceptor antagonists: β-blockers

Structures
Propranolol

OH
OCH$_2$CHCH$_2$NHCH(CH$_3$)$_2$

Others – general

OH
OCH$_2$CHCH$_2$NHCH(CH$_3$)$_2$
R$_1$
R$_2$

Examples

	R$_1$	R$_2$
Oxprenolol	OCH$_2$CH=CH$_2$	H
Atenolol	H	CH$_2$OCNH$_2$
Metoprolol	H	CH$_2$CH$_2$OCH$_3$
Practolol	H	NHOCCH$_3$
Bisoprolol	H	CH$_2$OCH$_2$CH$_2$OCH(CH$_3$)$_2$

Uses

In certain aspects of ischaemic heart disease:
(1) prophylaxis of angina pectoris;
(2) in acute myocardial infarction to limit extension of the infarct;
(3) following myocardial infarction to prevent recurrence ('secondary prevention').

Treatment of hypertension.
Treatment and prevention of supraventricular tachyarrhythmias.
Symptomatic relief in thyrotoxicosis.

Dosages

Oral:
Propranolol, 20–160 mg b.d.
Oxprenolol, 120–480 mg daily in two or three divided doses.
Atenolol, 100–200 mg o.d.
Metoprolol, 100–400 mg daily in two or three divided doses.
Bisoprolol, 5–20 mg daily.

Intravenous:
Practolol, 5–20 mg.

Mode of action

These drugs are competitive antagonists of adrenaline and noradrenaline at β-adrenoceptors, which are of two types (β_1 and β_2). Blockade of cardiac β_1 receptors slows the heart rate and reduces myocardial contractility (a negative inotropic effect). Clinically the degree of β-blockade can be assessed by the reduced response of the heart rate to exercise.

In angina pectoris these effects result in decreased cardiac work and decreased oxygen requirements, with less likelihood of the metabolic consequences of ischaemia. During exercise the prevention of tachycardia contributes to these effects.

In hypertension the mechanism of the hypotensive effect of β-blockers is difficult to explain. Most would agree that an effect of β-blockade on the heart is the first in a chain of events, that this leads to a variety of adaptive responses, for example changes in the sensitivity of baroreflex mechanisms, both central and peripheral, and perhaps to long-term changes in cardiac function, all of which compound to lower the blood pressure continuously. A decrease in renin secretion has also been invoked as playing a role.

The mechanism of the effect in supraventricular tachyarrhythmias is by a direct action on the heart.

In thyrotoxicosis, while β-blockade causes a clinically obvious reduction in sympathomimetic symptoms, it is not clear that the effect is by antagonism of sympathetic nervous system activity, since true increases in such activity in thyrotoxicosis have been difficult to demonstrate.

Blockade of β_2 receptors is mainly of importance in relation to adverse effects (see below). The different β-blockers have different effects on β_1 and β_2 receptors, some being relatively selective for β_1 receptors, others being non-selective. The order of selectivity of the relatively selective drugs listed above is bisoprolol > practolol > atenolol > metoprolol. In addition, some have partial agonist activity and penetration into the brain is variable. The differences are shown in the following table.

Drug	Receptor specificity	Partial agonist	Brain penetration
Propranolol	β_1 β_2	–	+
Oxprenolol	β_1 β_2	+	+
Atenolol	β_1	–	–
Metoprolol	β_1	–	+
Practolol	β_1	+	–
Bisoprolol	β_1	–	+

Kinetic data

Most β-blockers are well absorbed (atenolol is an exception at about 50 per cent). Propranolol and metoprolol are extensively metabolized during their first passage through the liver to active (hydroxylated) compounds, which are excreted in the urine. Bisoprolol is 50 per cent metabolized but without first-pass elimination. The other drugs are eliminated unchanged.

In angina pectoris, and probably in supraventricular tachyarrhythmias, it is likely that the degree of β-blockade is directly related to therapeutic efficacy, and that the $t_{1/2}$ of a β-blocker roughly correlates with its duration of action. Therefore propranolol is given b.d. or t.d.s. for angina, atenolol once daily. In hypertension, because of the complex mode of action (see above) the $t_{1/2}$ of a β-blocker is not related to

its duration of action, which is generally 12 h and often greater than 24 h. However, in practice, this has not resulted in dosage regimens different from those used in angina pectoris or arrhythmias.

Important adverse effects

Blockade of β_2 receptors in the lungs may cause bronchoconstriction in susceptible subjects and may lead to life-threatening acute severe asthma. Non-selective β-blockers should therefore not be given to asthmatics. Even relatively selective β-blockers should be used with caution if at all, since none is completely devoid of some β_2 receptor antagonism.

Because of their negative inotropic effects β-blockers may cause or worsen heart failure. It is therefore important to look out for the symptoms and signs of heart failure when using β-blockers in patients with cardiac disease.

Central nervous system effects (depression, hallucinations, sleep disturbances) can be reduced in frequency, although not completely avoided, by using a β-blocker which penetrates the brain poorly (see table).

Peripheral vasoconstriction, which results in Raynaud's phenomenon, and is particularly troublesome in the cold weather, is a common complaint; the precise mechanism is still not understood.

Practolol, in long-term oral use, causes a syndrome consisting of dry eyes (progressing to corneal ulceration and perforation), a skin rash, and peritoneal fibrosis. For this reason its use is restricted to intravenous short-term therapy of arrhythmias. There are reports of dry eyes in patients taking other β-blockers, but this complaint does not presage the occurrence of the practolol syndrome. It may, however, be sufficiently unpleasant to warrant withdrawal of therapy. There have also been reports of peritoneal fibrosis in patients on β-blockers, but so far it has not been proven that this occurs with greater frequency than in the untreated population.

The normal sympathetic response to hypoglycaemia is blocked by β-blockers. Sweating still occurs, however, since it is a sympathetic nervous function not served by adrenaline or noradrenaline.

If β-blocker therapy is to be withdrawn it should be withdrawn slowly, since abrupt withdrawal may result in a rebound increase in anginal symptoms or frank myocardial infarction, possibly related to adaptive β-adrenoceptor supersensitivity in response to chronic blockade.

Interactions

Cimetidine inhibits the first-pass metabolism of propranolol and metoprolol and the metabolism of bisoprolol. When β-blockers and verapamil are used concurrently there is an increased incidence of bradyarrhythmias and an increased risk of heart failure. There have also been reports of asystole attributed to the use of the combination (see p. 132).

The effects of insulin and oral hypoglycaemic drugs may be potentiated by β-blockers, with resulting hypoglycaemia. There is some evidence that this effect is more pronounced with non-cardioselective β-blockers. This interaction is distinct from the effects of β-blockers on the clinical *response* to hypoglycaemia (see above). B-blockers interact beneficially with some other drugs used in the treatment of cardiovascular disease. For example, the negative inotropic effects of β-blockers can be diminished by cardiac glycosides; the combination of α- and β-adrenoceptor antagonists is useful in the treatment of hypertension (see labetalol).

Alcohol

Alcohol is the name commonly given to ethyl alcohol or ethanol (C_2H_5OH). It is present in a wide range of drinks in a wide range of concentrations, for example in beers (2.5–11 per cent v/v), cider (3.5–5.0 per cent), table wines (9.5–15.5 per cent), fortified wines (16–23 per cent), and spirits (35–55 per cent).

In addition to alcohol, alcoholic drinks may contain other constituents called congeners, the commonest of which is fusel oil. Congeners may be present in quantities up to 0.3 per cent of the volume of alcohol, and they contribute to the taste of the drink.

Effects of alcohol

Alcohol has a wide range of effects on different tissues.

(a) Central nervous system

In the brain alcohol acts as a dose-dependent depressant, producing the well-known features of intoxication. At plasma concentrations of around 40 mg/dL (400 μg/mL or 8.7 mmol/L) learned skills are impaired, including the ability to maintain self-restraint. Other early effects include loss of attentiveness, loss of concentration, and impaired memory, and there may be lethargy.

At progressively higher concentrations there are further changes in mood, behaviour, and a variety of sensory and motor functions.

Mood

The effects of alcohol on mood depend on the individual's personality, mental state, and social environment. Commonly there is euphoria, but any kind of mood change can occur. Libido is often enhanced, but sexual performance impaired.

Behaviour

Alcohol generally increases confidence, often resulting in aggressive or silly behaviour; loss of self-restraint leads to increased loquacity with immoderate speech content, such as swearing or the use of lewd language.

Motor functions

Unsteadiness of gait, slurred speech, and difficulty in carrying out even simple tasks become obvious at plasma concentrations of about 80 mg/dL (the concentration above which driving is illegal in the UK and many other countries). Driving skills are therefore impaired, and are affected even at concentrations below 80 mg/dL. Impaired coordination leads to excessive movement of the steering wheel and inaccurate cornering; overconfidence leads to attempts at dangerous manoeuvres which, combined with impaired judgement and prolonged reaction time, may lead to accidents (see Fig. P1); sensory changes may

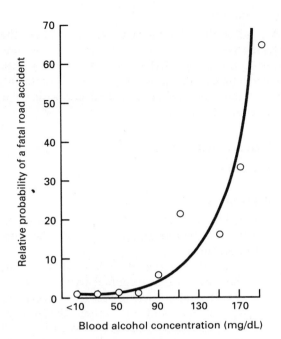

■ **Fig. P1** The relative probability among drivers of a fatal road accident in relation to the blood alcohol concentration. (Adapted from Perrine *et al.* (1971). Alcohol and highway safety: behavioural and medical aspects. *NHTSA Report*, DOS HS-800-599, with the permission of the US Department of Transport).

also contribute to impaired driving skills (see next section).

Sensory functions

Recovery from dazzle is delayed and this may impair night-time driving. Visual acuity and peripheral vision are reduced, and colour vision and visual tracking are impaired. Hearing and taste may also be impaired, and the pain threshold is increased. At high concentrations there may be vertigo and nystagmus.

Consciousness

Alcohol causes acute drowsiness and deep sleep, and in high concentrations may cause coma and respiratory depression. In some individuals sleep may later be impaired. On waking there is the characteristic 'hangover' which usually consists of irritability, headache, thirst, abdominal cramps, and bowel disturbance. The cause of hangover is not known.

Chronic effects

Alcohol may cause a variety of neurological abnormalities, including Wernicke's encephalopathy (due to thiamine deficiency), retrobulbar neuropathy (so-called alcohol amblyopia), cerebral atrophy, and polyneuropathy. Encephalopathy may occur as a result of chronic hepatic cirrhosis.

Dependence occurs during chronic ingestion, and withdrawal results in a typical syndrome, including delirium tremens (see Chapter 34).

(b) Cardiovascular system

In moderate amounts alcohol causes peripheral vasodilatation, resulting in skin flushing. At higher doses there may be hypotension. Chronic ingestion may cause a cardiomyopathy and hypertension.

(c) Skeletal muscle

Chronic ingestion can cause a skeletal myopathy.

(d) Gastrointestinal tract

In moderate doses alcohol stimulates gastric acid production and enhances the back-diffusion of hydrogen ions. At higher doses gastric acid output decreases, gastric mucus production increases, and the gastric mucosa becomes congested and hyperaemic. There may be vomiting and in severe cases acute gastritis. These effects are lessened by food.

Chronic ingestion may result in chronic atrophic gastritis, with hypochlorhydria.

(e) Metabolism and nutrition

Alcohol is oxidized in the liver at the expense of other compounds, such as those in the tricarboxylic acid (citric acid) cycle, which is thus inhibited. Blood glucose usually rises during acute alcohol ingestion, because of increased sympathetic nervous system activity. However, if glycogen stores are depleted because of malnutrition (for example in chronic alcholics) hypoglycaemia may occur, because of impaired gluconeogenesis, via the effects on the tricarboxylic acid cycle. Alcohol impairs fatty acid utilization and induces hepatic microsomal enzymes, causing increased lipoprotein synthesis. There may therefore be hyperlipoproteinaemia.

Alcohol may precipitate an acute attack of porphyria (see Chapter 8).

Chronic alcoholics tend to eat less than normal, partly because they prefer to spend their money on drink, and partly because chronic alcohol ingestion impairs the appetite. They do not lose weight, because alcohol provides all the energy they need, but may develop nutritional deficiencies. These include the following:

Wernicke's encephalopathy (or Wernicke–Korsakoff syndrome)

This is due to thiamine deficiency and the features include ocular disturbances (weakness of the lateral rectus muscles, nystagmus, and paralysis of conjugate gaze), ataxia, and impaired mental function, including Korsakoff's psychosis (a disorder of memory and other cognitive functions). There may also be delirium tremens.

Neuropathy

This is also due to thiamine deficiency, but may also be due in part to a direct effect of alcohol on peripheral nerves.

Anaemia

Alcoholics become anaemic through deficiency of iron, folate, or even vitamin B_{12}. However, the most common change in the blood is a macrocytosis without either megaloblastosis or anaemia; its cause is unknown.

(f) Renal function

Alcohol acts as a diuretic by decreasing water reabsorption in the renal tubules, perhaps by inhibiting ADH secretion in the pituitary.

Alcohol inhibits uric acid excretion and may cause hyperuricaemia or acute gout.

(g) Hepatic function

Acutely alcohol inhibits hepatic enzymes, but chronically may cause enzyme induction. However, if liver function is impaired because of chronic cirrhosis enzyme activity will become impaired.

Acutely alcohol causes fat deposition in the liver and this may be associated with an acute alcoholic hepatitis. Chronically it may cause cirrhosis, the pathogenesis of which is not fully understood.

(h) The fetus

Alcohol inhibits fetal growth, and may cause the 'fetal-alcohol' syndrome if taken in large amounts during pregnancy. Babies born to mothers with severe chronic alcoholism may have craniofacial, limb, and cleft deformities, and cardiovascular and brain defects.

Medical uses

Alcohol has a few medical uses:

(a) Local uses

Alcohol kills bacteria, and is therefore used to swab the skin before venepuncture or other surgical procedures.

It is rubefacient (i.e. it makes the skin red) and is therefore used as a counter-irritant in some liniments. It is also used to harden the skin to prevent bedsores, and to harden the nipples before breast-feeding. It decreases sweating, and is therefore incorporated into some antihidrotic solutions.

(b) Pain relief

Alcohol may be injected directly into nerve ganglia or around nerve trunks to destroy them and relieve severe or chronic pain (for example trigeminal neuralgia), but the results are generally short-lasting only.

(c) Treatment of acute methanol poisoning

Ethyl alcohol competes with methyl alcohol (methanol) for hepatic metabolism and is therefore used in the treatment of acute methanol poisoning (see Chapter 35, p. 499).

(d) Pharmaceutical uses

Alcohol is widely used as a solvent in pharmaceutical preparations.

Kinetic data

(a) Absorption

Alcohol is rapidly absorbed from all parts of the gut. The rate of absorption is concentration-dependent, for example in the stomach it is maximal at a concentration of about 30 per cent (v/v).

(b) Distribution

Alcohol is distributed throughout body tissues in an apparent volume of distribution roughly equal to that of total body water (i.e. about 0.6 L/kg), Thus, about 32 g of alcohol (about 2–3 pints of beer or two double measures of spirits) will produce a blood alcohol concentration of 80 mg/dL in a 70 kg individual. This figure, however, is calculated from mean data; it will vary greatly from individual to individual and may depend on the type of drink and whether or not food is taken with it. Women have a smaller distribution volume than men.

(c) Metabolism

Alcohol is metabolized 98 per cent by the route shown in Fig. P2. It is first oxidized to acetaldehyde by alcohol dehydrogenase, and this step is rate-limiting and has a K_m of about 10 mg/dL. Since blood alcohol concentrations are usually above 10 mg/dL the kinetics of alcohol metabolism are predominantly zero-order at most concentrations (see Chapter 3, p. 21 and Fig. 3.3). At whole blood concentrations over 10 mg/dL the clearance rate of alcohol is constant at about 6 g/h. For some drinks the clearance rate may be slower, since some congeners may compete with alcohol for metabolic sites.

The second step in alcohol metabolism is to acetate under the influence of aldehyde dehydrogenase. This step is rapid and blood aldehyde concentrations are usually low (below 2 mg/dL).

Alcohol does not induce the activity of its own metabolizing enzymes.

(d) Excretion

Most of the small amounts of alcohol which is not metabolized is excreted unchanged in the urine and breath. The concentration in the expired air is about 0.05 per cent of that in the blood, i.e. 0.04 mg/dL at a blood concentration of 80 mg/dL: sufficient for detection by a 'breathalyser'.

Interactions

(a) Pharmacodynamic

(i) Centrally-acting drugs

The most important interactions of drugs with alcohol are those with other centrally-acting drugs, such as the phenothiazines, butyrophenones, barbiturates, benzodiazepines, tricyclic antidepressants, antihistamines, and lithium. In all cases the effects of alcohol and the drug may be mutually enhanced, and patients taking centrally-acting drugs should be advised not to take any alcohol at all if they are going to drive or operate machinery.

(ii) Hypoglycaemic drugs

In about a third of patients taking chlorpropamide, alcohol causes facial flushing. The precise mechanism of this interaction is not known. It happens only rarely with other sulphonylureas.

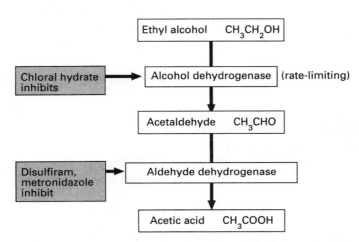

∎ **Fig. P2** The metabolism of alcohol and the sites of action of drugs which inhibit it.

Patients taking insulin should be advised not to drink, or to drink only small amounts of particular beverages (for example 'diabetic' lager, dry wine, or dry cider). This is because:

(1) alcohol impairs gluconeogenesis, which is the main source of blood glucose when glycogen stores are depleted;

(2) alcohol provides extra carbohydrate;

(3) if drunk diabetics may become careless about their general care and treatment.

(iii) Intravenous feeding

Alcohol and fructose should not be used together as energy sources in i.v. feeding, since alcohol encourages the formation of lactic acid by its effects on glucose metabolism and fructose is metabolized to lactic acid. There is thus an increased risk of lactic acidosis.

(b) Pharmacokinetic

(i) Inhibition of alcohol dehydrogenase

Chloral hydrate inhibits alcohol dehydrogenase and thus potentiates the effects of alcohol. It also has a potentiating pharmacodynamic effect as a sedative. The combination of alcohol and chloral hydrate or other sedatives has been called a 'Mickey Finn'.

(ii) Inhibition of aldehyde dehydrogenase

Disulfiram and metronidazole are inhibitors of aldehyde dehydrogenase and cause accumulation of acetaldehyde. This causes an unpleasant set of symptoms, including colic, flushing, dizziness, breathlessness, tachycardia, and vomiting. Disulfiram (Antabuse®) has therefore been use as aversion therapy in chronic alcoholism.

(iii) Hepatic microsomal enzyme induction

Chronic alcohol injection causes an increase in the activity of the mixed-function oxidative enzymes in the liver. This leads to an increased rate of metabolism of drugs such as phenytoin and warfarin. However, chronic liver damage due to alcohol may result in decreased drug metabolism and the changes in the kinetics of these drugs in chronic alcoholics may therefore be unpredictable.

Allopurinol

Structure

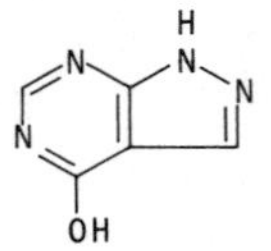

(Note the similarity to hypoxanthine.)

Mode of action

Both allopurinol and its metabolite, alloxanthine (oxypurinol), inhibit xanthine oxidase competitively. As shown below, this enzyme is involved in the production of uric acid from xanthines, as well as in the metabolism of allopurinol itself:

$$\text{Hypoxanthine} \xrightarrow[\text{oxidase}]{\text{Xanthine}} \text{Xanthine} \xrightarrow[\text{oxidase}]{\text{Xanthine}} \text{Uric acid}$$

$$\text{Allopurinol} \xrightarrow[\text{oxidase}]{\text{Xanthine}} \text{Alloxanthine (oxypurinol)}$$

There is therefore reduced production of uric acid and the purine load needing elimination is spread out amongst hypoxanthine, xanthine, and uric acid, the individual solubilities of which are not exceeded.

Uses

Treatment of chronic hyperuricaemia (both primary and secondary), and prevention of its complications (tophi, uric acid nephropathy, and acute attacks of gout).

Dosages

300–600 mg o.d., orally

Kinetic data

Well absorbed. The $t_{1/2}$ of allopurinol is 2 h, of alloxanthine 24 h. Thus, alloxanthine accumulates to a greater extent than allopurinol but, since it inhibits its own formation, the extent of its accumulation is dose-dependent. Both compounds are excreted in the urine.

Important adverse effects

During the first few days of treatment there is an increased risk of acute gout. This may be prevented by the concurrent use of colchicine (q.v.) or a non-steroidal anti-inflammatory drug. Allergic reactions are common, but generalized hypersensitivity reactions are rare. Skin rashes occur with an incidence of 2 per cent when allopurinol alone is given. However, when allopurinol is combined with ampicillin the incidence of skin rashes rises to 22 per cent (ampicillin alone 8 per cent). Renal failure, hepatitis, and eosinophilia have been occasionally reported.

Interactions

When 6-mercaptopurine is used in the treatment of leukaemia, the cell death which occurs results in the production of large amounts of purines, which are metabolized to uric acid with consequent hyperuricaemia and its attendant complications. Allopurinol is often used to guard against these, but allopurinol inhibits the metabolism of 6-mercaptopurine to 6-thiouric acid (by xanthine oxidase) and leads to accumulation of 6-mercaptopurine. For this reason the dosage requirements of 6-mercaptopurine are *reduced by 75 per cent* when allopurinol is also given. Because azathioprine is metabolized to 6-mercaptopurine it is also subject to this interaction.

The toxic effect of cyclophosphamide on the bone-marrow is potentiated by allopurinol.

The interaction between allopurinol and ampicillin is mentioned above under 'adverse effects'.

Amiloride

Structure

Mode of action

Amiloride acts in a manner similar to triamterene. It blocks sodium channels in the luminal membranes of cells in the late distal tubule, causing increased excretion of sodium, chloride, and water. This inhibition causes hyperpolarization of the apical plasma membrane, which discourages the secretion of potassium, an effect which is independent of aldosterone. Its use is therefore associated with potassium retention.

Uses

In combination with potassium-depleting diuretics (for example Moduretic®, a combination of hydrochlorothiazide and amiloride) in the treatment of oedema due to cardiac failure, liver disease, and the nephrotic syndrome.

Dosages

10–20 mg o.d. orally.

Kinetic data

Very poorly absorbed. Almost completely excreted unchanged in the urine. $t_{1/2} = 6$ h.

Important adverse effects

Hyperkalaemia, dehydration, and hyponatraemia are common. The incidence of hyperkalaemia (about 5 per cent) is the unaffected by concurrent administration of potassium-depleting diuretics. Nausea and vomiting occur occasionally.

Aminoglutethimide

Structure

Mode of action

Aminoglutethimide inhibits the first step in steroid synthesis, the conversion of cholesterol to pregnenolone. It thus reduces the production of all endogenous steroids, including cortisone, aldosterone, and the sex steroids (see Fig. 25.1).

Uses

1. To cause 'medical adrenalectomy' in women with metastatic breast cancer after the menopause or after oophorectomy.

2. To reduce adrenal steroid production in Cushing's syndrome due to adrenal tumours, ectopic ACTH production, or (in combination with metyrapone) excess pituitary ACTH production.

Dosages

250 mg o.d., orally for one week, increasing to 250 mg q.d.s. in the absence of severe adverse effects.

Supplementary therapy is discussed below.

Important adverse effects

Because aminoglutethimide inhibits steroid synthesis in general, supplementary steroid therapy is necessary to prevent Addison's disease, using oral hydrocortisone (15–60 mg orally o.d.) and fludrocortisone (50–300 micrograms orally o.d.).

Central nervous system effects are common and include dizziness, lethargy, and somnolence. Nausea, vomiting, and diarrhoea occur less often. All these effects are dose-related.

Drug rash with fever may occur after 1–2 weeks of treatment but is self-limiting and usually resolves within a further 1–2 weeks without withdrawal.

Occasionally aminoglutethimide may cause hypothyroidism.

Interactions

Aminoglutethimide increases the rate of metabolism (and therefore the dosage requirements) of warfarin, oral hypoglycaemics, and dexamethasone.

Aminoglycoside antibiotics

Structures

These drugs contain different amino sugars in glycosidic linkage. Gentamicin is shown as an example:

gentamicin C_1 : $R_1 = R_2 = CH_3$

C_2 : $R_1 = CH_3$; $R_2 = H$

C_{1a} : $R_1 = R_2 = H$

Gentamicin C_1: $R_1 = R_2 = CH_3$
$\quad\quad\quad\quad$ C_2: $R_1 = CH_3$: $R_2 = H$
$\quad\quad\quad\quad$ C_{1a}: $R_1 = R_2 = H$

Other aminoglycosides in common clinical use are streptomycin, neomycin, kanamycin, tobramycin, amikacin, and netilmicin.

Mode of action

The aminoglycosides inhibit protein synthesis in bacterial ribosomes and disrupt the translation process from RNA to DNA. This leads to a bacteriostatic effect, but the aminoglycosides are also bacteriocidal through a mechanism not yet fully understood. In hepatic encephalopathy neomycin may act by reducing the gut flora which possess urease activity, thus reducing ammonia production in the gut, but it may also inhibit protein absorption.

Uses

Below are listed some of the common examples of bacteria sensitive to the aminoglycosides and the associated diseases for which they are particularly used. Neomycin is also used in the treatment of hepatic encephalopathy.

Bacteria	Disease	Aminoglycoside
Gram-positive cocci	Streptococcal endocarditis	Gentamicin (in combination with penicillin G)
Gram-negative bacilli	Infections with *E. coli, Proteus, Pseudomonas,* and *Kl. pneumoniae*	Gentamicin Tobramycin Amikacin Netilmicin
Mycobacteria	Tuberculosis	Streptomycin
Various	Skin, ear, and eye infections	Neomycin

Dosages

Intramuscular or intravenous (assuming normal renal function):

Gentamicin, 2–2.5 mg/kg initially then 1–2 mg/kg eight-hourly; adjust doses according to plasma concentrations (see below). Dosages may need to be reduced after about a week of continuous therapy, because of slow accumulation.

Streptomycin (i.m. only), 7.5–15 mg/kg o.d.
Kanamycin, 10 mg/kg initially then 5–10 mg/kg b.d.; adjust dosages according to plasma concentrations.
Netilmicin, 4–6 mg/kg daily in 2 or 3 equal doses.

Intravenous doses of these drugs should be given by infusion over half an hour.

Oral:
Neomycin, 0.5–1 g four to six times daily.

Kinetic data

All are poorly absorbed and are therefore given parenterally or topically. Neomycin is given orally for its effect on the gastrointestinal tract.

Gentamicin, kanamycin, netilmicin, and streptomycin have an apparently short half-time of about 2 h, but long-term studies have shown that gentamicin has a terminal half-time of about 5 d, the plasma concentrations usually found during therapy being too low to detect this very long phase. Because of this long $t_{1/2}$, accumulation of gentamicin may become a problem after about 1–2 weeks of continuous treatment and dosage reductions should be anticipated.

Therapeutic plasma concentrations (see also Chapter 7) should be:

Gentamicin: less than 12 μg/mL about 1 h after an i.m. dose or 15 min after an i.v. dose ('peak' concentration) and less than 2 μg/mL just before the next dose ('trough' concentration).
Kanamycin: the corresponding values are 10 μg/mL and 40 μg/mL.
Netilmicin: the corresponding values are 4 μg/mL and 16 μg/mL.
Streptomycin: 15–20 μg/mL at steady rate.

The aminoglycosides are almost completely eliminated via the kidneys. For this reason dosages should be reduced in renal failure, using creatinine clearance as a guide. Dosages should be reduced in direct proportion to creatinine clearance (normal 80–120 mL/min); thus creatinine clearance = 50 mL/min, dose = 50 per cent of usual dose.

Important adverse effects

Hypersensitivity reactions are common, especially skin rashes (about 5 per cent). Streptomycin may cause dermatitis by a direct effect on the skin and it should be handled with gloves.

Auditory and vestibular dysfunction may occur as toxic effects. Gentamicin and streptomycin tend to affect vestibular function more commonly, resulting in nausea, vomiting, difficulty in standing, vertigo, and nystagmus. Kanamycin and amikacin, on the other hand, tend to affect auditory function more, resulting in tinnitus, reduction in high-tone perception, and deafness. The aminoglycosides have sometimes been used deliberately to produce these effects in patients with disabling Menière's disease. Netilmicin is less ototoxic and nephrotoxic than the other aminoglycosides.

Acute renal impairment due to tubular damage may occur as a toxic effect of the aminoglycosides. This is more likely to occur in patients who already have renal disease and in patients who are being treated with frusemide and ethacrynic acid.

The aminoglycosides have neuromuscular blocking effects and may exacerbate symptoms in patients with myasthenia gravis.

Neomycin may cause malabsorption and superinfection of the oropharynx with yeasts and fungi.

Interactions

Frusemide and ethacrynic acid may potentiate the ototoxic and nephrotoxic effects of the aminoglycosides. Other drugs which are also nephrotoxic should be avoided (for example polymixin, cisplatin, vancomycin).

The aminoglycosides potentiate the effects of neuromuscular blocking agents.

Neomycin inhibits the absorption of dietary vitamin K and destroys the bacteria in the gut which produce vitamin K; it may, therefore potentiate the effects of oral anticoagulants.

Amiodarone

Structure

Mode of action

Amiodarone is a class III antiarrhythmic drug. Its effects on the action potential (see lignocaine) resemble those of hypothyroidism. It prolongs the duration of action potential by slowing repolarization (phase 3). It does not prolong phase 4 depolarization, does not alter the threshold potential, and does not alter the rate of depolarization during phase 0 (cf. class I antiarrhythmics; see lignocaine).

Because it prolongs the action potential the refractory periods are also prolonged. These effects occur in the atria, ventricles, AV node, SA node, and conducting system. The QT interval is prolonged by amiodarone. These effects are probably mediated by actions on potassium channels.

Uses

Supraventricular and ventricular arrhythmias:

(1) Paroxysmal atrial fibrillation and flutter.

(2) Recurrent supraventricular tachycardias associated with the Wolff–Parkinson–White syndrome.

(3) Recurrent ventricular tachyarrhythmias.

Dosages

Intravenous: 5 mg/kg by infusion over 20–120 min in 250 ml of 5 per cent dextrose. Maximum dose 15 mg/kg (over 24 h).

Oral: initial dose, 20 mg t.d.s. for 1 week, followed by 200 mg b.d. for 1 week, then reducing to a maintenance dose. Average maintenance dose, 100–200 mg o.d.

Kinetic data

Amiodarone has a very long $t_{1/2}$ (of the order of a month or more), and its effects have been observed to last for weeks after its discontinuation. It is metabolized to an active metabolite desethylamiodarone.

Important adverse effects

In virtually all patients on long-term therapy amiodarone causes corneal microdeposits of lipofucsin, which can be seen with a slit lamp. They do not usually affect vision, but if central may cause visual haloes. They are not considered serious or requiring withdrawal of therapy. These microdeposits are reversible and disappear on withdrawal of amiodarone.

Photosensitization is very common and may cause reactions varying in intensity from an increased propensity to suntan to severe erythematous reactions requiring withdrawal. A slate-grey cosmetically undesirable pigmentation of the skin may also occur.

Amiodarone affects the thyroid in two ways. Firstly it decreases the peripheral conversion of T_4 to T_3 (see Fig. 25.2) causing an increase in serum T_4 and a decrease in serum T_3. Thyroid-binding globulin is unaffected and the secretion of TSH in response to TRH is usually, but not always, normal. These changes occur in the absence of functional thyroid disease, but amiodarone can also cause both hypothyroidism and hyperthyroidism in about 4 per cent of cases. However, routine monitoring of thyroid function is not recommended, and in patients in whom abnormal thyroid function is suspected clinically it may be difficult to interpret the results of thyroid function tests.

A reversible peripheral neuropathy has been described and attributed to demyelination.

Interstitial pneumonitis can occur and may be fatal. It is accompanied by a reduction in CO diffusing capacity. It responds to treatment with corticosteroids.

Hepatitis may occur, sometimes without premonitory changes in liver function tests.

Miscellaneous effects include constipation, headache, nausea, vomiting, fatigue, tremor, and nightmares.

Interactions

Amiodarone potentiates the effects of warfarin by inhibiting its metabolism.

Plasma concentrations of digoxin are increased by amiodarone because of reduced excretion. Digitalis toxicity may thus occur.

Amiodarone should not be used with other drugs which prolong the QT interval (for example quinidine, disopyramide, and procainamide).

Amphotericin B

Structure

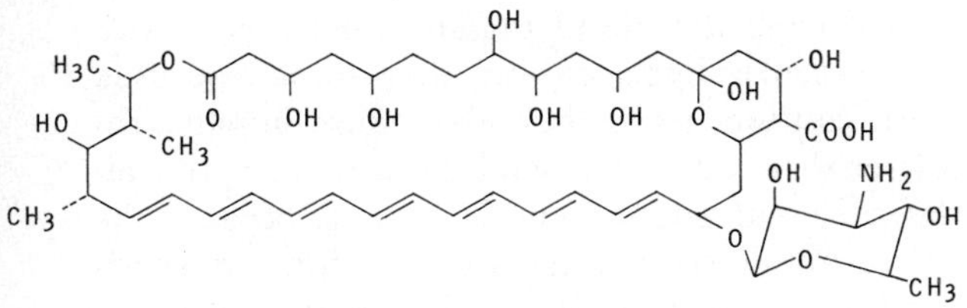

Mode of action

Amphotericin alters the permeability of cell membranes, leading to loss of essential cell constituents.

Uses

Local and systemic yeast and fungal infections (*Candida spp., Coccidioides, Histoplasma, Blastomyces, Mucor, Cryptococcus, Aspergillus*).

Dosages

Oropharyngeal infections: 10 mg lozenges q.d.s.

Intravenous therapy: 0.25–1.0 mg/kg daily by continuous infusion.

Kinetic data

Amphotericin is not absorbed after oral administration. $t_{1/2} = 1$ d. Almost completely metabolized.

Important adverse effects

Renal impairment is almost unavoidable, due to renal vasoconstriction and a direct effect on the tubules, resulting in diminished glomerular filtration rate and renal plasma flow, with consequent tubular acidosis and hypokalaemia. These effects can be reduced by concomitant mannitol infusion and are generally reversible, but they may become irreversible at total doses over 5 g.

Fever is common (50 per cent) and may be reduced by hydrocortisone.

A normochromic, normocytic anaemia occurs in most patients, because of bone-marrow depression.

The incidence of adverse effects may be reduced by alternate-day therapy of twice the dose.

Angiotensin converting enzyme (ACE) inhibitors

Structures

Captopril

Enalapril

Mode of action

The ACE inhibitors are competitive inhibitors of the angiotensin converting enzyme (ACE), which is a dipeptidyl carboxypeptidase, also known as kininase II. Inhibition of this enzyme results in a decrease in the conversion of angiotensin I to the vasoactive peptide angiotensin II and also in an accumulation of bradykinin, a vasodilator which is normally activated by kininase II.

The therapeutic effects of the ACE inhibitors in both hypertension and cardiac failure result from direct peripheral vasodilatation, due mainly to a decrease in the amount of circulating angiotensin II. Circulating aldosterone is also reduced because its release is reduced in the absence of angiotensin II.

Uses

Hypertension.

Congestive cardiac failure. The ACE inhibitors can be used to treat the signs and symptoms of congestive cardiac failure, and enalapril has been shown to reduce mortality rates in patients with severe congestive cardiac failure.

Dosages

Treatment should be started with low oral doses, and the dosage increased at 2 week intervals according to the patient's response.

Captopril: the initial oral dose is 6.25–12.5 mg b.d. Maintenance dosages are from 25 mg b.d. to a maximum of 50 mg t.d.s.

Enalapril: the initial oral dosage is 2.5–5 mg o.d. Maintenance dosages are 10–20 mg daily.

Kinetic data

Well absorbed, but absorption is reduced to 50 per cent by food.

Captopril is 50 per cent excreted unchanged and 50 per cent metabolized to inactive compounds.

Enalapril is metabolized to its active form enalaprilat, with a high first-pass effect. Enalaprilat is excreted unchanged in the urine.

The half-times of the ACE inhibitors are long because they bind to ACE in the plasma.

Although the ACE inhibitors are very effective in reducing the blood pressure in patients with renovascular hypertension, they should be used with caution, since they may cause impairment of renal function, particularly in those with unilateral renal artery stenosis. This is because the perfusion pressure in the affected kidney depends on the action of locally produced angiotensin.

Important adverse effects

Rashes are common (about 10 per cent) and may be accompanied by fever and eosinophilia. Rarely angio-oedema may occur.

Taste disturbance, which is usually transient, occurs in about 5 per cent of patients.

Proteinuria occurs in about 1 per cent of patients and the nephrotic syndrome in about 0.3

per cent. The latter is due to a membranous glomerulonephritis.

Neutropenia occurs in about 0.3 per cent of patients and may progress to agranulocytosis.

Interactions

Hypotension is common among patients treated with other antihypertensive drugs and particularly in patients who are volume-depleted by diuretics. This is especially a problem during the first few hours of administration of ACE inhibitors, and if patients are given an ACE inhibitor while also taking a diuretic they should take the first dose while lying down. Initiation of therapy in these cases is best done in hospital under careful supervision.

The ACE inhibitors cause an increase in the plasma potassium concentration, and the effects of other drugs with a similar action may be potentiated (for example potassium-sparing diuretics or potassium chloride supplements).

Cyclo-oxygenase inhibitors, such as indomethacin, may reduce the hypotensive effects of the ACE inhibitors.

Antifibrinolytic drugs

Structures

ε-aminocaproic acid

$$NH_2CH_2(CH_2)_4COOH$$

Tranexamic acid

Mode of action

ε-aminocaproic acid and tranexamic acid are antifibrinolytic agents which competitively inhibit the activation of plasminogen to plasmin (see Fig. P3, and compare with fibrinolytic drugs, which have the opposite actions).

Uses

These drugs are used in circumstances in which excessive bleeding cannot be controlled. They are best reserved for short-term use only, and the conditions in which they have been found to be valuable include post-operative haemorrhage, particularly after prostatectomy and bladder surgery, menorrhagia associated with intrauterine contraceptive devices, epistaxis, and dental extraction in haemophiliacs. Their usefulness in preventing rebleeding after subarachnoid haemorrhage is controversial and has not been proven satisfactory.

Tranexamic acid is also used to reverse the effects of fibrinolytic drugs if excessive (see p. 607), and in the treatment of hereditary angiooedema, as second choice after an anabolic steroid such as danazol.

Dosages

Intravenous: tranexamic acid, 1–2 g t.d.s. by infusion over at least 5 min.

Oral: tranexamic acid, 1–1.5 g, two to four times daily; ε-aminocaproic acid, 3 g four to six times daily.

Kinetic data

These drugs are well absorbed. They are mostly excreted unchanged by the kidneys and dosages should be reduced in renal failure. The $t_{1/2}$ of aminocaproic acid is 2 h, of tranexamic acid 14 h.

Important adverse effects

The incidence of adverse reactions to tranexamic acid is lower than for ε-aminocaproic acid, but the contra-indications are the same and are as follows:

1. Massive haematuria from the upper urinary tract, since these drugs promote clotting, which may cause ureteric obstruction.

2. A recent history of thromboembolism and in cases in which there is an increased risk of thrombosis, even in the presence of bleeding (for example disseminated intravascular coagulation).

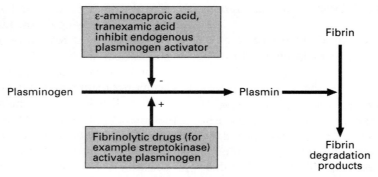

∎ **Fig. P3** The activation of plasminogen and the effects of drugs which activate it or inhibit its activation.

3. Pregnancy.

Adverse reactions to tranexamic acid are uncommon and consist mostly of nausea, vomiting, and diarrhoea, which are dose-related. Rarely giddiness may occur during over-rapid infusion.

ε-aminocaproic acid may cause nausea, vomiting, diarrhoea, nasal congestion, conjunctival suffusion, dizziness, hypotension, and skin rashes.

Rarely an acute myopathy may occur during long-term therapy (> 4 weeks) and cause muscle weakness, tenderness, and myoglobinuria, which may cause renal failure.

Interactions

The risk of thrombosis due to these drugs is increased by concomitant therapy with oral contraceptives.

Antifungal imidazoles

Structures

In common with metronidazole (q.v. p. 635) the antifungal imidazoles consist of an imidazole ring with different substituents attached. We give here miconazole as an example.

Other members of the group are clotrimazole, econazole, fluconazole, itraconazole, and keto-conazole.

Mode of action

The mode of action of the antifungal imidazoles has not been fully established, but several of their effects on fungal metabolism are known. For example, they increase membrane permeability by several mechanisms, including inhibition of membrane ATPase, inhibition of ergosterol synthesis, and an interaction with cell membrane phospholipids. They also inhibit cellular oxidative and peroxidative enzymes, leading to accumulation within the cell of toxic peroxides.

The effects of the antifungal imidazoles on fungal cells include leakage of essential cell constituents, swelling of the cells, and abnormalities of cell division.

Uses

The antifungal imidazoles are active against a wide variety of fungi, including mould fungi and yeast fungi. They are used in the treatment of the following infections:

1. Dermatophyte infections due to *Trichophyton, Microsporum,* and *Epidermophyton spp.,* for example *Tinea pedis, Tinea capitis, Tinea cruris.*

2. *Candida* infections, for example acute oral and vaginal candidiasis, intertrigo, paronychia, and chronic mucocutaneous candidiasis.

3. Vaginal trichomoniasis.

4. Certain systemic mycoses, including histoplasmosis, coccidioidomycosis, paracoccidioidomycosis, and systemic candidiasis.

Dosages

Intravenous: Miconazole, initially 600 mg eight-hourly by i.v. infusion in 200–500 mL of 5 per cent dextrose or isotonic saline over at least 30 min.

Fluconazole: initially 400 mg then 200 mg o.d., increasing if required to 400 mg o.d.

Oral: Ketoconazole, 200 mg o.d. until at least one week after symptoms have cleared and cultures have become negative.

Miconazole, 250 mg q.d.s., until at least two days after symptoms have cleared and cultures have become negative.

Fluconazole and itraconazole dosages vary with the infection.

Other routes: There is a wide variety of formulations of clotrimazole, econazole, and miconazole available for local application to the skin and vagina, for example creams, lotions, powders, vaginal creams, and pessaries. Miconazole may also be given intrathecally in fungal meningitis.

Kinetic data

Only small amounts of these drugs are absorbed after local application to the skin or vagina. They are poorly absorbed after oral administration, except itraconazole. They are widely distributed to body tissues, particularly the joints, skin, and eyes, but do not penetrate the CSF well. They are highly bound to plasma proteins and are mostly metabolized in the liver to inactive metabolites. Fluconazole is eliminated by the kidneys and dosages should be reduced in renal impairment. The $t_{1/2}$ for miconazole is 24 h, itraconazole 20 h, and ketoconazole 8 h.

Important adverse effects

There may be local irritation after local application of these drugs.

After intravenous infusion miconazole very commonly causes thrombophlebitis. Other common effects after i.v. infusion include pruritus, nausea and vomiting, fever, rashes, drowsiness, and hyponatraemia. Diarrhoea occurs occasionally and may also occur after oral administration. Rapid infusion may cause cardiac arrhythmias and should be avoided.

In addition there may be adverse reactions to the vehicle, a polyethoxylated castor oil (see also p. 708). These include hyperlipidaemia, blood abnormalities (for example erythrocyte clumping, thrombocytosis), and hypersensitivity reactions.

After oral administration of miconazole and ketoconazole there are a few adverse effects, but nausea, vomiting, diarrhoea, and pruritus occur occasionally. Ketoconazole may cause changes in liver function tests and may rarely cause hepatitis. Ketoconazole should be withdrawn if jaundice occurs.

Interactions

These drugs are enzyme inhibitors and enhance the effects of oral anticoagulants and phenytoin.

The absorption of ketoconazole is in part dependent on its dissolution in an acid medium. Concurrent administration of antacids or histamine (H₂) antagonists reduces its absorption.

Antihistamines (H₁ receptor antagonists)

Structures

The antihistamines form a heterogeneous group of compounds. Some (for example promethazine and trimeprazine) are related to the phenothiazines; others (for example buclizine, cinnarizine, and cyclizine) are related to piperazine; yet others are related to other compounds (for example mepyramine is an ethylenediamine). As examples we give here cinnarizine and promethazine.

Cinnarizine

Promethazine (cf. the phenothiazines)

Mode of action

The antihistamines inhibit the effects of histamine on H_1 receptors, particularly the effects of increased capillary permeability, vasodilatation, and itching, but in therapeutic doses they do not reverse them, once established. The H_1 antagonists do not block the effects of histamine on gastric acid secretion (see the H_2 receptor antagonists, p. 613). The adverse effects of the H_1 receptor antagonists are related mainly to their direct effects on the brain, causing sedation, and on muscarinic cholinergic receptors. Cinnarizine blocks transmembrane calcium ion transport in a manner similar to verapamil and nifedipine. It consequently has vasodilator properties but is not antiarrhythmic.

Uses

Treatment of allergic reactions, for example hay fever, urticaria, and angio-oedema, insect bites and stings, drug reactions, and transfusion reactions.

Prevention of motion sickness.

Symptomatic relief of Menière's disease and vertigo.

Symptomatic relief of pruritus.

Treatment of peripheral vascular disease (cinnarizine).

∎ **Table P1** Usual adult dosages and relative sedative and anticholinergic potencies of some antihistamines

	Dosages		Relative effects	
Drug	Oral	i.m. or i.v.	Sedative	Anticholinergic
Acrivastine	8 mg t.d.s.		−	−
Astemizole	10 mg o.d.		±	−
Betahistine	8–16 mg t.d.s.		+	+ +
Buclizine	25 mg t.d.s.		+	+ +
Chlorpheniramine	4 mg t.d.s.	10–20 mg	+ +	
Cinnarizine	15–30 mg t.d.s.		+	+
Cyclizine	50 mg t.d.s.	50 mg	+ +	+ +
Cyproheptadine	4–20 mg/d*		+ +	
Dimenhydrinate	50–100 mg 4-hourly (maximum 300 mg/d)	50mg	+ + +	
Diphenhydramine	50–200 mg/d		+ + +	+ +
Mebhydrolin	50–100 mg t.d.s.		+	
Mepyramine	100 mg t.d.s.		+ +	+
Oxatomide	30–60 mg b.d.		+	−
Promethazine	10–25 mg b.d. or t.d.s.	25–50 mg	+ + + +	+ + +
Terfenadine	60 mg b.d.		±	+
Trimeprazine	10–40 mg/d*		+ + + +	+ + +
Triprolidine	2.5–5 mg t.d.s.		+ +	

* In divided doses.

Dosages

The commonly used adult dosages are given in Table P1. If antihistamines are given by i.v. injection they should be given slowly and in dilute solution.

Kinetic data

All are well absorbed. Most are extensively metabolized with a $t_{1/2}$ of a few hours. Most enter the brain, but terfenadine and astemizole do so less than the rest.

Important adverse effects

Adverse effects occur in up to 50 per cent of cases. Sedation is common, but varies in severity from compound to compound (see Table P1) and from individual to individual. Patients should be warned of the hazards of driving or operating machinery while taking antihistamines. Rarely central nervous stimulation may occur, resulting in nervousness, tremor, insomnia, and convulsions.

Anticholinergic effects are common, including dry mouth, blurred vision, constipation, and urinary retention. Caution should be taken in patients with glaucoma or prostatic obstruction.

Direct application to the skin should be avoided, because of a high risk of sensitization.

Interactions

Antihistamines potentiate the effects of other drugs with central nervous depressant effects (for example alcohol, benzodiazepines, phenothiazines).

Azathioprine and 6-mercaptopurine

Structures

Azathioprine

Mercaptopurine, which is a metabolite of azathioprine, has SH instead of *S*-methylnitroimidazolyl.

Mode of action

Azathioprine has some therapeutic activity of its own but is almost completely metabolized to 6-mercaptopurine. Mercaptopurine is converted within cells to its 5-phosphate ribonucleotide, thioinosinate, which inhibits the synthesis of DNA from its purine precursors during S phase. The precise link between this effect and the cytotoxic and immunosuppressant effects of these drugs has not been fully worked out.

Uses

Azathioprine: immunosuppressant effects used in inhibiting rejection of transplanted organs (for example kidney) and in treating various autoimmune disorders, including systemic lupus erythematosus, dermatomyositis, polyarteritis nodosa, Wegener's granulomatosis, and rheumatoid arthritis.

Mercaptopurine is used in the treatment of acute leukaemias.

Dosages

Azathioprine: average daily oral dose is 2–5 mg/kg.

Mercaptopurine: initially 2.5 mg/kg o.d. orally, increasing to 5 mg/kg if required.

In both cases dosages should be altered depending on both the clinical responses and adverse effects.

Kinetic data

Both are well absorbed, azathioprine somewhat better than mercaptopurine. Azathioprine is converted to 6-mercaptopurine, which is further metabolized ($t_{1/2} = 1$ h) to inactive compounds.

Important adverse effects

Azathioprine: bone-marrow suppression is dose-related. Infections are common and may arise because of leucopenia and general immunosuppression. Long-term therapy with azathioprine, and indeed perhaps any effective immunosuppressant, is associated with an increased incidence of malignant tumours, particularly lymphoma. The effects of azathioprine on the fetus have not been firmly established, but it should not be used during pregnancy, if possible.

Mercaptopurine: nausea, vomiting, and diarrhoea are common with high dosages. Other adverse effects are similar to those of azathioprine.

Interactions

The metabolism of mercaptopurine and azathioprine is inhibited by allopurinol (for a full discussion see under allopurinol). Dosages of azathioprine and 6-mercaptopurine should be *reduced by 75 per cent* during treatment with allopurinol.

Baclofen

Structure

$$H_2NCH_2-CH-CH_2-COOH$$

Cl

Mode of action

Baclofen is the 4-chlorophenyl derivative of γ-aminobutyric acid (GABA), an inhibitory neurotransmitter. In the spinal cord GABA transmission would be expected to lead to muscle relaxation, and it was originally thought that the action of baclofen in relieving muscle spasm was as an agonist at postsynaptic $GABA_B$ receptors in the spinal cord. However, it is now thought that it acts as a GABA receptor *antagonist*, but at *pre*synaptic sites, where it reduces the release of excitatory neurotransmitters.

Uses

To alleviate muscle spasm in conditions of the spinal cord associated with spasticity, for example multiple sclerosis, spinal cord tumours, and transverse myelitis.

Dosages

Start with low dosages to reduce the incidence of adverse effects and increase slowly according to response. The initial oral dosage should be 5 mg t.d.s., increasing every 3 d by a total of 5 mg t.d.s. to 20 mg t.d.s. Occasionally higher dosages may be used, but the maximum daily dose should be 100 mg.

Kinetic data

Baclofen is well absorbed. It is mostly excreted unchanged by the kidney, $t_{1/2} = 4$ h.

Important adverse effects

The adverse effects of baclofen are dose-related. Nausea, vomiting, drowsiness, vertigo, confusion, and fatigue are all common. Nausea can be reduced by taking baclofen with food. As for other drugs used for muscle spasticity, baclofen can cause muscular hypotonia, especially in high dosages (60 mg per day or more).

Sudden withdrawal of baclofen should be avoided, since it can cause hallucinations.

Baclofen can cause convulsions, and it should be used with caution in patients with epilepsy or cerebrovascular disease.

Unpredictable psychiatric changes may occur, particularly in patients with psychiatric disease, in whom it should be used with caution.

The dosages of baclofen should be reduced in renal failure.

Interactions

Baclofen can cause hypotension and may therefore potentiate the effects of antihypertensive drugs.

Benzodiazepines

Structures

General

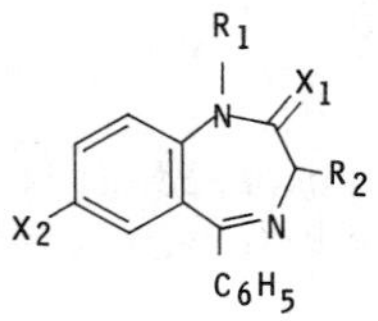

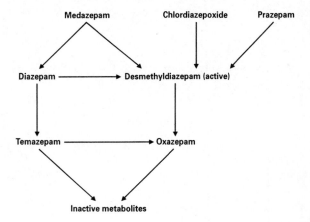

Examples

	R_1	R_2	X_1	X_2
Chlordiazepoxide	H	H	$NHCH_3$	Cl
Clonazepam*	H	H	O	NO
Diazepam	CH_3	H	O	Cl
Lorazepam*	H	H(OH)	O	Cl
Nitrazepam	H	H	O	NO_2
Oxazepam	H	H(OH)	O	Cl
Temazepam	CH_3	H(OH)	O	Cl

*These compounds have 5-o-chlorophenyl instead of 5-phenyl.
Midazolam has a related but slightly more complex structure.

Mode of action

Benzodiazepines bind to specific benzodiazepine receptors which are found in the nervous tissue in a complex with GABA receptors and a chloride channel. They facilitate GABA inhibitory neurotransmission via chloride influx, which tends to hyperpolarize the cell membrane. This action is presumed to result in their anxiolytic, sedative, and antiepileptic effects.

Uses

The relief of anxiety (particularly chlordiazepoxide, diazepam, oxazepam).

Night-time sedation (particularly nitrazepam, temazepam).

Epilepsy: status epilepticus (diazepam); myoclonic seizures (clonazepam).

Sedation for operative procedures (for example bone-marrow trephine, endoscopy) and in preoperative medication (midazolam).

Dosages

Anxiety:

Chlordiazepoxide, 10 mg t.d.s. orally.
Diazepam, 2–5 mg t.d.s. orally.
Oxazepam, 10–20 mg t.d.s. orally.

Night-time sedation:

Nitrazepam, 2.5–5 mg orally.
Temazepam, 10–20 mg orally.

Status epilepticus:

Diazepam, 10–20 mg i.v. initially, repeated if necessary after 30 min. If effective this is followed by a continuous i.v. infusion.

Myoclonic seizures:

Clonazepam, 2 mg t.d.s. orally.

Sedation for operative procedures:

Diazepam, 10–20 mg i.v.
Midazolam, 2 mg i.v. over 30 s, followed after 2 min if required by additional doses of 0.5–1 mg; usual range 2.5–7.5 mg.

Premedication:

Midazolam, 2.5–5 mg 30 min before surgery.

Kinetic data

Clonazepam, nitrazepam, and midazolam are metabolized to inactive compounds. The following diagram illustrates the metabolic interrelations of some of the benzodiazepines. For the half-times of the benzodiazepines see Table 31.3 (p. 449).

Important adverse effects

Drowsiness and ataxia are common adverse effects with day-time therapy, and patients should take care when operating dangerous machinery (for example when driving). Because of the cumulative effects of the long-acting benzodiazepines, adverse psychomotor effects may become marked after a week or two of continuous treatment. Disinhibitory effects may occur, causing behavioural abnormalities, such as aggression.

Psychological dependence is common. Physical dependence also occurs, and withdrawal results in anxiety, agitation, tremulousness, seizures, and rebound sleeplessness with EEG abnormalities. For this reason the benzodiazepines should generally only be used for a few weeks at a time. Intravenous administration of diazepam sometimes causes thrombophlebitis, but the risk can be minimized by using an i.v. emulsion formulation.

Interactions

The benzodiazepines potentiate the central nervous depressant effects of other drugs (for example alcohol, barbiturates). Cimetidine inhibits the metabolism of the benzodiazepines.

Bleomycin

Structure

R = terminal amine (variable)

Mode of action

Bleomycin acts on DNA in several ways: it inhibits DNA synthesis by inhibiting DNA polymerase; it forms an oxidizing complex with iron, which causes breakage of single-stranded and double-stranded DNA through the production of free oxygen radicals; it prevents repair of DNA, by inhibiting DNA ligase. It is specific to the G_2 phase of cell division but is also active during other phases.

Uses

In the cytotoxic chemotherapy of testicular carcinoma, Hodgkin's lymphoma, non-Hodgkin's lymphoma, and various squamous cell carcinomas.

Dosages

Dosages of bleomycin vary with the indication, and it is usually used in combination chemotherapy (see p. 511). For example, in testicular carcinoma it may be used in combination with cisplatin and etoposide in a dosage of 30 mg i.v. weekly, stopping at a total dose of 360 mg.

Kinetic data

Bleomycin is poorly absorbed and is not effective after oral administration. It is widely distributed in the body but does not readily penetrate the brain. It is rapidly inactivated enzymatically in most tissues, especially the lung and skin, $t_{1/2} = 4$ h.

Important adverse effects

Anorexia, nausea, and vomiting are relatively common but mild.

Stomatitis can occur.

Allergic reactions are frequent in patients with lymphoma, include fever and chills after injection and hypotension and cardiovascular collapse.

Effects on the skin are common and include hyperpigmentation, alopecia, and desquamation of the hands and feet and over areas subject to pressure.

The most serious adverse effect of bleomycin is pulmonary fibrosis, and lung function should be monitored during therapy. If impairment of lung function occurs, or if changes are seen in the chest X-ray, treatment should be immediately withheld.

Interactions

For the possible interaction with live vaccines see p. 251.

Bumetanide

Structure

$$CH_3(CH_2)_3HN \overset{COOH}{\underset{OC_6H_5}{\bigcirc}} SO_2NH_2$$

(Compare with frusemide.)

Mode of action

Bumetanide inhibits the reabsorption of sodium and potassium in the ascending limb of the loop of Henle, by inhibiting an Na/K/Cl co-transport there. It may also inhibit sodium reabsorption in the proximal convoluted tubule. It also increases the secretion of potassium in the distal convoluted tubule.

Uses

Oedema due to cardiac failure, liver disease, nephrotic syndrome, and drugs.

Dosages

1–5 mg o.d. orally or i.v.

Kinetic data

Bumetanide is well absorbed. It is excreted 60 per cent unchanged in the urine, $t_{1/2} = 1.5$ h. The rest is metabolized and excreted in the urine and bile.

Important adverse effects

Muscle pains and cramps are common. The other adverse effects of bumetanide are similar to those of frusemide (q.v.). However, bumetanide is said to have slightly less potassium-depleting and uric acid-retaining properties than frusemide and is not magnesium-depleting. It is much less ototoxic than frusemide in high doses.

Interactions

Hypokalaemia potentiates the effects of cardiac glycosides and alters the effects of anti-arrhythmic drugs, increasing the incidence of arrhythmias.

Busulphan

Structure

$$CH_3SO_2O(CH_2)_4OSO_2CH_3$$

Mode of action

Busulphan is an alkylating agent with specific effects on the myeloid series of cells. Alkylating agents react with guanine moieties in DNA, resulting in a variety of effects, which cause mismatching of base pairs during replication,

direct damage to the DNA molecule, or crosslinking of nucleic acid chains.

Uses

Myeloproliferative disorders, especially chronic myeloid leukaemia.

Dosages

Each case needs careful individualization of dosage according to response. However, a general formula for the treatment of chronic myeloid leukaemia might be as follows:

Induction of remission: 60 micrograms/kg o.d. orally until the white cell count falls to between 20 and 25x10^9/L.

Maintenance of remission: 0.5–2.0 mg o.d. orally.

Kinetic data

Busulphan is well absorbed. About 30 per cent appears in the urine in 24 h as metabolites, principally methanesulphonic acid, $t_{1/2} = 3$ h.

Important adverse effects

Bone-marrow suppression is dose-related, the main effect being on the myeloid cells and platelets. Care should be taken if the platelet count falls below 100×10^9/L during treatment. Hyperuricaemia is common and may be prevented by allopurinol (q.v.); busulphan should not be given to patients with hyperuricaemia. Increased skin pigmentation occurs in up to 10 per cent of cases and may occasionally accompany a syndrome similar to that of hypoadrenalism. Other rare adverse effects include pulmonary fibrosis, cataract, and pulmonary infection with *Pneumocystis carinii* and cytomegalovirus. Busulphan should not be used during pregnancy.

Interactions

The combination of busulphan with thioguanine may cause nodular hyperplasia in the liver and portal hypertension as a result. For the possible interaction of busulphan with live vaccines see p. 251.

Calcitonins

Structures

Calcitonin is a naturally-occurring single-chain polypeptide containing 32 amino acids (molecular weight 3600 daltons), which circulates in the plasma both as the monomer and in polymeric forms up to a molecular weight of about 60 000. Porcine calcitonin is used therapeutically and synthetic human calcitonin is now also available.

Salcatonin is synthetic calcitonin with the structure of salmon calcitonin.

Mode of action

Calcitonin is secreted in the parathyroid glands and in the parafollicular cells of the thyroid. It lowers plasma calcium and phosphate concentrations principally by a direct effect on bone, decreasing osteoclastic and osteocytic activity, thus decreasing bone resorption. This effect is most marked when bone turnover rate is high (for example in Paget's disease). It also increases urinary calcium and phosphate excretion and decreases calcium absorption from the gut, but these are minor effects.

Uses

Paget's disease with bone pain or hypercalcaemia.

To lower the plasma calcium concentration acutely in hypercalcaemia (calcitonin is not very effective and should be used in combination with other methods of treatment, see p. 377).

Dosages

Dosage units

100 i.u. (international units) of porcine calcitonin = 1 mg.

100 i.u. of salcatonin = 0.025 mg.

80 i.u. calcitonin (pork) = 50 i.u. salcatonin.

Paget's disease

Porcine calcitonin, s.c. or i.m., 80 i.u. 3 times weekly to 160 i.u. daily in single or divided doses; in patients with bone pain or nerve compression 80–160 i.u. daily for 3–6 months.

Hypercalcaemia

Porcine calcitonin, 4–8 i.u./kg daily s.c. or i.m.

Salcatonin, 400 i.u. every 6–8 h s.c. or i.m., adjusted according to clinical effect; maximum dosage 8 i.u./kg six-hourly.

Bone pain in neoplasia

Salcatonin, 200 i.u. 12-hourly for 48 h, s.c. or i.m.

Kinetic data

Human calcitonin has a half-time of about 5 h. Since its metabolism is mostly in the kidney the $t_{1/2}$ is prolonged in renal failure. Salcatonin has a longer duration of action than human and porcine calcitonins.

Important adverse effects

Calcitonins may cause nausea, vomiting, and flushing, effects which diminish with continued treatment. Unpleasant taste sensations, tingling of the hands, and pain at the site of injection may also occur.

Porcine calcitonin and salcatonin are immunogenic and antibodies may be formed. Thus, during long-term therapy there may be resistance to the pharmacological effects of these calcitonins.

Allergic reactions may also occur, and in patients with a history of allergy a skin test should first be carried out using a 1:100 dilution.

Salcatonin is less immunogenic than porcine calcitonin and is to be preferred in these patients, but a preliminary skin test is still necessary.

Calcitonins may impair glucose tolerance and lead to increased hypoglycaemic drug requirements in diabetes mellitus.

Calcium antagonists

Calcium antagonists fall into three broad categories.

(1) The dihydropyridines. Nifedipine is the most commonly used of these, but the group also includes amlodipine, isradipine, nicardipine, nimodipine, nisoldipine, and nitrendipine.

(2) The phenylalkylamines, typified by verapamil.

(3) The benzthiazepines, typified by diltiazem.

(a) Dihydropyridines

Structures

General

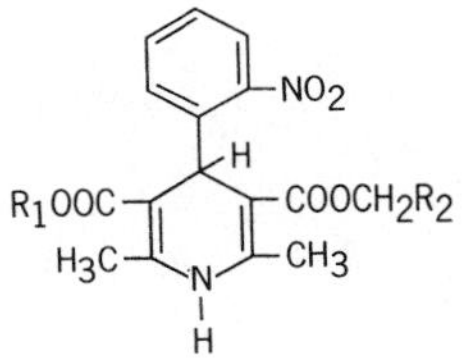

Examples

	R_1	R_2
Nifedipine	CH_3	H
Nicardipine	CH_3	$CH_2N(CH_3)CH_2C_6H_5$
Nimodipine	$CH(CH3)_2$	CH_2OCH_3

Mode of action

These drugs inhibit the transport of calcium into cells via L-type calcium channels. The dihydropyridines affect principally vascular smooth muscle, particularly in peripheral arterioles, causing a decrease in peripheral vascular resistance. They also affects normal coronary arteries, causing dilatation and preventing spasm.

Uses

Angina pectoris.
Hypertension.
Prevention and treatment of cerebral vasospasm in subarachnoid haemorrhage (nimodipine).

Kinetic data

The dihydropyridines are well absorbed after oral administration and more quickly after sublingual administration. However, they are extensively metabolized during the first passage through the liver to inactive metabolites with half-times of about 9 h (nifedipine 5 h). Because of a long side-chain at R_1 (see structure above), amlodipine has a longer duration of action than the other dihydropyridines, $t_{1/2} = 36$ h.

Dosages

Nifedipine, 5–20 mg t.d.s. orally, or 10–20 mg b.d. or a slow-release formulation.
Amlodipine, 5–10 mg o.d.
Isradipine, 1.25–2.5 mg b.d. initially, increasing as required to 5 mg b.d.
Nicardipine, 20 mg t.d.s. initially, increasing as required to 30 mg t.d.s.
Nimodipine: prevention of vasospasm in subarachnoid haemorrhage, 60 mg orally, 4-hourly; treatment of established vasospasm, 1 mg/h by i.v. infusion, increasing after 2 h to 2 mg/h if blood pressure satisfactory; start with 0.5 mg/h in small patients or those with an unstable blood pressure.

Important adverse effects

The commonest adverse effects are related to vasodilatation, and include headache, flushing, and oedema. In high dosages nifedipine may rarely exacerbate acute attacks of angina pectoris.

Interactions

Some of the dihydropyridines may increase plasma digoxin concentrations by an unknown mechanism. Digoxin dosage should be reduced if required, as assessed by plasma digoxin concentration measurements (see Chapter 7).

(b) Verapamil

Structure

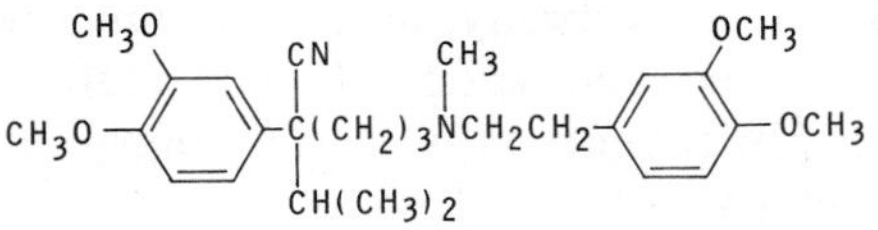

Mode of action

Verapamil is a calcium antagonist which has been categorized as a class IV antiarrhythmic drug. It impedes the transport of calcium across the myocardial and vascular smooth muscle cell membrane. It therefore prolongs the slow component of the action potential (phase 2, see lignocaine) and prolongs the effective refractory period. This effect occurs particularly in the SA and AV nodes, impairing conduction. It also results in a negative inotropic effect.

The effect on vascular smooth muscle results in peripheral vasodilatation and a reduction in the cardiac reload. This, coupled with the reduction in myocardial contractility, reduces myocardial oxygen requirements.

Uses

Supraventricular tachycardias, such as paroxysmal supraventricular tachycardia, and the reciprocating tachycardia of the Wolff–Parkinson–White syndrome.

Angina pectoris.

Dosages

Intravenous injection: 5–10 mg at a rate of 1 mg/min.

Intravenous infusion: 5–10 mg/h to a maximum of 100 mg/d.

Oral: 40–120 mg t.d.s.

Kinetic data

Verapamil is well absorbed orally, but is subject to 85 per cent first-pass metabolism in the liver. It is not known whether the metabolites have therapeutic activity. The $t_{1/2}$ of verapamil is 5 h and it is prolonged in liver disease.

Important adverse effects

The negative inotropic effect of verapamil may worsen cardiac failure.

Hypotension may result from both vasodilatation and the negative inotropic effect.

The effects on the SA and AV nodes may result in sinus bradycardia and impaired AV conduction. Verapamil should therefore be avoided in patients with the sick sinus syndrome, sinus bradycardia, and AV block.

Interactions

β-adrenoceptor antagonists may interact with verapamil: firstly, both are negatively inotropic and cardiac failure and hypotension may result from their combined use; secondly, there have been reports of asystole and an increased incidence of cardiac arrhythmias attributed to their concomitant use. Verapamil should not be used i.v. for at least 8 h after a β-adrenoceptor antagonist, but a β-adrenoceptor antagonist may be given within 30–60 min of an injection of verapamil.

Verapamil increases steady-state plasma digoxin concentrations by decreasing its renal clearance.

(c) Diltiazem

Structure

Mode of action

Diltiazem is a calcium antagonist which impedes the transport of calcium across the myocardial and vascular smooth muscle cell membrane. It therefore prolongs the slow component of the action potential (phase 2, see lignocaine) and prolongs the effective refractory period. This effect occurs particularly in the SA and AV nodes, impairing conduction. It has less of a negative inotropic effect than verapamil.

The effect on vascular smooth muscle results in peripheral vasodilatation and a reduction in the cardiac reload. This, coupled with the reduction in myocardial contractility, reduces myocardial oxygen requirements.

Uses

Angina pectoris.

Dosages

60–120 mg t.d.s. orally (b.d. in old people).

Kinetic data

Diltiazem is well absorbed orally, but is subject to 50 per cent first-pass metabolism in the liver and some of its metabolites have therapeutic activity. The $t_{1/2}$ of diltiazem is 5 h and it is prolonged in old people.

Important adverse effects

The effects of diltiazem on the SA and AV nodes may result in sinus bradycardia and impaired AV conduction. Diltiazem should therefore be avoided in patients with the sick sinus syndrome, sinus bradycardia, and AV block. It is teratogenic in animals and should therefore not be used in pregnancy.

Interactions

Diltiazem reduces the clearance of propranolol and the combination should be avoided.

Diltiazem increases steady-state plasma cyclosporin concentrations by inhibiting its metabolism and cyclosporin dosages should be reduced by about 40 per cent.

Diltiazem increases steady-state plasma digoxin concentrations by an unknown mechanism and digoxin dosages may need to be reduced.

Calcium salts

Uses

Chronic hypocalcaemia due to hypoparathyroidism or malabsorption (with vitamin D).

Acute hypocalcaemic tetany.

To stimulate myocardial contractility in cardiac arrest.

Kinetic data

Total body calcium in adults is about 500 mmol/kg (20 g/kg) of which nearly all is in the bony skeleton, about 25 mmol in all forming an exchangeable pool.

The normal plasma concentration is between 2.25 and 2.50 mmol/L, about 40 per cent of which is protein bound, 10 per cent in the form of diffusible salts (for example phosphate) and 50 per cent ionized. It is the ionized fraction which determines the amount of pharmacologically active calcium in the plasma.

Daily requirements of calcium are about 10–15 mmol (400–600 mg), increasing to 30 mmol (1200 mg) in pregnancy. The main sources of calcium in the normal diet are dairy products (milk, butter, cheese). Absorption of calcium is about 40 per cent but is very variable. Absorption is increased by parathyroid hormone and vitamin D and reduced by fatty acids and oxalates.

About 3 mmol (120 mg) of calcium are lost every day via the gastrointestinal tract and about 4 mmol (160 mg) via the urine. Renal tubular reabsorption is enhanced by parathyroid hormone in the distal renal tubules and by vitamin D in the proximal tubules.

Dosages

In the treatment of chronic hypocalcaemia dosages of calcium salts should be adjusted according to the response of the plasma calcium concentration. The maximum recommended dosage is 20 mmol/d. This can be given as one of a number of salts (for example calcium gluconate, 8.9 g; calcium lactate, 6 g).

In the treatment of acute hypocalcaemic tetany, i.v. calcium gluconate is used, 10–20 mL of a 10 per cent solution (i.e. 1–2 g of calcium gluconate, or 2.25–4.4 mmol of calcium) given over 10 min.

In cardiac arrest with electromechanical dissociation, especially in patients taking calcium antagonists and patients with hypocalcaemia or hyperkalaemia, i.v. calcium gluconate may be given (10 mL of a 10 per cent solution given over 10 min).

Important adverse effects

Excessive dosages may cause hypercalcaemia, resulting in general malaise, headache, anorexia, nausea and vomiting, muscle weakness, thirst, polyuria and nocturia, drowsiness, and confusion. In severe cases there may be psychosis and cardiac arrhythmias. Prolonged hypercalcaemia may cause tissue damage, with renal stone formation, nephrocalcinosis, and deposition of calcium in other tissues, such as skin, blood vessels, and eyes. In children hypercalcaemia may retard growth.

If calcium is given rapidly i.v. it can cause peripheral vasodilatation with consequent hypotension. Cardiac arrhythmias, nausea and vomiting, hot flushes, and sweating may also occur.

Interactions

Calcium salts should not be given i.v. in patients taking cardiac glycosides because of an increased risk of cardiac arrhythmias. They should not be given through the same i.v. line as bicarbonate salts (for example in cardiac arrest) because of precipitation of the insoluble salt calcium carbonate.

Carbamazepine

Structure

(Compare tricyclic antidepressants.)

Mode of action

The mechanism of action of carbamazepine is unknown, but it may act by stabilizing membrane potentials by encouraging the opening of potassium channels.

Uses

As an anticonvulsant (especially in the generalized tonic–clonic seizures of grand mal and the focal seizures of temporal lobe epilepsy).

Trigeminal neuralgia.

Relief of postherpetic neuralgia (in combination with a tricyclic antidepressant).

Dosages

100 mg o.d. orally, increasing at intervals of a few days up to 1600 mg if required. A controlled-release formulation is now available. This reduces the fluctuations in plasma concentrations and allows twice-daily administration and fewer adverse effects.

Kinetic data

Extensively metabolized; $t_{1/2} = 36$ h during chronic dosage. One metabolite may be active. Therapeutic plasma concentrations are in the range 13–42 μmol/L. Carbamazepine induces its own metabolism, and so plasma concentrations may fall after a week or two of initial therapy to a new steady state.

Important adverse effects

Visual symptoms are common at high doses (diplopia and blurred vision occurring at daily doses above 1200 mg). At all doses leucopenia may occur after a few months of treatment (6 per cent of all cases) but resolves after withdrawal. Central nervous effects, including drowsiness, loss of balance, and paraesthesiae, occur in up to 50 per cent of cases, depending on dose. Water retention may occur (inappropriate ADH syndrome).

Interactions

Carbamazepine may increase the metabolism of other drugs in the liver, for example other antiepileptic drugs and warfarin (see Chapter 10). It may thus increase the risk of pregnancy in women taking the oral contraceptive.

Alcohol potentiates the effects of carbamazepine on the brain and should be avoided.

Some drugs may increase plasma carbamazepine concentrations by inhibiting its metabolism. These include erythromycin, isoniazid, verapamil, diltiazem, and dextropropoxyphene.

Carbimazole

Structure

CH₃–N N–COOC₂H₅ (with S)

Mode of action

Carbimazole inhibits the iodination of tyrosine and perhaps also inhibits the coupling of iodo-tyrosines by inhibiting thyroid peroxidase. The end result is inhibition of the synthesis of triiodothyronine and thyroxine.

Use

To treat hyperthyroidism.

Dosages

Initially 30–60 mg daily orally, in single or divided doses, reducing the daily dose by 10–20 mg every 3–6 weeks to a maintenance dosage of 5–20 mg o.d. Continue treatment for 1–2 years (see the therapy of hyperthyroidism, p. 373).

Kinetic data

Carbimazole is rapidly metabolized to the active derivative methimazole, which has a $t_{1/2}$ of 6 h. Methimazole is mostly metabolized. Its duration of effect is longer than would be expected from its $t_{1/2}$.

Important adverse effects

Adverse effects occur in up to 7 per cent of cases, usually in the first 2 months of treatment. They are usually limited to gastrointestinal disturbances, headache, and skin rashes. In about 1 in 800 cases agranulocytosis occurs. When it occurs it usually comes on rapidly and patients should be warned to stop treatment and see their doctor if they develop a fever or sore throat. Over-treatment may result in hypothyroidism. Mothers should not breast-feed during treatment because of the risk of neonatal goitre.

Cardiac glycosides (digitalis)

Structures

General

Examples

	R₁	R₂	R₃	R₄	R₅
Digoxin	OH	H	CH₃	H	(Digitoxose)₃
Digitoxin	H	H	CH₃	H	(Digitoxose)₃
Ouabain	H	OH	CH₂OH	OH	Rhamnose

Mode of action

Cardiac glycosides inhibit the ATPase responsible for the sodium/potassium pump. Their electrophysiological effects and their effects on cardiac muscle are probably due to changes in intracellular free calcium concentration or disposition, secondary to the changes in intracellular sodium concentrations brought about by inhibition of sodium influx via the pump. The electrophysiological effects include slowing of the heart rate (*negative chronotropic effect*) due to decreased conduction velocity and prolongation of the effective refractory period in the AV node, in addition to effects on the other specialized conduction tissues and on various reflex arcs. The effect on cardiac muscles is that of increasing the rate of myocardial contractility (*positive inotropic effect*).

Uses

Treatment of atrial fibrillation (to slow the ventricular rate, although sometimes reversion to sinus rhythm occurs) and other supraventricular tachyarrhythmias (to slow the heart rate and to restore sinus rhythm). Treatment of cardiac failure, especially when due to ischaemic, valvular, and hypertensive heart disease.

Dosages

Oral

Digoxin: loading dose 15 micrograms/kg in three divided doses over 12 h, reducing the dose if evidence of toxicity occurs before the full dose has been given; the maintenance dosage depends on renal function, varying between 5 micrograms/kg o.d. with normal renal function and 2 micrograms/kg o.d. in the anephric state.

Digitoxin: loading dose 20 micrograms/kg given as described for digoxin; maintenance dosage 1–2 micrograms/kg o.d.

Intravenous

Digoxin, two-thirds of the oral doses.

Digitoxin, the same as oral doses.

Ouabain, 0.25–0.5 mg as the initial dose and continue with digoxin. When given i.v. digoxin and digitoxin should be infused over 0.5–1 h. Ouabain may be given over 5–10 min.

Important adverse effects

Adverse effects are dose-related. Common non-cardiac effects include anorexia, nausea, vomiting, and diarrhoea; confusion and acute psychiatric disturbances; visual disturbances (photophobia, blurring of vision, colour visual disturbances).

Virtually any cardiac arrhythmia may occur, the commonest being those which result from ventricular and supraventricular extra beats. AV nodal conduction may be impaired, leading to heart block. The combination of ectopic arrhythmias and heart block is particularly suggestive of glycoside toxicity. Bradycardia occurs occasionally.

The adverse effects of cardiac glycosides are enhanced by the following factors:

(1) electrolyte disturbances, especially *hypokalaemia*, hypercalcaemia, and hypomagnesaemia;

(2) hypoxia and acidosis;

(3) hypothyroidism;

(4) old age.

Patients with hyperthyroidism are relatively resistant to the therapeutic effects of cardiac glycosides.

Digitalis should not be used in the treatment of hypertrophic obstructive cardiomyopathy, since it increases the contraction of the left ventricle in the face of a fixed obstruction, thus worsening the condition. Its value in other cardiomyopathies and constrictive pericarditis is unclear.

It is of little value in the treatment of heart failure due to chronic cor pulmonale and may more readily cause toxicity because of the associated acidosis. It should not be used to treat arrhythmias associated with accessory conduction pathways (for example Wolff–Parkinson–White syndrome), since it impairs conduction through the normal conducting pathways without affecting the accessory pathways.

Kinetic data

	Absorption (%)	Elimination	$t_{1/2}$
Digoxin	67 (tablets) 80 (elixir) >90 (capsules)	Renal	40 h
Digitoxin	100	Metabolic	5 d
Ouabain	Virtually 0	Renal	20 h

Plasma concentrations should be below 3 ng/mL (digoxin) or 30 ng/mL (digitoxin) but toxicity may occur even below these concentrations (see Chapter 7).

Interactions

Hypokalaemia due to other drugs (for example diuretics) enhances the effects of cardiac glycosides.

Quinidine administration results in an increased incidence of adverse effects in patients on digoxin, because of diminished renal clearance and altered tissue distribution of digoxin.

Other drugs may cause an increase in plasma digoxin concentrations and increase the risk of toxicity. These include amiodarone and many of the calcium antagonists.

Cephalosporins and related compounds

Structures

The penicillins and cephalosporins share a common structure, the β-lactam ring, as seen in the following general structures:

Penicillins

Cephalosporins

R, R_1 and R_2 indicate a variety of different substituents. Cephamycins are related to the cephalosporins, having a methoxy group in the 7-position. Latamoxef is also related but has oxygen instead of sulphur in the general structure.

We shall refer here to the cephalosporins and related compounds collectively as 'cephalosporins'. The following are some of those available (see also Table 22.1):

Orally active: cephradine, cephalexin, cefaclor.
Injectable: cefuroxime (alternative cephamandole), cefotaxime, cefoxitin (a cephamycin), latamoxef (see 'structure' above).

The earlier cephalosporins, cephaloridine and cephalothin, have been supplanted by less toxic and more efficacious successors.

Mode of action

As for penicillin: inhibition of bacterial cell wall synthesis.

Bacterial resistance results mainly from bacterial production of β-lactamases (cephalosporinases), which open the β-lactam ring, destroying the activity. However, usually the β-lactam ring of the cephalosporins tends to be somewhat more stable than that of many penicillins toward the common β-lactamases. Nevertheless, with increasing use resistance to cephalosporins is emerging, and some bacteria now produce specific cephalosporinases.

Uses

In the treatment of infections caused by sensitive bacteria. The main bacterial sensitivities to cephalosporins and the usual indications for their use are shown in Tables P2 and P3.

Because new cephalosporins and related antibiotics with varying antibacterial spectra are continually being produced, there are changing opinions about the place of cephalosporins in the chemotherapy of infections. At the moment most authorities agree that the cephalosporins are usually second-choice antibiotics. They are seldom preferred to other first-line antibiotics on bacteriological grounds alone.

About 10 per cent of patients who give a history of an allergic reaction to penicillin will also be allergic to cephalosporins, so one cannot prescribe cephalosporins to penicillin-sensitive patients with absolute confidence, although they are in practice often used as alternatives to penicillin in penicillin-sensitive patients when the potential benefits outweigh the risks.

Dosages

Cephradine, 250–500 mg, 6-hourly orally or 0.5–1 g 6-hourly i.m. or i.v.

Cephalexin, 250–500 mg, 6-hourly orally.

Cefaclor, 250 mg 8-hourly orally.

Cefuroxime, 750 mg 8-hourly i.m.; up to 1.5 g 6-hourly i.v.

Cefotaxime, 1 g 6-hourly i.m. or i.v.

Latamoxef, 1 g, 8-hourly i.m. or i.v.

Cefoxitin, 1–2 g every 6–8 h i.m. or i.v.

Kinetic data

Elimination of the cephalosporins usually occurs by renal excretion. Cefotaxime is 40 per cent metabolized.

Because of preponderant renal excretion dosages should be reduced in renal failure. See Table P2 for values of $t_{1/2}$.

Important adverse effects

Allergic reactions occur in about 5 per cent of patients and are similar to those produced by the

∎ **Table P2** Sensitivities of various bacteria to some cephalosporins (see also Table 22.4)

Drug (Route; $t_{1/2}$	1	2	3	4	5	6	7	8	9	10	11	12
Cephradine (oral, i.m., i.v.; 0.9 h)	+ +	+ +	+ +	0	0	0	0	+ +	+ +	+ +	0	0
Cephalexin (oral; 0.9 h)	+ +	+ +	+ +	0	+	+	0	+ +	+ +	+	0	0
Cefaclor (oral; 0.6 h)	+ +	+ +	+ +	0	0	0	+ +	+ +	+ +	+ +	0	0
Cefuroxime (i.m., i.v.; 1.5 h)	+ + +	+ + +	+ + +	0	+ + +	+ + +	+ + +	+ + +	+ + +	+ + +	+	+ +
Cefotaxime (i.m., i.v.; 1.0 h)	+ +	+ +	+ +	±	+ +	+ +	+ + +	+ + +	+ + +	+ + +	+ +	+
Cefoxitin (i.m., i.v.; 0.7 h)	+ +	+ +	+ +	0	+ +	+ +	+ +	+ + +	+ + +	+ + +	0	+ +

+ + + Usually very sensitive.
+ + Quite sensitive.
+ Sensitive.
± Some activity but not useful.
⁰Usually resistant.

1. *Staphylococcus aureus*
2. *Streptococcus pyogenes*
3. *Streptococcus pneumoniae*
4. *Streptococcus faecalis*
5. *Neisseria meningitidis*
6. *Neisseria gonorrhoeae*
7. *Haemophilus influenzae*
8. *Escherischia coli*
9. *Klebsiella spp.*
10. *Proteus spp.*
11. *Pseudomonas aeruginosa*
12. *Bacteroides fragilis*

∎ **Table P3** Some infections in which cephalosporins would be commonly used as second-line agents

Infection	First line antibiotic	Cephalosporin
Acute otitis media (*Strep. pyogenes, H. influenzae*)	Amoxycillin	Cefaclor
Pneumonia (*H. influenzae* and *Strep. pneumoniae*)	Amoxycillin	Cefuroxime
Hospital-acquired urinary infections (resistant enterobacteria)	Gentamicin	Cefotaxime
Intra-abdominal infection (anaerobic bacteria: *Bacteroides fragilis*)	Metronidazole	Cefoxitin
Skin and soft tissue infections:		
Strep. pyogenes	Benzylpenicillin	Cephalexin or
Staph. aureus	Flucloxacillin	Cephradine
Gram-negative septicaemia:		
E. coli	⎰ Azlocillin +	Cefotaxime
Klebsiella spp.	⎱ Gentamicin	

penicillins. Some patients allergic to penicillins may also be allergic to cephalosporins (see above). Thrombophlebitis at the site of an i.v. infusion can be a problem. Infrequently the cephalosporins produce a positive Coombs' test, but haemolytic anaemia is very rare.

The older cephalosporins, for example cephaloridine, were undoubtedly nephrotoxic, but this does not seem to be a problem with the cephalosporins listed here.

Interactions

The nephrotoxicity of the older cephalosporins was enhanced by frusemide, ethacrynic acid, and aminoglycosides. It is doubtful that this is likely to be a problem with the cephalosporins discussed here, but it is still probably wise to be cautious about the use of large doses of cephalosporins in very ill patients receiving gentamicin, frusemide, or ethacrynic acid.

Chloral derivatives

Structures

General

$$Cl_3C - CH - R_1$$
$$R_2$$

Examples

	R_1	R_2
Chloral hydrate	OH	OH
Dichloralphenazone*	OH	OH
(Trichloroethanol	H	OH)

*Two molecules of chloral hydrate combined with one of antipyrine.

Mode of action

Cerebral depressant of unknown mechanism.

Use

Hypnotic.

Dosages

Chloral hydrate: 500–1000 mg orally.
Dichloralphenazone: 650–1300 mg orally.

Kinetic data

Well absorbed. Completely hydrolyzed to the active compound trichloroethanol which is in turn partly metabolized to the therapeutically inactive compound trichloroacetic acid, which does, however, participate in some drug interactions (see below). $t_{1/2}$ of trichloroethanol = 6 h.

Important adverse effects

The commonest adverse effect is the sensation of an unpleasant taste. This may be trivial but may sometimes be severe enough to require withdrawal of therapy. Gastric irritation with nausea and vomiting are also common.

Interactions

Stimulation of drug metabolism may result in reduced effects of oral anticoagulants.

Trichloroacetic acid displaces other drugs from protein binding sites, and this particularly affects phenytoin, warfarin, and tolbutamide. For a discussion of the clinical relevance of this effect see Chapter 10. The antipyrine in dichloralphenazone stimulates warfarin metabolism.

Alcohol potentiates the effect of chloral derivatives (for example 'Mickey Finn').

Chlorambucil

Structure

$$(ClCH_2CH_2)_2N - \langle \rangle - CH_2CH_2CH_2COOH$$

(Compare cyclophosphamide, melphalan.)

Mode of action

Alkylating agent (see busulphan).

Uses

Chronic lymphatic leukaemia.
Primary (Waldenström's) macroglobulinaemia.

Dosages

A general formula for the treatment of chronic lymphatic leukaemia might be as follows: Induction of a remission: 0.1–0.2 mg/kg o.d. orally for 3–6 weeks, monitoring the peripheral white cell count as a guide. Maintenance of a remission: 2 mg o.d. orally. However, each case needs careful individualization of dosage according to response.

Kinetic data

Well absorbed. $t_{1/2} = 1.5$ h. Mostly metabolized to phenylacetic acid mustard.

Important adverse effects

The most important adverse effects of chlorambucil are on the bone-marrow and on spermatogen-esis. Bone-marrow suppression is dose-related and is potentiated by concurrent radiotherapy or other cytotoxic chemotherapy. All alkylating agents may inhibit spermatogenesis; this results in oligospermia, which may be reversible but which may progress to irreversible azoospermia with sterility. Chlorambucil should not be used during pregnancy, because it is potentially teratogenic.

Interaction

For the possible interaction with live vaccines see p. 251.

Chloramphenicol

Structure

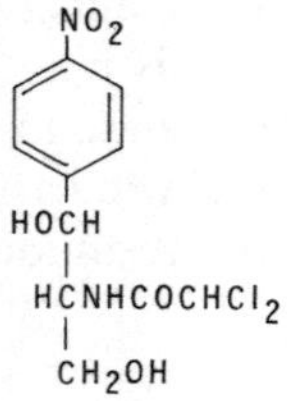

$$NO_2$$

HOCH

HCNHCOCHCl$_2$

CH$_2$OH

Mode of action

Inhibition of bacterial protein synthesis by an effect on the 50S ribosomal subunit.

Uses

Infections due to:
Gram-positive cocci (anaerobic streptococci, *Strep. pneumoniae*).
Gram-negative cocci (*N. meningitidis*).
Gram-negative bacilli (*E. coli*; *Kl. pneumoniae*, *S. typhi*, *Serratia*, *H. influenzae*, *Brucella abortus*).
Rickettsiae.
Chlamydiae.
The use of chloramphenicol should be severely restricted in therapeutic practice because of its adverse effects. However, it is still drug of first choice in meningitis due to *H. influenzae* and in acute typhoid fever. It is also the first alternative in penicillin-sensitive patients who have meningococcal or pneumococcal meningitis, and in Rickettsial infections in patients in whom tetracyclines are contra-indicated (for example pregnant women). It is very commonly used in bacterial infections of the eye.

Dosages

25–50 mg/kg in four divided doses, orally or i.v. Dosages should be adjusted if salts such as the palmitate are used, to allow for different molecular weights (for example 1.7 g palmitate = 1 g base).

Kinetic data

Well absorbed after oral administration but poorly absorbed after i.m. administration; for this reason the i.m. route is better avoided. Extensively metabolized by the liver. $t_{1/2} = 2$ h.

Important adverse effects

Neonates, who are unable to metabolize chloramphenicol as well as adults, may develop the 'grey syndrome' if ordinary dosages are used. The syndrome consists of peripheral circulatory collapse with cyanosis, vomiting, irregular respiration, abdominal distension, and diarrhoea. Neonates should either not be given chloramphenicol or given it only in low dosages (less than 25 mg/kg/d).

Chloramphenicol has two effects on the bone-marrow:

(1) A dose-related inhibition of erythropoiesis and other marrow functions. This effect usually occurs at high dosages (over 50 mg/kg/d) or after prolonged therapy (over 2 weeks), and is probably due to the same mechanism involved in the effect of chloramphenicol on bacterial protein synthesis. There is also inhibition of incorporation of iron into haem.

(2) A hypersensitivity reaction resulting in granulocytopenia, agranulocytosis, aplastic or hypoplastic anaemia, or thrombocytopenia. This adverse effect is uncommon (occurring in between 1 in 20 000 and 1 in 400 000 patients) but carries a high mortality, particularly if the clinical onset of the reaction is more than 2 months after the course of treatment.

Because of these effects blood test should be carried out regularly in patients taking chloramphenicol, and treatment courses should not be prolonged beyond 1 or 2 weeks.

Interactions

Chloramphenicol inhibits hepatic microsomal drug-metabolizing enzymes. It thereby increases the effects of oral anticoagulants.

Chlormethiazole

Structure

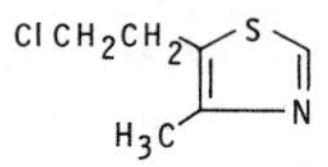

Mode of action

Although chlormethiazole is structurally related to vitamin B_1 (aneurine or thiamine) there is no evidence that its mode of action is exerted through an effect involving that vitamin. Its mode of action is not yet understood.

Uses

As a hypnotic and anxiolytic, especially in old people.

To treat the symptoms of acute alcohol withdrawal.

As an antiepileptic in status epilepticus (i.v. use).

Dosages

Chlormethiazole edisylate 250 mg = chlormethiazole (base) 192 mg. The dosages that follow are for the edisylate.

Oral:
Sedation: 250–500 mg at night.
Anxiety: 250 mg t.d.s.
Acute alcohol withdrawal: 1 g initially followed by 750 mg six-hourly for 2 d, 500 mg six-hourly for 3 d, and 250 mg six-hourly for 4 d. Do not continue for more than 9 d in all.

Intravenous (chlormethiazole edisylate solution contains 8 mg/mL (i.e. 0.8 per cent).):

Status epilepticus and acute alcohol withdrawal: 40–100 mL (i.e. 320–800 mg) at a rate of 4 mL/min initially, followed by continuous infusion at a rate of 1 mL/min, adjusting the rate subsequently to a rate sufficient to stop convulsions.

Kinetic data

Chlormethiazole is well absorbed, but is subject to extensive first-pass metabolism by the liver. Its systemic availability is therefore reduced in chronic liver disease, in which oral (but not i.v.) dosages should be reduced. $t_{1/2} = 4$ h.

Important adverse effects

The most common adverse effect is nasal irritation, causing sneezing soon after administration. Conjunctival irritation, headache, nausea, and vomiting may also occur.

Sedation is common with regular daytime dosages and patients should be warned to take care when driving or operating machinery.

There is a risk of dependence of the barbiturate-alcohol type (see Chapter 31), especially in patients being treated for alcohol withdrawal symptoms, and in those patients treatment should be restricted to 9 d, as detailed above.

When given i.v. chlormethiazole may cause a superficial phlebitis. Other adverse effects during i.v. administration occur with high dosages, and constant observation of the patient is necessary during continuous i.v. infusion. These effects include sedation and respiratory depression.

Interactions

The effects of chlormethiazole are potentiated by other drugs which act on the central nervous system (for example alcohol, benzodiazepines).

Cimetidine inhibits the metabolism of chlormethiazole, reducing dosage requirements.

Chloroquine

Structure

Mode of action

Chloroquine has many actions, listed below.

As an antimalarial

(1) Interference with plasmodial DNA replication.
(2) Possibly metabolic effects upon plasmodia (chloroquine is concentrated in infected erythrocytes).

As an anti-inflammatory agent

The mechanism by which chloroquine exerts its effect in rheumatoid arthritis is uncertain. While chloroquine probably has a direct anti-inflammatory effect by stabilizing lysosomes, thereby inhibiting the release of lysosomal enzymes and preventing their inflammatory actions, the drug seems to have a more profound effect upon the disease process, more like penicillamine or gold (qq.v.).

Uses

1. Treatment of malaria due to chloroquine-sensitive *Plasmodium vivax*, *P. ovale*, *P. falciparum*, or *P. malariae*.
2. Rheumatoid arthritis and lupus erythematosus (especially of the discoid variety).

Dosages

Dosages here are expressed in terms of chloroquine base (150 mg chloroquine base = 200 mg chloroquine sulphate = 250 mg chloroquine phosphate).

Malaria

See therapy of malaria, p. 242 for details:

(1) Acute uncomplicated attack: 5–10 mg/kg daily.
(2) Acute complicated attack (chloroquine-sensitive *P. falciparum*): 10 mg/kg over 8 h then 15 mg/kg over next 24 h.
(3) Prophylactic dose: 300 mg weekly.

Rheumatoid arthritis and lupus erythematosus

150–300 mg orally daily (see 'adverse effects').

Kinetic data

Rapidly and completely absorbed. Chloroquine is concentrated in erythrocytes, liver, spleen, kidney, heart, and lung. It binds to melanin, and may be deposited in the cornea, forming characteristic opacities, and in the retina, causing retinal damage (see below). It is mainly (75 per cent) metabolized in the liver, the rest being excreted unchanged in the urine. $t_{1/2} = 5$ d. The long $t_{1/2}$ is mainly due to extensive tissue binding.

Important adverse effects

In the doses used in the treatment of malaria serious adverse effects are rare. Mild headaches, nausea and vomiting, pruritus, and skin rashes occur occasionally.

The larger doses used in rheumatoid arthritis and lupus erythematosus may cause corneal opacities and, more seriously, a retinopathy associated with visual loss (see p. 114). All patients taking long-term chloroquine treatment should be carefully monitored for ophthalmic changes.

Other effects of prolonged treatment include bleaching of the hair, bluish pigmentation of the skin and mucous membranes, lichenoid skin lesions, and ototoxicity. Occasionally thrombocytopenia occurs. Chloroquine may cause haemolysis in subjects with G6PD (glucose 6-phosphate dehydrogenase) deficiency (see Chapter 8).

Chloroquine is best avoided during pregnancy because of the danger of ototoxicity in the fetus, a hazard which is probably dose-related. However, it may be used in pregnant women with acute malaria, when the benefit outweighs the risk.

Some patients are hypersensitive to chloroquine and they should not be given it. Chloroquine may precipitate psoriasis in susceptible patients and is best avoided in patients with psoriasis.

Because it is cleared by both liver and kidney dosages should be reduced in patients with hepatic or renal disease.

Interactions

There is an increased risk of exfoliative dermatitis when chloroquine is used together with gold or phenylbutazone, and these combinations should not be used.

The risk of retinopathy is increased in patients also taking probenecid.

Cholestyramine

Structure

Typified structure of main polymeric groups.

Mode of action

Cholestyramine is an exchange resin. It sequesters bile acids in the gut, leading to a reduction in the amount of bile acids subject to enterohepatic recirculation. Because bile acids inhibit the breakdown of cholesterol, their reduction results in increased breakdown of cholesterol and consequent lowering of plasma cholesterol concentrations. Furthermore, removal of bile acids from the gut may reduce cholesterol absorption.

However, these effects may be offset by an increase in cholesterol synthesis.

Cholestyramine increases plasma triglyceride concentrations.

Uses

Familial hypercholesterolaemia (type IIa).
Pruritus of obstructive jaundice (due to accumulation of bile acids in the skin).

Diarrhoea due to ileal disease or resection (due to excess bile acids).
Digitoxin toxicity.
It should not be used in patients with hypertriglyceridaemia.

Dosages

Cholesterol reduction and diarrhoea: 12–24 g o.d. or in divided doses orally.
Pruritus: 4–8 g o.d. orally.

Kinetic data

Cholestyramine is not absorbed and is excreted unchanged in the faeces.

Important adverse effects

Constipation occurs in up to 50 per cent of cases and patients may complain of other gastrointestinal symptoms, such as nausea and heartburn. The absorption of vitamins A and K may be impaired.

Interactions

Cholestyramine inhibits the absorption of warfarin, thyroxine, and digitoxin.

Cholic acids (chenodeoxycholic and ursodeoxycholic acids)

Structure

Mode of action

Chenodeoxycholic acid (illustrated) is a naturally-occurring bile acid. Ursodeoxycholic acid is its 7β-epimer. They are used to dissolve gallstones and they act by at least two mechanisms:

1. By increasing the proportion of bile salts in the bile. This reduces the proportion of cholesterol in the bile below the value at which cholesterol precipitation occurs. Cholesterol reabsorption from formed cholesterol stones then results in dissolution of the stones.

2. By reducing cholesterol synthesis. The cholic acids inhibit microsomal 3-hydroxy-3-methyl-glutaryl coenzyme A (HMG CoA) reductase which converts HMG CoA to mevalonate, which is in turn metabolized to cholesterol. This is probably their main mode of action.

Use

In the treatment of radiotranslucent cholesterol-containing gallstones. Other types of stones are not affected.

Dosages

Chenodeoxycholic acid, 10–15 mg/kg daily as a single night-time dose or in two divided doses if more than 500 mg; continue treatment for up to 2 years, depending on the size of the stone.

Ursodeoxycholic acid, 8–10 mg/kg daily in two doses for up to two years, depending on the size of the stone.

In both cases treatment should be continued for 3 months after the stones have dissolved.

Kinetic data

In common with other bile salts these drugs are 95 per cent absorbed via the terminal ileum. Absorption is saturable and reduced at single doses of more than 500 mg. They are conjugated with taurine and glycine in the liver and are excreted into the bile. The conjugates are reabsorbed in the terminal ileum, but about 5 per cent is deconjugated by intestinal bacteria and converted to lithocholic acid, which is excreted in the faeces. The normal daily endogenous production of bile salts (the sodium salts of the bile acids) is about 10 mg/kg.

Important adverse effects

The major adverse effect is diarrhoea due to impaired intestinal water and electrolyte reabsorption. Tolerance to this effect occurs with prolonged treatment. Ursodeoxycholic acid causes less diarrhoea than chenodeoxycholic acid. Chenodeoxycholic acid may impair liver function.

The cholic acids should not be used in patients who have alimentary disorders which interfere with bile salt deposition (for example regional ileitis, cholestasis, a non-functioning gall-bladder, and severe chronic liver disease).

These drugs may exacerbate peptic ulceration and should not therefore be used in patients with peptic ulcers.

Interactions

Drugs which lower blood cholesterol (for example clofibrate) and drugs which increase cholesterol elimination in the bile (for example oestrogen) oppose the effects of the cholic acids.

Cisplatin

Structure

Cisplatin is a platinum complex *cis*-diammine-dichloroplatinum:

$$(NH_3)_2PtCl_2$$

Mode of action

Cisplatin inhibits DNA synthesis by cross-linking complementary strands of DNA, particularly at guanine residues. It is not specific for any particular phase of the cell cycle.

Uses

In the combination therapy of various malignancies, such as testicular carcinoma, ovarian carcinoma, and carcinomas of the head and neck.

Dosages

Dosage regimens vary with indication. For example, in testicular carcinoma cisplatin may be used, in combination with etoposide and bleomycin, in a dose of 20 mg/m^2 of body surface area, given i.v. for 5 d every 3 weeks and for four courses.

Because it is nephrotoxic cisplatin must be given only after hydration of the patient with 1–2 L of i.v. fluid 8–12 h beforehand. Hydration must also be maintained for 24 h thereafter, since vomiting is common.

Kinetic data

Not absorbed after oral administration. It is rapidly cleared from the plasma but the metabolites are extensively bound to tissues and consequently the overall $t_{1/2}$ of platinum in the body is long (about 3 d). Platinum may be detected in tissues 4 months or more after a dose. Platinum is excreted in the urine, and dosages of cisplatin should be reduced in renal failure.

Important adverse effects

Severe nausea and vomiting often occur after treatment starting within a few hours and usually lasting for a day, but sometimes up to a week. Bone-marrow toxicity is dose-related (see Chapter 36, p. 512).

Nephrotoxicity is important and results in reduced creatinine clearance and necrotic changes in the kidney. Patients with renal failure are more at risk because of accumulation, and the toxicity is therefore self-perpetuating.

Ototoxicity is common and results in tinnitus and deafness. Formal audiometry should be carried out before each dose. When high dosages are used a peripheral neuropathy can occur.

Hypomagnesaemia can occur but can usually be prevented by the prophylactic administration of parenteral magnesium.

Interactions

Gentamicin may potentiate the nephrotoxic effects of cisplatin. For the possible interactions with live vaccines see p. 251.

Colchicine

Structure

Mode of action

A plausible explanation of the action of colchicine in gout is that it inhibits the migration of phagocytes to gouty tissue and thereby prevents both the phagocytosis of urate crystals and the subsequent increase in local lactate release following phagocytosis, which is responsible for further urate deposition.

Uses

Acute gout.

Prevention of acute gout during the early phases of treatment of hyperuricaemia (for example with allopurinol, q.v.).

Dosage

Acute gout: 1 mg orally initially, then 0.5 mg every 2–3 h until the pain subsides, *or* vomiting or diarrhoea occur, *or* until a total dose of 10 mg has been given. Colchicine should then not be given for a further 3 d.

Prophylaxis of acute gout: 0.5 mg b.d. orally.

Dosages should be reduced in hepatic failure and severe renal failure.

Kinetic data

Although colchicine is said to have a short $t_{1/2}$ (about 1 h), in leucocytes it may be detectable for several *days* after a single dose, and clearly accumulation occurs. It is mostly metabolized (80 per cent) in the liver and its metabolites are excreted in the bile.

Important adverse effects

Gastrointestinal symptoms are dose-related and include abdominal pain, diarrhoea, nausea, and vomiting, and in severe poisoning an enteritis resembling cholera.

Rarely bone-marrow suppression, resulting in leucopenia and thrombocytopenia, may occur during chronic administration, as may steatorrhoea, and peripheral neuropathy or myopathy.

Corticosteroids

1. Glucocorticoids

Structures

The general structure of the glucocorticoids is illustrated here by hydrocortisone.

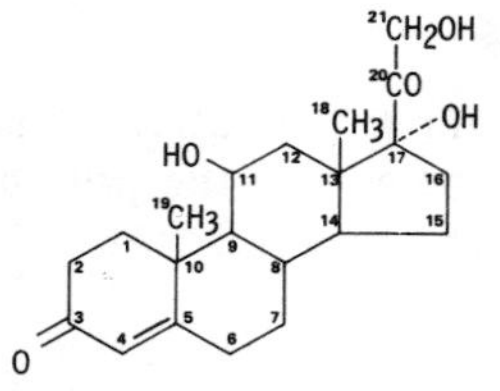

Various groups in this general structure can be substituted to form compounds with greater or lesser glucocorticoid or mineralocorticoid activity. For example, hydroxylation or methylation at the C16 position decreases mineralocorticoid activity, while α-fluoro-substitution of the C9 position increase mineralocorticoid activity. Thus, betamethasone and dexamethasone are potent glucocorticoids with little mineralocorticoid activity, whereas 9-α-fluorohydrocortisone (fludrocortisone) is a potent mineralocorticoid (see p. 587) with little glucocorticoid activity.

Mode of action

Glucocorticoids have the following effects:

1. *Effects on protein and carbohydrate metabolism* Glucocorticoids induce the mobilization of proteins and amino acids from skeletal muscle, skin and bone. Enzymes involved in gluconeogenesis are induced by glucocorticoids, the mobilized amino acids are converted in the liver to glucose, and glycogen stores are built up. There is therefore a negative nitrogen balance. Large doses of glucocorticoids cause high blood glucose concentrations and diabetes mellitus may occur.

2. *Effects on fat metabolism* Body fat is redistributed, leading to truncal obesity and the so-called 'buffalo hump' and 'moon face'. Glucocorticoids also facilitate the actions of lipolytic agents, such as adrenaline, glucagon, ACTH, and TSH.

3. *Mineralocorticoid effects (see below)* The extent of mineralocorticoid effects varies from glucocorticoid to glucocorticoid.

4. *Anti-inflammatory and immunosuppressive actions* Glucocorticoids are widely used for these effects. They prevent the vascular response (i.e. capillary dilatation) and increased vascular permeability which normally lead to tissue oedema and swelling. They have inhibitory effects on the cellular components of the acute inflammatory response, inhibiting the migration of leucocytes and their phagocytic activity. They also inhibit certain aspects of chronic inflammation, for example capillary and fibroblast proliferation and the deposition of collagen. The precise mechanisms by which these effects are produced are unknown.

Glucocorticoids have immunosuppressive effects. They inhibit lymphocyte functions: the responses of both B-cells and T-cells to antigens are suppressed and this results in impairment of humoral and cellular immunity. Again the precise mechanisms underlying these effects are unknown.

Although from the above discussion it would appear that nothing is known about the mechanisms by which glucocorticoids exert their effects, that is not quite true. It *is* known that corticosteroids combine with cytosolic receptor proteins, and that this complex then binds to chromatin in the cell nucleus. RNA polymerases are activated and the transcription of specific mRNAs occurs. This results in the synthesis of protein in the ribosomes. Thus, many of the actions of glucocorticoids depend on protein synthesis, and one must presume that such proteins, either as enzymes or as regulatory factors, control the appropriate cell functions which result in the pharmacological effects described above.

Some of the anti-inflammatory actions of the corticosteroids may come about through their inhibitory effects on prostaglandin synthesis. This is also mediated by protein synthesis, since corticosteroids cause the synthesis of transcortin and macrocortin, proteins which inhibit prostaglandin synthesis through inhibition of phospholipase A_2. Cell-mediated responses may be indirectly inhibited by inhibition of the production of certain growth factors, including tumour necrosis factor and interleukins.

Uses

Replacement therapy

In hypopituitarism and hypoadrenalism.

Anti-inflammatory and immunosuppressive therapy

1. Diseases characterized by vasculitis (for example lupus erythematosus, polyarteritis nodosa, dermatomyositis, polymyalgia rheumatica, giant cell arteritis, Wegener's granulomatosis).
2. Sarcoidosis.
3. Rheumatoid arthritis.
4. Bronchial asthma.
5. Skin diseases of various kinds (especially eczema and psoriasis: local treatment; pemphigus: systemic treatment).
6. Eye diseases of inflammatory origin (but not *Herpes simplex*).
7. Some gastrointestinal disorders (ulcerative colitis, Crohn's disease).
8. Liver diseases, especially chronic active hepatitis.
9. Renal diseases, especially minimal change glomerulonephritis.
10. Prevention of transplant rejection.
11. Blood disorders, especially some haemolytic anaemias, idiopathic thrombocytopenia, and some haematological malignancies (acute leukaemias and lymphomas).
12. Septicaemic shock.
13. Cerebral oedema.

Malignancies

In patients with terminal illness prednisolone may for a short time induce a general sense of well-being.

Dosages

The relative potencies of available glucocorticoids are as follows, with hydrocortisone as reference:

Cortisone	0.8
Hydrocortisone	1
Prednisolone	4
Methylprednisolone	5

Triamcinolone	5
Betamethasone	25
Dexamethasone	25
Beclomethasone	50

The following are examples of commonly used dosages for the relevant conditions. There is a wide dosage variation for many of the conditions.

Oral therapy

Replacement: hydrocortisone 20–30 mg daily.

Anti-inflammatory and immunosuppressive treatment: prednisolone, initially 40–60 mg daily in two divided doses for a few days, then reducing gradually over a week or two to a maintenance dosage (usually 5–15 mg once daily in the morning), In some conditions (for example acute severe asthma) it may be possible to treat the acute condition without continuing with a maintenance dose simply by tailing off the dose completely.

Parenteral therapy

Addisonian crisis. An Addisonian crisis may be precipitated, in susceptible patients, by stress such as infection, trauma, or a gastrointestinal disturbance. In such circumstances replacement therapy should be given at high dosage, for example hydrocortisone 100 mg 8 hourly.

Substitution for oral therapy. There will be occasions (for example during surgical procedures) when patients taking oral corticosteroids need to have treatment continued i.v. One would then use hydrocortisone in a dose equipotent with the therapy being replaced (see examples of relative potencies above). Often, however, higher doses may be required because of the clinical circumstances (for example increased stress during surgical procedures).

Septicaemic shock. The use of corticosteroids in septicaemic shock is controversial, but if they are to be used the dose should be high, for example hydrocortisone i.v. in doses up to 500 mg repeated at 4-hourly intervals for a short period. During short-term therapy the risk of serious adverse effects, even with such high doses, is minimal.

Cerebral oedema. Dexamethasone, 10 mg i.m., then 4 mg 6-hourly until a clinical response occurs. The dosage should then be gradually reduced over the next week and oral therapy may be used where possible.

Rectal therapy

Ulcerative colitis. Prednisolone, 20 mg enema once nightly until a clinical response occurs.

Inhalation therapy

Asthma. Betamethasone, one puff (100 micrograms) or beclomethasone, two puffs (100 micrograms) by aerosol q.d.s.; budesonide, one puff (200 micrograms) o.d. or b.d.

Kinetic data

All are well absorbed. Cortisone and hydrocortisone are extensively metabolized ($t_{1/2} = 30$ min and 1.5 h respectively). The others are also metabolized, but at a slower rate, for example prednisolone $t_{1/2} = 3$ h, dexamethasone $t_{1/2} = 4$ h.

Important adverse effects
Oral therapy

The appearance of adverse effects is related to the duration of treatment and the dosage used. The following effects are common.

Suppression of the pituitary–adrenal axis occurs inevitably to a greater or lesser extent, depending on the duration of treatment. Steroid withdrawal will then result in hypoadrenalism, which may cause an Addisonian crisis. Withdrawal of steroids after long-term treatment should be very slow to allow recovery of normal adrenocortical function. Sometimes total withdrawal is not possible. The inhibitory effects of corticosteroids on adrenal secretion are greater at night than during the day. They can therefore be minimized by giving the dose all in the morning or half in the morning and half at lunchtime.

Oral steroids may cause all the features of Cushing's syndrome, i.e. moon-face, bruising, hirsutism, impaired glucose tolerance, hypertension, acne, weight gain, and osteoporosis with an increased risk of spontaneous fractures.

Gastrointestinal disturbances are common. At daily doses of prednisolone of 15 mg and over there is an increased incidence of peptic ulceration, the risk being related to dose and duration of treatment and being especially high in patients with a predisposition to ulceration (for example patients with rheumatoid arthritis, cirrhosis, and previous ulceration).

Corticosteroids may interfere with the normal inflammatory responses. This may result in the suppression of the clinical signs and symptoms of perforation of a peptic ulcer, or of any abdominal viscus ('silent abdomen'). The signs or symptoms of septicaemia or tuberculosis may be suppressed, and fever may be absent in conditions in which it would ordinarily provide useful information.

Salt and water retention may result in peripheral oedema which, in combination with hypertension, may cause heart failure. Mental disturbance can occur, including any kind of mood change. Ischaemic necrosis of the femoral head occurs commonly and is often bilateral.

Hypokalaemia may require potassium supplementation. Muscle weakness is common and may be accompanied by a myopathy. Glaucoma may occasionally be precipitated during systemic therapy. Cataracts are common and usually posterior in position.

In children retardation of growth occurs and epiphyseal closure may be delayed. Corticosteroid administration during pregnancy may suppress fetal adrenal function and cause cleft palate.

Inhalation therapy

Local irritation of the oropharynx and fungal infections of the upper respiratory tract occur. Long-term use may cause a reversible dysphonia, due to weakening of the adductors of the vocal cords.

Local application to the skin

This may cause atrophy with scarring and telangiectasia. Systemic effects from local treatment are uncommon, but may occur if large areas are treated under occlusive dressings.

Local application to the eyes

Infections may be exacerbated, with resultant corneal damage. This is particularly important in herpetic infections. Glaucoma may occur and is unpredictable; it is due to a genetic susceptibility and is usually reversible. Cataracts occur occasionally.

Interactions

Enzyme-inducing drugs may enhance the rate of metabolism of corticosteroids.

Hypokalaemia due to corticosteroids potentiates the effects of cardiac glycosides and alters the effects of class I antiarrhythmic drugs (see lignocaine). Other drugs causing potassium depletion may potentiate the hypokalaemic effects of corticosteroids.

The effects of antihypertensive and hypoglycaemic drugs may be attenuated by corticosteroids.

Corticosteroids may potentiate the effects of warfarin.

2. Mineralocorticoids

Structures

For fludrocortisone see under glucocorticoids.

Mode of action

Mineralocorticoids act on the distal convoluted tubule of the kidney, enhancing the reabsorption of sodium and the secretion of potassium and hydrogen ions. Water is retained along with the sodium. Aldosterone is the most potent naturally occurring mineralocorticoid (500 times more potent that hydrocortisone), but the semi-synthetic compound 9-α-fluorohydrocortisone (fludrocortisone), which is less potent, is used in therapy.

Uses

Replacement therapy in adrenocortical or pituitary insufficiency.

Postural hypotension. Temporary benefit, probably due to an increase in intravascular volume, may be gained in the treatment of postural hypotension. However, the danger of fluid overload in these circumstances is considerable.

Dosages

Fludrocortisone:

Replacement therapy: 50–300 micrograms orally o.d.

Postural hypotension: 50 micrograms orally o.d.

Kinetic data

Well absorbed. Extensively metabolized; $t_{1/2} = 30$ min.

Important adverse effects

Sodium and water retention result in oedema and cardiac failure in susceptible individuals.

Corticotrophins (ACTH and tetracosactrin)

Structure

```
  1   2   3   4   5   6   7   8   9  10  11  12  13  14  15
Ser-Tyr-Ser-Met-Glu-His-Phe-Arg-Trp-Gly-Lys-Pro-Val-Gly-Lys
                                                            |
                                                           16
                                                           Lys
                                                            |
                                                           17
                                                           Arg
                                                            |
 32  31  30  29  28  27  26  25  24  23  22  21  20  19  18
Ala-Ser-Glu-Asp-Glu-Ala-Gly-Asn-Pro-Tyr-Val-Lys-Val-Pro-Arg
 |
 33
Glu
 |
 34  35  36  37  38  39
Ala-Phe-Pro-Leu-Glu-Phe        Human ACTH
```

ACTH is a single-chain polypeptide containing 39 amino acids, of which the first 24 are identical in all species. Tetracosactrin (Synacthen®) is a synthetic, single-chain polypeptide containing those 24 amino acids. It has the same pharmacological effects as ACTH but a shorter duration of action.

Mode of action

ACTH is the endogenous adrenocortical-stimulating hormone synthesized in cells of the anterior pituitary. Its release is stimulated by the action of the corticotrophin-releasing factor (CRF) synthesized in the hypothalamus.

ACTH acts on the adrenal gland, stimulating the production of glucocorticoids, but has little effect on the production of aldosterone. Increases in circulating corticosteroid concentration decrease the secretion of ACTH (negative feedback).

Uses

In the diagnosis of adrenocortical insufficiency. As a short-term alternative to corticosteroids.

Dosages

Note: 1 mg of tetracosactrin i.v. is equivalent to 100 international units (i.u.) of ACTH.

(a) Short ACTH test of adrenal gland responsiveness to ACTH

(i) Tetracosactrin (Synacthen®)

0.25 mg i.m., with blood samples immediately before and 30 min after for measurement of plasma cortisol concentrations.

(ii) ACTH

40 i.u. i.m., with blood samples immediately before and 4 h after for measurement of plasma cortisol concentrations.

(b) As a short-term alternative to corticosteroids

(i) Tetracosactrin

As Synacthen Depot®, a slow-release formulation of tetracosactrin with a zinc phosphate complex, initially 1 mg daily (or 12 hourly) in acute cases, then 0.5–1 mg i.m. once or twice a week.

(ii) ACTH

Initial dose 40–80 i.u. i.m. o.d. After a few days the dose and dosage interval should be altered according to the individual patient's response, in order to achieve a therapeutic effect with as low a dose as possible.

Important adverse effects

The corticotrophins are polypeptides and may therefore cause allergic reactions, including (rarely) fatal anaphylactic reactions. Even a mild allergic reaction should be a sign to withhold treatment.

Overtreatment can result in Cushing's syndrome, hypoglycaemia, and hypokalaemia.

The contra-indications to the use of corticotrophins are the same as those for the glucocorticosteroids (see p. 520).

Interactions

As for glucocorticosteroids (p. 587).

Co-trimoxazole (trimethoprim + sulphamethoxazole)

Structures

Sulphamethoxazole

See sulphonamides.

Trimethoprim

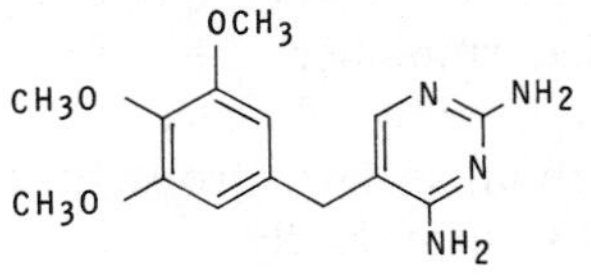

Mode of action

The original aim of this combination was to interfere with two different metabolic steps in folic acid metabolism, essential for bacterial integrity. The sequence is as follows:

2-amino-4-hydroxy-6-
hydroxymethyldihydropteridine
+
para-aminobenzoic acid

|
1
↓

dihydrofolic acid

|
2   dihydrofolate reducatase
↓

tetrahydrofolic acid

Sulphonamides inhibit the production of dihydropteroic acid at step 1. Trimethoprim is a dihydrofolate reductase inhibitor, decreasing the production of tetrahydrofolate at step 2.

Uses

Co-trimoxazole is used in infections due to bacteria sensitive to these agents (see sulphonamides). The combination is used most frequently in Gram-negative infections of the urinary tract (for example *E. coli*, *Proteus*) and chest (for example *H. influenzae*). It may also be of value in the treatment of typhoid fever, brucellosis, and infections with *Pneumocystis carinii* and *Nocardia*.

However, trimethoprim alone is as clinically efficacious as co-trimoxazole for most indications, especially for urinary tract infections and chronic bronchitis.

Dosages

Co-trimoxazole, 2 tablets b.d. orally (each tablet contains 480 mg of co-trimoxazole as 400 mg of sulphamethoxazole and 80 mg of trimethoprim).

Trimethoprim, 200 mg b.d., orally.

Kinetic data

Trimethoprim is rapidly absorbed, but both are well absorbed. $t_{1/2} = 10$ h (trimethoprim) and 9 h (sulphamethoxazole). The resulting steady-state concentrations are in the ratio 20:1 (trimethoprim:sulphamethoxazole), which is said to be the optimum ratio. Both are excreted mainly in the urine, and dosages should be reduced in renal failure.

Important adverse effects

Those attributable to sulphonamides (qq.v) but crystalluria does not occur. Folate deficiency may occur in those who are already relatively folate depleted. Bone-marrow toxicity is rare, but elderly people are more susceptible.

Cromoglycate and nedocromil

Structures
Cromoglycate

Nedocromil

Mode of action

Cromoglycate and nedocromil may act by inhibiting the release of histamine and the slow-reacting substance of anaphylaxis from mast cells in the mucosa of the bronchial tree, nose, and eye. It has also been suggested that cromoglycate may act by inhibiting local axon reflexes in the bronchial tree.

Uses

Prophylaxis of asthma and reversible aspects of chronic obstructive lung disease, allergic rhinitis, and allergic conjunctivitis.

Dosages
Cromoglycate

Asthma: 20 mg powder q.d.s., by inhalation via a so-called 'spinhaler'; 2 mg q.d.s. by aerosol; or 20 mg q.d.s. via a nebulizer.

Allergic rhinitis: Two drops of a 2 per cent solution q.d.s. intranasally.

Allergic conjunctivitis: One or two drops of a 2 per cent solution q.d.s. to the eyes.

Nedocromil

Asthma: 2 puffs (4 mg) b.d. by aerosol inhalation.

Important adverse effects

The common adverse effects of cromoglycate are trivial, but occasionally bronchiolar irritation, causing bronchoconstriction, may follow inhalation. This may be overcome by the use of 0.2 mg of isoprenaline incorporated into the powder formulation.

Nedocromil may occasionally cause headache, nausea, and a bitter taste.

Cyclophosphamide

Structure

(Compare melphalan, chlorambucil.)

Mode of action

Cyclophosphamide is an alkylating agent (see busulphan).

Uses

A wide variety of malignant diseases, including Hodgkin's and non-Hodgkin's lymphomas and multiple myeloma. It is also used in the treatment of various forms of necrotizing vasculitis, for example Wegener's granulomatosis, in which it acts as an immunosuppressive.

Dosages

Dosages vary widely and, as with all cytotoxic agents, specialist advice on dosage regimens should be sought.

Kinetic data

Cyclophosphamide itself is relatively inactive. In the liver it is metabolized to aldophosphamide, which circulates to other tissues where it is converted to cytotoxic alkylating derivatives, $t_{1/2} = 7\,h$. Cyclophosphamide and its metabolites are filtered by the renal glomerulus but undergo extensive passage tubular reabsorption; thus, only about 10 per cent of the administered dose is excreted unchanged in the urine. The polar metabolites may be toxic (see below).

Important adverse effects

Bone-marrow suppression is dose-related. Hair loss is common. Anorexia, nausea, and vomiting occur at higher dosages.

A haemorrhagic cystitis occurs in about 10 per cent of cases and bladder fibrosis may occur. This effect is thought to be due to toxic polar metabolites of cyclophosphamide, particularly acrolein. Measures taken to try to reduce its incidence include increasing fluid intake, alkalinizing the urine, bladder irrigation, and the administration of mesna (sodium-2-mercaptoethane sulphonate), which forms a non-toxic compound with acrolein and thus detoxifies it. Because mesna has a shorter half-time than cyclophosphamide ($1.5\,h$) it has to be given several times after each dose. Its use does not prevent the other adverse effects of cyclophosphamide.

Water retention and hyponatraemia may occur at high dosages, probably through an effect on the distal renal tubule.

Cyclophosphamide should not be used during pregnancy. Dosages may have to be reduced in patients with severe liver disease.

Infertility, caused by a testicular effect, resulting in diminished numbers of normal spermatozoa, may occur during long-term therapy and may not be reversible.

Interactions

Cyclophosphamide inhibits pseudocholinesterase and prolongs the neuromuscular blocking effect of suxamethonium. An alternative muscle relaxant should be used in patients taking cyclophosphamide and perhaps other alkylating agents (see p. 467).

Allopurinol potentiates the toxic effect of cyclophosphamide on the bone-marrow.

For the possible interaction of cytotoxic drugs with live vaccines see p. 251.

Cyclosporin

Structure

Cyclosporin is a fungal metabolite and is an unusual cyclic polypeptide.

Mode of action

Cyclosporin is predominantly active against T lymphocytes, preventing their activation and reducing lymphokine release. It binds to intracellular proteins (cyclophilins) and also to the intracellular calcium-binding protein calmodulin. Its binding to cyclophilins correlates with its immunosuppressive activity.

Uses

As an immunosuppressive agent in organ transplantation, in combination with corticosteroids and azathioprine. Also in the treatment of graft-versus-host disease and of autoimmune diseases involving T cell activation (uveitis, Behçet's disease, and Crohn's disease).

Dosages

The initial oral dosage in renal transplantation is $15\,mg/kg$ daily, reducing to a maintenance dosage of $3–10\,mg/kg/d$, but guided by trough whole blood concentrations. Intravenous dosages should be one-third of oral dosages.

Kinetic data

Cyclosporin is soluble in water and is given in an oily solution, with a systemic availability of 20–50; $t_{1/2} = 6\,h$. It binds to erythrocytes and lipoproteins. It is metabolized in the liver and excreted in the bile. Blood concentrations rise in liver disease. Some metabolites may also be immunosuppressive. For monitoring of blood concentrations see p. 93.

Important adverse effects

May be nephrotoxic in therapeutic doses. Hirsutism, gum hypertrophy, abnormal liver function tests, fits, hypertension, and muscle weakness may occur.

Secondary lymphomas due to Epstein–Barr B virus occur with increased frequency, because of impaired immune surveillance. In bone-marrow transplant recipients a haemolytic–uraemic syndrome has been reported. The intravenous formulation is dissolved in polyethoxylated castor oil and this is associated with anaphylactoid reactions.

Interactions

The metabolism of cyclosporin is enhanced by activators of the P450 cytochrome pathway (rifampicin, phenytoin); prednisolone competes with cyclosporin for this metabolic pathway. Aminoglycosides, ketoconazole, trimethoprim, diltiazem, and amphotericin all increase blood cyclosporin concentrations.

Cytarabine

Structure

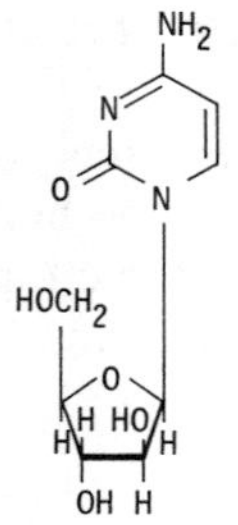

NH$_2$

HOCH$_2$

O

H HO

H H

OH H

Mode of action

Cytarabine (cytosine arabinoside or Ara-C) is converted within the cell to phosphorylated derivatives which competitively inhibit DNA polymerase, thus inhibiting the synthesis of DNA. This effect is specific to the S phase of cell division.

Uses

Acute leukaemias.

Dosages

Cytarabine is given i.v., usually in combination therapy (see Chapter 35). Recommended dosages vary, but an example would be 2 mg/kg by rapid i.v. injection daily until a response or toxicity occurs. Cytarabine may also be given by i.v. infusion, the total dose being infused over 24 h.

Kinetic data

Cytarabine is rapidly metabolized in the liver and many other cells, $t_{1/2} = 3$ h. It is mostly (90 per cent) excreted in the urine as the inactive metabolite, uracil arabinoside (Ara-U).

Important adverse effects

Anorexia, nausea, and vomiting are common, especially after rapid i.v. injection.

Stomatitis is uncommon.

Bone-marrow suppression is dose-related.

Interaction

For the possible interaction with live vaccines see p. 251.

Dantrolene

Structure

O_2N—⟨benzene ring⟩—furan—$CH{=}N$—(hydantoin ring with O, NH, O)

Mode of action

Dantrolene relieves muscle spasticity by a direct effect on skeletal muscle. This effect may be related to a decrease in the amount of calcium released from the sarcoplasmic reticulum, leading to a dissociation of excitation–contraction coupling.

Uses

To alleviate muscle spasm in spasticity, for example in multiple sclerosis, spinal cord injury, and cerebral palsy.

In the treatment of malignant hyperpyrexia (see Chapter 8).

Dosages

Oral: in order to minimize adverse effects start treatment with a low dosage, increasing according to response. Initial oral dosage should be 25 mg o.d., increasing at weekly intervals to 25 mg b.d., 50 mg b.d., 50 mg t.d.s., and 75 mg t.d.s. In a few cases up to 100 mg q.d.s. may be required.

Intravenous: in malignant hyperpyrexia, after discontinuing anaesthetic drugs give 1 mg/kg dantrolene and repeat as required up to a maximum of 10 mg/kg.

Kinetic data

Dantrolene is slowly and incompletely absorbed. It is mostly metabolized in the liver and excreted in the bile (50 per cent) and urine (25 per cent); $t_{1/2} = 9$ h.

Important adverse effects

Adverse effects are most common during prolonged oral treatment, and rarely occur after i.v. administration. The main effects are on the muscles and nervous system. Dantrolene causes muscle weakness and hypotonia, and that tends to reduce its efficacy as a treatment for spasticity. Common central nervous system effects include drowsiness, dizziness, vertigo, and nervousness. Patients should be warned to take care when driving or operating machinery.

Dantrolene may rarely cause liver damage, usually after prolonged treatment with high dosages. Furthermore, because it is mostly metabolized by the liver caution must be taken in patients with liver disease. Liver function should be monitored before and during therapy. Dantrolene should not be used in patients with *active* liver disease.

Dantrolene should be used with caution in patients with cardiac or pulmonary disease.

Interactions

Other drugs acting on the central nervous system (for example alcohol, tranquillizers) potentiate the central effects of dantrolene. The risk of liver damage may be increased in patients taking oestrogens.

Dapsone

Structure

H_2N—⟨benzene ring⟩—SO_2—⟨benzene ring⟩—NH_2

(Compare sulphonamides.)

Mode of action

Dapsone has the same antibacterial action as the sulphonamides (qq.v.).

Its mode of action in dermatitis herpetiformis is unknown.

Uses

Malaria prophylaxis (with pyrimethamine).
Leprosy.
Dermatitis herpetiformis.

Dosages

Malaria prophylaxis: given as Maloprim® tablets, one tablet each week (one tablet contains 100 mg dapsone and 12.5 mg pyrimethamine).

Kinetic data

Dapsone is slowly but well absorbed. It is poly-morphically acetylated (cf. sulphonamides), $t_{1/2} = 24$ h.

Important adverse effects

Allergic reactions are common, particularly skin reactions, but fever and hepatitis may also occur.

A dose-related, reversible, haemolytic anaemia may occur, due to a metabolite, and is more pronounced in patients with G6PD deficiency (see Chapter 8).

Interactions

Enzyme inducers increase the rate of metabolism of dapsone and shorten its half-time.

Debrisoquine

Structure

Use

The adrenergic neurone blocking drugs (for example debrisoquine, bethanidine, and guanethidine) are no longer used as antihypertensive drugs. However, debrisoquine is used as a marker for polymorphic drug hydroxylation of the type indicated by cytochrome P450IID6.

Dosages

A single dose of 10 mg is given before bed and the morning urine is collected for the measurement of the ratio of debrisoquine to 4-hydroxyde-brisoquine.

Important adverse effects

Adverse effects are rare after a single dose.

Desferrioxamine (deferoxamine)

Structure

Mode of action

Desferrioxamine is an iron-chelating drug which chelates iron mole for mole (i.e. 1 g of desferrioxamine chelates a maximum of 85 mg of iron). It removes all the iron bound to ferritin and haemosiderin, but much less from transferrin and none from haemoglobin, myoglobin, and iron-containing enzymes such as the cytochromes.

Uses

Acute iron poisoning.
Chronic iron overload secondary to repeated blood transfusion (for example in thalassaemia).

Dosages

Acute iron poisoning

Gastric lavage with desferrioxamine 2 g/L. Leave 10 g in 50 mL of water in the stomach. Give 2 g i.m. and repeat after 12 h (1 g in a child). Give 15 mg/kg/h by continuous i.v. infusion to a maximum of 80 mg/kg/day.

Chronic iron overload

Intramuscular: 25 mg/kg/d.

Subcutaneous: initially 2 g daily by continuous s.c. infusion over 6–12 h. In most patients this will produce a maximum effect on urinary iron excretion, which should be checked. However, higher dosages should be tried in all patients, since in some cases greater effects may be obtained from daily dosages of up to 16 g.

Kinetic data

Desferrioxamine is poorly absorbed and must be given parenterally. It is metabolized by enzymes in the plasma and also excreted unchanged in the urine.

Important adverse effects

The most important adverse effect during i.v. infusion of desferrioxamine is hypotension, perhaps because of histamine release. It should therefore not be injected rapidly when given i.v. Other adverse effects are rare and include skin rashes, dizziness and convulsions, pain after i.m. injections, and gastrointestinal irritation after oral administration. It is not yet known if there are serious adverse effects associated with the long-term subcutaneous administration of high dosages in chronic iron overload.

Interactions

Vitamin C (100–200 mg orally o.d.) improves the therapeutic effect of desferrioxamine in chronic iron overload, perhaps through its action as an antioxidant.

Dipyridamole

Structure

Mode of action

Dipyridamole inhibits ADP-induced platelet aggregation *in vitro*, and is thought to have a similar effect *in vivo*, thus inhibiting intravascular clot formation.

Uses

Prevention of emboli from prosthetic heart valves (in combination with warfarin).

Dosages

100–200 mg t.d.s. or q.d.s. orally.

Kinetic data

Well absorbed.

Important adverse effects

The most common effects are headache and diarrhoea. Peripheral vasodilatation may result in facial flushing.

Interactions

Because of its effects on platelets, dipyridamole may impair haemostasis in patients who bleed while taking anticoagulants.

Disopyramide

Structure

Mode of action

Disopyramide is a class I antiarrhythmic drug whose direct actions on the cardiac conducting tissues are virtually identical to those of quinidine and procainamide. These effects are discussed under lignocaine.

In addition, and in common with quinidine, disopyramide has potent anticholinergic effects. It also has a negative inotropic action.

Uses

Although it has been shown that disopyramide can be of use in the treatment of both supraventricular and ventricular arrhythmias, it is more useful in the latter.

Dosages

Intravenous: loading dose 2 mg/kg over 30 min followed by an i.v. infusion of 400 micrograms/kg/h to a total of 800 mg daily.
Oral: 100–200 mg 6-hourly.

Kinetic data

Disopyramide is moderately well absorbed. About 50 per cent of a dose is eliminated unchanged by renal excretion, and 20 per cent as the mono-*N*-dealkylated metabolite. $t_{1/2} = 6$ h. The clearance is reduced in renal failure and dosages should be reduced.

At therapeutic plasma concentrations the percentage of disopyramide bound to plasma proteins varies between 30 and 80 per cent, because its binding to plasma proteins is saturable. Thus, the unbound fraction of drug in the plasma is increased at higher concentrations and this results in a higher renal and metabolic clearance. The exact clinical significance of this has not yet been worked out.

Important adverse effects

Cardiac

The negative inotropic effect of disopyramide may cause hypotension and aggravate cardiac failure. This is particularly important during i.v. treatment and it is important to avoid too rapid infusion during the loading phase. Disopyramide prolongs the QT interval, although less so than quinidine, and ventricular arrhythmias as a result are also less common.

Anticholinergic

Dry mouth, blurred vision, and constipation are common. Disopyramide may exacerbate glaucoma.

Other

Nausea, vomiting, and diarrhoea sometimes occur. Hypoglycaemia has been reported.

Interactions

Disopyramide should not be used with other drugs which prolong the QT interval (for example quinidine, procainamide, and amiodarone).

The anticholinergic effects of other drugs (for example tricyclic antidepressants) will add to the anticholinergic effects of disopyramide.

The negative inotropic effects of other drugs (for example β-adrenoceptor antagonists) will be potentiated.

Hypokalaemia, for example due to diuretics, alters the effects of class I antiarrhythmic drugs on the cardiac action potential, and the hypokalaemia should be corrected when using disopyramide.

Domperidone

Structure

Mode of action

Domperidone is a selective antagonist at dopamine (D_2) receptors. It penetrates the nervous system poorly, but since the floor of the fourth ventricle, in which the chemoreceptor trigger zone is located, is accessible without penetration of the blood–brain barrier, domperidone has antiemetic effects without entering the brain. It also has effects on dopamine receptors in the stomach, where it increases oesophageal tone, increases pyloric contraction, and enhances the rate of gastric and duodenal emptying.

Uses

In the treatment of acute nausea and vomiting. It may be particularly helpful in treating nausea and vomiting due to L-dopa or dopamine agonists, since it will not prevent their beneficial effects, which are centrally mediated.

Dosages

Orally: 10–20 mg at 4–8 hourly intervals, depending on response.

Rectally: 1 or 2 30 mg suppositories at 4–8 hourly intervals, depending on response.

Kinetic data

Domperidone is well absorbed but extensively metabolized during its first passage through the gut and liver, $t_{1/2} = 8$ h.

Important adverse effects

In common with other dopamine receptor antagonists domperidone stimulates the release of prolactin from the pituitary and may cause galactorrhoea. It only rarely causes dystonic reactions (see metoclopramide) through inhibition of central dopamine receptors.

Interactions

The systemic availability of domperidone is reduced by food, antacids, and histamine (H_2) antagonists).

Its effects on the gut may be antagonized by anticholinergic drugs and opioids.

Dopamine

Structure

Mode of action

In low dosages (1–5 micrograms/kg/min) dopamine is active on dopamine receptors in renal arterioles and causes renal vasodilatation, which results in increased renal flow and diuresis. This action is useful in circumstances in which poor renal perfusion has led to the vicious circle of oliguria and worsening renal function.

In higher dosages (5–20 micrograms/kg/min) dopamine acts on cardiac β_1-adrenoceptors and produces a positive inotropic effect.

Very large dosages of dopamine (above 20 micrograms/kg/min) act on α-adrenoceptors, causing tachycardia, cardiac arrhythmias, and vasoconstriction, with deleterious effects, such as hypertension, angina, and even renal vasoconstriction.

Uses

Dopamine is used in the treatment of shock accompanied by poor perfusion, low cardiac output, and impending renal failure associated with such conditions as myocardial infarction (cardiogenic shock), severe trauma, septicaemia, and after cardiac surgery. It has also been used in the treatment of severe heart failure.

Because of its tendency to decrease peripheral resistance in low to medium doses, and also to reduce intravascular volume, the blood volume should be restored with plasma expanders when necessary before dopamine is used.

Dosages

The mode of administration of dopamine is important. It is infused i.v. generally in a final concentration of 1600 micrograms/mL (i.e. 800 mg of dopamine in 500 mL of physiological saline or 5 per cent dextrose). Infusion is usually started at 2 micrograms/kg/min and the dosage should be increased in increments of 5 micrograms/kg/min according to the patient's response, monitored by measuring urine output, blood pressure, vascular perfusion, heart rate, and (if available) central venous pressure. The maximum dose should usually be 20 micrograms/kg/min. Higher dosages have been used, but careful monitoring for adverse effects is necessary.

Kinetic data

Dopamine is eliminated mainly by metabolism (oxidative deamination, conjugation, and other routes). Its $t_{1/2}$ is short (2 min) and it is therefore given by continuous i.v. infusion.

Important adverse effects

In high dosages (see 'Mode of action' above) sinus tachycardia, extra beats and other arrhythmias, and vasoconstriction (with the risks of angina, hypertension, and renal impairment) are almost inevitable. Other common adverse effects include nausea, vomiting, and dyspnoea. If accidental overdosage occurs the α-adrenergic effects, such as hypertension, can be quickly controlled by discontinuing the infusion and administering the α-adrenoceptor antagonist phentolamine intravenously.

Interactions

Dopamine should not be used in patients taking MAO inhibitors, since they inhibit its metabolism. It should not be infused in alkaline solutions, which inactivate it.

Dopamine receptor agonists

Structures

Bromocriptine (illustrated here) is structurally related to ergotamine (q.v.). Lisuride is a structurally dissimilar dopamine agonist.

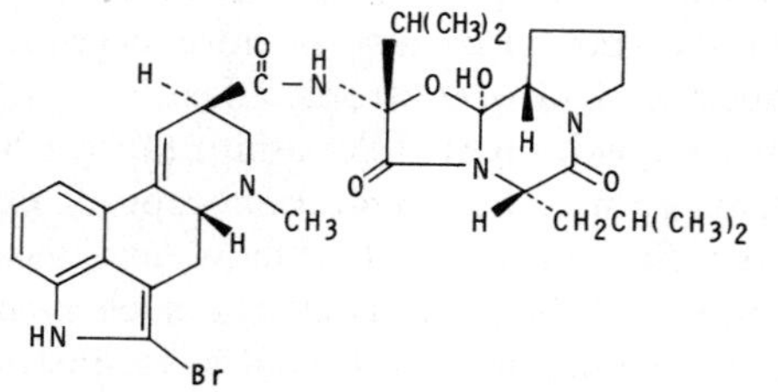

Mode of action

In Parkinson's disease the dopamine receptor agonists directly stimulate nigrostriatal dopamine receptors, to some extent replacing the effects of the deficient dopamine. This is currently the only indication for lisuride in the UK, but bromocriptine has other uses.

In hyperprolactinaemia bromocriptine inhibits the release of prolactin from the pituitary. It also inhibits lactation by this mechanism in healthy women.

The action of bromocriptine in acromegaly is paradoxical: in healthy individuals dopamine causes an increase in the release of growth hormone from the pituitary, as does bromocriptine; however, in acromegaly bromocriptine *inhibits* the release of growth hormone.

Uses

Parkinson's disease (idiopathic Parkinsonism).

The prevention and suppression of lactation after pregnancy.

Hyperprolactinaemia.

Acromegaly.

Cyclical breast disease and cyclical menstrual disorders.

Dosages

Note the wide differences in the dosages of bromocriptine in different conditions.

Parkinson's disease

Bromocriptine, initially 1.25 mg orally at night with food; increase as required by 2.5 mg every 2–3 d to a total of 40–100 mg per day in divided doses with food.

Lisuride, initially 200 micrograms orally at night with food; increase as required at weekly intervals to 200 micrograms b.d. then 200 micrograms t.d.s. Further increments can be made by adding 200 micrograms to each dose in turn. The maximum total daily dose is 5 mg.

Prevention of lactation

2.5 mg orally on the day of delivery, then 2.5 mg b.d. for 14 days.

Suppression of lactation

2.5 mg orally on the first day, increasing after 2–3 days to 2.5 mg b.d. for 14 days.

Hypogonadism with galactorrhoea (hyperprolactinaemia)

As for Parkinson's disease initially. The usual daily maintenance dose is 7.5 mg, but up to 30 mg may be required.

Acromegaly

As for Parkinson's disease initially. The usual daily maintenance dose is 20–60 mg.

Cyclical breast and menstrual disorders

As for Parkinson's disease initially, increasing to a maintenance dosage of 2.5 mg b.d.

Kinetic data

Bromocriptine is poorly absorbed and has extensive first-pass metabolism; $t_{1/2} = 15$ h. It is excreted in the bile. Lisuride is well absorbed but is subject to extensive first-pass metabolism; $t_{1/2} = 8$ h. It is excreted in the bile.

Important adverse effects

Adverse effects with these drugs are numerous, frequent, and dose-related. They can be minimized by slow introduction of dosage (see the regimens above) and by taking the drugs in divided doses through the day and with food.

Nausea, vomiting, and constipation are common. Hypotensive reactions can occur during the first few days of treatment, and patients should exercise care while driving or operating machinery. However, tolerance occurs.

Treatment of hyperprolactinaemia may make a woman fertile; for contraception a barrier method should be used, not oestrogens, since they may stimulate prolactin secretion.

In acromegaly there is an increased risk of peptic ulceration and bromocriptine increases that risk.

With the high dosages used in acromegaly and Parkinson's disease adverse effects are common and include drowsiness, confusion, dyskinetic reactions (particularly in patients also taking L-dopa), dry mouth, and leg cramps. Hallucinations, spasm of digital arteries, and cardiac arrhythmias can also occur, and care should be taken in patients with a history of psychosis or cardiovascular disease.

Interactions

The dopamine antagonists oppose the actions of the dopamine agonists and the dopamine agonists should not be used to treat neuroleptic drug-induced Parkinsonism. The combination of a dopamine agonist with L-dopa may be beneficial in Parkinsonism and may allow a reduction in the dosage of L-dopa.

Doxapram

Structure

Mode of action

Doxapram is an analeptic drug, i.e. it is a non-specific stimulant of the central nervous system. However, in low doses it is relatively specific in stimulating respiration, principally by stimulating carotid chemoreceptors, but also by stimulating the respiratory centre in the medulla oblongata (cf. nikethamide).

Uses

Respiratory stimulants have a limited role in the short-term management of ventilatory failure in patients with chronic obstructive airways disease. A doxapram infusion may be of use to stimulate respiration in those patients with hypoxia and hypercapnia who cannot tolerate even as low a concentration of inspired oxygen as 24 per cent without worsening CO_2 narcosis, and in whom artificial ventilation is contra-indicated. A single i.v. dose of a respiratory stimulant may also be useful in rousing patients for long enough to help them to cough up bronchial secretions.

Respiratory stimulants should not be used if there is no retention of carbon dioxide, or in patients with respiratory failure secondary to neurological or muscle disease, or in overdose. They are of no value in the long-term treatment of chronic respiratory failure.

Dosages

0.5–4 mg/min by continuous i.v. infusion, depending on response. Monitor progress frequently with arterial blood gas and pH measurements.

Kinetic data

Doxapram has a half-time after i.v. injection of about 3 h in adults and about 8 h in premature babies.

Important adverse effects

Adverse effects are common and dose-related. They include tachycardia and cardiac arrhythmias, nausea and vomiting, dizziness, restlessness, tremor, and convulsions.

Doxapram should not be given to patients with respiratory failure in association with neurological disease (including cerebral oedema), or to patients with acute severe asthma, coronary artery disease, hyperthyroidism, or severe hypertension. It should be given only with great care to patients with a history of epilepsy.

It is not helpful, and may be dangerous, in patients with respiratory depression due to overdose with hypnotics or sedatives. However, it may be used to treat respiratory depression due to buprenorphine if naloxone has not proved successful.

Interaction

The effects of doxapram are potentiated by MAO inhibitors, and the combination should be avoided.

Doxorubicin

Structure

Mode of action

Doxorubicin (former generic name adriamycin) is a cytotoxic antibiotic. It inhibits DNA-dependent RNA and DNA synthesis, by intercalating between DNA base pairs. It is known to affect topoisomerase II activity, has effects on the plasma membrane, and also generates free radicals. It is not specific for any phase of the cell cycle.

Uses

Acute leukaemias.
Many different malignant tumours, including breast cancer, sarcomas, and lymphomas.

Dosages

Doxorubicin is frequently used in combination therapy (see Chapter 36). A typical i.v. dose is 60 mg/m^2 body surface area given once every 3 weeks. It should be given through a fast-running infusion line in order to avoid thrombophlebitis and local extravasation. The total dose should not normally exceed 600 mg/m^2, because of adverse effects on the heart.

Kinetic data

Doxorubicin is poorly absorbed and is therefore not used orally. It is highly bound to tissues, which results in a long $t_{1/2}$ (17 h). It is metabolized by the liver, with 75 per cent excretion in bile as drug and active metabolite (adriamycinol). Dosages should be reduced if liver function is poor. Urine excretion accounts for about 10 per cent.

Important adverse effects

Nausea and vomiting and alopecia are common and usually moderate in severity. Diarrhoea and stomatitis may also occur. Bone-marrow suppression is dose-related (see Chapter 33). Doxorubicin is cardiotoxic and can cause a cardiomyopathy. This effect is dose-related (see dosages above). Treatment should be withheld if there is any evidence of a cardiomyopathy or of ECG changes (for example sinus tachycardia or other arrhythmias, T-wave flattening or inversion, ST segment depression). Doxorubicin should not be used in patients with pre-existing heart disease.

Interactions

For the possible interaction with live vaccines see p. 251. Doxorubicin may enhance the hepatotoxicity of mercaptopurine and azathioprine.

Ergotamine

Structure

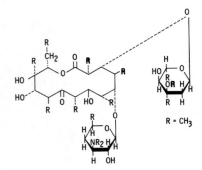

Mode of action

Ergot compounds cause vascular constriction and contraction of uterine muscle. The mode of action of ergotamine in migraine is uncertain (see p. 437).

Uses

Migraine.

Dosages

2 mg orally or sublingually at the onset of an attack, and repeated in 30–60 min if required. Not more than 6 mg in one day or 16 mg in one week.

In severe attacks parenteral ergotamine may be used: 125– 500 micrograms i.m. or s.c.

Aerosol: one puff (360 micrograms), repeated after 5 min if required; maximum 6 puffs in a day and 15 in a week.

Rectal: one suppository (2 mg), repeated after 30 min if required; maximum 3 per day and 6 per week.

Kinetic data

Ergotamine is poorly absorbed, especially during an attack of migraine. It is mostly metabolized during its first passage through the liver, which accounts for its routes of administration; $t_{1/2} =$ 3 h.

Important adverse effects

Peripheral vasoconstriction is common and ergotamine is contra-indicated in patients with established arterial disease. Overdosage is extremely dangerous and patients should be properly instructed as to the correct dosage. Even in those without vascular disease overdosage may lead to severe peripheral vasoconstriction and gangrene of toes and feet. Vasoconstriction may be relieved by the use of an α-adrenoceptor antagonist (for example phenoxybenzamine) or by a directly acting vasodilator (for example sodium nitroprusside).

The use of ergotamine is contra-indicated in pregnancy, because of its direct effect on the uterus, and during breast-feeding, because it enters the milk.

Nausea and vomiting are common during prolonged used and withdrawal may result in a headache.

Erythromycin

Structure

Mode of action

Inhibition of bacterial protein synthesis by binding to 50S ribosomal subunits.

Uses

Erythromycin is active against Gram-positive cocci, Gram-negative cocci, *Haemophilus influenzae, Mycoplasma pneumoniae, Legionella pneumophila,* and Gram-positive rods, such as *Clostridium perfringens* and *Corynebacterium diphtheriae.*

It is used in many infections with the above organisms in which penicillin would be the treatment of choice but where the patient is penicillin-sensitive. The most important exception is meningococcal meningitis, in which chloramphenicol is the best alternative to penicillin. Erythromycin is the treatment of choice in Legionnaires' disease.

Dosage

250–1000 mg q.d.s. orally or i.v.

Kinetic data

The absorption of erythromycin is variable and dependent on the salt form used: the estolate is best absorbed (the stearate and ethylsuccinate being the two other available salts). Erythromycin is 50 per cent metabolized and most of the remainder is excreted unchanged in the bile, $t_{1/2} = 2$ h.

Important adverse effects

It was once thought that intrahepatic cholestasis due to erythromycin was generally due to the estolate. However, jaundice probably occurs equally frequently with all the salts of erythromycin, and the estolate may be preferable for some patients and for children, who may find that other salts cause nausea, vomiting, or anorexia.

Intravenous administration often results in thrombophlebitis, particularly if high doses are used. Otherwise the most frequent adverse effects are gastrointestinal, and include nausea, vomiting, epigastric pain, and diarrhoea. Allergic reactions, particularly skin rashes, occur rarely.

Interactions

Erythromycin inhibits the metabolism of some other drugs, including theophylline and carbamazepine.

In a few patients it may inhibit the bacterial metabolism of digoxin in the gut, increasing its systemic availability.

Erythromycin may prolong the actions of warfarin.

Ethambutol

Structure

$$CH_3CH_2\overset{\displaystyle CH_2OH}{\underset{\displaystyle |}{C}}HNHCH_2CH_2NH\overset{\displaystyle CH_2OH}{\underset{\displaystyle |}{C}}HCH_2CH_3$$

Mode of action

Bacteriostatic to Mycobacteria by an unknown mechanism.

Uses

Tuberculosis.

Dosages

Initially 25 mg/kg/d given as a single oral dose. After a few weeks the dose is usually reduced to 15 mg/kg/d.

Kinetic data

Well absorbed. $t_{1/2} = 4$ h. Mostly excreted unchanged by the kidney.

Important adverse effects

Optic neuritis frequently occurs at dosages of over 25 mg/kg/d. It may result in loss of visual acuity, ocular scotomata, or colour vision defects.

Ethosuximide

Structure

Mode of action

Although the precise mode of action of ethosuximide is not understood, in animals it raises seizure thresholds to various convulsant stimuli.

Uses

Generalized absence seizures (petit mal).

Dosages

Adults and children over 6 years of age: 500 mg orally o.d. initially, increasing no more often than weekly to the minimal effective dose (usually no more than 1.5–2.0 g).

Kinetic data

Ethosuximide is well absorbed and mostly metabolized. $t_{1/2} = 60$ h. Optimal control of absence seizures is attained at serum concentrations of 280–700 µmol/L (40–100 g/mL).

Important adverse effects

Adverse effects are few and usually limited to gastrointestinal disturbances and CNS effects such as drowsiness, mood change, and dizziness.

Fibrates

General structure

X—⬡—R₃, R₁, R₂

Mode of action

The fibrates are isobutyric acid derivatives which inhibit cholesterol synthesis in the liver and increase the rate of removal of VLDL from the blood. As a result, there are falls in the plasma concentrations of triglycerides and (to a lesser extent) cholesterol.

Uses

Hyperlipoproteinaemias, particularly of types IIb, III, and IV, or in the presence of xanthomata.

Dosages

Clofibrate, 30 mg/kg daily orally in two divided doses.

Bezafibrate, 200 mg t.d.s.; 400 mg orally at night.

Gemfibrozil, 300–600 mg b.d. orally.

Fenofibrate, 200–400 mg daily in divided doses orally.

Kinetic data

All are well absorbed. The protein binding of clofibrate is saturable leading to non-linear kinetics at high doses or in the presence of hypoalbumi-naemia (see below). It therefore has a very variable 'half-time' (about 20 h at low doses). It is about 60 per cent metabolized by glucuronidation but otherwise excreted unchanged in the urine. The other fibrates have shorter half-times.

Important adverse effects

The incidence of gallstones is increased two- to three-fold in patients taking clofibrate because of altered bile composition. The other fibrates do not seem to do this, Clofibrate should be used only in patients without a gall bladder.

The fibrates may cause a myositis, with muscle pain, stiffness, and weakness. This is most commonly seen with clofibrate, particularly in patients with hypoalbuminaemia, for example in the nephrotic syndrome. The risk of myositis is also increased in patients taking an HMG CoA reductase inhibitor and this combination should not be used. Use the fibrates with caution in patients with renal impairment. Check the lenses annually for cataracts in patients taking gemfibrozil.

Interactions

Fibrates potentiate the anticoagulant effects of warfarin by increasing the turnover rate of factors II and X, and by displacing warfarin from its plasma protein binding sites. They reduce the adhesiveness of platelets and this may contribute to impaired haemostasis if bleeding occurs. The adverse interaction with the HMG CoA reductase inhibitors is noted above.

Fibrinolytic drugs

Mode of action

Streptokinase, alteplase, anistreplase, and urokinase are all activators of plasminogen and thus cause fibrinolysis (see Fig. P4).

Streptokinase is an enzyme isolated from haemolytic streptococci. It combines with plasminogen to form an activator complex which converts plasminogen to plasmin.

Urokinase is an enzyme similar to streptokinase, but obtained from human urine or cultures of kidney cells.

Alteplase is a plasminogen activator produced by recombinant DNA technology from human tissue cultures. It activates plasminogen already bound to fibrin and its action on circulating plasminogen is limited.

Anistreplase is *p*-anisoylated (human) lys-

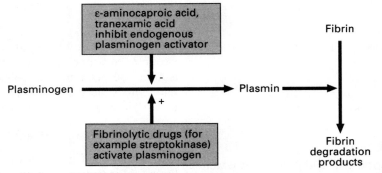

■ **Fig. P4** The activation of plasminogen and the effects of drugs which activate it or inhibit it.

plasminogen-streptokinase active complex. It is not active in plasma. It binds to fibrin, deacylation occurs, and plasminogen activator complex is formed, with some localization to the thrombus.

Uses

Myocardial infarction.
Thromboembolic disease of major vessels.
Major pulmonary embolism.
Thrombosis of large arteries.
Thrombosis of arteriovenous shunts (dialysis patients).
Studies are proceeding on the effect of the fibrinolytic drugs in cerebral thrombosis.

Dosages

Intravenous dosage in myocardial infarction

Thrombolytic treatment should be given as soon as possible (see Chapter 26 for details).
Streptokinase 1–5 million units by intravenous infusion over one hour.
Alteplase: a total dose of alteplase of 100 mg should be given intravenously over three hours: 10 per cent of the dose as a bolus over 1–2 min; 50 per cent of the dose as an infusion over 1 h, and 40 per cent of the dose by infusion over the next 2 h.
Anistreplase is given as a single dose of 30 units by slow intravenous injection over 5 min.

Intravascular dissolution of thrombi and emboli

Streptokinase 250 000 units are infused intravenously over 30 min, followed by a maintenance infusion of 100 000 units/h for 1–3 d, depending on the site of the thrombus or embolus.

Urokinase

1. *Thrombosed arteriovenous shunts*
   3000–37 500 units in 2–3 mL of 0.9 per cent sodium chloride by i.v. infusion into the shunt.

2. *Pulmonary embolism and deep venous thrombosis*
   Intravenous infusion of 4400 U/kg over 10 min then 4400 U/kg for 12 h in pulmonary embolism or 12–24 h in deep venous thrombosis.

Contra-indications and cautions

Recent or existing haemorrhage.
Recent severe trauma.
Recent surgery (including dental extraction).
Coagulation defects, bleeding disorders.
Active or recent peptic ulceration.
Severe hypertension.
Severe liver damage.
Oesophageal varices.
Recent abortion or delivery.
Recent puncture of large arteries.
Recent stroke, partcularly cerebral haemorrhage.
Severe diabetes mellitus with diabetic retinopathy.
Care in pregnancy: abortion or fetal death may occur.

In the case of streptokinase, previous allergic reactions to the drug, recent streptococcal infection, and streptokinase therapy within the last year should prompt the use of alteplase as an alternative.

Important adverse effects

Bleeding, particularly oozing at puncture sites. If bleeding is severe, the thrombolytic should be stopped and antifibrinolytic drugs (aprotinin or tranexamic acid) should be given with fresh frozen plasma. Other adverse effects include headache, pain in the back, allergic or anaphylactic reactions, vasculitic purpura, and vasculitic glomerulonephritis.

Fluorouracil

Structure

Mode of action

Fluorouracil (5-fluorouracil) inhibits thymidylate synthetase and hence decreases the production of thymidylic acid, the deoxyribonucleotide of thymine (5-methyluracil), a DNA pyrimidine base. Thus, DNA synthesis is blocked. It is specific to the S phase of the cell cycle.

Uses

Carcinomas of breast, ovary, and skin. Adenocarcinomas of the gastrointestinal tract.

Dosages

Fluorouracil may be given i.v. or topically. There is a variety of different regimens; an example is the palliative treatment of colorectal carcinoma, in which fluorouracil may be given in a dose of 12 mg/kg i.v. daily for 5 d every 4 weeks.

Kinetic data

Fluorouracil is poorly absorbed. After i.v. administration the apparent $t_{1/2}$ is about 20 min, but intracellular concentrations persist for much longer. It is converted inside the cell to its deoxynucleotide, 5-fluorodeoxyuridylate, which is pharmacologically active. Further metabolism occurs in the liver and the inactive products are excreted in the urine (10–15 per cent) and as CO_2 in the breath (60–90 per cent).

Important adverse effects

Anorexia, nausea, and vomiting are common. Stomatitis and diarrhoea are less common but are indications for withholding treatment. Bone-marrow suppression is dose-related (see Chapter 36). Alopecia and dermatitis can occur. Cerebellar ataxia occurs rarely.

Interaction

For the possible interaction with live vaccines see p. 251.

Folic acid (pteroylglutamic acid)

Structure

Mode of action

Folic acid is converted to several congeners of tetrahydrofolic acid, each of which plays an essential role in intracellular metabolism. The metabolic processes involved are as follows: the synthesis of purines and thymidylate; the conversion of serine to glycine and of homocysteine to methionine; the metabolism of histidine; and the utilization and generation of formate.

Uses

Folate deficiency (prevention and treatment).

Dosages

Prevention of folate deficiency: the daily requirement of folate is 50 micrograms but in pregnancy this increases to 200 micrograms or more. Because dietary folate intake may not be sufficient, folate is given in a usual daily oral dose of 200–500 micrograms during pregnancy, in combination with an iron salt.

Treatment of folate deficiency: 10–20 mg o.d., orally for a week or two, followed by a maintenance dose of 5 mg o.d.

Kinetic data

Folic acid is mostly absorbed in the upper jejunum. Its metabolism to active compounds (for example tetrahydrofolate) is dose-dependent, being almost complete at low doses (100 micrograms) but only 10–50 per cent at high doses (5–15 mg). If folate does not enter the body the total stores are depleted within four months (contrast vitamin B_{12}).

Important adverse effects

Folic acid is well tolerated, even in high doses, and adverse effects are exceedingly rare and limited to hypersensitivity reactions. It should never be given to patients with pernicious anaemia without concurrent administration of vitamin B_{12} since it does not prevent, and may precipitate, the onset of subacute combined degeneration of the spinal cord.

Frusemide

Structure

Mode of action

Frusemide is a loop diuretic, capable of producing a greater diuresis than diuretics which act elsewhere in the nephron. Its efficacy is similar to that of bumetanide (q.v.). It is called a loop diuretic because it inhibits sodium and chloride reabsorption in the ascending limb of the loop of Henle, with a resulting increase in sodium excretion and a decrease in free water clearance. It does this by inhibiting a Na/K/Cl co-transport system. In addition potassium secretion in the distal convoluted tubule is increased, because of exchange of potassium for sodium, under the influence of aldosterone and the increased intraluminal sodium concentration. This leads to increased potassium excretion.

The action of frusemide in the treatment of acute pulmonary oedema is complex. Intravenously administered frusemide will reduce pulmonary vascular congestion and pulmonary venous pressure within a few minutes, well before it has an appreciable diuretic effect. This action is thought to be due to systemic venous dilatation (i.e. a reduction in cardiac preload).

Uses

Oedema due to cardiac failure, hepatic disease, nephrotic syndrome, and drugs.
Acute pulmonary oedema.
Acute and chronic renal failure (note dose).

Dosages

As a diuretic

Orally: 40–160 mg o.d.
i.v.: 20–160 mg (also acute pulmonary oedema).

In renal failure:

i.v. infusion 250–2000 mg at a rate not exceeding 4 mg/min.
Orally: 250–2000 mg/d.

Kinetic data

Frusemide is poorly absorbed (about 50 per cent) and its absorption may be impaired in severe cardiac failure. It is mainly excreted unchanged in the urine, $t_{1/2} = 1$ h.

Important adverse effects

Hypokalaemia, hyponatraemia, and dehydration are the most important. Hypokalaemia may be prevented or treated with potassium supplements (q.v.) or potassium-sparing diuretics (for example spironolactone, amiloride, or triamterene). Hypomagnesaemia may also occur.

Hyperglycaemia is usually not of clinical importance, although in diabetes increased doses of oral hypoglycaemics may be needed.

Hyperuricaemia occurs but rarely causes frank gout.

In patients with prostatic hypertrophy acute urinary retention may be precipitated.

In hepatic insufficiency encephalopathy may be precipitated, particularly if hypokalaemia occurs.

Rapid intravenous injection of high doses may result in cochlear damage (usually reversible).

Interactions

Frusemide reduces the excretion of lithium. The dose of lithium should be halved.

Hypokalaemia potentiates the effects of cardiac glycosides. It alters the effects of anti-arrhythmic drugs such as procainamide and quinidine and there is a greater risk of cardiac arrhythmias, particularly polymorphous ventricular tachycardias.

The nephrotoxic and ototoxic effects of the aminoglycoside antibiotics are potentiated by frusemide.

Fusidic acid (sodium fusidate)

Structure

Mode of action

Fusidic acid is bactericidal to staphylococci and acts by inhibition of bacterial protein synthesis.

Uses

Infections due to penicillin-resistant staphylococci, particularly osteomyelitis.

Dosages

Fusidic acid 250 mg = sodium fusidate 175 mg. The dosages given here are for sodium fusidate.
Oral: 500 mg 8-hourly.

Intravenous: 500 mg by infusion over 6 h t.d.s.

Local applications: formulations contain 2 per cent fusidic acid or sodium fusidate and are applied up to four times a day.

Kinetic data

Fusidic acid is well absorbed. It is widely distributed to body tissues, including bone, but does not normally penetrate into the CSF. It is mostly metabolized in the liver and excreted in the bile; $t_{1/2} = 9$ h.

Important adverse effects

After oral therapy adverse effects are usually limited to nausea, vomiting, and skin rashes. Rarely reversible liver damage may occur.

After i.v. infusion thrombophlebitis can occur and infusion ideally should be via a large cannula in a large vein and at a slow rate (see dosages above). Liver damage is more likely after high dosages of i.v. fusidic acid than after oral therapy.

Gold salts

Structures

Sodium aurothiomalate

$$CH_2COONa$$
$$|$$
$$AuSCHCOONa$$

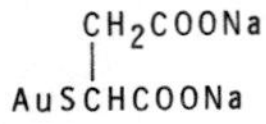

Auranofin

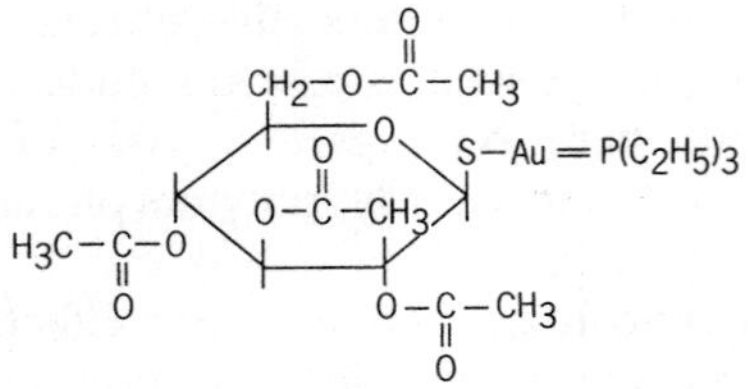

Mode of action

Although the detailed pharmacological actions of gold in rheumatoid and related types of arthritis are unknown, broadly speaking it suppresses inflammatory and immune responses. It is taken up by macrophages and inhibits phagocytosis and lysosomal enzyme activity; it reduces the concentrations of rheumatoid factor and immunoglobulins; and it suppresses cell-mediated immune reactions.

Uses

Severe active rheumatoid arthritis. Gold is toxic and its use should be restricted to cases particularly likely to benefit from its use; this usually needs specialist opinion.

Dosages

Sodium aurothiomalate

The patient's tolerance should first be tested by an i.m. dose of 10 mg. If no adverse effects occur, 50 mg is given i.m. once weekly until a therapeutic response occurs, after which the frequency of dosing may be reduced according to the clinical response. Many patients can be managed on 50 mg i.m. every 4–6 weeks.

If the patient relapses the dose should be increased to 50 mg i.m. weekly then readjusted as above. Treatment should be continued indefinitely.

Auranofin

6 mg daily increasing if necessary after 6 months to 9 mg daily. Discontinue if no response after another three months.

Kinetic data

Sodium aurothiomalate

Erratically absorbed after i.m. injection (time to peak plasma concentrations = 4–6 h). Eliminated unchanged in the urine. $t_{1/2} = 6$ d.

Auranofin

Poorly absorbed, mostly excreted via the faeces. $t_{1/2} = 21$ d.

Important adverse effects

Adverse effects are common, occurring in up to 40 per cent of cases. They may be serious in about 10 per cent. Skin rashes occur in about 25 per cent of cases. Blood disorders occur occasionally, and may be severe and fatal. They consist of thrombocytopenia, agranulocytosis, and aplastic anaemia. Traces of proteinuria are common and unimportant, but heavy proteinuria indicates more serious renal damage, and may be associated with the nephrotic syndrome due to a membranous glomerulonephritis. Stomatitis with oral ulceration and other gastrointestinal symptoms, such as nausea, vomiting, and abdominal discomfort, are common. Diarrhoea is common with oral gold.

Severe reactions to gold therapy may be controlled by the use of corticosteroids, with or without the addition of dimercaprol or penicillamine to hasten elimination.

Interaction

When gold salts are used in combination with chloroquine there is an increased risk of exfoliative dermatitis; this combination should not be used.

Griseofulvin

Structure

Mode of action

Griseofulvin binds to keratin and makes it resistant to fungal infections. It interacts with fungal microtubules and disrupts the mitotic spindle. New growths of skin, hair, and nails are the first to become free of infection, then as the fungus-infected tissues are shed they are replaced by uninfected tissues. It follows that treatment should be continued until the diseased tissue has been shed (see below under 'Dosages').

Uses

Griseofulvin is used in the treatment of ringworm (*Tinea*) infections of the skin, hair, and nails, particularly when these are widespread and intractable.

Dosages

0.5–1 g o.d. orally for at least 4 weeks (hair and skin infections), 6 months (fingernails), or 12 months (toenails). Griseofulvin should be taken after meals, when its absorption is improved.

Kinetic data

Griseofulvin is almost completely metabolized by the liver. $t_{1/2} = 15$ h.

Important adverse effects

Headache is the most common adverse effect and may be severe. Griseofulvin may precipitate an attack of acute intermittent porphyria (see Chapter 8).

Interactions

Griseofulvin induces the metabolism of warfarin by the liver and may reduce its effects.

Heparin

Structure

The value of n is variable, yielding molecular weights in the range 5000–20 000.

Mode of action

Heparin is a mucopolysaccharide which is acidic and carries a negative charge at physiological pH. It enhances the interaction between antithrombin III and both thrombin and the factors which are involved in the intrinsic clotting cascade. It also inhibits fibrin-induced platelet aggregation.

Uses

As an anticoagulant in the treatment of deep venous thrombosis and pulmonary embolism or in the prevention of deep venous thrombosis.

Dosages

Prophylaxis: 5000 i.u. every 8–12 h s.c.

Treatment: loading dose, 10 000 i.u. i.v.; maintenance dose 1000–1500 i.u./h by i.v. infusion.

These are usual doses; adjustments may be made on the basis of the partial thromboplastin time.

Kinetic data

Heparin is mostly metabolized in the liver. Its $t_{1/2}$ is dose-dependent: at low doses (< 5000 i.u. i.v.) it is about 1 h and increases to 2–6 h at higher doses.

Important adverse effects

Haemorrhage is a common complication. The effects of heparin may be reversed by an injection of protamine sulphate: 1 mg of protamine neutralizes 100 i.u. of heparin and the dose of protamine can be calculated on this basis within 15 min of a single dose of heparin. Obviously the longer the time after a single dose of heparin, the less heparin there will be in the blood, and the less protamine will be necessary to neutralize its effects. Protamine sulphate should not be given in doses greater than 50 mg and it should be given slowly i.v. (over 10 min) to avoid hypotension, bradycardia, flushing, nausea, and vomiting. Occasionally allergic reactions occur.

Thrombocytopenia is now a well-recognized complication of full-dose heparin therapy. There is an early transient thrombocytopenia due to a direct aggregatory effect of heparin on platelets; this usually improves. However, there also appears to be an immune mechanism which occurs 6–12 d after the start of heparin therapy; this is heparin-associated immune-mediated platelet aggregation, with the release of adenosine diphosphate. The activated platelets have themselves potent aggregating activity and may initiate thrombus and disseminated intravascular coagulation as well as thrombocytopenia. The risk depends on the duration of heparin therapy and it appears to be more common with bovine than with porcine heparin. Severe thrombocytopenia may necessitate withdrawal of heparin to prevent bleeding.

Low molecular weight heparin

The anticoagulant activity of heparin is a function of its molecular size. Low molecular weight heparin can be prepared by depolymerization or fractionation of commercial heparin and has a lower net molecular weight (approximately 5000 daltons) than the parent heparin. This low molecular weight heparin has a greater capacity to potentiate the inhibition of factor Xa than it does to potentiate the inhibition of thrombin or overall clotting, as measured by the partial thromboplastin time (PTT). Low molecular weight heparin therefore has little effect on the PTT but seems to have its effects higher up the cascade by inhibition of activated factor X. Possible advantages from this are lower risks of thrombocytopenia and bleeding. The other advantages are that is is not necessary to monitor the PTT, and that daily or twice daily subcutaneous injection is sufficient. Low molecular weight heparin has been particularly promoted for the prophylaxis of venous thrombosis, both pre- and post-operatively.

Histamine (H$_2$) antagonists

Structures

Cimetidine

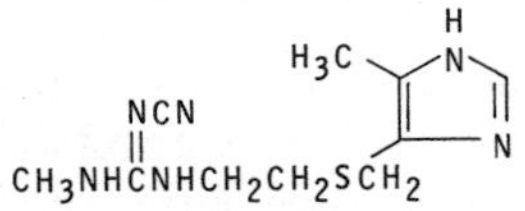

$$CH_3NHCNHCH_2CH_2SCH_2$$
$$NCN$$
$$H_3C$$
$$H$$
$$N$$
$$N$$

Ranitidine

$$(CH_3)_2NCH_2 \quad O \quad CH_2SCH_2CH_2NHCNHCH_3$$
$$CHNO_2$$

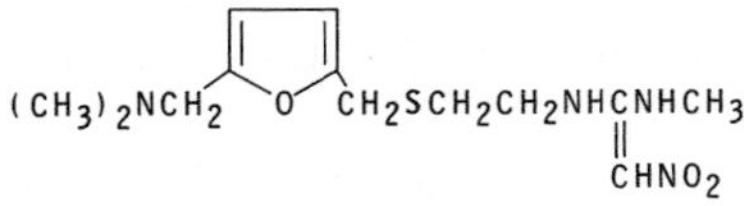

Other H$_2$ antagonists include famotidine and nizatidine.

Mode of action

These drugs are specific antagonists of histamine (H$_2$) receptors in the stomach and thereby reduce gastric acid secretion.

Uses

Gastric ulceration.
Duodenal ulceration.
Reflux oesophagitis.

Dosages

Cimetidine

Gastric and duodenal ulceration: 200 mg t.d.s. and 400 mg at night orally for 4–6 weeks; maintenance therapy: 400 mg nightly for 6 months;

Reflux oesophagitis: 400 mg q.d.s., orally for 6 weeks.

Ranitidine

150 mg b.d. orally for 4–6 weeks; maintenance therapy, 150 mg at night.

Kinetic data

	Cimetidine	Ranitidine
Absorption	Well absorbed	50 per cent
$t_{1/2}$	2 h	2 h
Elimination	Both are mostly excreted unchanged in the urine	

Important adverse effects

These drugs have few adverse effects during short-term treatment. Cimetidine causes an increase in plasma prolactin concentrations and has an antiandrogenic action by binding to androgen receptors. It may therefore sometimes cause gynaecomastia; ranitidine does not do this.

Although the question has been raised of the potential of these drugs to cause gastric carcinoma, there is no evidence that this happens. The suggestion that nitrosamine formation in the stomach, either from the drugs themselves, or from dietary nitrates because of the raised pH of gastric juices, might result in gastric carcinoma is purely speculative.

Interactions

There are two mechanisms whereby cimetidine interacts with other drugs:

Inhibition of hepatic drug-metabolizing enzymes. Interactions of this type with cimetidine have been described for warfarin, benzodiazepines, phenytoin, theophylline, lignocaine, and fluorouracil.

Decrease in liver blood flow. By decreasing liver blood flow cimetidine can reduce the clearance of drugs with a high extraction ratio (see Chapter 3). Interactions of this type have been described for propranolol and labetalol, whose systemic availability is increased.

Ranitidine has been reported not to interact in either of these ways with other drugs.

HMG CoA reductase inhibitors

Structures

Simvastatin is illustrated here. Lovastatin (not currently available in the UK) and pravastatin are closely related to it.

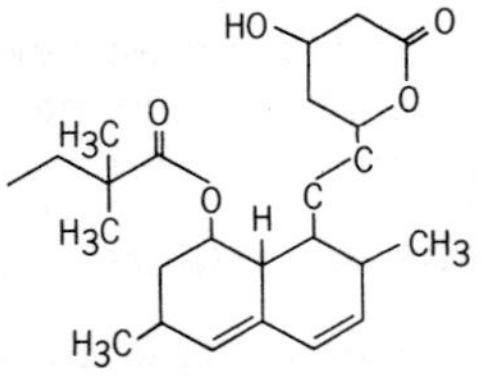

Mode of action

These drugs inhibit the action of hydroxy-methyl-glutaryl co-enzyme A (HMG CoA), the rate-limiting enzyme in the endogenous synthesis of cholesterol in the liver. This leads to upregulation of LDL receptors in the liver, which in turn causes increased clearance of LDL-cholesterol from the blood. They also increase HDL-cholesterol concentrations by an unknown mechanism.

Uses

Primary and secondary hyperlipoproteinaemias.

Dosages

Pravastatin and simvastatin, 10 mg o.d. at night, increasing if required in 10 mg increments at no less than 4-weekly intervals to a maximum of 40 mg o.d.

Kinetic data

Simvastatin is well absorbed, the others poorly. All are extensively metabolized by first-pass metabolism, $t_{1/2}$ about 2 h, with excretion in the bile. All are highly bound to plasma proteins.

Important adverse effects

The major adverse effect of the HMG CoA reductase inhibitors is a reversible myopathy, associated with muscle pain and/or weakness, raised plasma creatine kinase activity, and myoglobinuria; it occurs in about 0.5 per cent of patients. More commonly there is an asymptomatic increase in plasma creatinine kinase activity.

Liver function tests should be carried out regularly, since increases in liver transaminase activities are common. These are usually small and are often transient, but persistent increases occur in about 2 per cent of cases. If the rise is progressive and if activities reach three times normal the drug should be withdrawn.

Regular checks of the lenses of the eyes are recommended, because of reports of cataracts in animals, although this has not been reported in humans.

A variety of other minor adverse effects have also been reported, including insomnia, headache, nausea, dyspepsia, constipation, diarrhoea, and abdominal cramps.

Interactions

The myopathy due to the HMG CoA reductase inhibitors is exacerbated by concurrent use of the fibrates, niacin, and cyclosporin; these combinations should not be used.

Hydralazine

Structure

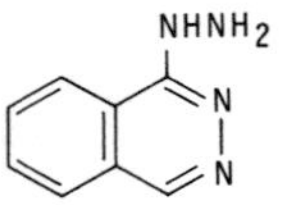

Mode of action

Hydralazine causes peripheral arteriolar dilatation by a direct relaxing effect on vascular smooth muscle, perhaps mediated by an action on potassium channels. This peripheral dilatation causes a fall in blood pressure with a resultant reflex tachycardia, which can nullify the fall in blood pressure. The reflex tachycardia is prevented by β-adrenoceptor antagonists which therefore potentiate the effect of hydralazine. For this reason hydralazine has been used in combination with a β-adrenoceptor antagonist in the treatment of hypertension. In the treatment of heart failure, on the other hand, peripheral vasodilatation lessens cardiac afterload with a resultant increase in cardiac output and little change in blood pressure; no appreciable reflex tachycardia occurs and the heart rate may slow because of improvement in cardiac function.

Uses

Hypertension.
Cardiac failure.

Dosages

Oral: 25–50 mg t.d.s. or q.d.s.
Intravenous or i.m.: 10–20 mg.

Kinetic data

Hydralazine is well absorbed and extensively metabolized, principally by acetylation, with a bimodal distribution in the general population (see Chapter 8). The $t_{1/2}$ is about 4 h and because the acetylation of hydralazine occurs mainly during the first passage through the liver, the subsequent rate of clearance is not appreciably related to the rate of acetylation, and is therefore unaffected by the patient's acetylator status. Thus, the $t_{1/2}$ does not much differ between slow and fast acetylators. The hydralazine which is not acetylated is hydroxylated.

Important adverse effects

Palpitation and tachycardia, nausea, vomiting, diarrhoea, and postural hypotension are all common.

In dosages over 200 mg daily an arthropathy resembling rheumatoid arthritis or a syndrome similar to that of systemic lupus erythematosus (so-called LE or lupus-like syndrome) may occur, especially in slow acetylators. Hydralazine-induced lupus is more common in patients with the HLA phenotype DR4.

Idoxuridine

Structure

Mode of action

Incorporation into viral DNA of idoxuridine results in faulty transcription, leading to failure of viral replication.

Uses

Infections with DNA viruses, particularly of the herpes group, for example superficial *Herpes simplex* keratitis (dendritic keratitis) and *Herpes zoster* infections (shingles).

Dosages

Skin: application of a 5 per cent solution in dimethylsulphoxide q.d.s.

Eyes: application of a 0.5 per cent ointment five times daily.

Important adverse effects

When applied locally idoxuridine has few adverse effects. Pain or stinging at the site of application occurs transiently, and inflammatory reactions may occur in the eye.

Immunoglobulin

Structure

Immunoglobulin for intravenous administration comprises 90 per cent monomeric IgG, with variable amounts of IgA and IgG dimers and fragments. The subclass distribution of IgG approximates to that of normal serum. Available products differ in their exact composition, because of differences in manufacturing techniques, and they should not be used interchangeably.

Mode of action

Immunoglobulin replaces absent antibodies in humoral immune deficiency. When used in high doses it reduces autoantibody production by B lymphocytes and blocks IgG Fc receptors on the phagocytic cells of the reticuloendothelial system. It may have other effects on T lymphocytes.

Uses

As replacement therapy for primary antibody deficiency and as an immunomodulatory agent in autoimmune thrombocytopenia, autoimmune haemolytic anaemia, and Kawasaki syndrome.

Normal immunoglobulin and specific immunoglobulins are used intramuscularly in passive immunization (see p. 251).

Dosages

Replacement therapy 200–600 mg/kg i.v. every week. As an immunosuppressive 400 mg/kg/d i.v. for 5 d or 2 g/kg i.v. as a single dose.

Kinetic data

$t_{1/2} = 21$–24 d. This is reduced in hypercatabolic states.

Important adverse effects

Immunoglobulin may produce immune-complex reactions with complement activation if it is infused into actively infected patients, leading to chills, shivering, headaches, and loin pain. Severe reactions cause bronchospasm and hypotension. Treatment is with antihistamines, corticosteroids, and if severe with colloids and adrenaline i.m.

(see the treatment of anaphylaxis, p. 524). Patients with renal impairment may develop transient worsening of renal function. IgA deficient patients (1 in 400 to 1 in 800 of the population) are at risk of developing anti-IgA antibodies, and may have anaphylactic reactions to intravenous immunoglobulin. Such patients should only be treated under the guidance of a specialist. Transmission of non-A, non-B hepatitis has occurred, but not of HIV.

Interactions

There are no specific drug interactions. False positive serology for viral and bacterial infections may occur after infusion.

Insulin

Structure

Human insulin

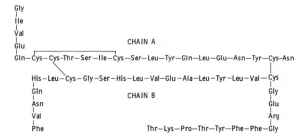

Mode of action

Insulin has multiple effects on the metabolism of carbohydrates, fats, and proteins, and acts on specific receptors on cell membranes to regulate various processes as follows:

1. It promotes the transport of glucose into cells and its utilization therein.

2. It increases hepatic glycogen formation and inhibits gluconeogenesis.

3. It inhibits lipolysis.

4. It increases protein synthesis and decreases protein breakdown.

When insulin promotes glucose uptake by cells, potassium influx is also enhanced. This is important, because during treatment of diabetic ketoacidosis with insulin the plasma potassium concentration may fall to dangerously low values unless intravenous potassium is given (see p. 379). This principle is also applied in the treatment of hyperkalaemia with insulin and glucose.

Uses

Diabetes mellitus.

Dosages and formulations

The dosage of insulin varies widely from individual to individual (see the treatment of diabetic mellitus, Chapter 27).

Insulin is formulated in solutions of strength 100 i.u./mL.

Kinetic data

Insulin is not absorbed from the gut, because it is metabolized by the proteolytic enzymes in the gut and the liver. It is therefore administered parenterally, usually subcutaneously, but in emergencies intravenously or intramuscularly.

One must distinguish between insulin itself (so-called 'soluble' insulin), which is a clear liquid, and the various formulations of insulin, which are designed to alter the absorption characteristics of insulin after s.c. injection, and which are always cloudy in appearance. After intravenous injection soluble insulin is rapidly metabolized by the liver and kidney with a $t_{1/2}$ of about 6 min. Other formulations are prepared by, for example, the addition of protamines to form isophane insulins, zinc to form zinc suspensions, differences in crystalline structure and suspension, and mixtures of these approaches. These changes alter the rate of absorption of insulin from subcutaneous injection sites, and it is the $t_{1/2}$ of *release* of insulin from these formulations which is the prime determinant of the duration of action. Some examples of types of insulin are shown in Table P4.

∎ **Table P4** Brand names of formulations of insulins available in the UK (all are in U100 (100 i.u./ml) strength)

(a) Human insulins

Type of insulin	Novo Nordisk Wellcome	Novo Nordisk	Fisons	Lilly
Soluble insulin (neutral)	Human Velosulin	Human Actrapid	Pur-in Neutral	Humulin S
Isophane insulin	Human Insulatard	Human Protaphane	Pur-in Isophane	Humulin I
Insulin zinc suspension (lente)	–	Human Monotard	–	Humulin Lente
Insulin zinc suspension (ultralente)	–	Human Ultratard	–	Humulin Zn
Biphasic neutral/ crystalline	Human Initard 50/50 Human Mixtard 30/70	Human Actraphane Penmix 10/90 Penmix 20/80 Penmix 30/70 Penmix 40/60 Penmix 50/50	Pur-in Mix 15/85 Pur-in Mix 25/75 Pur-in Mix 50/50	Humulin M1 Humulin M2 Humulin M3 Humulin M4

(b) Porcine and bovine insulins

Type of insulin	Novo Nordisk Wellcome	Evans	CP Pharm	Novo Nordisk
Soluble insulin (neutral)	Velosulin	No brand name	Hypurin Neutral	–
Isophane insulin	Insulatard	No brand name	Hypurin Isophane	–
Insulin zinc suspension (lente)	–	No brand name	Hypurin Lente	Lentard MC
Insulin zinc suspension (semilente)	–	–	–	Semitard MC
Protamine zinc insulin	–	–	Hypurin Protamine Zinc	–
Biphasic Neutral/ crystalline	Initard 50/50 Mixtard 30/70	–	–	Rapitard MC

Although the time of onset and duration of action of insulins (for example fast-, intermediate-, and long-acting) are related to the rate of release of insulin from its injection site, many other factors can influence this. As little as 50 per cent or as much as 80 per cent of a dose of isophane insulin may be left at the subcutaneous injection site by 6 h after injection. By 24 h the amount remaining varies from none to 50 per cent. Absorption is usually faster from the abdomen or arms, if the injection site is heated (for example in a hot bath), if the muscles underneath are exercising, or if the volume injected is small. Absorption is usually slower if insulin is injected into the legs or buttocks, if the injection site is damaged (for example fat hypertrophy), if the injection is cooled (this is useful in the treatment of insulin overdose), if the muscles underneath are at rest, and if the volume injected is large.

It should be remembered that if injections are given at intervals of less than about four half-times of release of a preparation (for example daily for ultralente, or twice daily for soluble insulin), a steady state will not occur until four or five half-times of release have elapsed. For example, in the case of ultralente a steady state will not be reached for about 5–7 d. Thus the effect of insulin treatment will be cumulative over that period of time.

The subcutaneous absorption kinetics of the commonly used insulin preparations are given in Table P5. Human insulins are prepared either semi-synthetically (by altering a single amino acid in the structure of porcine insulin) or biosynthetically (by introducing genetic material coding for the production of insulin into *E. coli* or yeasts). Some patients still take porcine insulin but bovine insulin is rarely used. Human insulin is used by 80 per cent of insulin-treated diabetics.

Important adverse effects

Acute hypoglycaemic reactions are common and result from either insulin overdose, mismanagement of the diet, or exercise. Chronic hypoglycaemia may result in neurological or psychiatric disturbances. A few patients who take human insulin report reduced awareness of hypoglycaemia compared with animal insulins.

Allergy occurs occasionally, resulting in local skin reactions at the site of injection or, less commonly, generalized reactions.

Lipodystrophy (either atrophy or hypertrophy) may occur at the site of injection. It may be avoided by the use of the modern purified

■ **Table P5** The characteristics of commonly used formulations of insulins

1. Short-acting insulins
Subcutaneous kinetics
  Time to peak action 2–4 h
  Duration of action 6–12 h
Formulations
  Neutral insulin

2. Intermediate-acting insulins
Subcutaneous kinetics
  Time to peak action 3–8 h
  Duration of action 12–20 h
Formulations
  Insulin zinc suspension (amorphous), semilente
  Isophane insulin
  Globin zinc insulin
  Biphasic insulin (neutral + crystalline)

3. Long-acting insulins
Subcutaneous kinetics
  Time to peak action 6–12 h
  Duration of action 16–30 h
Formulations
  Insulin zinc suspension (crystalline), ultralente
  Insulin zinc suspension (mixed), lente
  Protamine zinc insulin

preparations and by careful rotation of injection sites. Lipodystrophy may be reversed by changing from an old-fashioned insulin formulation to a purified variety.

Insulin resistance may occur, necessitating increased doses. This happens to a lesser extent with the use of purified preparations.

Interactions

Numerous hormones and drugs antagonize the effects of insulin, including β-adrenoceptor agonists, corticosteroids, growth hormone, thyroxine, glucagon, diazoxide, and thiazide diuretics.

Non-selective β-adrenoceptor antagonists (for example propranolol) may worsen hypoglycaemia, because they block the glycogenolytic effects of adrenaline. They also block most of the clinical manifestations of an attack of hypoglycaemia, but sweating is preserved.

Iron salts

Uses

Iron deficiency anaemia (treatment and prevention).

Dosages

Normal daily iron requirements are 1–2 mg, the average daily dietary intake in the UK being 10–20 mg.

Oral iron

In pregnancy daily requirements increase to 3–4 mg and dietary intake should be increased to 30–40 mg daily. This can be achieved using one tablet or capsule of any formulation available in the UK containing a mixture of a ferrous salt and folic acid (see Table 26.2).

Oral treatment of iron deficiency anaemia usually requires between 120–180 mg of elemental iron daily. Examples of commonly used dosages are:

Ferrous sulphate, 200 mg t.d.s. (= 60 mg of iron t.d.s.).

Ferrous fumarate, 200 mg t.d.s. (= 65 mg of iron t.d.s.).

Ferrous succinate, 200 mg b.d. (= 70 mg of iron b.d.).

Ferrous gluconate, 600 mg b.d. (= 70 mg of iron b.d.).

Numerous slow-release formulations are available for those who cannot tolerate ordinary formulations.

Parenteral iron

Calculate the total body deficit of iron from the following equation (see p. 399 for a discussion of its derivation).

iron deficit (mg) = Hb deficit (g/dL)

$$\times \text{ body weight (kg)} \times 2.21$$

Thus, a 50 kg woman with a haemoglobin of 8 g/dL (normal 14) will require $(14 - 8) \times 50 \times 2.21 = 663$ mg of iron.

Intravenous therapy

Note that the intravenous route is hazardous, because of the risk of allergic reactions. It is therefore reserved for special cases (for example women with severe anaemia in the third trimester of pregnancy). Intravenous iron is given as iron dextran (50 mg/mL), the total doses required being made up in 500–1000 mL of saline and infused over 6–8 h. It is important to give first a test dose of 50 mg over 10 min for signs of allergy before continuing with the infusion. Careful observation is necessary throughout the infusion and for an hour after. Be prepared to stop the infusion and to treat allergic reactions (see pp. 522–4).

Intramuscular therapy

Iron dextran (50 mg of iron/mL), 1 mL on the first day, 2 mL on subsequent days.

Iron sorbitol (50 mg of iron/mL), 1.5 mL/kg up to a maximum of 100 mg daily or on alternate days.

The number of injections likely to be required can be calculated from the calculated deficit (see above).

Because staining at the i.m. injection site can occur due to leakage of iron along the needle track, a special injection technique is required: draw back the skin over the intended injection site in the buttock as far as it will go; inject deeply into the muscle using a long (5 cm) long-bevelled needle; after injection and removal of the needle the tissues which have been drawn back over the injection point will fall back and create a zigzag needle track. In this way staining can be reduced, although not completely eliminated.

Kinetic data

Medicinal iron behaves in the same way as dietary iron. Normally about 10 per cent of oral intake is absorbed, but absorption increases in iron deficiency and decreases in iron overload. In haemochromatosis iron absorption is abnormally increased. Absorption from slow-release formulations is less reliable than from ordinary formulations.

Of the daily losses of 1–2 mg from a total load of 3–5 g most is lost via the epithelial sloughing of the gastrointestinal tract, and via the urine and skin, but in small amounts.

After i.m. injection iron dextran is very slowly absorbed (about 50 per cent in 3 d) and 20 per cent may remain after 1 month. Iron sorbitol, on the other hand, is rapidly absorbed (about 80 per cent within 12 h).

Important adverse effects

The commonest adverse effects with oral iron are gastrointestinal symptoms: nausea, abdominal discomfort, vomiting, and constipation or diarrhoea. These effects are dose-related and are reduced by using slow-release formulations.

Iron salts make the faeces black, which may cause alarm because it may be mistaken for melaena. However, stools which are black because of iron are negative for occult blood and look and smell differently from melaena.

After parenteral injection allergic reactions can occur. They are rare but may be severe and great care must be taken, especially in patients with a history of allergy of any sort (see dosage recommendations above). Do not give i.v. iron to patients with a history of asthma. Allergic reactions are more likely after i.v. injection but can also occur after i.m. injection, especially with the rapidly absorbed form, iron sorbitol.

Staining of the skin after i.m. injection has been mentioned above.

Other adverse effects after parenteral injection include thrombophlebitis after i.v. infusion, a metallic taste in the mouth, hypotension and bradycardia, abdominal pain, lymph node enlargement, arthralgia, and myalgia.

Parenteral iron should not be given to patients with severe hepatic or renal disease or to patients with active renal infection.

Interactions

Iron absorption is enhanced by vitamin C, but the addition of vitamin C to oral iron formulations does not influence the therapy of iron deficiency.

A chelating interaction of iron with tetracycline results in the formation of an insoluble precipitate and the absorption of both compounds is impaired.

Isoniazid

Structure

CONHNH$_2$

Mode of action

Isoniazid is an antituberculous drug, and may act by inhibiting the synthesis of long-chain mycolic acids, which are unique to mycobacteria.

Uses

All forms of tuberculosis, in combination with other antituberculous drugs.

Dosages

5 mg/kg/d, usually up to 300 mg/d, commonly given as a single daily dose. Extensive caseous disease, tuberculous meningitis, and isoniazid-resistant infections may require higher dosages, when pyridoxine (10–20 mg o.d.) will also be needed (see below).

Kinetic data

Isoniazid is well absorbed. It is metabolized principally by acetylation, with a bimodal distribution in the general population (see Chapter 8). $t_{1/2} = 1$ h in fast acetylators, 3 h in slow acetylators.

Important adverse effects

Peripheral neuropathy is common with high dosages, is more frequent among slow acetylators, and may be prevented or treated by administration of pyridoxine, which should always be given when the dosage is 5 mg/kg/d or more. Other neurological effects include optic neuritis or atrophy, various mental disturbances, dizziness, paraesthesiae, ataxia, and convulsions, all of which may be prevented or reduced by pyridoxine. Hepatic damage occurs occasionally, and although it has been linked to fast acetylation, suggesting that it may be due to a toxic metabolite, this is contentious.

Labetalol

Structure

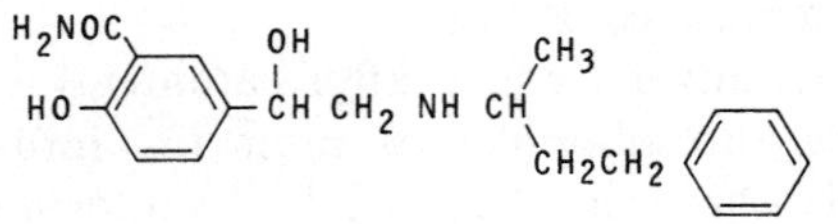

H_2NOC — , OH , CH_3
HO — CH CH_2 NH CH
CH_2CH_2 ⬡

Mode of action

Labetalol combines the actions of a non-selective β (i.e. β_1 and β_2)-adrenoceptor antagonist and an α-adrenoceptor antagonist. It is about three times more potent as a β-antagonist than as an α-antagonist and causes peripheral arteriolar vasodilatation without reflex tachycardia. It has no sympathetic agonist effects.

Use

Hypertension

Dosages

Oral: 100–800 mg t.d.s. Start with a low dosage and increase gradually in order to minimize adverse effects. Increases in dosage may be made every 1–2 weeks if required.

Intravenous: 1–4 mg/min by continuous infusion to a maximum of 200 mg. Alternatively give 50 mg i.v. over 1 min and repeat if necessary at 15 min intervals to a maximum total of 200 mg.

Kinetic data

Labetalol is well absorbed, but subject to extensive first-pass metabolism in the liver (hence the large difference between oral and i.v. dosages). It is almost completely metabolized, $t_{1/2} = 4$ h. Dosages should be reduced in liver disease.

Important adverse effects

Labetalol commonly causes postural hypotension, probably because of its α-antagonist effect.

Other adverse effects are uncommon, but include a lichenoid skin rash, tingling of the scalp, and difficulty in ejaculation and micturition.

Care should be taken in patients with heart block, heart failure, and asthma.

Interactions

The effects of labetalol are enhanced by other antihypertensive drugs, such as diuretics, and labetalol is best used in combination therapy.

Cimetidine increases the systemic availability of labetalol after oral administration from about 40 per cent to about 80 per cent.

L-dopa and decarboxylase inhibitors

Structures

General

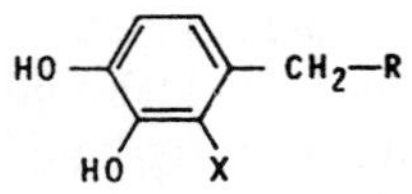

HO — ⬡ — CH_2—R
HO X

L-dopa (levodopa) and the decarboxylase inhibitors share similar structures.

Mode of action

Exogenously administered L-dopa crosses the blood–brain barrier and is assumed to enter dopaminergic nerve-endings in the basal ganglia.

	R	X
L-dopa	-CHCOOH | NH_2	H
Carbidopa	-CH_3 | -CCOOH | $NHNH_2$	H
Benserazide	-NHNHCOCHCH$_2$OH | NH	OH

There it is converted to dopamine, which is released by nerve impulse. This can only occur in viable dopaminergic neurones, but it is presumed that this sequence corrects the dysfunction brought about by the dopamine deficiency accompanying the loss of normally functioning dopaminergic neurones in Parkinsonism.

Dopa decarboxylase inhibitors inhibit the metabolism of L-dopa outside the brain, thus allowing more L-dopa to enter the brain. They do not themselves enter the brain and thus do not inhibit the production of dopamine there. This allows the use of lower doses of L-dopa, with fewer peripheral adverse effects.

Uses

Parkinsonism, but not that associated with the use of neuroleptic drugs (for example phenothiazines, thioxanthenes, and butyrophenones).

Dosages

Several formulations of L-dopa plus a decarboxylase inhibitor are available. L-dopa plus carbidopa is called co-careldopa and L-dopa plus benserazide is called co-beneldopa:

	L-dopa (mg)	Decarboxylase inhibitor (mg)
(a) Co-careldopa		
Sinemet® 110	100	10
Sinemet® LS	50	12.5
Sinemet-Plus®	100	25
Sinemet® 275	250	25
(b) Co-beneldopa		
Madopar® 62.5		
(tablets and capsules)	50	12.5
Madopar® 125		
(capsules and tablets)	100	25
Madopar® CR		
(slow-release	100	25
capsules)		
Madopar® 250		
(capsules and tabs)	200	50

Some formulations containing L-dopa alone are also available.

Generally, treatment is begun with 50 or 100 mg of L-dopa t.d.s. or q.d.s. The dosage is then increased every few days in increments of 100 mg of L-dopa until a satisfactory response is achieved. Most patients achieve a therapeutic response and can be maintained on an L-dopa dosage for Sinemet® of 750–1500 mg daily and for Madopar® of 400–800 mg daily. The large range of dosage forms available gives flexibility in producing the best response.

Kinetic data

L-dopa is poorly absorbed and delays its own absorption by delaying gastric emptying. It is completely metabolized with a $t_{1/2}$ of 3 h, but when given with a decarboxylase inhibitor its metabolism is 80 per cent reduced ($t_{1/2} = 15$ h).

Important adverse effects

Common important adverse effects include: changes in bowel habit; epigastric and abdominal pain; anorexia, nausea, and vomiting; cardiac arrhythmias; orthostatic hypotension; dizziness; polyuria, difficulty with micturition, incontinence, discolouration of the urine and other body fluids (for example sweat); unpleasant body odour.

These adverse effects are reduced by using a decarboxylase inhibitor.

Common mental symptoms include euphoria, excitement, confusion, hallucinations and delusions, agitation, and anxiety.

Abnormal movements may limit dosage. The 'on-off' effect, characterized by fluctuations in the patient's ability to perform voluntary movements, may be troublesome. It usually occurs suddenly and may be so frequent as to be as disabling as the original illness (see p. 431).

L-dopa is contra-indicated in patients with glaucoma, and caution should be taken in patients with a history of psychiatric illness or dementia and in patients with a history of myocardial ischaemia or cardiac arrhythmias.

Interactions

The effects of L-dopa are potentiated by MAO inhibitors, which should be withdrawn at least 2 weeks before L-dopa is started.

Neuroleptic drugs reduce the effects of L-dopa by blocking its action on dopamine receptors.

Pyridoxine is a co-factor for dopa decarboxylase and enhances its activity. It may therefore increase the dosage requirements of L-dopa if a decarboxylase inhibitor is not used.

Active transport of L-dopa across the gut and into the brain is inhibited by some dietary amino acids. A low protein diet may therefore improve the efficacy of L-dopa therapy.

Lignocaine (lidocaine)

Structure

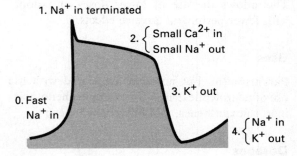

Mode of action

Lignocaine is a class I antiarrhythmic drug which is grouped together with a number of other antiarrhythmic drugs because they have similar effects on the action potential of cardiac conducting tissues. Other drugs in class I are quinidine, procainamide, disopyramide, and phenytoin. Other classes of action are discussed under amiodarone and verapamil (in the section on calcium antagonists).

To understand the actions of these drugs it is necessary first to examine the cardiac action potential itself. In Figs. P5 and P6 is shown an example of a fast action potential recorded in a Purkinje fibre. The action potential is divided into five phases:

■ **Fig. P6** The cationic changes which take place during the period of an action potential in a Purkinje fibre. The numbers 0–4 correspond to the defined phases of the action potential (see Fig. P5).

Phase 4

In cells normally capable of spontaneous depolarization, for example cells in the sinoatrial (SA) node, atrioventricular (AV) node, and His–Purkinje system, there is a slow drift during the resting phase (phase 4) from the maximum negative

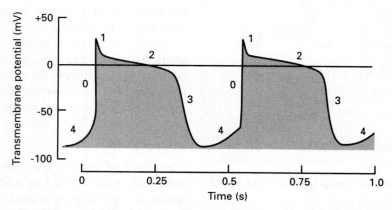

■ **Fig. P5** An example of two consecutive action potentials recorded from a single cardiac Purkinje fibre. The phases of the action potential are numbered 0–4 (see text).

potential (around -90 mV in Purkinje fibres, although in the SA node the potential is never less than -60 mV), to a more positive potential (around -70 mV in Purkinje fibres). This slow drift of potential during phase 4 is due to a small influx of sodium ions and efflux of potassium ions. This spontaneous depolarization to the threshold at which the action potential is initiated confers automaticity on these tissues. In contrast, atrial and ventricular myocardial cells no not normally exhibit spontaneous depolarization and are therefore at rest until stimulated by a propagatory impulse.

Phase 0

When the threshold potential is reached there is then a fast inward flux of sodium ions, causing a rapid rise in transmembrane potential to positive values (i.e. depolarization).

Phase 1

When the transmembrane potential reaches a given positive value (for example about $+20$ mV in Purkinje fibres) the fast inward sodium flux is rapidly terminated. The potential then starts to fall towards zero.

Phase 2

During this phase, called the plateau phase of the action potential, the transmembrane potential remains relatively stable, due to low conductance of ions. There is a small inward current of calcium ions which is balanced by a small outward current of potassium ions. Eventually the small inward calcium current is slowly terminated. The time taken before the slow inward calcium current is terminated is a factor determining the duration of phase 2 and therefore the time of onset of repolarization (phase 3).

Phase 3

The major portion of repolarization to the maximum negative potential occurs during this phase and is primarily due to outward flux of potassium through a large number of different types of potassium channels. As the transmembrane potential falls to its maximum negative value there may be slight hyperpolarization and this outward flux is terminated. Phase 4 then begins again with a small influx of sodium ions and efflux of potassium ions.

Refractory periods

During the phases of *re*polarization (phases 1–3) the fibres are refractory to further *de*polarization, although when about 50 per cent of repolarization has occurred a larger than normal stimulus *can* cause depolarization. The period during which depolarization cannot normally occur is called the *effective* refractory period, and the period during which depolarization cannot occur, no matter how large a stimulus occurs, it is called the *absolute* refractory period.

The effects of the class I antiarrhythmic drugs on the action potential are of three types, which can be compared by considering the effects of quinidine, lignocaine, and flecainide separately. The effects are summarized in Table P6.

(a) Quinidine

Quinidine is categorized as having class Ia activity.

(i) Automaticity

Quinidine slows the rate of depolarization during phase 4 and increases the threshold at which phase 0 depolarization occurs. Automaticity is thus suppressed.

(ii) Rate of depolarization and conduction velocity

There is a decrease in the rate of the fast inward sodium current during phase 0 and thus a slowing of depolarization. This results in a reduction in conduction velocity in both normal and ischaemic tissues.

(iii) Effective refractory period and total action potential duration

Quinidine slightly increases the duration of action potential. It also increases the effective refractory period, but to a greater extent. Thus, the proportion of the total action potential duration during which the fibres are effectively refractory (i.e. the ratio ERP/APD) is *increased*.

These effects of quinidine occur in normal Purkinje fibres, ventricular muscle fibres, and ventricular ectopic foci, and also in the fibres of the AV node, atrial muscle fibres, and atrial ectopic foci. Quinidine prolongs the QRS complex and QT interval of the ECG.

■ **Table P6** The actions of different subclasses of class I antiarrhythmic drugs

Class	Phase 0	APD	ERP	ERP/APD	Effect on Myocardial conduction velocity	PR interval	QRS interval	QT interval
Ia	+ +	↑↑	↑↑	↓	↓	⇔↑	⇔↑	↑↑↑
Ib	+	↓	↓	↓	⇔	⇔	⇔	⇔↓
Ic	+ + +	↓⇔	↑	↓	↓↓	↑↑	↑↑	↑

↑ Increased; ↓ Reduced; ⇔ Unchanged.

Procainamide and disopyramide have effects similar to those of quinidine, but disopyramide has greater effects on atrial and ventricular muscles and lesser effects on Purkinje fibres. These compounds also differ in the potency of their anticholinergic effects: lignocaine, phenytoin, and procainamide have no anticholinergic properties in contrast to quinidine and disopyramide.

(b) Lignocaine

Lignocaine is categorized as having class Ib activity.

(i) Automaticity

Lignocaine slows the rate of depolarization during phase 4, but in contrast to quinidine it does not change the threshold at which phase 0 depolarization occurs. Automaticity is thus suppressed to a lesser extent.

(ii) Rate of depolarization and conduction velocity

There is a reduction in the rate of the fast inward sodium current during phase 0, and thus a slowing of the rate of depolarization. In contrast to quinidine this effect does not result in a change in conduction velocity in normal conducting tissues; however, in ischaemic conduction tissues conduction velocity is reduced.

(iii) Effective refractory period and total action potential duration

There is enhancement of the outward potassium flux during phase 3, with an increase in the rate of repolarization and shortening of the total action potential duration (APD). The effective refractory period (ERP) is also shortened, but to a lesser extent. Thus the *proportion* of the total duration of the action potential during which the fibres are effectively refractory (i.e. the ration ERP/APD) is *increased*. This means that during the period of the action potential the conduction tissue is refractory to new depolarizing stimuli for a relatively longer period of time.

These effects of lignocaine are exerted principally on normal Purkinje fibres, ventricular muscle fibres, and ventricular ectopic foci. The SA node, AV node, atrial muscle fibres, and atrial ectopic foci are generally unaffected. The ECG is usually unaffected by lignocaine.

Phenytoin and tocainide have effects similar to those of lignocaine, but phenytoin tends to *increase* conduction velocity in ischaemic tissue.

(c) Flecainide

Flecainide is categorized as having Class Ic activity.

In common with lignocaine and quinidine, flecainide slows the rate of depolarization by reducing the rate of the fast inward sodium current during phase 0. However, in contrast to lignocaine and quinidine it has little or no effect on the action potential duration. Flecainide affects the SA and AV nodes, accessory pathways, and atrial and intraventricular fibres. It broadens the QRS complex on the ECG. Lorcainide, encainide, and propafenone are other drugs with similar properties.

Despite the detailed knowledge about the actions of these drugs on cardiac electrophysiological events, it is still difficult to relate these actions in any precise way to their therapeutic effects on various arrhythmias. Likewise there is still much to be learned about the precise molecular events by which these drugs produce their electrophysiological effects.

Local anaesthetic action of lignocaine

In common with other local anaesthetics, such as procaine, amethocaine, cocaine, bupivacaine, mepivacaine, and prilocaine, lignocaine acts by decreasing the large transient increase of sodium permeability resulting from slight depolarization of the membrane and thereafter by increasing the threshold for electrical excitability. This results in blockade of the nervous impulse.

Uses

Lignocaine is used in the treatment and prevention of acute ventricular arrhythmias (ventricular extrasystoles, ventricular tachycardia, and ventricular fibrillation), for example after myocardial infarction and cardiac surgery. It is also used as a local anaesthetic.

Dosages

(a) Antiarrhythmic dosages

Lignocaine is given by i.v. injection in an initial dose of 100 mg, given as 10 mL of a 1 per cent solution over 2 min. In order to maintain therapeutic plasma concentrations thereafter, it is usual to continue treatment with an i.v. infusion, starting at a high rate and gradually decreasing to a maintenance rate. This is because lignocaine has a short half-time and the initial bolus dose will be subject to elimination which is too rapid for a low fixed rate maintenance infusion to replace. A suggested regimen after the initial bolus is: 4 mg/kg/h for 0.5 h; 2 mg/kg/h for 2 h; 1 mg/kg/h thereafter for 24 h (see Fig. 6.1, p. 69).

Lignocaine has also been used by the i.m. route (50–100 mg) in prophylaxis against cardiac arrhythmias outside hospital before admission of the patient to hospital. The therapeutic value of this approach is uncertain.

(b) Local anaesthetic dosages

There are two important matters here. The first is to appreciate the general toxicity of lignocaine and related local anaesthetics, and therefore to limit the total dosage given in a single injection or infiltration. Under these circumstances the total dose of lignocaine should not exceed 200 mg, or 500 mg when given with adrenaline.

The second is to appreciate that some formulations of lignocaine and other local anaesthetics contain adrenaline. For instance, lignocaine is available in solutions of 0.5 per cent, 1 per cent, and 2 per cent, both alone and in combination with adrenaline 1 in 200 000 (i.e. 500 micrograms/100 mL). The maximum dose of adrenaline at any one time is 500 micrograms.

Kinetic data

After oral administration lignocaine is almost completely metabolized on its first passage through the liver. For this reason it has to be given i.v. Metabolism ($t_{1/2} = 1.5$ h) is to two active metabolites, monoethylglycinexylidide (MEGX) and glycinexylidide (GX), both of which have less antiarrhythmic activity than lignocaine but which are more toxic and are probably responsible for CNS toxicity. Since the half-times of these metabolites are longer than that of lignocaine, continuous i.v. infusion of lignocaine should be limited to 24–48 h to limit the extent of their accumulation.

In liver disease the metabolism of lignocaine may be decreased and dosages must be reduced. In patients with heart failure there may be reduced clearance because of hepatic congestion and the apparent volume of distribution may also be reduced; these changes result in lower dosage requirements.

Plasma concentration measurements

The therapeutic range of plasma lignocaine concentrations is 1–5 µg/mL, although in some patients concentrations of up to 9 µg/mL may be required. Routine plasma lignocaine concentration measurement has not been proved useful.

Important adverse effects

The adverse effects of lignocaine are dose-related and occur in about 6 per cent of patients treated by i.v. infusion. The common effects are central nervous system toxicity, (including nausea, vomiting, drowsiness, convulsions, and coma) and cardiac effects (including sinus bradycardia, tachyarrhythmias, asystole, and hypotension). Lignocaine should be used with caution in patients with pre-existing impairment of conduction in the AV node and bundle of His and in patients with the sick sinus syndrome, in whom it may further impair sinus nodal function.

Interactions

Since lignocaine has a high hepatic extraction ratio (see Chapter 3) its clearance by the liver is reduced by drugs which reduce liver blood flow, for example cimetidine and propranolol.

Hypokalaemia, for example due to diuretics, alters the effects of class I antiarrhythmic drugs on the action potential and their arrhythmogenic effects may be more pronounced. Hypokalaemia should be corrected when using lignocaine.

Lincomycin and clindamycin

Structures

General

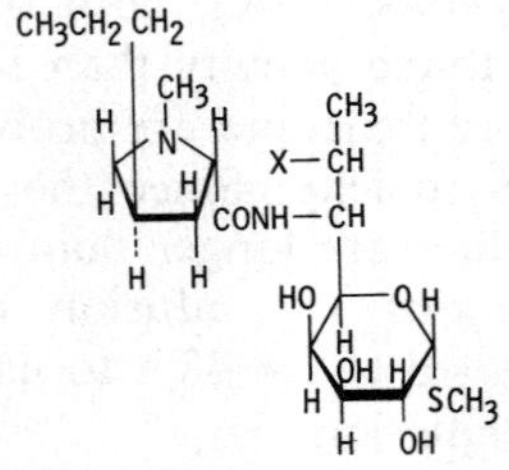

Lincomycin: X = OH
Clindamycin: X = Cl

Mode of action

Inhibition of bacterial protein synthesis by an effect on ribosomal RNA.

Uses

The following organisms are generally sensitive to these antibiotics:

Gram-positive cocci (streptococci, penicillin-resistant staphylococci).
Gram-negative bacilli (*Bacteroides*).
Gram-positive bacilli (*Corynebacterium diphtheriae, Clostridium spp.*).

Because of their adverse effects these antibiotics are generally reserved for infections in bones and joints, for severe intra-abdominal sepsis, and for severe infections of the skin.

Dosages

Oral therapy:

Lincomycin 500 mg every 6 to 8 h.
Clindamycin 150–300 mg every 6 h.

Parenteral therapy:
Note that intravenous infusion of these drugs should be carried out over 1 h in 250 mL of a solution of 5 per cent dextrose or physiological saline. Rapid infusion carries a risk of cardiopulmonary arrest.

Lincomycin i.m. 600 mg every 12 or 24 h; i.v. 600 mg every 8 or 12 h.
Clindamycin i.m. or i.v., 0.6–2.4 g daily in 2–4 divided doses.

Kinetic data

	Lincomycin	Clindamycin
Absorption	20–40%	90–100%
$t_{1/2}$	5 h	2 h
Metabolism	80%	90%
Excretion	20% unchanged in urine	10% unchanged in urine

Important adverse effects

Diarrhoea is common (up to 50 per cent) and may occasionally be due to pseudomembranous colitis, which is a serious complication and which has a high mortality if untreated. Pseudomembranous colitis may present as mild diarrhoea or as an acute fulminant colitis with profuse bloody diarrhoea. Sigmoidoscopy shows raised white plaques on the colonic mucosa. It is caused by overgrowth in the colon of *Clostridium difficile*, which produces a necrotizing toxin. Treatment is with oral vancomycin (500 mg 6-hourly).

Pseudomembranous colitis may occur with other antibiotics, including ampicillin, the cephalosporins, chloramphenicol, co-trimox- azole, gentamicin, kanamycin, metronidazole, and tetracycline. The incidence is lower with these antibiotics than with lincomycin and clinda- mycin.

Interactions

Lincomycin and clindamycin may potentiate the effects of neuromuscular blocking drugs.

Lithium

Mode of action

Lithium is an element which exists as a cation in solution. It has several pharmacological effects on the function of brain monoamines, and these may be due to its effects on transmembrane sodium fluxes or to its effect in inhibiting the function of the second messenger system linked to the turnover of cellular phophatidylinositides. However, the relation of these effects to its thera- peutic action is unknown.

Uses

1. Manic depression: prevention of mood swings.
2. Unipolar depression: prevention of recurrent depressive episodes. Also used as an adjunct to other antidepressant treatment in patients with resistant symptoms.
3. Mania: lithium is effective in the treatment of acute mania but its slow onset of action is a disadvantage; for this reason acute manic epis- odes are usually treated with a neuroleptic drug.

Dosages

Lithium salts are available in both conventional formulations and in sustained-release formula- tions. The latter have been devised in order to reduce the frequency of dosage. The following are available:

Lithium carbonate (300 mg = 8 mm Li$^+$):

Camcolit® 250 (250 mg)
Camcolit® 400 (400 mg)
Liskonum® (450 mg, sustained-release)

Phasal® (300 mg sustained-release)
Priadel® (400 mg sustained-release);

Lithium citrate (564 mg = 6 mmol Li$^+$):

Litarex® (564 mg).

The initial dose of lithium is 6 mmol orally daily (i.e. lithium carbonate 250 mg, lithium cit- rate 564 mg). The dose is then gradually increased, depending on the plasma concentra- tion, to a final maintenance dose which varies among individuals, usually in the range of 16–40 mmol of lithium daily.

Kinetic data

Lithium is well absorbed. It is eliminated unchanged in the urine and its $t_{1/2}$ therefore varies with age, being about 20 h in young adults and up to 36 h in old people. Therapeutic plasma concentrations measured in blood samples taken 12 h after the last dose of lithium vary between 0.4 and 0.8 mmol/L. At concentrations above 1.5 mmol/L adverse effects become common (see Chapter 7).

Important adverse effects

The effects of lithium intoxication are gastrointes- tinal disturbances (anorexia, nausea, vomiting, and diarrhoea) and CNS disturbances (drowsi- ness, lethargy, giddiness, ataxia, tremor, lack of co-ordination, and dysarthria). Severe overdose (plasma concentrations about 3 mmol/L) may cause coma, fits, toxic psychoses, oliguria, circu- latory failure, and occasionally death.

Less serious adverse effects commonly experi- enced are mild gastrointestinal disturbances, tremor, and either fluid retention with weight gain and oedema or polyuria and polydipsia.

In the long term nephrogenic diabetes insipidus may occur, due to competitive inhibition of the action of ADH on the renal tubules, and hypothyroidism is not uncommon.

Interactions

Diuretics, such as thiazides and frusemide, cause lithium retention, and care should be taken to avoid lithium intoxication in patients taking this combination. Lithium dosages should be halved if diuretic therapy is prescribed and the dosage of lithium should then be adjusted according to its plasma concentration.

A neurotoxic syndrome has been described when lithium is used in combination with high doses of antipsychotic drugs (butyrophenones and phenothiazines).

Loperamide

Structure

(Compare haloperidol.)

Mode of action

Loperamide binds to opioid receptors in the gastrointestinal tract, where it has morphine-like effects. It also has anticholinergic effects on the bowel. It does not penetrate the brain well and is therefore relatively free of central opiate effects.

Use

Symptomatic relief of diarrhoea.

Dosages

4 mg initially, followed by 2 mg after each loose stool. During long-term treatment the total dose, titrated against the effect on bowel movement, may be given in two divided doses. The maximum daily dose is 16 mg.

Kinetic data

Loperamide is poorly absorbed, partly because it decreases gastrointestinal motility, and it is therefore mostly excreted unchanged in the faeces.

Important adverse effects

Constipation will occur with over-treatment. Tolerance does not develop to the constipating effect during long-term therapy. Loperamide occasionally causes abdominal pain, dry mouth, dizziness, headache, and rashes.

Melphalan

Structure

$$HOOCCHCH_2 - \langle \rangle - N(CH_2CH_2Cl)_2$$
$$\quad\quad | $$
$$\quad\quad NH_2$$

(Compare chlorambucil, cyclophosphamide.)

Mode of action

Alkylating agent (see busulphan).

Uses

Multiple myeloma.
Some solid tumours, for example malignant melanoma and advanced carcinoma of the breast.

Dosages

0.15 mg/kg o.d. orally for 7 d repeated at 6-weekly intervals, according to the response.

Kinetic data

Melphalan is variably absorbed. It is mostly metabolized, $t_{1/2} = 1.5$ h.

Important adverse effects

Bone-marrow suppression is dose-related. Prolonged therapy results in an increased incidence of leukaemia.

Melphalan should not be used during pregnancy. dosages should be reduced in old people and people with renal impairment.

Interaction

For the possible interaction with live vaccines see p. 251.

Metformin

Structure

$$CH_3 \backslash$$
$$\quad\quad N - C - NH - C - NH_4$$
$$CH_3 \diagup \quad \| \quad\quad \|$$
$$\quad\quad\quad NH \quad\quad NH$$

Mode of action

Metformin is a biguanide which inhibits the intestinal absorption of glucose, increases peripheral glucose utilization by enhancing the actions of insulin at its receptors, increases muscle glucose uptake, and reduces gluconeogenesis. It may produce these effects by binding to membrane phospholipids. It does not have an effect on insulin release (cf. sulphonylureas). Phenformin and buformin, related drugs, are no longer used, because of adverse effects.

Use

Diabetes mellitus of mature onset type.

Dosage

500 mg t.d.s. orally. Maximum 850 mg b.d.

Kinetic data

Metformin is about 60 per cent absorbed. It is excreted mostly unchanged in the urine, $t_{1/2} = 9$ h.

Important adverse effects

Nausea, vomiting, and diarrhoea are common. Lactic acidosis may occasionally occur. It is thought to be due to inhibition of electron transport and tissue oxidation at the levels of succinic dehydrogenase and cytochrome oxidase. The presentation consists of nausea, vomiting, abdominal pain, hyperventilation or dyspnoea, drowsiness, and, in severe cases, coma. The risk of lactic acidosis with metformin is increased in patients with renal impairment.

Methotrexate

Structure

Mode of action

Methotrexate inhibits the activity of dihydrofolate reductase (see co-trimoxazole). This leads to decreased production of tetrahydrofolic acid which is required for the synthesis of thymidylic acid and purine nucleotides. This effect prevents the synthesis of nuclear material in the S phase and causes cell death.

Uses

Acute lymphoblastic leukaemia: to maintain remission and to prevent or treat CNS infiltration.

Choriocarcinoma.

Other solid tumours, such as those of head, neck, breast, and lung.

Severe psoriasis not responding to other treatment.

Rheumatoid arthritis (as immunosuppressive therapy).

Dosages

Dosage regimens vary with the indication:

1. Maintenance therapy during remission in acute leukaemia is carried out with low dosages, for example 15 mg/m^2 once weekly.

2. Intrathecal methotrexate is given in doses up to 15 mg at weekly intervals for the prevention and treatment of CNS infiltration in lymphoblastic leukaemia.

3. High dose regimens: it is possible to give methotrexate in higher doses for the treatment of certain solid tumours and to avoid bone-marrow suppression by giving folinic acid (so-called 'rescue'). For example, in the treatment of choriocarcinoma, methotrexate is given in a dose of up to 60 mg i.m. every 48 h for four doses. This is followed by an intravenous infusion of folinic acid in a dose of up to 120 mg, followed by 12–15 mg i.m. every 6 h for eight doses.

The idea behind this regimen is that because the cells of the tumour are turning over very rapidly the methotrexate affects them before it affects the cells of the bone-marrow. The effect on the tumour occurs early and then the actions of methotrexate are reversed by the folinic acid before the full effect occurs on the bone-marrow.

4. Psoriasis: 10–25 mg orally once weekly.

Kinetic data

The absorption of methotrexate is saturable. It is mostly excreted unchanged in the urine and is subject to active tubular secretion. $t_{1/2} = 4$ h.

Important adverse effects

Bone-marrow suppression is dose-related and may be prevented by the use of folinic acid (see above).

Oral ulceration, stomatitis, pharyngitis, glossitis, and gingivitis are common (up to 30 per cent of cases), as are gastrointestinal disturbances, including anorexia, nausea, vomiting, and diarrhoea.

During prolonged treatment (for example in psoriasis) hepatotoxicity is common. In about 20 per cent of cases it may result in hepatic fibrosis.

The use of intrathecal methotrexate is often accompanied by headache and vomiting and occasionally neurological disturbances may occur.

Methotrexate should not be used in pregnancy because of its teratogenic effects. Contraceptive precautions should be taken during and for 3 months after its use, because of its effects on spermatogenesis and oogenesis.

Dosages should be reduced by half in patients with renal failure and methotrexate should not be used in patients with liver damage.

Interactions

Methotrexate potentiates the effects of other dihydrofolate reductase inhibitors.

Aspirin and probenecid inhibit the tubular secretion of methotrexate and thus enhance its effects.

Asparaginase may reduce the risk of methotrexate toxicity by inhibiting protein synthesis.

Methyldopa

Structure

(Compare adrenoceptor agonists, L-dopa, dopamine.)

Mode of action

Methyldopa (α-methyldopa) enters the brain and neurones. In noradrenergic neurones it is decarboxylated to α-methylnoradrenaline. It is thought that this potent α_2-adrenoceptor agonist is then released by inhibitory noradrenergic neurones in vasomotor centres controlling sympathetic outflow. The net result is central inhibition of peripheral sympathetic nervous system function.

Use

Hypertension.

Dosages

Initially 250 mg b.d. orally, increasing as required in increments of 250 mg to a maximum of 3 g daily.

Kinetic data

The systemic availability of methyldopa is variable, because it is metabolized in the gut wall. It is extensively metabolized and the metabolites are excreted in the urine. Very little of the drug actually enters the brain to produce a pharmacological effect; $t_{1/2} = 2$ h.

Important adverse effects

The commonest adverse effects are on the central nervous system: depression, drowsiness, sleep disturbances, and dizziness. Other important effects are postural hypotension and erectile impotence.

Although a positive Coombs' test occurs in about 20 per cent of patients, autoimmune haemolytic anaemia occurs in only 0.02 per cent.

Methyldopa should be used with caution in patients with active liver disease, since it can cause liver damage. In patients with severe renal impairment dosages should be reduced.

If treatment is being stopped methyldopa dosage should be tailed off gradually, since sudden withdrawal may result in severe rebound hypertension.

Metoclopramide

Structure

Mode of action

Metoclopramide has several different effects at different sites, all of which contribute to its antiemetic action.

1. Its most important effects are directly on the gastrointestinal tract. It increases oesophageal tone, increases pyloric contraction, and enhances the rate of gastric and duodenal emptying. These effects may be mediated by both cholinergic and antidopaminergic effects.

2. It is a central dopamine antagonist and may block the action of dopamine released within the chemoreceptor trigger zone in the floor of the fourth ventricle, which is thought to

be one of the neurotransmitter functions involved in the process of emesis.

3. It may also decrease afferent impulses to the brain from emetic foci, for example gastric mucosa.

Its major adverse effects are caused by its antidopaminergic effects on the brain.

Uses

As an antiemetic in the following conditions:

gastroduodenal disorders;
drug-induced nausea and vomiting (but not with cytotoxic drugs);
postoperatively;
in migraine, in which it also increases the rate of absorption of analgesics.

It is also used to increase gastroduodenal transit time during radiological procedures.

Dosages

Antiemetic: 10 mg orally, i.m. or i.v. May be given t.d.s. if required.

In radiology: 10 mg i.m. or i.v.

Migraine: 10 mg orally at the onset of the attack, repeated twice at most if required (i.e. a total of 30 mg). Metoclopramide is available in proprietary formulations suitable for use in migraine: Migravess® (metoclopramide 5 mg, aspirin 325 mg) and Paramax® (metoclopramide 5 mg, paracetamol 500 mg).

Note that all these dosages refer to adults over 20 years of age. The dosages in other age groups corresponding to an adult dosage of 10 mg t.d.s. are:

children under 1 year old, 1 mg b.d.;
children 1–3 years, 1 mg b.d. or t.d.s.;
children 4–5 years, 2 mg b.d. or t.d.s.;
children 6–14 years, 2.25–5 mg t.d.s.;
young adults 15–20 years, 5–10 mg t.d.s.

Always start at the lower end of the dosage range, increasing only if required.

Kinetic data

Metoclopramide is well absorbed. It is extensively metabolized in the liver to inactive metabolites, $t_{1/2} = 4$ h.

Important adverse effects

The most important adverse effects of metoclopramide are extrapyramidal reactions caused by its antidopaminergic action in the nigrostriatal tracts. These reactions occur in about 1 per cent of patients and are usually dystonic in nature, including facial muscle spasm, trismus, titubation, extraocular muscle spasm and oculogyric crisis, torticollis, and opisthotonos. Parkinsonian features occur during chronic therapy and metoclopramide should be avoided in patients with Parkinsonism. These reactions are dose-dependent and dosages should be reduced in children and young adults (see above). In old people start with doses of 5 mg, increasing to 10 mg only if necessary. Dystonic reactions should be treated with procyclidine 5 mg i.v. or diazepam 10 mg i.v.

Metoclopramide may also occasionally cause central nervous symptoms, such as dizziness and drowsiness.

In common with other dopamine receptor antagonists it stimulates the release of prolactin from the pituitary and may cause galactorrhoea.

Interactions

Metoclopramide potentiates the antidopaminergic actions of other dopamine receptor antagonists (phenothiazines, thioxanthenes, and butyrophenones), with an increased risk of dystonic reactions.

Anticholinergic drugs antagonize its effects on the gastrointestinal tract and L-dopa its effects on the oesophagus.

Because it increases gastric emptying rate metoclopramide may increase the *rate* of absorption of some drugs. This is important in the treatment of migraine where a rapid analgesic effect is required but gastric stasis prevents the absorption of analgesic drugs (see dosages above). It is probably of little importance in other circumstances, since the *extent* of absorption of drugs is usually not affected.

Metronidazole

Structure

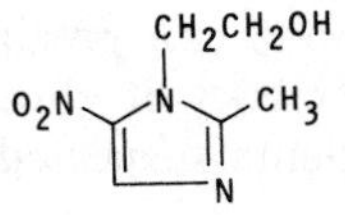

CH₂CH₂OH
O₂N — CH₃ — N

Mode of action

Metronidazole kills bacteria and protozoa whose metabolism is anaerobic or microaerophilic. In such organisms it is reduced to active metabolites which interfere with nucleic acid function.

Uses

Infections due to:

Trichomonas (genital);
Anaerobic bacteria (for example Bacteroides);
Amoeba enterohepatica (amoebiasis);
Giardia lamblia (giardiasis);
Vincent's organisms (acute ulcerative gingivitis).

Dosages

Trichomoniasis: 20 mg t.d.s. orally to each sexual partner for 7 d.

Anaerobic infections: 400 mg t.d.s. orally for 7 ds, or 1 g t.d.s. by suppository for 3 d followed by oral therapy.

Amoebiasis: 400–800 mg t.d.s. orally for 5–10 d depending on the form of the infection.

Giardiasis: 2 g o.d. orally for 3 d.

Acute ulcerative gingivitis (Vincent's angina): 200 mg t.d.s. orally for 3 d.

In severe sepsis due to sensitive organisms i.v. administration may be necessary.

Kinetic data

Metronidazole is well absorbed after oral and rectal administration. It is mostly metabolized. $t_{1/2} = 9$ h.

Important adverse effects

Adverse effects are infrequent. During long-term therapy a peripheral neuropathy may occur.

Interactions

Metronidazole inhibits hepatic microsomal drug-metabolizing enzymes. It thus enhances the effect of warfarin (see Chapter 10) and may cause a disulfiram-like reaction to alcohol. Cimetidine inhibits the metabolism of metronidazole.

Metyrapone

Structure

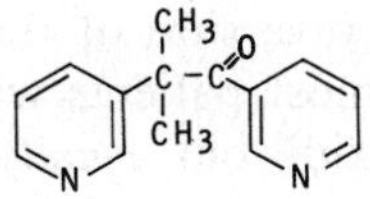

CH₃
C — C
CH₃

Mode of action

Metyrapone inhibits the 11-hydroxylation of 17, 21-hydroxyprogesterone to cortisol (hydrocortisone). It is thus more selective in its inhibition of steroid biosynthesis than aminoglutethimide, which inhibits synthesis at an early stage and thus inhibits the synthesis of other steroids (see Fig. 27.1). Metyrapone also inhibits the synthesis of aldosterone, but that is a relatively small effect.

Inhibition of cortisol synthesis should normally cause the release of ACTH from the pituitary, resulting in increased formation of the 11-desoxycorticosteroids (17-hydroxycorticoids), precursors of cortisol. The changes in concentrations of those steroids in the urine after metyrapone forms the basis of the use of metyrapone to test hypothalamic–pituitary axis function. For example, in Cushing's syndrome due to pituitary overactivity there is an exaggerated response to metyrapone, while in ectopic ACTH production there is no response.

Uses

Assessment of anterior pituitary function.
Suppression of adrenal corticosteroid produc-

tion in Cushing's syndrome and in metastatic breast carcinoma ('medical adrenalectomy').

Dosages

Diagnostic: 750 mg orally 4-hourly for six doses. Measure urinary 17-oxogenic steroids before, during, and after metyrapone.

Therapeutic (for example Cushing's syndrome): 0.25–6 g daily in divided doses, depending on the response to plasma cortisol concentrations.

Important adverse effects

Because metyrapone can precipitate acute adrenocorticol insufficiency it should be used with great care in patients suspected of having hypopituitarism.

Metyrapone can cause nausea and vomiting. These can be lessened by taking it with food.

Minoxidil

Structure

Mode of action

Minoxidil has a direct effect on arteriolar smooth muscle causing vasodilatation. It does not affect venules. Most of its adverse effects are due to vasodilatation, but it causes fluid retention both by reducing renal blood flow and by inhibition of sodium reabsorption in the proximal tubule.

Use

Hypertension.

Dosages

Initially 5 mg o.d. orally, increasing to 10 mg and then in increments of 10 mg every 3 d as required to a maximum of 50 mg daily.

Kinetic data

Minoxidil is well absorbed. It is mostly metabolized in the liver to relatively inactive compounds; the $t_{1/2}$ of minoxidil is 4 h but its therapeutic effects last for at least 16 h, perhaps because it remains bound to arteriolar smooth muscle or perhaps because of active metabolites.

Important adverse effects

Adverse effects are common and mostly attributable to vasodilatation. Reflex tachycardia and fluid retention necessitate the use of minoxidil only in combination with other antihypertensive drugs, namely a β-adrenoceptor antagonist and a diuretic. Although a thiazide diuretic may suffice, fluid retention may be severe enough to warrant the use of frusemide or bumetanide. Reflex tachycardia due to minoxidil may sometimes precipitate an acute attack of angina.

Increased hair growth (hypertrichosis) is common after about 3 weeks of treatment. It is reversible on withdrawing therapy, but may be cosmetically unacceptable, particularly in dark-haired women.

Flattening or inversion of the T wave in the ECG occurs in most patients within a few days of starting minoxidil but usually resolves within a few weeks. This may make interpretation of the ECG difficult. Cardiac ischaemic pain irrespective of ECG changes should be a sign to withhold the drug. Rarely minoxidil may cause pericardial effusion.

Interaction

Neuroleptic drugs may enhance the hypotensive effect of minoxidil. The beneficial effects of using β-adrenoceptor antagonists and diuretics with minoxidil have been mentioned above.

Misoprostol

Structure

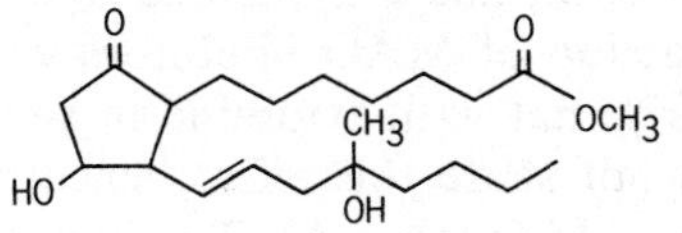

Mode of action

Misoprostol is an ester of prostaglandin E_1 and it binds to prostaglandin receptors on the parietal cell. It has several pharmacological properties, including reduction of gastric acid production and increases in gastric mucus production, mucosal blood flow, and duodenal bicarbonate secretion.

Uses

The prevention and treatment of peptic (especially gastric) ulceration caused by non-steroidal anti-inflammatory drugs. It can be used prophylactically against mucosal injury by non-steroidal anti-inflammatory drugs, but this is probably best reserved for patients in high-risk groups, such as old people and patients with a previous history of peptic ulceration.

Dosage

200 micrograms q.d.s. orally.

Kinetic data

Misoprostol is well absorbed and is subsequently de-esterified to the active free acid. Following further fatty acid oxidation to inactive metabolites it is excreted in the urine; $t_{1/2} = 0.5$ h. Renal failure and old age impair drug excretion to a limited extent, but dosage alterations are not usually necessary.

Important adverse effects

Diarrhoea may occur and is sometimes severe enough to necessitate withdrawal. Nausea, vomiting, and abdominal pain may occur and can be reduced by taking misoprostol with food. Abnormal vaginal bleeding occurs occasionally. Misoprostol causes uterine contraction and should not be used in pregnancy.

Monoamine oxidase (MAO) inhibitors

Structures

The MAO inhibitors form a group of compounds of differing structures: some are hydrazines (for example phenelzine, isocarboxazid, and iproniazid), and others are not (for example tranylcypromine, which is a derivative of amphetamine). We give here phenelzine as an example:

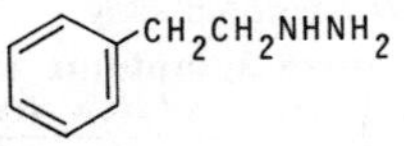

Mode of action

MAO has isoenzymes which have been classified as type A (present in the gut and liver) and type B (present in the brain). The commonly used MAO inhibitors, phenelzine, isocarboxazid, tranylcypromine, and iproniazid are non-selective inhibitors of MAO types A and B. Pargyline is a selective inhibitor of MAO type A at low doses but is non-selective in clinically effective doses. Selegiline (deprenyl) is a relatively selective inhibitor of MAO type B.

These different isoenzymes have different selectivities for amine substrates, but the physiological importance of this is not clear. Since MAO is one of the two main enzymes involved in the metabolism of 5-hydroxytryptamine (5-HT) and catecholamines (for example adrenaline, noradrenaline, and dopamine), the MAO inhibitors cause an increase in 5-HT and catecholamine concentrations in the brain and other nervous tissues. It is this effect that is thought to be the primary action leading to the therapeutic effect of the MAO inhibitors in relieving depression, although how this is achieved is as yet unknown.

In Parkinson's disease selegiline acts by inhibiting the breakdown of dopamine in the nigrostriatal region. There is also evidence that it may arrest the progress of the disease, perhaps by inhibiting the formation of toxic substances involved in its pathogenesis.

Uses

Phobic anxiety states with depression.

Because of drug and food interactions with MAO inhibitors (see below) they are less popular currently in the treatment of endogenous depression than the tricyclic and other antidepressants. They are usually reserved for patients who have failed to respond to other forms of drug therapy.

Selegiline is used in the treatment of Parkinson's disease.

Dosages

Depression

Phenelzine, 15 mg orally t.d.s. initially, increasing to q.d.s. after 2 weeks if necessary, then reducing gradually to the lowest effective maintenance dosage.

Isocarboxazid, 10–20 mg orally o.d.

Tranylcypromine, 10 mg orally b.d. initially, increasing if required to t.d.s. after 1 week, then reducing to a maintenance dosage (usually 10 mg o.d.).

Iproniazid, 100–150 mg orally o.d. initially, reducing gradually to a maintenance dosage of 25–50 mg o.d.

Parkinson's disease

Selegiline, 5–10 mg orally o.d.

Kinetic data

The MAO inhibitors are all well absorbed. The hydrazine derivatives (for example phenelzine) are metabolized by acetylation, which is generally polymorphic (see Chapter 8). The duration of action of the hydrazine derivatives does not depend on their half-times, since they cause irreversible inhibition of MAO, and after withdrawal their effects last for as long as it takes for MAO stores to be repleted by fresh synthesis (i.e. about 2 weeks).

Tranylcypromine is extensively metabolized. Its inhibitory effect on MAO is reversible and its duration of action after withdrawal is about 4 d.

Selegiline is extensively metabolized, $t_{1/2} = 40$ h.

Important adverse effects and interactions

The most important adverse effect of the MAO inhibitors is an acute hypertensive crisis due to the interaction of MAO inhibitors with amines, particularly that with tyramine in foods. Selegiline does not share this effect, since it does not inhibit gut MAO (type A). The important interactions of MAO inhibitors can be classified as follows:

(a) Monoamines

(i) Tyramine

MAO inhibitors interact with tyramine in foods and the interaction can result in a serious, potentially fatal reaction consisting of severe hypertension associated with severe headache, sweating, flushing, nausea, vomiting, and palpitation. The mechanism of this interaction (the so-called

---

TREATMENT CARD

Carry this card with you at all times. Show it to any doctor who may treat you other than the doctor who prescribed this medicine, and to your dentist if you require dental treatment.

INSTRUCTIONS TO PATIENTS

Please read carefully

While taking this medicine and for 10 days after your treatment finishes you must observe the following simple instructions:-

1 Do not eat CHEESE, PICKLED HERRING OR BROAD BEAN PODS.

2 Do not eat or drink BOVRIL, OXO, MARMITE or ANY SIMILAR MEAT OR YEAST EXTRACT.

3 Do not take any other MEDICINES (including tablets, capsules, nose drops, inhalations or suppositories) whether purchased by you or previously prescribed by your doctor, without first consulting him.

NB *Cough and cold cures, pain relievers and tonics are medicines.*

4 Drink ALCOHOL only in moderation and avoid CHIANTI WINE completely.

Report any severe symptoms to your doctor and follow any other advice given by him.

Prepared by The Pharmaceutical Society and the British Medical Association on behalf of the Health Departments of the United Kingdom.

11530/1963 R16S 568906 250m 11/77 AG 3640/4

■ **Fig. P7** An example of the kind of warning card which should be given to a patient taking MAO inhibitors. (Reproduced with the permission of The Pharmaceutical Society of Great Britain and the British Medical Association.)

'cheese reaction') is discussed in Chapter 10 and a list of foods particularly to be avoided is given in Table 10.3. Patients should be warned about such interactions and should be given a warning card of the type illustrated in Fig. P7. Treatment of the hypertension is these cases is with i.v. phentolamine (see pp. 129 and 264).

(ii) Other indirectly-acting amines

The effects of other amines, such as ephedrine, pseudoephedrine, phenylpropanolamine, and amphetamines, which release noradrenaline from nerve-endings, may be potentiated by MAO inhibitors, since the amount of noradrenaline in nerve-endings is increased by MAO inhibitors, and the increased amount of noradrenaline so released is less well metabolized. A severe hypertensive reaction may result. Since indirectly-acting amines are found in proprietary cold and cough 'cures', which can be bought at pharmacists' shops over the counter, patients should be warned not to use such medicines (see Fig. P6).

(iii) Dopamine receptor agonists

L-dopa and dopamine may cause similar hypertensive reactions in patients taking non-selective MAO inhibitors and generally should be avoided. Selegiline may be combined with L-dopa (see uses above).

(iv) Directly-acting adrenoceptor agonists

For the same reasons, exogenously administered catecholamines, such as adrenaline, noradrenaline, and isoprenaline, should not be given to patients taking MAO inhibitors. This is particularly important when using local anaesthetics, such as lignocaine, which may also contain adrenaline (see p. 475).

(b) Tricyclic antidepressants

Since tricyclic antidepressants inhibit monoamine reuptake by nerve-endings, the combination of tricyclic antidepressants and MAO inhibitors is theoretically hazardous and sometimes is so in practice.

Adverse effects of this interaction include flushing, sweating, hyperpyrexia, restlessness, excitement, tremor, muscle twitching, muscle rigidity, convulsions, and coma.

However, there are also reports of the successful and safe use of this combination by some psychiatrists. Nevertheless, such treatment requires experience and care, and should be used only by those expert in the treatment of psychiatric disorders.

(c) Pethidine

The combination of pethidine with MAO inhibitors is a serious and potentially fatal one and should be avoided. The mechanism of the interaction is not known, but it can result in flushing, sweating, hyperpyrexia, restlessness, increased muscle tone, muscle rigidity, respiratory depression, severe hypotension, and coma. Other narcotic analgesics do not seem to be involved in this type of interaction.

(d) Oral hypoglycaemic drugs

For unknown reasons MAO inhibitors may potentiate the effect of oral hypoglycaemic drugs.

(e) Others

It is generally unwise to combine MAO inhibitors with other drugs which in some way affect monoamine function, for example methyldopa and reserpine.

Apart from the adverse effects attributable to these interactions, MAO inhibitors have mild adverse effects, which usually consist of central nervous system and autonomic effects, including dizziness, drowsiness, weakness, dry mouth, blurred vision, and postural hypotension. Over-stimulation can occur, particularly with tranylcypromine, and can lead to insomnia, acute anxiety, and agitation. Patients with cerebrovascular disease are more susceptible to these effects and should not be given MAO inhibitors.

The MAO inhibitors are contra-indicated in patients with liver disease, mainly because they are metabolized in the liver. The hydrazine derivatives have been reported to cause liver damage rarely, but with a high mortality rate (20 per cent).

Oedema and gastrointestinal effects (nausea, vomiting, and constipation) may occur.

Mustine

Structure

$$CH_3N(CH_2CH_2Cl)_2$$

Mode of action

Mustine (other names nitrogen mustard, meth-chloroethamine, chlorethazine) is an alkylating agent (see busulphan).

Uses

Bronchogenic carcinoma.
Non-Hodgkin's lymphoma.

Dosages

The usual dose is 0.4 mg/kg i.v. as a single dose. Because it is a powerful tissue irritant mustine should be given into the tubing of a fast-running i.v. infusion to avoid thrombophlebitis at the site of injection.

Kinetic data

After i.v. injection mustine disappears from the blood within 10 min and is metabolized to the reactive ethyleneimmonium ion.

Important adverse effects

Anorexia, nausea, and vomiting are common. Bone-marrow suppression is dose-related. Local irritation occurs at the site of injection if there is extravasation or if a fast-running infusion technique is not used (see above). If extravasation occurs infiltrate the area with 3 per cent sodium thiosulphate and apply icepacks intermittently for 6–12 h thereafter; lignocaine may also be infused locally to relieve pain.

Interaction

For the possible interaction with live vaccines see p. 251.

Narcotic analgesics

Narcotic analgesics may be classified as follows:

1. Opiate analgesics

(a) derived from opium alkaloids (morphine, codeine);

(b) semi-synthetic congeners of morphine (diamorphine, dihydrocodeine, pholcodine).

2. Non-opiate morphine-like analgesics

pethidine (meperidine);
methadone;
dipipanone;
dextromoramide;
dextropropoxyphene;
pentazocine;
diphenoxylate;
buprenorphine.

1. Opiate analgesics and opiate antagonists

Structures

General

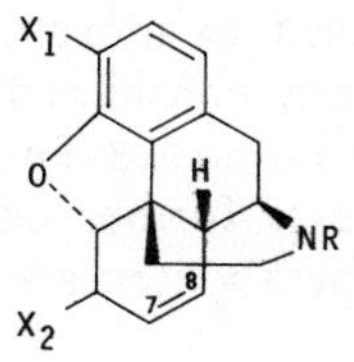

Examples

	X_1	X_2	R
Agonists			
Morphine	OH	OH	CH_3
Diamorphine (heroin)	$COOCH_3$	$COOCH_3$	CH_3
Codeine	OCH_3	OH	CH_3
Dihydrocodeine*	OCH_3	OH	CH_3
(other related agonists include buprenorphine and pholcodine.)			
Antagonists			
Naloxone*	OH	= O	$CH_2CH = CH_2$

*Single bond at C7–8.

Mode of action

In the central nervous system opiate analgesics bind to specific opioid receptors and act as partial and complete agonists, mimicking the effects of the endogenous opioids which normally bind to those receptors. This results in a variety of effects, each of which depends on the area of the brain affected and the physiological function of that area. For example, the analgesic effects are thought to be mediated by the binding of opiate analgesics to those areas involved in the perception of pain in the spinal cord, spinal trigeminal nucleus, periaqueductal and periventricular grey matter, and medullary raphe nuclei.

There is a multiplicity of CNS effects resulting from the actions of opiates on various areas of the brain and spinal cord. In addition to the desired effect of analgesia, these cause the following unwanted effects;

nausea and vomiting;
pupillary constriction;
drowsiness and sleep;
respiratory depression and suppression of the cough reflex;
mood change: usually euphoria, occasionally dysphoria;
decreased sympathetic outflow, urinary retention, and constipation;
lowering of temperature.

The peripheral effects of the opiate analgesics are also mediated by their effects on opioid receptors. These include a decrease in gastrointestinal motility with constipation, spasm of the sphincter of Oddi, and increased pressure in the biliary tract (which may result in biliary colic).

Morphine and diamorphine are vasodilators, an action which may be due to their effects in releasing histamine and in suppressing central sympathetic outflow.

The mechanisms by which tolerance and addiction to opiates occur are still unclear, despite the discovery of the enkephalins and endorphins.

Opiate antagonists are competitive antagonists at opioid receptors and reverse the pharmacological effects of the opiate agonists.

Uses

Severe pain: particularly effective in visceral pain (morphine, diamorphine, and buprenorphine).

Moderate pain (codeine, dihydrocodeine, buprenorphine).

Acute pulmonary oedema due to left ventricular failure (morphine, diamorphine).

Symptomatic relief of diarrhoea (codeine).

Suppression of cough (morphine, codeine, pholcodine).

Preoperative medication (morphine).

Naloxone is used to reverse the adverse effects of the opiate analgesics, but is only partially effective in reversing the effects of buprenorphine. Naloxone also reverses the effects of other narcotic analgesics, such as pethidine, dextropropoxyphene, and methadone.

Dosages

There are many different dosage formulations of the opiate analgesics, and individual patients' needs will dictate the use of one or another. A selection of commonly used dosages and formulations is given below. Other formulations are listed in more comprehensive formularies.

(i) Parenteral

Relief of pain (see also p. 463), treatment of pulmonary oedema, preoperative medication (morphine):

Morphine, 10–20 mg i.v., i.m., or s.c.
Diamorphine, 5–10 mg i.v., i.m., or s.c.
Dihydrocodeine, 25–50 mg i.m. or by deep s.c. injection.
Buprenorphine, 300–600 micrograms i.m. or by slow i.v. injection.

(ii) Oral, sublingual, and rectal formulations for severe pain

Morphine sulphate, sustained-release tablets (MST-1 Continus® tablets) contain morphine 10 mg or 30 mg; initial dose 10–20 mg b.d.

Buprenorphine, 2 sublingual tablets (0.4 mg each) every 6–8 h as required.

Morphine hydrochloride or sulphate, 1 to 2 suppositories (15 mg each).

(iii) Oral or sublingual formulations for the treatment of moderate pain

Codeine phosphate, 10–60 mg 4-hourly when required, to a maximum of 200 mg daily.

Dihydrocodeine, 30–60 mg every 4–6 h as required.

Buprenorphine, as for severe pain.

(iv) Oral formulations for other indications

Diarrhoea: opium tincture (morphine 10 mg/ml), 1–2 mL; codeine phosphate, 45–120 mg daily in 3–6 divided doses.

Cough suppression: linctus codeine, 15 mg/5 mL, adults 5–20 mL; linctus pholcodine, 5 mg/mL; up to 10 mL 4-hourly.

(v) Opiate antagonists

Naloxone, 0.4 mg i.v., repeated once or twice at 2–3 min intervals if respiratory function does not improve after a single dose. Further doses may be required if the effects of naloxone wear off.

Kinetic data

Morphine and diamorphine are extensively metabolized by the liver and after oral administration their systemic availability is about 25 per cent, because of marked first-pass metabolism. Diamorphine is said to enter the brain more readily than morphine, and its earlier effects after parenteral injection may be due to this, but it is rapidly metabolized to morphine ($t_{1/2} = 2$ min) and is not generally considered to be preferable to morphine for routine use. The $t_{1/2}$ of morphine is 3 h. Morphine is further extensively metabolized and its metabolites are excreted in the urine.

The systemic availability of codeine is probably more than that of morphine and diamorphine and it is metabolized by the liver, 10 per cent being demethylated to morphine, $t_{1/2} = 3$ h.

Naloxone has a $t_{1/2}$ of 1 h. Note that this is shorter than that of morphine.

Important adverse effects

Nausea and vomiting are dose-related. However in clinical practice with judicious dosing it is often possible to achieve good analgesic effects with minimal emetic effects. Because in many acute clinical situations routine dosage regimens have to be used, for example acute myocardial infarction and postoperative pain, antiemetics are often given routinely with opiates (for example cyclizine in Cyclimorph®, chlorpromazine in elixirs, and metoclopramide).

Hypotension is not infrequent due to vasodilatation and may cause concern after myocardial infarction. Confusion, dizziness, and mental clouding often occur, particularly in old people. Micturition may be difficult because of effects on the bladder. Dry mouth and constipation are common.

Occasionally, instead of euphoria and sedation, dysphoria, restlessness, and even psychiatric mental excitement can occur.

Urticaria may occur because of the histamine-releasing effects, as may pruritus and itching of the nose.

Physical drug dependence can occur quite quickly, but under usual clinical circumstances, when narcotic analgesics are being given for the relief of pain, addiction is not a problem. However, *tolerance*, which is pharmacologically related to dependence, does occur and may result in the need for higher doses. Tolerance to and physical dependence on opiate analgesics occurs at different rates for the different opiates, but typically begins to occur after about 2 weeks of continuous treatment with morphine or diamorphine. Abrupt withdrawal of the opiate, or administration of an opiate antagonist such as naloxone, then results in a typical withdrawal syndrome. The first signs of withdrawal are yawning, sweating, lachrymation, and rhinorrhoea, occurring at about 12 h after withdrawal. These are followed by restlessness, insomnia, irritability, tremor, anorexia, dilated pupils, and gooseflesh (so-called 'cold turkey'). All of these symptoms become progressively worse and the syndrome reaches its peak of intensity at about 2–3 d after withdrawal. At that time other symptoms occur, including nausea and vomiting, abdominal cramps, diarrhoea, muscle spasms, sexual orgasm, and an increase in heart rate and blood pressure. Treatment is by giving the patient his usual dose of opiate, but some have found that clonidine is effective in treating the syndrome. Untreated the syndrome disappears in about a week, but during that time may be complicated by dehydration with all its consequences.

The syndrome which follows the withdrawal of methadone takes longer to occur and is less severe than that which follows the withdrawal of morphine or diamorphine. For this reason it is possible to treat physical dependence on morphine or diamorphine by substituting methadone in a suitable dose and then slowly withdrawing the methadone. A dose of methadone of 1 mg for every 4 mg of morphine or 2 mg of diamorphine is usually adequate, and withdrawal of methadone can be carried out by small daily reductions in dose over a period of about 2–3 weeks. It is important that this procedure be carried out in hospital, so that one may observe any acute withdrawal symptoms which require treatment. During methadone withdrawal minor withdrawal symptoms may be treated symptomatically. Alternatively, withdrawal of methadone may be carried out on an out-patient basis very gradually over several months.

Special problems may arise with the use of opiate analgesics in patients with respiratory or hepatic disease.

(i) Respiratory disease

In acute asthma and chronic obstructive airways disease opiate analgesics can be dangerous, because they reduce respiratory drive, diminish ventilation, and exacerbate hypoxia and hypercapnia. Catastrophic impairment of respiratory function may then result. Opioids should only be used to relieve pain (and not distress) in these patients and doses must be titrated carefully against pain relief.

(ii) Hepatic disease

Opiate analgesics are dangerous in severe hepatic disease for two reasons. Firstly, their metabolism by the liver may be reduced and their $t_{1/2}$ prolonged. Secondly, in hepatic failure incipient hepatic encephalopathy may render the brain more sensitive to the effects of opiates and coma and respiratory depression may result.

Naloxone has virtually no adverse effects, apart from producing an acute withdrawal syndrome in subjects with physical dependence on opiates.

Interactions

Opiate analgesics and other centrally depressant drugs have additive effects. This is important for the co-administration of, for example, phenothiazines.

2. Non-opiate narcotic analgesics

Structures

Methadone, dextropropoxyphene, dipipanone, and dextromoramide have related structures. Dextropropoxyphene is shown here as an example:

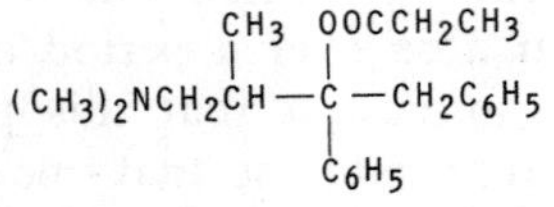

$$(CH_3)_2NCH_2CH-\underset{\underset{C_6H_5}{|}}{\overset{\overset{CH_3}{|}}{C}}-CH_2C_6H_5 \quad OOCCH_2CH_3$$

Pethidine and diphenoxylate are related. Pethidine (meperidine) is shown here:

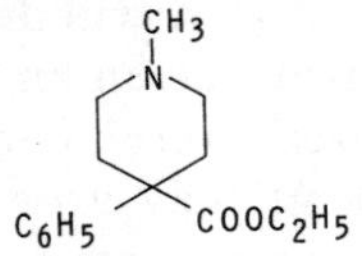

Mode of action

See opiate analgesics.

Uses

Analgesia:

Severe pain: particularly effective in visceral pain (pethidine, methadone, dipipanone, and dextromoramide).

Mild to moderate pain (dextropropoxyphene, often combined with paracetamol or aspirin).

Diarrhoea (diphenoxylate, combined with atropine sulphate).

Pre-operative medication (pethidine).

Treatment of opiate addiction (methadone).

Dosages

Parenteral

Pethidine, 25–100 mg i.m. or s.c. 4-hourly as required.

Methadone, 5–10 mg i.m. or s.c. 4-hourly as required.

Oral

Pethidine, 50–100 mg 4-hourly as required.

Methadone, 5–10 mg 4-hourly as required.

Dipipanone, 10 mg initially, increasing to 30 mg every 4 h as required.

Dextromoramide, 5 mg initially, increasing to 20 mg six-hourly as required.

Dextropropoxyphene. This is commonly used in combination with paracetamol, the combination being called co-proxamol, which is dextropropoxyphene 32.5 mg with paracetamol 325 mg. Dose 1–2 tablets every 6–8 h.

Diphenoxylate. This is commonly used in combination with atropine sulphate, the combination being called co-phenotrope, which is diphenoxylate 2.5 mg with atropine sulphate 25 micrograms in each tablet or 5 mL of elixir. Dose, four tablets or 20 mL of elixir initially, followed by two tablets or 10 mL of elixir 6-hourly.

Kinetic data

	Absorption	Metabolism	$t_{1/2}$
Pethidine	55%	Liver + + +	3 h
Methadone	Well absorbed		1–2 d
Dipipanone		Liver + + +	
Dextromoramide			
Dextropropoxyphene	Well absorbed	Liver + + +	12 h

Important adverse effects

The adverse effects of the non-opiate narcotic analgesics are similar to those of the opiate analgesics. However, dextropropoxyphene and diphenoxylate do not commonly cause adverse effects in short courses of therapeutic doses. However, chronic usage can lead to constipation and overdosage has the same effects as morphine.

Interactions

As for opiate analgesics.

Neuroleptic drugs

Structures

The neuroleptic drugs are of three chemical types, the phenothiazines and thioxanthenes, which are structurally related, and the butyrophenones. Domperidone and metoclopramide, dopamine receptor antagonists which are used to treat nausea and vomiting, are dealt with in separate monographs.

Phenothiazines, general

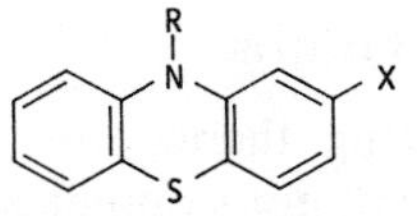

(Compare tricyclic antidepressants.)

Phenothiazines in common use are chlorpromazine, fluphenazine, perphenazine, prochlorperazine, thioridazine, and trifluoperazine.

Thioxanthenes, general

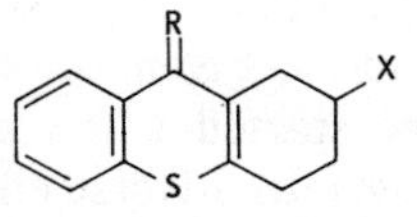

Thioxanthenes in common use are flupenthixol and clopenthixol.

The substitution of chemical groups at position R determines the pharmacological actions of both of these types of drugs and substitution at position X determines their potency.

Butyrophenones

Haloperidol is illustrated here. Other butyrophenones (for example droperidol) share the 4-fluorobutyrophenone structure, but have different substituents at the fourth carbon of the butyrate moiety.

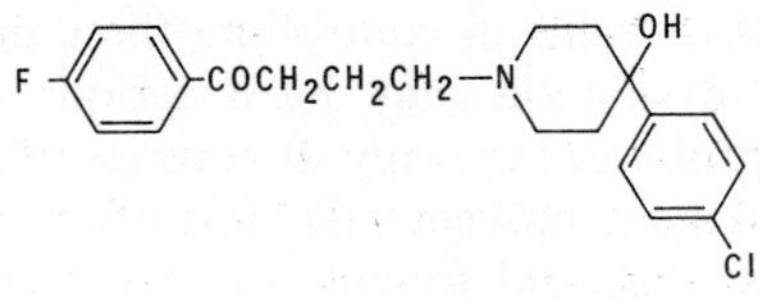

Mode of action

The neuroleptic drugs are antagonists at dopamine receptors in the brain. It is probable that this effect is the basis of their mode of action in the treatment of the acute psychoses (mania and schizophrenia), of acute confusional states, and as antiemetics. However, the development of adaptive pharmacological responses to the acute dopamine inhibitory effects are also likely to be an important part of their antipsychotic action.

Some of these drugs also have anticholinergic and antihistaminic effects and block the actions of 5-hydroxytryptamine and the α-adrenergic actions of noradrenaline; the contribution of these effects to their therapeutic efficacy is at present unclear, but may be important for adverse effects. Their effect in inhibiting dopamine receptors is responsible for their extrapyramidal adverse effects.

These classes of compounds are often called 'neuroleptics' (Greek νευρον = a string or cord, and by extension, a nerve; ληψομαι, from λαμβανειν = to seize). This is a term which has been coined to describe their effects of tranquillizing and causing psychomotor slowing.

Uses

As sedatives and tranquillizers.

In the treatment of acute psychotic and confusional states and in the chronic treatment of schizophrenia.

As an adjunct to narcotic analgesia in the pain of terminal illness.

In the treatment and prevention of nausea and vomiting, particularly during radiotherapy and cancer chemotherapy.

In premedication before general anaesthesia (droperidol).

Dosages

Dosages vary according to the indication, severity of illness, and the individual. The following dosage recommendations are only a rough guide.

Antiemetic

Chlorpromazine, a single i.m. dose of 25–50 mg; orally 25 mg t.d.s.

Prochlorperazine, a single i.m. dose of 12.5–25 mg or 5–25 mg t.d.s. orally.

Trifluoperazine, 1–3 mg daily in divided doses i.m. or 2–4 mg daily in divided doses orally.

Droperidol, 5–15 mg i.v., 5–10 mg i.m., or 5–20 mg orally as a single dose, repeated 6-hourly if required.

Ranges of dosages for acute psychoses

Chlorpromazine, 25–100 mg 4–6 hourly i.m.

Perphenazine, initially 5–10 mg i.m., followed by 5 mg 6-hourly, to a maximum of 15 mg daily.

Prochlorperazine, 12.5–25 mg two to three times daily orally.

Thioridazine, 200 mg orally, followed by up to 600 mg daily.

Trifluoperazine, 1–3 mg daily in divided doses i.m.

Haloperidol, 10–30 mg i.m. as a single dose, repeated 6-hourly if required.

Ranges of dosages and treatment regimens for long-term use in psychotic illness

Chlorpromazine, 25 mg t.d.s. orally, adjusted according to response to 1 g daily or more.

Fluphenazine HCl, 2.5–10 mg o.d. orally, adjusted according to response to a maximum of 20 mg daily.

Fluphenazine decanoate and enanthate (i.m. depot injections), test dose 12.5 mg; maintenance dosage 25–50 mg every 2–6 weeks (decanoate) or 10–28 d (enanthate).

Perphenazine, 4 mg t.d.s. orally, adjusted according to response by 5 mg daily every 3 d.

Thioridazine, up to 600 mg daily orally.

Trifluoperazine, 5 mg b.d. orally, adjusted according to response by 5 mg daily every 3 d.

Flupenthixol decanoate (i.m. depot injection), test dose 20 mg; maintenance dosage 20–40 mg every 2–4 weeks.

Clopenthixol decanoate (i.m. injection), test dose 100 mg; maintenance dosage 200–400 mg every 2–4 weeks.

Haloperidol, initially 10 mg daily, increasing as required to 200 mg daily in divided doses; some patients may respond to less than 10 mg daily; whenever a theraputic effect is achieved the dosage should be reduced gradually to the minimum effective dose.

Premedication

Droperidol, 5–15 mg i.v. or 5–10 mg i.m.

Kinetic data

The phenothiazines have variable systemic availability, because of extensive metabolism during their first passage through the gut wall and liver. Numerous metabolites of varying degrees of therapeutic activity and toxicity are formed and persist in the body for weeks or even months.

The butyrophenones are mostly metabolized in the liver to inactive compounds. Their half-times are 20 h (haloperidol) and 3 h (droperidol), but the effect of droperidol lasts much longer (up to 48 h).

Depot formulations

The chronic drug therapy of schizophrenia is dogged by patient non-compliance, and formulations have been developed which provide low but adequate plasma concentrations for several weeks after injection (see dosage regimens above). These formulations contain esters of the parent drug in vegetable oil, from which the drug is slowly absorbed after intramuscular injection. Because of the prolonged effect of these formulations a test dose should be given initially and regular therapy may be started a few days later if the patient has no serious adverse effects. A practical point of management is that the patient is seen every 2–6 weeks or so for the injection and progress can be assessed at the same time.

Important adverse effects

Sedation is common early on, but tolerance develops rapidly.

Extrapyramidal signs and symptoms occur commonly, trifluoperazine and perphenazine being more potent in this respect than chlorpromazine or thioridazine. These may result in Parkinsonism, akathisia, and various acute dystonic reactions. Anticholinergic drugs, such as procyclidine, are of value in controlling these problems. Tardive dyskinesia may be a serious problem during prolonged therapy. It consists of involuntary dyskinetic movements, most often involving the jaws, lips, and tongue, but the face, limbs, and trunk may also be affected. Such movement disorders may persist despite withdrawal of therapy. A serious adverse reaction is the neuroleptic malignant syndrome (see p. 457).

Anticholinergic effects occur and include dry mouth, blurred vision, urinary retention, and constipation.

Hypotension may occur (particularly with chlorpromazine) in the critically ill patient with organic confusion who is also hypovolaemic, and care should be taken in these circumstances. The butyrophenones can cause cardiac arrhythmias.

Hypersensitivity reactions occur occasionally. Skin rashes are common and photosensitivity is a particular problem. Cholestatic jaundice is caused by chlorpromazine and has been reported in up to 2 per cent of cases.

In the elderly hypothermia may be a problem.

Endocrine disturbances may be associated with increased prolactin secretion, because of dopamine receptor inhibition. These include gynaecomastia, galactorrhoea, and menstrual disturbances.

Prolonged high dosages may cause corneal and lens opacities and pigmentation of the cornea, conjunctiva, and retina.

Blood dyscrasias are rare. Leucopenia and agranulocytosis have been reported.

Interactions

The sedative effects of these drugs are potentiated by alcohol and other sedative drugs. The effects of hypotensive agents are potentiated.

Neuromuscular blocking drugs (muscle relaxants)

1. Non-depolarizing muscle relaxants

Structures

Tubocurarine (as chloride)

Metocurine (as chloride)

Pancuronium (as bromide)

Other drugs of this type include alcuronium, metocurine, atracurium, and vecuronium.

Mode of action

The non-depolarizing neuromuscular blocking drugs act by competitive inhibition of the action of acetylcholine at the motor end-plate. They thus cause paralysis of voluntary muscle without first causing depolarization (cf. depolarizing agents below).

Their actions are reversible by acetylcholinesterase inhibitors such as neostigmine.

Uses

For the production of muscle relaxation during surgical anaesthesia.

Dosages

Tubocurarine, 10–15 mg i.v. initially, followed by additional doses of 5 mg i.v.

Pancuronium, 60–100 micrograms/kg initially, followed by supplementary doses of 10–40 micrograms/kg according to response.

Alcuronium, 200 micrograms/kg as the initial dose, followed by supplementary doses of $\frac{1}{4}$ to $\frac{1}{6}$ of the initial dose.

Metocurine, initial dose 0.25–0.4 mg/kg for intubation; additive doses of 2–5 mg i.v.

Atracurium, doses of 0.4–0.5 mg/kg are needed for intubation, with increments of 0.08–0.1 mg/kg. As an alternative, maintenance by be provided by an infusion of atracurium (6–8 micrograms/min) when given during nitrous oxide-narcotic anaesthesia. The use of volatile agents to supplement nitrous oxide will reduce maintenance requirements by about 30 per cent.

Vecuronium, doses of 80–100 micrograms/kg are used for intubation, with maintenance dosing by increments of 10–15 micrograms/kg or by infusion (1–2 micrograms/kg/min). For procedures of short duration (for example laparoscopy) doses of vecuronium as low as 0.06 mg/kg may be used to allow prompt antagonism of paralysis.

Kinetic data

The rate of onset, time to peak, and total duration of effect of these drugs are dose-dependent. The following data pertain to usual dosages.

Tubocurarine

The onset of paralysis is rapid, with a peak at 3–5 min and a duration of 20–30 min. Tubocurarine does not cross the blood-brain barrier. Placental transfer is poor and so there is little effect on the fetus. Renal excretion accounts for 30 per cent of the total elimination of the drug. $t_{1/2} = 125$–500 min.

Pancuronium

The onset of paralysis is rapid, with a peak at 3 min and a duration of action of 20–30 min. Pancuronium does not cross the blood–brain barrier. Placental transfer is poor and so there is little effect on the fetus. Pancuronium is metabolized by the liver and excreted by the kidney and in the bile. $t_{1/2} = 90$–200 min. Pancuronium is excreted 35 per cent unchanged by the kidney. One of the metabolites of pancuronium (3-hydroxypancuronium) is pharmacologically active, with a potency about 50 per cent that of the parent compound.

Alcuronium

The onset of paralysis occurs within 2–4 min, with a peak effect after 4–8 min. The duration of action of an intubation dose is 20–40 min. Alcuronium does not cross the blood-brain barrier; although it crosses the placenta. About 80–85 per cent of the relaxant dose is excreted unchanged, and hence efficacy is prolonged in renal failure. $t_{1/2} = 3$ h.

Metocurine

Metocurine is similar to tubocurarine, but is about 50 per cent more potent. In addition, it has no effect on the vagus and does not block sympathetic ganglia. It therefore has fewer cardiovascular effects than tubocurarine. About 50 per cent of the dose is excreted unchanged via the kidney, $t_{1/2} = 4$ h.

Atracurium

Intubation doses of atracurium produce a maximal effect within 2–4 min, although intubation may be achievable before this. The duration of action is 20–30 min. Atracurium is metabolized by two separate mechanisms: chemical degradation of the Hofmann pathway (which is pH- and temperature-dependent) and ester hydrolysis. Although the former route was originally thought to be the main pathway, recent work has shown that over 60 per cent of the clearance of atracurium is organ-dependent (i.e. via the liver and kidney). Ester hydrolysis is not reduced in patients with plasma pseudocholinesterase deficiency. Hofmann breakdown results in two metabolites, laudanosine and the monoquaternary alcohol. Neither is clinically active as a muscle relaxant; however, high concentrations of laudanosine cause CNS stimulation and have seizure-like activity in animals. The $t_{1/2}$ of atracurium is 20 min.

Vecuronium

Maximum neuromuscular blockade blockade occurs with vecuronium within 3–5 min and lasts for 20–30 min. In contrast to its quaternary congener, pancuronium, vecuronium undergoes only 10–25 per cent renal elimination unchanged. The rest of the drug is metabolized by esterases, which hydrolyse acetoxy groups at positions 3 and 17. The 3-hydroxy, 17-hydroxy, and 3,17-dihydroxy metabolites are probably pharmacologically inactive in humans. Deacetylation occurs at a rate 2–3 times that of pancuronium.

$t_{1/2} = 30–90$ min. The duration of effect of vecuronium is prolonged in both severe liver disease and in renal failure.

Important adverse effects during anaesthesia

Tubocurarine causes some degree of autonomic ganglion blockade and histamine release. It may therefore cause slight hypotension, occasional bradycardia, and a transient erythematous rash. Bronchospasm occurs rarely.

Pancuronium does not cause autonomic ganglion blockade and causes little histamine release. Thus, hypotension is less of a problem than with tubocurarine.

Vecuronium has no blocking activity on the cardiac vagus or sympathetic ganglia, and there is therefore a tendency for bradycardia to occur in association with surgical stimulation of parasympathetically innervated organs, and with use of opioid analgesics or halothane anaesthesia. Bradycardia may be more pronounced in patients whose compensatory sympathetic reflexes are impaired by β-blockers. Vecuronium does not release histamine.

Atracurium is a weak histamine releaser, with a potency less than one-third of that of tubocurarine. Reactions usually take the form of cutaneous eruptions, without cardiovascular or other untoward effects. However, cases of bronchospasm and cardiovascular collapse have been reported. The cutaneous reactions can be minimized if atracurium is given into large veins and separate from the induction agent. A second adverse effect associated with atracurium is bradycardia. However, since neither atracurium nor its breakdown products have significant effects on the heart or autonomic nervous system, it seems that these episodes of bradycardia are due to the effects of concurrently administered anaesthetic agents (fentanyl, halothane) and vagal stimulation during surgery.

Interactions

The effects of the non-depolarizing muscle relaxants are reversed by acetylcholinesterase inhibitors (qq.v.).

Some drugs with direct neuromuscular blocking effects may potentiate the effects of the non-depolarizing muscle relaxants. They include aminoglycosides, polymixins A and B, clindamycin and lincomycin, colistin, and quinine and quinidine. Magnesium salts also potentiate the effects of these muscle relaxants.

2. Depolarizing muscle relaxants

Structures

Suxamethonium (succinylcholine) is the most commonly used drug of this type:

$$CH_2COOCH_2CH_2\overset{+}{N}(CH_3)_3$$
$$|$$
$$CH_2COOCH_2CH_2\underset{+}{N}(CH_3)_3$$

Mode of action

Suxamethonium produces a prolonged depolarization of the motor end-plate and thus prevents any response to acetylcholine. This action is *not* reversible by acetylcholinesterase inhibitors (cf. non-depolarizing muscle relaxants).

Uses

For the production of muscle relaxation during anaesthesia, particularly when only short-term effects are required (i.e. to effect intubation).

Dosages

20–100 mg i.v., according to the patient's needs and response.

Kinetic data

The onset of action of suxamethonium occurs within 30 s, and its duration of action is 3–5 min in normal individuals. It is rapidly hydrolysed by pseudocholinesterase in the plasma and tissues. $t_{1/2} = 2–4$ min. However, in patients with pseudocholinesterase deficiency the metabolism is lowed and the $t_{1/2}$ and duration of effect are prolonged (see Chapter 8).

Important adverse effects

Muscle fasciculation occurs during the onset of muscle relaxation because of depolarization, and muscle pains are common after the procedure.

Prolonged apnoea occurs when there is pseudocholinesterase deficiency, either acquired (for example due to liver disease, malnutrition, or severe anaemia) or congenital (hereditary pseudocholinesterase deficiency, discussed in Chapter 8).

Suxamethonium has some muscarinic activity, causing a transient rise in intraocular pressure, salivary gland enlargement, increased bowel motility, and increased gastric and salivary secretions. For these reasons premedication with atropine is desirable before suxamethonium is used. It should not be used in patients with glaucoma and during ophthalmic operations.

Dual block may occur with non-depolarizing block (see Chapter 30).

Repeated doses may produce cardiac slowing.

A small rise in plasma potassium concentration (about 0.2–0.4 mmol/L) may occur, due to potassium release from muscle; larger increases may occur following denervation or in muscle diseases or damage.

There is increased pseudocholinesterase activity, and hence a shortened duration of action of suxamethonium, in patients with the genetic C_5 isoenzyme variant and in a number of diseases, including nodular goitre, essential hypertension, thyrotoxicosis, alcoholism, schizophrenia, obesity, and some hyperlipidaemias.

Interactions

Potentiation of suxamethonium may occur with drugs which have direct neuromuscular blocking effects, including aminoglycosides, clindamycin and lincomycin, colistin, and quinine and quinidine. Magnesium salts also potentiate the muscle relaxant effects of suxamethonium metabolism.

Drugs which inhibit the activity of pseudocholinesterase decrease suxamethonium metabolism and thus enhance its effects; these include cyclophosphamide, mustine, thiotepa, MAO inhibitors, oral contraceptives, chlorpromazine, pancuronium, ester-type local anaesthetics, trimethoprim, glucocorticoids, esmolol, and inhibitors of acetylcholinesterase. Included in the last group are long-acting acetylcholinesterase inhibitors such as ecothiopate, which is used in eye drops in the treatment of glaucoma, and organophosphorus insecticides.

Malignant hyperthermia (see Chapter 8) may occur in susceptible patients when suxamethonium is used in combination with some inhalational anaesthetics.

Suxamethonium may potentiate the effects of cardiac glycosides by an unknown mechanism.

Nikethamide

Structure

Mode of action

Nikethamide is an analeptic, i.e. it is a stimulant of various central nervous system functions. It stimulates respiration by a direct effect on the respiratory centre in the medulla oblongata and does not stimulate carotid chemoreceptors (cf. doxapram).

Uses

For a discussion of the uses of respiratory stimulants see under doxapram.

Dosages

0.5–2 g i.v. repeated as necessary every 15–30 min. Frequent monitoring of arterial blood gases and pH are required to allow regulation of the dosage.

Important adverse effects

Adverse effects are common and are dose-related. They include nausea and vomiting, tachycardia and cardiac arrhythmias, dizziness, restlessness, tremor and convulsions.

Nikethamide should not be given to patients with respiratory depression in association with neurological disease (including cerebral oedema), or to patients with status asthmaticus, coronary artery disease, hyperthyroidism, or severe hypertension. It should be given only with great care to patients with a history of epilepsy.

It is not helpful, and may be dangerous, in patients with respiratory depression due to overdose with hypnotics or sedatives.

Nitrates

Structures

Glyceryl trinitrate

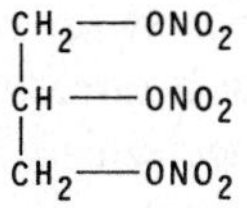

Isosorbide dinitrate (sorbide nitrate)

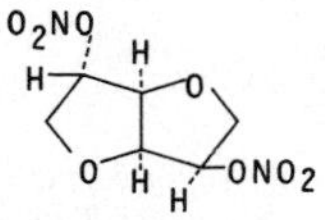

Isosorbide mononitrate:

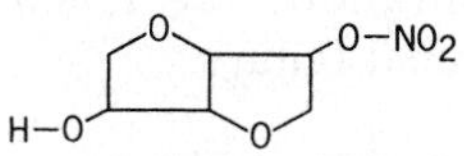

Mode of action

The actions of the nitrates in relieving angina pectoris are complex. Three main mechanisms are involved:

1. Peripheral arteriolar vasodilatation with reduction in peripheral resistance and lowering of blood pressure. This leads to a decrease in cardiac work and a reduction in myocardial oxygen requirements.

2. Peripheral venous vasodilatation results in peripheral venous pooling, a reduction in left ventricular end-diastolic pressure, and a reduction in resistance to coronary blood flow during diastole.

3. The vasodilatory effects of the nitrates may also affect certain areas of the coronary arteriolar bed, redistributing blood flow to areas of myocardial ischaemia. This may be of particular importance in angina due to coronary arterial spasm.

The actions of the nitrates in heart failure depend on venous and arterial vasodilatation, with consequent reductions in preload and afterload.

Uses

Angina pectoris.
Cardiac failure.

Dosages

Glyceryl trinitrate

Angina, one or two 0.5 mg tablets sublingually when pain occurs or in immediate anticipation of the pain (for example before exercise or an expected emotional stress); ointment, 1–2 inches of a 2 per cent ointment rubbed into the skin, usually of the anterior chest.

Buccal tablets, 1–3 mg t.d.s.

Transdermal patches, one 5 mg or 10 mg patch applied once a day (removed for a few hours each day, in order to reduce the risk of tolerance, see below).

Isosorbide dinitrate

Angina, 5–20 mg orally b.d., t.d.s., or q.d.s.
Heart failure: 10–30 mg q.d.s. orally.

Isosorbide mononitrate

20–120 mg orally daily in divided doses.
For i.v. doses of nitrates see p. 274.

Kinetic data

Because glyceryl trinitrate undergoes extensive first-pass metabolism in the liver it is usually given sublingually and is well and rapidly absorbed through the oral mucosa, whence it enters the systemic circulation. Buccal administration has a similar effect, although this route is used for a more prolonged action over a few hours. Absorption via the skin is slow, and this route can therefore be used for a sustained effect over several hours.

Isosorbide is absorbed from the gut and is extensively metabolized to active metabolites, especially isosorbide mononitrate, which is itself metabolized. Isosorbide dinitrate and mononitrate are therefore active after oral administration.

The $t_{1/2}$ of glyceryl trinitrate is a few minutes and of isosorbide dinitrate 1 h. Isosorbide mononitrate has a $t_{1/2}$ of 4 h and this rate-limits the kinetics of the dinitrate.

Important adverse effects

Vasodilatation may result in throbbing headache, sinus tachycardia, and hypotension. Tolerance to headache may develop with prolonged use, particularly of the transdermal formulations. Patients should be advised to swallow any remnants of a sublingual tablet of glyceryl trinitrate once relief of anginal pain has occurred, to try to minimize the acute adverse effects.

Tolerance to the therapeutic actions of the nitrates occurs with prolonged administration, and this is especially the case with the transdermal patches, if they are left on the skin continuously. This can be minimized or avoided by removing the patch for a few hours each day (for example overnight). The mechanism of this tolerance is discussed in Chapter 4.

Nitrofurantoin

Structure

Mode of action

Nitrofurantoin is converted by bacterial nitrofuran reductases to active metabolites which alter nucleic acid function.

Uses

Urinary infections due to Gram-negative organisms, particularly *E. coli*.

Dosage

100 mg q.d.s. orally.

Kinetic data

Nitrofurantoin is well absorbed. About 40 per cent of the dose of nitrofurantoin is secreted unchanged into the urine ($t_{1/2} = 30$ min) in concentrations two to four times the usual minimal inhibitory concentration for sensitive bacteria. Blood concentrations are much lower but are increased in renal failure.

Important adverse effects

Nausea and vomiting are common, Mild allergic reactions occur in about 4 per cent of patients. They are usually unimportant in themselves, but their occurrence is a warning to stop treatment, since they may herald more serious forms of allergy, resulting in lung or liver damage.

Long-term therapy occasionally results in a peripheral neuropathy, which is dose-related.

Nitrofurantoin may cause haemolysis in patients with G6PD deficiency (see Chapter 8).

Nitrofurantoin should not be used in patients with renal failure.

Interactions

Magnesium trisilicate reduces the absorption of nitrofurantoin. Probenecid and sulphinpyrazone inhibit its urinary secretion and may reduce its effect. Acidification of the urine increases the secretion of nitrofurantoin, as does pyridoxine.

The quinolones and nitrofurantoin have an antagonistic interaction *in vitro* and should not be used together.

Non-steroidal anti-inflammatory drugs

The non-steroidal anti-inflammatory drugs are of four broad chemical types: the arylalkanoic acids (derivatives of acetic, propionic, and butyric acids), the anthranilic acids (derivatives of phenylanthranilic acid), the pyrazolones (azapropazone, phenylbutazone, and oxyphenbutazone), and the salicylates. The pyrazolones and the salicylates are dealt with in separate monographs.

Structures

1. Arylalkanoic acids

(a) Acetic acid derivatives

Example:

Indomethacin

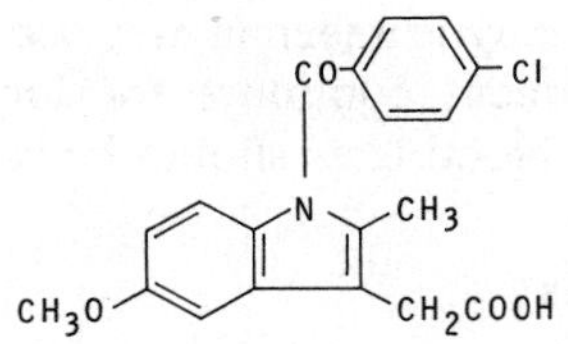

(b) Propionic acid derivatives

General

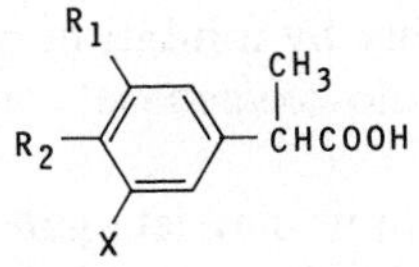

Examples

	R_1	R_2	X
Fenoprofen	C_6H_5O	H	H
Flurbiprofen	H	C_6H_5	F
Ibuprofen	H	$(CH_3)_2CHCH_2$	H
Ketoprofen	H	H	COC_6H_5

(c) Butyric acid derivatives

Example:

Fenbufen

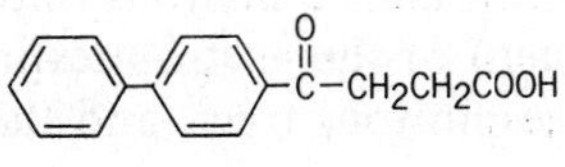

2. Anthranilic acids

General

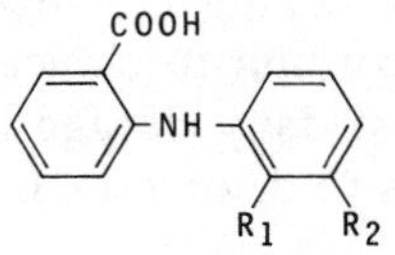

Examples

	R_1	R_2
Mefenamic acid	CH_3	CH_3
Flufenamic acid	H	CF_3

Mode of action

The non-steroidal anti-inflammatory agents have analgesic, antipyretic, and anti-inflammatory properties. Their total mode of action is unknown, but inhibition of prostaglandin synthesis is thought to play an important part.

Uses

All may be used as analgesic and anti-inflammatory agents in the treatment of rheumatoid arthritis, osteoarthritis, ankylosing spondylitis, and acute musculoskeletal disorders. Ibuprofen may be used in Still's disease (juvenile rheumatoid arthritis) and in seronegative (non-rheumatoid) arthropathies. Naproxen and diclofenac may be used in the symptomatic treatment of acute gout. Indomethacin is used to treat patent ductus arteriosus in premature babies; this is a specialist indication and needs careful supervision.

Mefenamic acid is used in the relief of menorrhagia due to dysfunctional causes and the presence of an intrauterine contraceptive device.

Dosages

Fenoprofen, 300–600 mg q.d.s.
Flurbiprofen, 50–100 mg t.d.s.
Ibuprofen, 200–400 mg t.d.s. or q.d.s.
Ketoprofen, 50 mg b.d. to q.d.s.

Naproxen, 250–500 mg b.d. (acute gout, 750 mg initially and 250 mg 8-hourly until relief is obtained).

Diclofenac, 25–50 mg b.d. or t.d.s. (75 mg o.d. or b.d. i.m.).

Indomethacin, 25 mg b.d. initially increasing gradually according to clinical response. The usual range of daily dosage is 50–200 mg in divided doses (b.d. or t.d.s.). Rectal therapy, 100 mg b.d.

Fenbufen, 300 mg in the morning and 600 mg at bedtime, or 450 mg b.d.

Nabumetone, 1 g at night plus 0.5–1 g in the morning also if required.

Mefenamic acid, 500 mg t.d.s. orally.

Flufenamic acid, 200 mg t.d.s. orally.

Kinetic data

These drugs share similar kinetic properties. They are well absorbed, the anthranilic acids slowly. All are extensively metabolized to inactive compounds and have half-times of 2–14 h (diclofenac 2 h, naproxen 14 h). Excretion is via the urine and bile (the latter up to 50 per cent) with some enterohepatic recycling. All are highly bound to plasma proteins.

Important adverse effects

Gastrointestinal adverse effects occur in up to 50 per cent of patients, and include nausea, vomiting, symptoms of 'dyspepsia', and diarrhoea. Some of these symptoms can be reduced by taking the tablets with or just after food. Gastrointestinal bleeding occurs with a frequency and severity varying from compound to compound.

Ibuprofen is the least likely to cause gastrointestinal bleeding; naproxen also causes gastrointestinal bleeding less frequently than some of the other drugs, but when bleeding occurs it may be very severe; this is a particular problem in old people. In general, however, daily occult blood loss is less than with aspirin.

Allergic reactions (rashes, angio-oedema, and bronchospasm) occur occasionally. Some patients with hypersensitivity to aspirin may have cross-sensitivity to an arylalkanoic acid (see p. 111).

Fluid retention occurs and may occasionally cause peripheral oedema; hypertension has been reported.

Indomethacin commonly causes headache, which may be associated with other central nervous system effects such as vertigo, sleep disturbance, and psychiatric problems.

Leucopenia, thrombocytopenia, and an auto-immune haemolytic anaemia may occur occasionally. If treatment continues for longer than 7 days regular blood tests should be carried out.

Interactions

The non-steroidal anti-inflammatory drugs may counteract the effects of diuretics because they cause fluid retention.

They antagonize the hypotensive effect of propranolol, possibly by inhibition of prostaglandin synthetase (cyclo-oxygenase) activity in the kidney.

Since they inhibit platelet aggregation and may cause peptic ulceration, they should be used with care in patients who are also taking anticoagulants.

Nystatin

Structure

(Compare amphotericin B.)

Mode of action

Nystatin alters the permeability of cell membranes leading to loss of essential cell constituents.

Uses

Infections with *Candida albicans* (moniliasis, candidiasis, thrush) of the gastrointestinal tract, the vagina, the respiratory tract, and the skin.

Dosages

Dosages depend on the formulation and route of administration, e.g.:
oral thrush: nystatin suspension 100 000 i.u. t.d.s.;
vaginal thrush: nystatin pessaries 100 000 200 000 i.u. o.d.

Kinetic data

Nystatin is not absorbed after oral or topical administration.

Important adverse effects

Adverse effects are rare and generally unimportant.

Omeprazole

Structure

Mode of action

Omeprazole causes a dose-dependent inhibition of gastric acid secretion by inhibiting the proton pump in the gastric parietal cell. This is achieved by an active metabolite of omeprazole which binds to and inhibits the enzyme H^+/K^+ ATPase. Omeprazole suppresses acid production with much greater efficacy and a longer duration than the histamine (H_2) antagonists.

Uses

Erosive reflux oesophagitis and peptic ulceration resistant to other medical therapy.

Zollinger–Ellison syndrome.

Dosages

20–40 mg daily orally for 4–8 weeks. Higher dosages may be required in the Zollinger–Ellison syndrome.

Kinetic data

Omeprazole is activated at low pH. It is absorbed in the small intestine before being concentrated in the acidic compartment of the parietal cell. Unbound drug is rapidly metabolized and excreted in the urine. Its $t_{1/2}$ is about 1 h, but its effects last for more than 24 h, because of irreversible binding at the site of action, the maximum effect being reached after 3–5 d of therapy.

Important adverse effects

Omeprazole is generally well tolerated. Occasional nausea, headache, diarrhoea, constipation, and skin rashes have been reported.

The main concern regarding omeprazole comes from studies in animals in which it significantly raises serum gastrin concentrations. In animals given long-term omeprazole there is an increased incidence of gastrin-dependent hyperplasia of enterochromaffin-like cells and of gastric carcinoid tumours. Omeprazole is therefore only licensed for use in short courses.

Interactions

Omeprazole inhibits hepatic cytochrome P450 and can delay the elimination of diazepam, phenytoin, and warfarin. Although this effect is a minor one at therapeutic dosages it is wise to monitor phenytoin concentrations and the prothrombin time in patients taking phenytoin and warfarin respectively.

Paracetamol (acetaminophen)

Structure

$$CH_3CONH-\!\!\langle\ \rangle\!\!-OH$$

Mode of action

Paracetamol has analgesic and antipyretic properties but little anti-inflammatory activity. The mechanism of these effects is unknown, but may be related to selective inhibition of prostaglandin synthesis in certain tissues.

Uses

For the treatment of mild pain, particularly in musculoskeletal conditions, headache, and dysmenorrhoea.

Dosages

0.5–1 g every 4–6 h orally as required. Maximum 4 g daily.

Kinetic data

Paracetamol is well absorbed. It is almost completely converted ($t_{1/2} = 3$ h) to metabolites which are excreted in the urine. The route of metabolism is important in understanding the reason for the occurrence of hepatic damage in overdose and in providing the rationale for its prevention (see Fig. 35.1). About 80 per cent of an administered dose of paracetamol is normally conjugated as glucuronide and sulphate, but these pathways are easily saturated; of the remainder about 15 per cent is metabolized to a hydroxylamine derivative, which is non-toxic at concentrations resulting from conventional doses, since it reacts with hepatic glutathione intracellularly and is detoxified. However, when the concentration rises the hepatic stores of glutathione are exhausted and the hydroxylamine combines with cell structures, causing cellular damage that results in hepatic necrosis. Because of saturation of metabolism in overdose the $t_{1/2}$ is prolonged.

Prevention of hepatic necrosis in paracetamol overdose can be achieved by providing sulphydryl groups which replenish hepatocellular glutathione, thus detoxifying the hydroxylamine. *N*-acetylcysteine and methionine are examples of compounds which are used for this purpose (see p. 494).

Important adverse effects

Adverse effects are rare with therapeutic doses. In overdose hepatic necrosis is the most important effect and when it occurs hepatic enzymes are usually raised by 48 h after overdose. Rarely acute tubular necrosis also occurs, sometimes in the absence of hepatic damage.

Penicillamine

Structure

$$\underset{(CH_3)_2C-CHCOOH}{\overset{SH\quad NH_2}{|\quad\quad|}}$$

(Prepared by the hydrolytic degradation of penicillin, q.v.)

Mode of action

Penicillamine is a chelating agent, and that forms the basis of its mode of action in the treatment of heavy metal poisoning (for example lead) and of Wilson's disease, in which there is accumulation of copper. In cystinuria it probably acts by forming a soluble disulphide complex with cystine. The complexes with heavy metals and with cystine are excreted in the urine. The mode of action in rheumatoid arthritis and its variants is unknown.

Uses

Wilson's disease (hepatolenticular degeneration).

Chronic lead poisoning.

Active rheumatoid arthritis.

Cystinuria.

Dosages

Wilson's disease: initially 250 mg b.d. orally, increasing to a total of 2 g daily as required, depending on urinary copper excretion.

Lead poisoning: up to 1 g daily orally, the dose being adjusted according to urinary lead excretion.

Rheumatoid arthritis: initially 125–250 mg o.d. orally, increasing every 4–8 weeks by 125–250 mg. Some patients need as little as 250 mg daily, while others need as much as 1 g daily. It takes up to 12 weeks to see improvement, and if improvement occurs therapy should be continued for 6 months, after which the dose should be gradually reduced.

Cystinuria: initially 500 mg at night orally, increasing in increments of 250 mg to 2 g daily (range 1–4 g), depending on urinary cystine excretion. An adequate fluid intake should be ensured.

Kinetic data

Penicillamine is poorly absorbed (about 40 per cent) and is metabolized about 50 per cent in the liver. It is excreted in the urine both as free penicillamine and as disulphide derivatives and its sulphoxidation is polymorphic (see p. 96). Following oral and i.v. administration it disappears from the plasma with a $t_{1/2}$ of a few hours, but continues to be excreted for several days after. Dosages should be reduced in renal failure.

Important adverse effects

Adverse effects are common, and on average 30 per cent of patients suffer serious adverse effects. The risk of adverse effects is higher in patients who are poor sulphoxidizers and in individuals of certain HLA phenotypes (see p. 110).

Allergic reactions include fever (usually transient); syndromes mimicking pemphigus, myositis, systemic lupus erythematosus, and the muscle weakness of myasthenia gravis; nephritis (see below); and skin rashes. Early rashes (morbilliform) may necessitate decreased dosages and late rashes (pemphigus-like) may necessitate the withdrawal of treatment altogether.

Proteinuria occurs in up to 15 per cent of cases and may herald an immune-complex nephritis, which may proceed to the nephrotic syndrome. Treatment may be continued in the presence of proteinuria as long as daily proteinuria is no greater than 2 g, oedema is absent, and other indices of renal function remain normal.

Haematological complications may occur. Thrombocytopenia has been seen in up to 4 per cent of cases and leucopenia in up to 2 per cent. More rarely aplastic anaemia and agranulocytosis occur.

In high doses penicillamine impairs collagen synthesis and may cause thinning of the skin. Haemorrhage into the skin may then occur.

Anorexia, nausea, and vomiting are common during the early stages of treatment, but may be reduced by taking the drug with food and by very gradual introduction of dosage. Impaired taste occurs during the first few weeks of treatment but subsequently recovers. Occasionally mouth ulcers may occur.

Because of these adverse effects blood and urine testing must be carried out at least monthly intervals and patients should be carefully observed.

Penicillins

Structures

General

Penicillinase acts here

(Compare cephalosporins.)

Various side chains at R alter resistance to gastric acid, resistance to penicillinase, and antibacterial spectrum.

Mode of action

Penicillins are bacteriocidal and act by inhibition of bacterial cell wall synthesis through inhibition of a membrane-bound transpeptidase. Weakening of the cell wall and consequent lysis and cell death result.

Bacterial resistance to penicillin occurs among organisms which produce an enzyme, penicillinase (β-lactamase), which splits the β-lactam ring of the penicillin nucleus (see general structure). The chief organisms which produce penicillinase include *Staph. aureus* (especially those found in hospitals) and some *E. coli*, *Proteus mirabilis*, and *Pseudomonas aeruginosa*. Some penicillins are resistant to the effects of penicillinase, and they are indicated in the classification below.

Classification

The penicillins may be empirically classified, principally according to certain bacteriological criteria, as follows:

Group 1: Penicillinase-sensitive penicillins

(a) Benzylpenicillin (penicillin G), i.v. and i.m. Benzylpenicillin is also formulated as salts to provide slow release from i.m. injection sites and therefore a longer duration of action. These salts include procaine penicillin (i.m. 1–2 times daily) and benethamine penicillin (i.m. once every 2–3 d).

(b) Phenoxymethylpenicillin (penicillin V), oral.

Group 2: Penicillinase-resistant penicillins

Cloxacillin, i.m. and i.v.
Flucloxacillin, oral, i.m., and i.v.
(Antipseudomonal penicillins: see below.)

Group 3: Broad-spectrum penicillins

Amoxycillin, oral, i.m., and i.v.
Ampicillin, oral, i.m., and i.v. Ampicillin is also formulated as esters (prodrugs, see Chapter 2), which have better absorption after oral administration and which are then completed converted to ampicillin. These esters include talampicillin and pivampicillin (both for oral use only).

Group 4: Antipseudomonal penicillins

Carbenicillin, i.m. and i.v.
Carfecillin, oral (a prodrug ester of carbenicillin).
Ticarcillin, i.m. and i.v.
Azlocillin, i.v.

Group 5: Amidinopenicillins

Mecillinam, i.m. and i.v.
Pivmecillinam, oral (a prodrug ester of mecillinam).

Uses

In Table P7 are listed some of the common examples of bacteria which are sensitive to the penicillins and the associated diseases for which they are particularly used.

Kinetic data

Many of the orally administered penicillins are poorly absorbed. The exceptions are the various prodrug esters, which have been specifically designed to improve absorption (see classification above), and amoxycillin. The penicillins are mostly excreted unchanged by filtration and secretion into the urine, but phenoxymethylpenicillin, cloxacillin, and flucloxacillin are about 60 per cent metabolized. Half-times vary between 30 and 60 min, but are generally prolonged in renal failure, when dosages should be reduced.

Dosages

Dosages vary widely, depending on the clinical indication. Some common dosages are given below:

Group 1: Penicillinase-sensitive penicillins

Benzylpenicillin (penicillin G), 0.3–6.0 g daily i.m.; up to 24 g by i.v. infusion. For example, pneumococcal pneumonia, 1.2 g 6-hourly i.m. (Note: 600 mg = 1 million i.u. = 1 megaunit).

Procaine penicillin, 300 mg 1–2 times daily i.m.

Phenoxymethylpenicillin (penicillin V), 250 mg q.d.s. orally.

Group 2: Penicillinase-resistant penicillins

Flucloxacillin, 250 mg 6-hourly orally, i.m., or i.v.

Group 3: Broad-spectrum penicillins

Amoxycillin, 250 mg t.d.s. orally.

Group 4: Antipseudomonal penicillins

Carbenicillin, 5 g every 4–6 h by i.v. infusion.
Carfecillin, 500–1000 mg t.d.s. orally.

■ **Table P7** The main indications for the use of penicillins

Bacteria	Disease	Penicillin
Gram-positive cocci		
Streptococci pyogenes	Tonsillitis Pharyngitis Otitis media Prophylaxis of rheumatic fever Puerperal sepsis	Penicillinase-sensitive penicillins (Group 1), for example penicillin V
Streptococcus viridans *Streptococcus faecalis* *Streptococcus bovis* Anaerobic streptococci	Bacterial endocarditis	Penicillin G + gentamicin
Staphylococcus aureus (presumed penicillinase-producing)	Boils Pneumonia Endocarditis Osteomyelitis	Penicillinase-resistant penicillins (Group 2), for example flucloxacillin
Streptococcus pneumoniae	Pneumococcal lobar pneumonia Pneumococcal meningitis	Penicillin G
Gram-negative cocci		
Neisseria meningitidis	Meningococcal meningitis	Penicillin G
Neisseria gonorrhoeae	Gonorrhoea	Penicillinase-sensitive penicillins (Group 1), for example procaine penicillin + probenecid (q.v.)
Gram-negative bacilli		
Pseudomonas aeruginosa	Urinary tract infection	Antipseudomonal penicillins (Group 4) (may be combined with an aminoglycoside)
Haemophilus influenzae	Acute or chronic bronchitis Bronchopneumonia Otitis media Sinusitis	Broad-spectrum penicillins (Group 3), for example amoxycillin
Salmonella spp.	Invasive salmonellosis (typhoid, paratyphoid)	Broad-spectrum penicillins (Group 3: probably not first choice)
Vincent's organisms	Acute ulcerative oropharyngitis	Penicillinase-sensitive penicillins (Group 1), e.g. penicillin G.
Gram-positive bacilli		
Bacillus anthracis	Anthrax	Penicillin G
Corynebacterium diphtheriae	Diphtheria	Penicillin G
Clostridium perfringens	Gas gangrene	Penicillin G
Clostridium tetani	Tetanus	Penicillin G
Others		
Treponema pallidum	Syphilis	Penicillin G
Actinomyces israeli	Actinomycosis	Penicillin G
Leptospira spp.	Leptospirosis	Penicillin G
Treponema pertenue Yaws	Penicillin G	

Ticarcillin, 15–20 g daily in divided doses i.m. or i.v.

Azlocillin, 2–5 g 8-hourly i.v.

In severe infections dosages may be adjusted by measuring the bacterial inhibitory activity of penicillin in the blood against the infecting organism *in vitro*.

Important adverse effects

Although the penicillins are very safe antibiotics they have important adverse effects.

Hypersensitivity reactions

Anaphylactic shock is a very serious adverse effect which may be fatal, and it is vital to find out if a patient is known to be allergic to penicillin before administering or prescribing any penicillin. The incidence is between 1 in 2500 and 1 in 10 000, with a fatality rate in those affected of about 10 per cent.

Serum sickness and Stevens–Johnson syndrome occur in up to 5 per cent of patients and usually present 1–3 weeks after starting treatment.

Skin rashes are common (about 10 per cent) and range in severity from mild maculopapular or urticarial eruptions to the Stevens–Johnson syndrome. The usual onset of these rashes is at between 3 and 10 d. With ampicillin and amoxycillin a specific maculopapular rash, usually of later onset and apparently not related to true penicillin hypersensitivity, occurs in up to 18 per cent of patients but in about 90 per cent of those with infectious mononucleosis. It is also common among patients with infections with some other viruses, such as cytomegalovirus, and in patients with lymphoid malignancies. The ampicillin/amoxycillin rash is not a contra-indication to treatment with penicillins at a later date.

If a patient gives a history of penicillin allergy (and that information should always be sought), a complete history should be taken to confirm that that is so. It may be possible to thus distinguish the late-onset ampicillin/amoxycillin rash from that due to true penicillin hypersensitivity, but if there is any doubt it is usually best to assume that hypersensitivity exists. In such cases an alternative antibiotic should be used. Skin testing for penicillin hypersensitivity is unreliable and sometimes dangerous and has not found a place in clinical practice.

The problem of whether or not to give a patient with known penicillin hypersensitivity a cephalosporin is a difficult one. About 10 per cent of all patients with penicillin hypersensitivity will develop skin rashes with cephalosporins, and sometimes this risk has to be taken. However, there is some evidence that the likelihood of a hypersensitive reaction to cephalosporins is greater in patients with a history of severe penicillin hypersensitivity reaction (for example anaphylaxis), and the cephalosporins should be avoided in such patients.

Other adverse effects

Diarrhoea occurs commonly with oral penicillin formulations, but is less frequent with those which are well absorbed (for example amoxycillin). Rarely ampicillin and other penicillins may cause a pseudomembranous colitis (see lincomycin and clindamycin).

Superinfection of the oropharynx with, for example, *Candida albicans*, may occur particularly in old and debilitated people.

Hyperkalaemia and hypernatraemia with fluid retention may occur as a consequence of high intravenous dosages of certain penicillins, because of the salt form, for example potassium and sodium benzylpenicillin and disodium carbenicillin.

Penicillin is neurotoxic in high doses and may cause myoclonic jerks, generalized seizures, or coma. This is a particular hazard with intrathecal therapy.

Acute interstitial nephritis and blood dyscrasias, such as haemolytic anaemia (Coombs' positive), thrombocytopenia, and leucopenia, are all rare complications.

Interactions

Drugs which inhibit renal tubular secretion of the penicillins reduce their excretion and may thus cause accumulation with increased plasma concentrations. Commonly used drugs which have this effect are probenecid, sulphinpyrazone, phenylbutazone, and indomethacin.

Advantage is taken of this interaction in the concurrent use of probenecid with penicillin to enhance the therapeutic efficacy of the antibiotic in the treatment of gonorrhoea and of infective endocarditis. The dosage of probenecid (q.v.) is 500 mg q.d.s.

Co-amoxiclav

Co-amoxiclav is a combination of clavulanic acid with amoxycillin. It may be used in the treatment of infections with bacteria usually sensitive to amoxycillin, but producing penicillinase, and particularly to infections of the urinary and respiratory tracts. Clavulanic acid is an inhibitor of penicillinase. It will not therefore be of value in treating infections by organisms whose resistance to penicillin is not mediated by penicillinase, such as penicillin-resistant pneumococci or gonococci, or cloxacillin-resistant staphylococci.

Phenobarbitone and primidone

Structures

Phenobarbitone

Primidone

Mode of action

The exact mode of action of these drugs at the molecular level is unknown, although the barbiturates probably act by modulating GABA inhibitory neurotransmission by opening chloride channels and thus causing membrane hyperpolarization At the neurophysiological level they limit the spread of seizure activity and increase seizure threshold.

Uses

Anticonvulsants in generalized tonic-clonic seizures (grand mal epilepsy). By general agreement phenobarbitone is now restricted to this indication in the UK.

Dosages

Phenobarbitone, 90–360 mg o.d. orally at night is the usual dosage range, but higher dosages, to a maximum of 600 mg daily, may occasionally be required.

Primidone, initially 125 mg o.d. orally at night, increasing the dose as required at 3-d intervals by 125 mg daily to a dose of 500 mg daily. Then, if necessary, the daily dose should be increased by 250 mg at 3-d intervals until a therapeutic effect is achieved or a maximum daily dose of 1.5 g is reached. The higher dosages should be divided into two or three equal doses.

Kinetic data

Both are well absorbed, phenobarbitone more slowly than primidone (time to peak concentrations 6–18 h and 2–4 h respectively).

Primidone is slowly metabolized ($t_{1/2} = 8$ h) to phenobarbitone (about 20 per cent) and phenylethylmalonic acid. However, the extent of its metabolism is very variable and this results in the large variability in dosages. Increases in dosage should not be made more frequently than every three days.

Phenobarbitone is mostly metabolized (80 per cent) by parahydroxylation and conjugation ($t_{1/2} = 4$ d). Its metabolism is saturable in overdose.

Important adverse effects

Effects on the brain are common and include drowsiness, dizziness, headache, and ataxia. Old people are particularly susceptible. Occasionally allergic skin reactions occur. Barbiturates may precipitate an attack of acute intermittent porphyria (see Chapter 8).

Interactions

Phenobarbitone and primidone both induce the hepatic microsomal enzymes involved in drug metabolism. Phenobarbitone therefore induces the metabolism (i.e. increases the rate of clearance) of several drugs, including warfarin, prednisone, digitoxin, and phenytoin. The interaction with phenytoin is complicated by the fact that phenytoin is also an inducer of hepatic microsomal drug-metabolizing enzymes. The resultant effect on the clearance of each drug in the individual patient is unpredictable.

Chloramphenicol inhibits the metabolism of phenobarbitone, resulting in increased plasma phenobarbitone concentrations. Conversely phenobarbitone induces chloramphenicol metabolism.

There are pharmacodynamic interactions with other CNS depressant drugs. For example, the effects of alcohol, hypnotics, tranquillizers, and antihistamines are all potentiated. In addition the CNS adverse effects of phenytoin may be enhanced, increasing the complexity of this interaction.

Phenytoin (diphenylhydantoin)

Structure

Mode of action

At the neurophysiological level phenytoin prevents the spread of the epileptic discharge rather than suppressing the activity of the primary focus or altering the seizure threshold. The molecular events which result in these effects are still obscure. Phenytoin alters transmembrane fluxes of sodium and potassium, but the relationship of this action to its anticonvulsant effect is unknown. It also has various effects on the functions of some neurotransmitters (for example GABA and 5-hydroxytryptamine), but equally the link between these effects and its anticonvulsant effect is unclear. Phenytoin also possesses a membrane stabilizing effect not unlike that of lignocaine (q.v.), and this may at least account for its actions in the treatment of cardiac arrhythmias, although its role in the anticonvulsant effect is not clear. However, unlike lignocaine and other class 1 antiarrhythmic drugs, it does not decrease the rate of conduction through the AV node, and this makes it of particular value in the treatment of arrhythmias due to digitalis intoxication.

Uses

Epilepsy: generalized tonic–clonic seizures (grand mal epilepsy); partial seizures (for example psychomotor and temporal lobe epilepsy).

Ventricular arrhythmias: particularly those induced by digitalis.

Dosages

Epilepsy: dosages vary widely from individual to individual, because of the variability of phenytoin's pharmacokinetics (see below). A typical dosage would be 300 mg o.d. orally.

Cardiac arrhythmias: 4 mg/kg given by slow i.v. infusion with ECG monitoring. If chronic oral treatment is required anticonvulsant dosages should be used.

Kinetic data

Phenytoin is well, but slowly, absorbed (time to peak plasma concentrations 3–10 h). The intramuscular route should be avoided if possible, because of crystallization at the site of injection and consequent unpredictable systemic availability.

Phenytoin is almost completely metabolized by the liver and its major metabolite is *para*-hydroxyphenytoin. This oxidative metabolism is saturable within the range of therapeutic doses, and because the point of saturability varies from individual to individual, it is necessary to adjust the dosage in each case according to the plasma concentration and the clinical response (see Chapter 7). The metabolism of phenytoin is also bimodally distributed in the population, about 9 per cent of subjects being poor hydroxylators (see Chapter 8).

Because of its saturable metabolism the $t_{1/2}$ of phenytoin varies with dose, being longer at high doses (up to 60 h or more).

Plasma phenytoin concentrations should generally be within the range 40–80 μmol/L (see Chapter 7, p. 88). The plasma concentration should be measured at steady state, i.e. after at least one week of continuous treatment. If it is found necessary to increase the dose this should be done in increments of no more than 50 mg before further measurements are made.

In renal failure the therapeutic plasma concentration falls, because of reduced protein binding of the drug. This also happens during the last trimester of pregnancy and in other states producing hypoalbuminaemia, and if there is displacement of phenytoin from its plasma protein binding sites by another drug (see Chapter 10).

Important adverse effects

At plasma concentrations above the therapeutic range toxic effects increase in incidence, and are mostly due to effects on the brain. They consist of nystagmus, ataxia, tremor, lethargy, dysarthria, psychological disturbances, seizures, and ultimately coma. Increasing plasma concentrations have been related in rising sequence to nystagmus (80–120 μmol/L), ataxia (120–160 μmol/L), and mental changes (> 160 μmol/L).

There are other adverse effects which are not clearly related to dose and which occur during long-term therapy. These include: gum hypertrophy and changes in facial features owing to increased collagen thickness; hirsutism or acne; megaloblastic anaemia (due to folate deficiency, the reason for which is still not clear); osteomalacia (due to increased vitamin D metabolism); and lupus erythematosus, erythema multiforme, and other skin rashes; and lymphadenopathy. After prolonged administration there appears to be an increased incidence of lymphoma.

There are certain risks associated with the use of phenytoin in pregnancy. There may be an increased risk of cleft lip and palate and of digital hypoplasia in the fetus, and the neonate may suffer vitamin K deficiency with haemorrhagic consequences. The mother should be treated with vitamin K during the last month of pregnancy.

Interactions

Drugs which induce or inhibit the activity of the hepatic mixed-function oxidases will alter the metabolism of phenytoin (see Chapter 10). Phenytoin itself induces the activity of those oxidases and this effect results in increased metabolism of some drugs. Phenytoin alters the action of warfarin by complex mechanisms and unpredictably in a given patient. The oestrogen in the combined oral contraceptive is metabolized more rapidly and the contraceptive may therefore become ineffective. This is usually signalled by mid-cycle spotting, and if that occurs the dose of oral contraceptive should be doubled.

Folic acid, in the doses taken during pregnancy, increases phenytoin clearance by an unknown mechanism and thus lowers plasma phenytoin concentrations.

Vigabatrin increases plasma phenytoin concentrations by an unknown mechanism.

Pizotifen

Structure

Mode of action

Pizotifen is a 5-hydroxytryptamine (5-HT) antagonist. The role of 5-HT in migraine is not fully understood, but there is evidence that during the early part of an attack of migraine there is release of 5-HT from platelets, with precipitation of vasoconstriction in the cerebral blood vessels. The aim of pizotifen is to prevent this sequence.

Use

Migraine prophylaxis.

Dosages

Initially 0.5 mg o.d. orally, increasing to 0.5 mg t.d.s. in 0.5 mg increments every few days. In severe cases up to 2 mg t.d.s. may be required.

Kinetic data

Well absorbed. $t_{1/2} = 1$ d.

Important adverse effects

Mild drowsiness occurs in up to 60 per cent of cases, but tolerance develops within a few weeks. Increased appetite and weight gain are common. Dizziness, nausea, and vomiting may occur.

Interactions

The effects of drugs acting on the brain (for example alcohol) may be potentiated.

Potassium chloride

Uses

Treatment or prevention of potassium depletion from any cause, for example in patients taking diuretics, corticosteroids, or carbenoxolone. This is of especial importance in patients taking digitalis preparations, in patients receiving insulin therapy for diabetic ketoacidosis, and in old people, who are particularly prone to potassium depletion. Potassium chloride is the salt of choice in treating or preventing potassium depletion, since retention of potassium will not occur unless the concomitant chloride depletion is also corrected.

Formulations

There are numerous formulations of potassium chloride available for oral and i.v. use and formulations containing potassium chloride and a diuretic.

(a) Oral formulations

(i) Sustained-release formulations

Leo K® (tablets), Nu-K® (capsules), Slow-K® (tablets). Each tablet or capsule contains 8 mmol of potassium as the chloride salt.

(ii) Effervescent formulations

Potassium chloride tablets, effervescent (6.5 mmol of potassium as the chloride salt in each tablet): Kloref® (6.7 mmol of potassium as the chloride salt in each tablet); Sando-K® (8 mmol of potassium as the chloride salt in each tablet); Kloref-S® (20 mmol of potassium as the chloride salt in each sachet of granules).

(iii) Liquid formulations

Kay-Cee-L® (1 mmol of potassium as the chloride salt in each 1 mL).

(iv) Combinations of potassium chloride with a diuretic

There is a large number of such formulations, containing 6.7–10 mmol of potassium as the chloride salt in each tablet. However, it should be noted that in some of these formulations the dose of diuretic is half the usual dose found in the corresponding formulation without potassium. For example, Burinex® (bumetanide) is formulated as a 1000 microgram tablet while Burinex-K® tablets contain 500 micrograms of bumetanide with 7.7 mmol of potassium chloride. This is obviously important when considering the required dose of diuretic.

(b) Intravenous formulations

There are two types of formulation of potassium chloride for i.v. use: those which can be added to i.v. infusion solutions and those which are already made up for direct infusion.

Because of the hazard of cardiac arrhythmias due to too rapid infusion, solutions containing more than 40 mmol of potassium per litre should not be used. When potassium solutions are infused the rate generally should be about 10 mmol/h and should not exceed 20 mmol/h.

(i) 'Undiluted' solutions

There are several formulations of various strengths, but a commonly used formulation contains 20 mmol of potassium as the chloride salt in 10 mL. This solution must be diluted to a volume of at least 500 mL before administration.

NB Because of the hazards of infusing too large a dose of potassium, which may be fatal, great care must be taken in making up and mixing potassium solutions for infusion. For preference potassium solutions should be used which have already been prepared pharmaceutically.

(ii) Ready-prepared solutions

Potassium chloride in sodium chloride solution for i.v. infusion. This solution contains K^+ 40 mmol, Na^+ 150 mmol, and Cl^- 190 mmol in 1 L.

Potassium chloride in dextrose solution for i.v. infusion. This solution contains K^+ 40 mmol and Cl^- 40 mmol in 1 L of 5 per cent dextrose.

Dosages

The total body potassium is about 3500 mmol, of which 90 per cent is intracellular. Daily intake is 60–80 mmol, most of which is eliminated in the urine. A singe dose of frusemide or a thiazide diuretic causes the loss of about 16 mmol during the resultant sodium diuresis in a patient who has not previously received a diuretic. However, during repeated administration of these diuretics, at least in patients with hypertension, there is evidence that total body potassium stores are not depleted by the usual antihypertensive diuretic dosages. In these patients potassium supplements are often not necessary, but it is advisable to check the plasma potassium concentration occasionally.

In patients with oedema due to heart failure, hepatic cirrhosis, and the nephrotic syndrome, the administration of diuretics often leads to potassium depletion and it is wise to use potassium chloride in a dose of 16–48 mmol per day in divided doses to prevent this. In such circumstances a potassium-sparing diuretic may be a useful alternative to potassium chloride.

Intravenous potassium therapy may be indicated to prevent potassium depletion when patients are unable to take oral potassium; this requires about 80 mmol/d.

In the treatment of severe hypokalaemia and the prevention of hypokalaemia during insulin therapy of diabetic ketoacidosis intravenous potassium chloride administration is indicated and should be monitored by frequent plasma potassium concentration measurements.

Important adverse effects

These occur in about 12 per cent of patients taking potassium supplements, and include *hyperkalaemia* (particularly in old people), nausea, vomiting, diarrhoea, and abdominal cramps.

Intestinal ulceration is a hazard of using enteric-coated potassium formulations, and such formulations should no longer be used.

Oesophageal ulceration has been reported with the slow-release oral formulations listed above in patients with oesophageal obstruction (for example due to left atrial enlargement in mitral stenosis).

Interactions

The risk of hyperkalaemia is greatly increased if potassium supplements are combined with a potassium-sparing diuretic or an ACE inhibitor, and in general these combinations should not be used.

Care should be taken not to make the careless mistake of unwittingly prescribing potassium for a patient being treated with a combination formulation of a thiazide diuretic and a potassium-sparing diuretic, for example Aldactide® (containing spironolactone), Dyazide® (containing triamterene), or Moduretic® (containing amiloride).

Probenecid

Structure

$$(CH_3CH_2CH_2)_2NSO_2-\!\!\!\!\bigcirc\!\!\!\!-COOH$$

Mode of action

Probenecid inhibits the renal tubular transport of organic acids, such as uric acid and penicillin. Since the renal excretion of penicillin is mainly by tubular secretion its elimination is blocked by probenecid. However, uric acid is not only excreted by active tubular secretion but is also subject to active tubular reabsorption; probenecid in low dosages blocks the active secretion and causes *retention* of uric acid; in higher (therapeutic) dosages it also blocks the active reabsorption and the net effect is an *increase in elimination* of uric acid (see Fig. 29.4). This dual dose-dependent effect on uric acid excretion is shared by aspirin and sulphinpyrazone.

Uses

Gout and hyperuricaemia.

To increase the blood concentrations of penicillins and cephalosporins.

Dosages

Gout and hyperuricaemia: 250–500 mg b.d. orally.

As an adjunct to penicillin therapy: 500 mg q.d.s. orally.

Kinetic data

Probenecid is well absorbed. Its $t_{1/2}$ is dose-dependent (usually 6–12 h). It is metabolized 95 per cent to active and inactive compounds, which are excreted in the urine.

Important adverse effects

Adverse effects are uncommon and generally mild. Gastrointestinal disturbances (about 2 per cent) and skin rashes (about 3 per cent) are the most frequent.

Probenecid may precipitate haemolytic anaemia in patients with G6PD deficiency (see Chapter 8).

Interactions

Probenecid inhibits the tubular secretion of penicillin and has therefore been used as an adjunct to penicillin therapy to cause retention of penicillin.

By a similar mechanism it causes retention of methotrexate and thereby enhances its toxicity.

The risk of chloroquine-induced eye damage is increased in patients taking probenecid.

For the interaction of probenecid with aspirin see under sulphinpyrazone.

Procainamide and acecainide

Structures

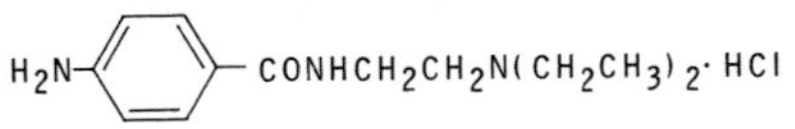

$$H_2N-\text{[benzene ring]}-CONHCH_2CH_2N(CH_2CH_3)_2 \cdot HCl$$

Procainamide is shown here. Acecainide is *N*-acetylprocainamide.

Mode of action

Procainamide is a class Ia antiarrhythmic drug with direct actions on cardiac conducting tissues similar to those of quinidine. These effects are discussed under lignocaine. However, in contrast to quinidine, procainamide has no anticholinergic or α-adrenoceptor antagonist properties. In contrast, acecainide is a class III antiarrhythmic drug (see amiodarone)

Uses

Acute and chronic ventricular arrhythmias.

Dosages

Procainamide, i.v. 100 mg every 5 min with ECG and blood pressure monitoring until the arrhythmia is controlled or a maximum dose of 1 g is reached. If it is considered necessary to continue with oral or i.v. therapy this would be considered the loading dose. Maintenance i.v. infusion 0.25–2 mg/min; oral: procainamide is available as ordinary or sustained-release formulations.

Ordinary formulations

Loading dose 1 g, followed by 250–500 mg 4-hourly.

Sustained-release formulations

Loading dose 2 g, followed by 1.5 g 8-hourly.

Acecainide, i.v. 18 mg/kg over 30 min; orally 1.0–1.5 g 8-hourly. (Note that acecainide is not available in the UK.)

Kinetic data

Procainamide is well absorbed orally. It is metabolized about 50 per cent to acecainide and inactive metabolites, the remaining 50 per cent being excreted by the kidneys. The amount of acecainide produced depends on whether the patient is a slow or fast acetylator (see Chapter 8). Procainamide $t_{1/2} = 3$ h, acecainide $t_{1/2} = 6$ h. Acecainide is excreted unchanged in the urine.

In renal failure excretion of both procainamide and acecainide is impaired and dosages should be reduced.

In hepatic disease the metabolism of procainamide is decreased and dosages should be reduced. In congestive cardiac failure metabolism may be reduced because of hepatic congestion, but the apparent volume of distribution is also reduced and both loading and maintenance dosages should be reduced.

The therapeutic range of plasma concentrations of procainamide is 4–10 µg/mL, but this does not take into account the fact that acecainide also has therapeutic activity. Since the production of acecainide varies from individual to individual the interpretation of plasma procainamide concentrations alone is difficult. The therapeutic range of plasma concentrations of acecainide is 15–30 µg/mL.

Important adverse effects

Cardiac effects

These are common with both drugs and include hypotension (particularly after fast i.v. administration), heart block, and ventricular arrhythmias. These effects are commonly dose-related.

Non-cardiac effects

Lupus-like syndrome (see also Chapter 9)

In common with some other drugs (for example hydralazine) procainamide may produce a syndrome like systemic lupus erythematosus, characterized by arthralgia, arthritis, fever, pleurisy, pulmonary involvement, pericarditis, and rashes. Renal involvement is uncommon. Tests for anti-nuclear factor (ANF) are usually positive in patients with the syndrome. However, procainamide therapy is associated with a positive ANF in 60–70 per cent of patients, of whom only 20–30 per cent develop the clinical syndrome if therapy is continued. In patients who are slow acetylators the rate of development of a positive ANF is faster.

Usually the syndrome resolves when the drug is stopped, but it may take months and occasionally years to do so.

It is thought that the syndrome is due to procainamide itself or to some non-acetylated metabolite since it resolves on substituting acecainide and since it does not occur with acecainide itself. Occasionally patients taking acecainide may develop a positive ANF, possibly due to back-conversion of acecainide to procainamide.

Other non-cardiac effects

Anorexia, nausea, and vomiting may occur with both procainamide and acecainide. Rarely procainamide may cause giddiness and mental symptoms, while acecainide can cause blurred vision, insomnia, and fatigue.

Procainamide can cause hypersensitivity reactions, resulting in fever and blood disorders, including agranulocytosis. This may be more common with slow-release formulations of procainamide.

Interactions

Procainamide and acecainide should not be given together with other drugs which prolong the QT interval (for example quinidine, amiodarone, and disopyramide).

Hypokalaemia, for example due to diuretics, alters the effects of antiarrhythmic drugs on the cardiac action potential, and the hypokalaemia should be corrected when using procainamide.

Propylthiouracil

Structure

$$CH_3CH_2CH_2$$ — [pyrimidine-2-thione ring structure with N–H, S, NH, O substituents]

Mode of action

Inhibition of the synthesis of thyroid hormones by interfering with the incorporation of iodine into tyrosyl residues, and possibly with the coupling of those residues into iodothyronines.

Use

Hyperthyroidism.

Dosages

Initially 100–200 mg 8-hourly orally. As a response is obtained reduce the dose gradually to a maintenance dosage of 50–150 mg daily in one or two divided doses. Treatment is usually continued for 1–2 y.

Kinetic data

Propylthiouracil is well absorbed. It is partly metabolized ($t_{1/2} = 2$ h).

Important adverse effects

Adverse reactions occur in up to 3 per cent of cases and resemble those of carbimazole (q.v.). However, the incidence of agranulocytosis is higher (up to 1:250).

Pyrazolones

Structures
General

[chemical structure with C_6H_5, O, N, N, R, $CH_3CH_2CH_2CH_2$, O substituents]

Phenylbutazone: $R = C_6H_5$. Oxyphenbutazone: $R = C_6H_4OH$.

Azapropazone also belongs to this class of non-steroidal anti-inflammatory drugs.

Mode of action

The pyrazolones have analgesic, antipyretic, and anti-inflammatory properties, actions which may be related to their inhibitory effects on prostaglandin synthesis. Their uricosuric effect is due to inhibition of tubular reabsorption of uric acid.

Uses

Because of the high incidence of adverse effects during prolonged dosage, the use of phenylbutazone and oxyphenbutazone is now limited to ankylosing spondylitis which has not responded to other agents.

Azapropazone has similar indications to the arylalkanoic acids (qq.v.).

Dosages

Azapropazone, 300–600 mg b.d., t.d.s., or q.d.s.

Phenylbutazone, 200 mg t.d.s., orally for 2 d, then 100 mg t.d.s.; rectal route, 250 mg b.d.

Oxyphenbutazone: as for phenylbutazone.

These drugs should be taken with food if possible to minimize gastrointestinal adverse effects.

Kinetic data

All are well absorbed. Phenylbutazone is metabolized to its active metabolite, oxyphenbutazone and both compounds are excreted in the urine, $t_{1/2} = 3$ d. A second metabolite, γ-hydroxyphenbutazone has uricosuric effects only and a shorter $t_{1/2}$ (12 h). Azapropazone is excreted unchanged by the kidney. All are highly bound to plasma proteins.

Important adverse effects

Both phenylbutazone and oxyphenbutazone can cause bone-marrow suppression, resulting in aplastic anaemia, agranulocytosis, or thrombocytopenia. The incidence of aplastic anaemia is about 1:50 000.

All can cause gastrointestinal effects, including nausea, vomiting, symptoms of 'dyspepsia', and peptic ulceration, which may result in anaemia from blood loss or serious haematemesis.

Fluid retention may occur, causing peripheral oedema, which may be relieved by diuretics. In severe cases cardiac failure may occur.

Dosages of azapropazone should be reduced in patients with renal impairment.

Interactions

These drugs should not be used in conjunction with warfarin because of direct and indirect interactions by the following mechanisms:

(1) inhibition of the metabolism of s-warfarin;

(2) peptic ulceration;

(3) inhibition of platelet aggregation;

(4) thrombocytopenia;

(5) displacement of warfarin from protein binding sites.

The effects of sulphonylureas are increased by the pyrazolones, because of inhibition of metabolism and inhibition of renal excretion. The metabolism of phenytoin is inhibited by the pyrazolones.

Phenylbutazone and azapropazone increase the risk of methotrexate toxicity, probably by inhibiting its renal secretion.

The pyrazolones may offset the effects of antihypertensive drugs by causing fluid retention.

When phenylbutazone is used in combination with chloroquine there is an increased risk of exfoliative dermatitis and this combination should not be used.

Quinidine

Structure

(Quinidine is the dextrorotatory diastereomer of quinine.)

Mode of action

Quinidine is a class Ia antiarrhythmic drug, and has direct actions on cardiac conducting tissues. Those effects are discussed in detail under lignocaine. (p. 624)

Quinidine differs from lignocaine in some aspects of its actions on the cardiac action potential and in that it has a more pronounced negative inotropic effect on the heart and a greater propensity to produce heart block and cardiac arrhythmias.

In addition to its Class I antiarrhythmic actions it has anticholinergic and α-adrenoceptor antagonist properties.

Uses

Acute and chronic supraventricular and ventricular arrhythmias. Although quinidine is effective in the treatment of supraventricular arrhythmias, such as paroxysmal SVT and atrial flutter, its use in these conditions has largely been superseded by other drugs (see the treatment of arrhythmias, p. 276) and by cardioversion, partly because of the toxicity of quinidine. It is still sometimes of value in the treatment of recurrent atrial flutter, when it is generally combined with digitalis (but see interactions below). It also has a place in the treatment of acute and chronic ventricular tachyarrhythmias.

Dosages

Quinidine is available either as quinidine sulphate in ordinary tablets, or as quinidine bisulphate in sustained-release formulations. The latter are to be preferred, because of the reduced frequency of administration and reduced fluctuations of plasma concentrations. Quinidine sulphate 200 mg is equivalent to quinidine bisulphate 250 mg.

Before embarking on chronic quinidine therapy a single *test* dose of quinidine sulphate 200 mg should be given.

Chronic oral dosages: quinidine sulphate, 200–400 mg, 3–4 times daily; quinidine bisulphate, 500 mg every 12 h, increasing as required to 1.25 g every 12 h.

Kinetic data

Quinidine is well absorbed. It is mostly metabolized, but about 20 per cent is excreted unchanged in the urine and its rate of renal elimination is increased by acidification of the urine. The usual $t_{1/2}$ is 6 h. The clearance of quinidine is reduced in liver disease. In congestive heart failure not only is its clearance reduced because of hepatic congestion, but the apparent volume of distribution is also reduced. Dosages should therefore be reduced by about 25 per cent in patients with hepatic disease or congestive cardiac failure. The therapeutic range of plasma quinidine concentrations is 3–6 µg/mL. Routine plasma quinidine concentration measurement has not been proved useful.

Important adverse effects

Adverse effects with quinidine are very common indeed and have limited its usefulness.

Dose-related effects
Cardiac

Quinidine may cause ventricular arrhythmias, particularly ventricular tachycardia, which may cause syncope. Patients with a prolonged QT interval are particularly susceptible to ventricular arrhythmias, and in such patients quinidine should be avoided. Quinidine may also impair sinus nodal function, producing sinus bradycardia and predisposing to supraventricular tachyarrhythmias. This occurs particularly in patients with the sick sinus syndrome. It can also cause atrioventricular block and worsen pre-existing conduction defects. It should not, therefore, be used in patients with pre-existing AV block. Quinidine may cause postural hypotension by α-adrenoceptor antagonism.

Non-cardiac

Overdose with quinidine has long been known to produce a syndrome called *cinchonism*. The manifestations of this syndrome are tinnitus, deafness, blurring of vision, vomiting, diarrhoea, and abdominal pain. In severe toxicity there may also be headache, diplopia, photophobia, altered colour vision, flushing, confusion, delirium, and psychosis.

Quinidine may cause hypoglycaemia during the treatment of malaria.

Hypersensitivity reactions

Thrombocytopenia is an uncommon but serious effect. Rarely haemolytic anaemia may occur. In addition to these effects nausea, diarrhoea, and vomiting are very common with quinidine in therapeutic doses.

Interactions

Quinidine inhibits the renal tubular secretion of digoxin and doubles steady-state plasma digoxin concentrations. It may also reduce the positive inotropic effects of digoxin, and the combination is better avoided in heart failure. If the combination of digoxin and quinidine is used in the treatment of atrial tachyarrhythmias the dose of digoxin should be halved.

Phenobarbitone, phenytoin, and rifampicin increase the dosage requirements of quinidine by increasing its metabolism.

Quinidine should not be used in combination with other drugs which prolong the QT interval (for example procainamide, amiodarone, and disopyramide).

Hypokalaemia, for example due to diuretics, alters the effects of antiarrhythmic drugs on the cardiac action potential and the hypokalaemia should be corrected when using quinidine.

Quinidine potentiates the anticoagulant effect of warfarin in some patients by an unknown mechanism.

Quinine

Structure

(Quinine is the laevorotatory diastereomer of quinidine.)

Mode of action

As an antimalarial quinine probably binds to plasmodial DNA and prevents its replication.

In nocturnal leg cramps quinine reduces the excitability of the motor end-plate and reduces its response to acetylcholine and tetanic stimulation.

Uses

In the treatment of chloroquine-resistant *P. falciparum* malaria.
Nocturnal leg cramps.

Dosages

P. falciparum malaria (see therapy of malaria, p. 242)

Oral, 600 mg every 12 h for a total of six doses; i.v. (complicated *P. falciparum* infections), 5–10 mg/kg of base infused over 4 h, repeated every 12–24 h to a total of four doses or until oral therapy is possible.

The longer dosage interval should be used in patients with liver damage.

Nocturnal leg cramps

Quinine bisulphate, 200–300 mg at bedtime for two weeks. In some cases cramps do not recur after a single course, but long-term treatment may be necessary.

Kinetic data

Quinine is almost completely absorbed. It is metabolized 95 per cent in the liver, $t_{1/2} = 10$ h. In severe malaria the $t_{1/2}$ is prolonged to about 20 h.

Important adverse effects

Toxic effects include tinnitus, deafness, headache, nausea, and visual disturbances. This cluster of symptoms has been called 'cinchonism' (see also quinidine, p. 672).

Hypersensitivity reactions, such as angiooedema, and acute idiosyncratic reactions, such as flushing, dyspnoea, and feeling 'peculiar', also occur.

Intravenous infusions can be associated with CNS toxicity, such as tremor, delirium, fits, and coma.

Haemolytic anaemia may occur, especially in patients with G6PD deficiency (see Chapter 8). Thrombocytopenia occurs occasionally, usually as a type II allergic reaction (see p. 111).

The effects of quinine on the heart are similar to those of quinidine, and care should be taken in patients with cardiac arrhythmias and heart block.

Interactions

In antimalarial doses quinine may inhibit the renal elimination of digoxin in a fashion similar to quinidine. It also potentiates the anticoagulant effect of warfarin and has itself some hypoprothrombinaemic effect.

Quinolones

Structures

We illustrate here ciprofloxacin. The other quinolones share its piperazine structure.

Other quinolones available include acrosoxacin, cinoxacin, enoxacin, nalidixic acid, norfloxacin, and ofloxacin.

Mode of action

The quinolones act by inhibiting bacterial DNA gyrase (topoisomerase), which is involved in the super coiling of DNA. This impairs DNA replication and protein synthesis.

Uses

The quinolones are effective against Grampositive and Gram-negative organisms, including *S. aureus*, *N. gonorrhoea*, *E. coli*, *H. influenzae*, *Ps. aeruginosa*, *Campylobacter*, *Shigella*, and *Salmonella*.

Ciprofloxacin is used in the treatment of urinary, respiratory, and gastrointestinal infections, gonorrhoea, and septicaemia. Enoxacin is used for urinary and skin infections and gonorrhoea. Cinoxacin, nalidixic acid, and norfloxacin are used for urinary tract infections. Acrosoxacin is used to treat gonorrhoea in patients with penicillin allergy or when the organism is resistant to other antibiotics.

Dosages

Acrosoxacin, orally 300 mg as a single dose on an empty stomach.

Cinoxacin, orally 500 mg b.d.

Ciprofloxacin, orally 250–750 mg b.d. (a single dose of 250 mg orally for gonorrhoea); by i.v. infusion (over 30–60 min) 200 mg b.d.

Enoxacin, orally 200–400 mg b.d.

Nalidixic acid, orally 1 g 6-hourly.

Norfloxacin, orally 400 mg b.d.

Kinetic data

The quinolones are moderately well (for example ciprofloxacin) or very well absorbed. Most of them are eliminated unchanged in the urine, but nalidixic acid is extensively metabolized and one of its metabolites is active and appears in the urine. Their half-times vary from about 1 h (cinoxacin) to about 6 h (enoxacin and ofloxacin).

Important adverse effects

Adverse effects common to all the quinolones include gastrointestinal disturbances in up to 8 per cent (nausea, vomiting, diarrhoea, abdominal pain), CNS disturbances occasionally (headache, dizziness, tiredness, restlessness), and skin rashes in 1–2 per cent. Liver function tests are abnormal in up to 5 per cent of cases and hepatitis and jaundice may occur occasionally. Anaphylactoid reactions and psychiatric disturbances have been reported with some of the quinolones. Dosages should be reduced in moderate to severe renal impairment.

The quinolones cause arthropathy in animals and they should not be given to infants or pregnant women. They can cause haemolysis in patients with G6PD deficiency (see Chapter 8). They lower the seizure threshold and should not be used in patients with epilepsy.

Ciprofloxacin may cause crystalluria, and a good urine flow must be ensured by a high fluid intake.

Interactions

Several of the quinolones (ciprofloxacin, enoxacin, and norfloxacin) inhibit the metabolism of theophylline, whose dosages should be reduced; ofloxacin does not do this.

Antacids reduce the absorption of the quinolones.

Retinoids

Structures

The retinoids, etretinate, isotretinoin, and tretinoin, are analogues of vitamin A (retinoic acid); isotretinoin is 13-*cis*-retinoic acid and tretinoin is all-*trans*-retinoic acid. Etretinate is shown here.

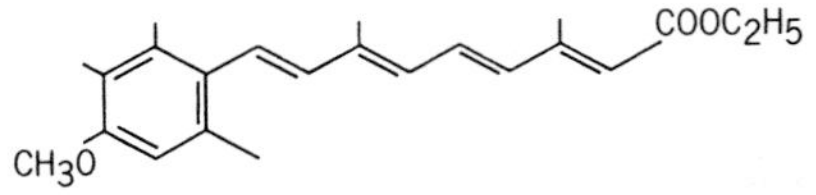

Mode of action

The mechanisms of action of the retinoids are not fully understood, but they alter epithelial differentiation, keratinization, and sebum production.

Uses

The retinoids are used in the specialist treatment of a variety of skin disorders.

Etretinate is used for severe extensive psoriasis, palmoplantar pustular psoriasis, severe congenital ichthyosis, and severe keratosis follicularis (Darrier's disease).

Isotretinoin, and tretinoin are used (orally and topically respectively) in the treatment of severe acne vulgaris.

Dosages

Etretinate dosages vary widely because of variable kinetics from individual to individual. The initial dosage is up to 0.75 mg/kg/d orally in divided doses for 2–4 weeks. The dosage may be increased if required to 1 mg/kg/d (maximum total daily dose 75 mg). Improvement can be expected to start at around 3 weeks and be maximal at 6–8 weeks, when the dosage should be reduced to a usual maintenance dosage of 250–500 micrograms/kg/d.

Isotretinoin dosages also vary widely because of variable kinetics. The initial dosage is 0.5 mg/kg/d orally for 4 weeks. Those who respond can continue to take isotretinoin for up to 16 weeks in all. In those who do not respond initially the dosage may be increased to 1 mg/kg/d for a further 8–12 weeks. If adverse effects occur with the initial dosage it can be reduced to 0.1–0.2 mg/kg/d.

Tretinoin is applied sparingly once or twice a day in a cream (0.025 or 0.5 per cent), a lotion (0.025 per cent) strength, or a gel (0.01–0.025 per cent). It is used for 6–8 weeks, after which occasional application may be sufficient.

Kinetic data

Isotretinoin is well absorbed and extensively metabolized, $t_{1/2} = 90$ h; the metabolites are eliminated via the faeces and bile. Etretinate is poorly and variably absorbed. It is partly metabolized and excreted via the faeces, $t_{1/2} = 3$ months.

Important adverse effects

The retinoids have many contra-indications and serious adverse effects. They should not be used in patients with hepatic or renal disease, nor during pregnancy (because of teratogenicity) or in breast-feeding mothers. They should only be used in premenopausal women if they have severe disabling skin disease resistant to other treatments and if pregnancy has been excluded. Treatment should be started only during the second or third day of a menstrual cycle and contraceptive precautions should be taken during treatment and for some time after the end of treatment (at least 4 weeks for isotretinoin and 1 year for etretinate).

The retinoids can cause impaired liver function, and liver function tests should be monitored before and during therapy. Serum lipids should be monitored similarly because of increases in serum triglyceride concentrations.

During the first few weeks of treatment acne may get worse with both systemic and topical treatment. Most patients develop a dry skin with cheilitis, facial erythema, and pruritus, dry eyes, a dry nose, sometimes, with mild bleeding, a dry throat with hoarseness, and some hair loss.

Occasionally muscle stiffness and pain may occur, particularly after exercise. Benign intracranial hypertension (pseudotumor cerebri) may occur.

Because the retinoids persist in the blood patients should not donate blood while taking the retinoids, nor afterwards for 4 weeks (isotretinoin) or 1 year (etretinate).

Interactions

Tetracyclines and corticosteroids increase the risk of benign intracranial hypertension.

Solutions containing alcohol, menthol, or other astringents (for example perfumes and aftershave lotions) should not be used during topical tretinoin administration.

Rifampicin (rifampin)

Structure

Mode of action

Rifampicin acts by inhibiting the DNA-dependent RNA polymerase in bacteria, but not in mammalian cells.

Uses

Despite its wide and effective antibacterial spectrum, rifampicin is largely restricted to the treatment of tuberculosis in combination with other antituberculous drugs.

Other uses include the prevention of meningococcal infection in contacts of a proven case of meningococcal meningitis and the treatment of leprosy.

Dosage

450–600 mg o.d. orally.

Kinetic data

Rifampicin is well absorbed. It is partly metabolized to inactive metabolites (35 per cent), and partly excreted into the bile unchanged (35 per cent), with consequent recirculation. The rest is eliminated unchanged in the urine, $t_{1/2} = 3$ h. Biliary excretion increases progressively during the first 2 weeks of treatment and the $t_{1/2}$ shortens. Rifampicin is also excreted in tears and sweat and these, as well as the urine, may turn red as a result.

Important adverse effects

Liver damage can occur occasionally and liver function tests should be monitored regularly, especially in patients with pre-existing liver disease, which is associated with an increased risk of adverse liver reactions. This is partly important because of the association of alcoholic cirrhosis with tuberculosis.

A flu-like illness may occur initially if high doses are used. Thrombocytopenia, a mild leucopenia, and skin rashes are rare.

Interactions

Rifampicin induces hepatic drug-metabolizing enzymes. This is especially important with regard to warfarin and the oral contraceptive, whose effects may be diminished. For advice on the dosage of oral contraceptive see under phenytoin.

Salicylates

Structures

Aspirin (acetylsalicylic acid)

Other salicylates include benorylate, which is a compound in which aspirin is linked with paracetamol, and diflunisal, which is a difluorophenyl derivative.

Mode of action

Salicylates have analgesic, antipyretic, and anti-inflammatory actions. At the molecular level the main known action of salicylates is inhibition of the enzyme cyclo-oxygenase with a resultant reduction in prostaglandin synthesis. This action may account for some of the therapeutic and adverse effects of the salicylates, but the total spectrum of their pharmacological actions is difficult to explain on this basis alone. The action of inhibiting platelet aggregation is mediated by inhibition of prostaglandin synthesis.

The effects of aspirin in inhibiting prostaglandin synthesis differ for different prostaglandins. Thus, while low doses of aspirin inhibit only the production of thromboxane in platelets, higher doses inhibit the production of both thromboxane in platelets and prostacyclin in vessel walls. This is why low-dose aspirin is of value in the prevention of myocardial infarction (see below).

Uses

Anti-inflammatory: in rheumatoid arthritis and osteoarthritis; in acute rheumatic fever; in Dressler's syndrome; it is particularly effective in these last two.

Analgesic: as a mild analgesic, for instance in musculoskeletal pain, simple headache, and dysmenorrhoea.

Antipyretic: for symptomatic relief of fever in viral infections such as influenza and infectious mononucleosis, and sometimes in bacterial infections.

Because of its effects on thromboxane synthesis by platelets low dosages of aspirin are used in the treatment of transient ischaemic episodes, the prevention of occlusive stroke, and the prevention of myocardial infarction in patients with angina pectoris or a previous myocardial infarction. Aspirin also augments the beneficial effects of streptokinase in reducing mortality immediately after an acute myocardial infarction.

Dosages

Acute rheumatic fever

Aspirin, 0.9–1.2 g every 4 h to a maximum of 8 g daily. In this condition plasma salicylate concentrations of about 1 mmol/L are effectively anti-inflammatory.

Chronic rheumatoid arthritis and osteoarthritis

Aspirin, 900 mg orally every 4–6 h.
Benorylate, 1.5 g t.d.s. orally (tablets) or 4 g b.d. orally (elixir).
Diflunisal, 250–500 mg b.d. orally.

Analgesia

Aspirin, 300–900 mg every 4–6 h orally, to a maximum of 4 g daily.
Diflunisal, 250–500 mg b.d. orally (limit 750 mg daily during chronic therapy).

Effects on platelets

Prevention of stroke and myocardial infarction and treatment of transient ischaemic attacks: aspirin, 300 mg o.d.
Prevention of coronary graft occlusion: aspirin, 100 mg o.d.
After acute myocardial infarction: aspirin, 150 mg o.d.

Kinetic data

All these salicylates are well absorbed.

Aspirin has a short $t_{1/2}$ (about 15 min) in the plasma, but is metabolized to an active metabolite, salicylic acid, whose elimination is saturable. The apparent $t_{1/2}$ of salicylic acid is 3–6 h at low therapeutic doses but at higher doses the apparent $t_{1/2}$ lengthens and in overdose may be as long as

20 h. This underlines the need to monitor plasma salicylate concentrations during treatment with very high dosages, because of the variability of metabolism from patient to patient. The optimum range of plasma salicylate concentrations for anti-inflammatory effects is 0.7–2.3 mmol/L (100–300 µg/mL). Salicylic acid itself is further metabolized by the liver and is also excreted in the urine.

Benorylate is metabolized, after absorption, to salicylic acid and paracetamol.

Diflunisal is excreted unchanged by the kidney ($t_{1/2} = 8$ h).

Important adverse effects

The commonest adverse effects of the salicylates are gastrointestinal. Occult blood loss of the order of a few mL per day occurs during aspirin therapy in the majority of patients but is less during treatment with both benorylate and diflunisal. Aspirin may also cause acute gastrointestinal blood loss. In patients with a predisposition to gastrointestinal haemorrhage (for example patients with oesophagitis, gastritis, peptic ulceration) the risk of bleeding is increased. When it occurs bleeding is generally from small gastric erosions, but occasionally larger ulcers may occur. The risk of bleeding may be reduced by using soluble, buffered, or enteric-coated forms of aspirin.

In patients who tend to bleed for other reasons (for example patients with haemophilia or von Willebrand's disease, or those taking anticoagulants), this tendency is enhanced by salicylates.

Aspirin hypersensitivity is not common. However, in patients with a history of asthma or hypersensitivity reactions to other drugs, the incidence of hypersensitivity to aspirin is increased. Wheezing and urticaria may result, and such patients often also have nasal polyps. A history of ingestion of proprietary medicines (of which there is a large number) which, unknown to patient, contain aspirin, should be sought in all patients with gastrointestinal bleeding or unexplained allergic reactions.

Uric acid renal tubular secretion is lowered by low dosages of salicylate and gout may occur. Higher (analgesic) dosages reduce the active reabsorption of uric acid and the net result is increased uric acid secretion (see Fig. 27.4).

Tinnitus is a common toxic effect of salicylates and is usually the first sign that the dosage is too high.

Aspirin should not be given to children under 12 years of age, because of the risk of Reye's syndrome.

For a discussion of salicylate poisoning see p. 493.

Interactions

The risk of bleeding in patients taking anticoagulants is increased by aspirin for two reasons: firstly, because of the increased risk of gastrointestinal bleeding and secondly, because of the inhibition of platelet aggregation, which leads to measurable and long-lasting (5 days) impairment of haemostasis. In addition, salicylate displaces warfarin from protein binding sites in the plasma, leading to a transient increase in warfarin effect (see Chapter 10 for discussion).

Aspirin inhibits the tubular secretion of methotrexate and methotrexate dosage requirements are reduced by about one-third. However, this is a potentially fatal interaction and the combination is best avoided altogether.

For the interaction of aspirin with sulphinpyrazone and probenecid see under sulphinpyrazone.

Sex hormones (polypeptide and steroid)

1. Gonadotrophins

Structures

The gonadotrophins are glycoproteins of large molecular weight. FSH (follicle stimulating hormone) and LH (luteinizing hormone) are of pituitary origin, while HCG (human chorionic gonadotrophin) and CFSH (chorionic follicle stimulating hormone) are of placental origin. ICSH (interstitial cell stimulating hormone) was the term used to describe the gonadotrophin in men now recognized to be identical with LH.

Mode of action

Endogenous FSH and LH are produced in the same cell type in the pituitary in response to the effects of the hypothalamic gonadotrophin-releasing hormone (gonadorelin, or GnRH, formerly called LHRH). It is thought that it is the steroid composition of the circulating plasma which determines whether it is FSH or LH which is released in response to gonadorelin.

Following i.v. gonadorelin there is a large rise in serum LH within 2 min and a smaller and more delayed rise in serum FSH. The changes in serum concentrations of FSH and LH in relation to the normal menstrual cycle are shown in Fig. P8.

During the first 14 days of the cycle (the menstrual and follicular phases) there is an increase in serum FSH concentration, which in turn promotes ovarian follicular maturation and stimulates oestradiol secretion. Oestradiol inhibits FSH secretion, but stimulates LH secretion through release of gonadorelin, and this in turn induces ovulation. The follicle differentiates

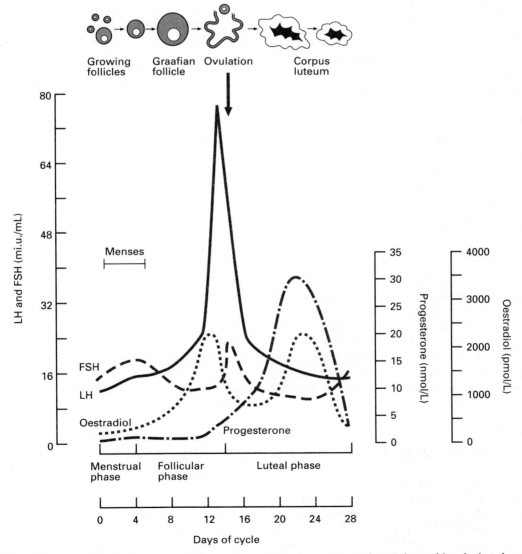

∎ **Fig. P8** Changes in circulating concentrations of steroid sex hormones and gonadotrophins during the normal menstrual cycle. (Adapted from Marshall (1981). Amenorrhoea. *Med. Int.* **1**, 291, with permission.)

into the corpus luteum, which secretes oestradiol and progesterone during the latter half of the cycle (the luteal phase). As the corpus luteum degenerates oestradiol and progesterone concentrations fall and the cycle starts again.

In men serum FSH and LH concentrations do not fluctuate. FSH stimulates the growth of testicular seminiferous tubules, leading to an increase in testicular weight during maturation. It also stimulates spermatogenesis. LH stimulates androgen production by the interstitial cells of the testis.

HCG is secreted by the placenta and has LH-like actions. During pregnancy it stimulates the corpus luteum which then continues to secrete oestradiol and progesterone until the third month of pregnancy, when placental oestrogen and progesterone secretion takes over.

The role of CFSH is not known.

Uses

Infertility secondary to hypopituitarism (FSH and LH).

Cryptorchidism (LH).

Diagnostic tests of hypothalamic–pituitary–gonadal function (GnRH).

Prostatic carcinoma (buserelin and goserelin, semi-synthetic analogues of gonadorelin).

Formulations

Pituitary FSH and LH formulations are now available but are very expensive. Alternatives are HCG, with its LH-like properties, prepared from pregnant women's urine, and HMG (human menopausal gonadotrophin or menotrophin) prepared from the urine of post-menopausal women, which contains approximately equal amounts of FSH and LH, but is used principally for its FSH content.

Dosages

The use of these drugs should be limited to specialists.

Gonadorelin, 100 micrograms.

FSH and LH in infertility. Various regimens are described, of which the following is one: one i.m. dose of HMG (75 i.u. of FSH + 75 i.u. of LH) on alternate days for three doses, followed by a single dose of HCG (5000 i.u. i.m.) 2 d later.

Cryptorchidism. HCG 500–4000 i.u. i.m. three times a week.

Prostatic cancer. Buserelin, intranasally 200 micrograms six times a day. Goserelin, 3.5 mg by s.c. implant monthly.

Kinetic data

The gonadotrophins must be given parenterally and are generally given i.m. when used therapeutically. Gonadorelin is given i.v. for diagnostic purposes. After i.v. injection FSH, LH, and HCG disappear from the serum with half-times of 20 min, 4 h, and 11 h respectively. However, their eventual half-times are longer (4, 70, and 23 h respectively). HCG is partly excreted unchanged in the urine, but little FSH or LH is so excreted. The half-time of buserelin is 20 min. The half-time of goserelin is rate-limited by its route of administration and is therefore very long.

Important adverse effects

Gonadorelin and goserelin may cause nausea, abdominal pain, headache, and menorrhagia.

HCG can cause precocious puberty when used in cryptorchidism. It can also cause gynaecomastia, ovarian hyperstimulation (causing abdominal discomfort due to mild ovarian enlargement, or even ovarian rupture and haemoperitoneum), fluid retention, changes in mood, headache, and tiredness. Occasionally allergic reactions may occur.

HMG can cause ovarian hyperstimulation (see HCG above), fluid retention, arterial thromboembolic disease, hypotension, and oliguria. Occasionally it may cause allergic reactions. Pituitary tumours may increase in size. There is an increased risk of multiple births, which are common.

2. Female sex hormones: oestrogens and progestogens

Structures

Naturally occurring oestrogens (oestradiol, oestrone, and oestriol) are synthesized mostly in the ovary under the control of FSH. However, the oestrogens commonly used therapeutically are semisynthetic and include ethinyloestradiol, mestranol, and diethylstilboestrol (dealt with separately, p. 687). Ethinyloestradiol is the most commonly used.

The naturally-occurring progestogen, progesterone, is synthesized mostly in the ovary under the control of LH. There are several semi-synthetic progestogens in use, including norethisterone, levonorgestrel, ethynodiol, lynoestrenol, and desogestrel. Norethisterone is the most commonly used.

Modes of action

Oestrogens

Feminizing effects

Oestrogens cause the changes which occur at puberty: growth and development of the vagina, uterus, and Fallopian tubes; breast formation; the pubertal growth spurt and eventual fusion of the bony epiphyses; and other secondary sexual characteristics. such as growth of axillary and pubic hair and pigmentation of the nipples, areolae, and external genitalia.

Cyclical ovulation

Oestrogens cause the release of LH at the end of the follicular phase of the menstrual cycle (see Fig. P8) and that in turn lead to ovulation. An increase in circulating oestrogen concentrations in the blood inhibits the release of FSH from the pituitary and this mechanism acts as a negative feedback for the control of oestrogen release (see also gonadotrophins above).

Pregnancy

During pregnancy oestrogens, the major source of which is the placenta, have a variety of effects. They promote uterine growth by increasing the size and number of myometrial cells; they inhibit LH and FSH production, thus preventing ovarian follicle development and ovulation; they cause changes in the uterine cervix which allow dilatation at the time of labour; and they stimulate breast development in preparation for lactation. They may also be responsible for the increased skin pigmentation in pregnancy and cause changes in haemostatic mechanisms which may help limit blood loss at time of delivery (increased synthesis of clotting factors, increased platelet aggregability, and decreased fibrinolytic activity).

Metabolic effects

Oestrogens have effects on metabolism, including sodium and water retention, and an anabolic effect on tissue proteins similar to that of the androgens (see below). They may also impair glucose tolerance in patients with or without a predisposition to diabetes mellitus.

Contraceptive actions

See Chapter 12 (p. 147).

Progestogens

Endometrial effects

Progesterone has direct effects on the endometrium, causing it to become secretory during the luteal phase of the menstrual cycle (see Fig. P8). The sharp fall in circulating progesterone at the end of the cycle is principally responsible for the onset of menstruation. In contrast to the oestrogens, progesterone has no feedback effects on FSH or LH.

Effects during pregnancy

During pregnancy progesterone prevents uterine contractions and may have effects in preventing the immunological rejection of the fetus. Together with oestrogens it causes breast enlargement in preparation for lactation after delivery.

Contraceptive actions

See Chapter 12 (p. 147).

Uses

Oestrogens alone

Primary amenorrhoea.
Breast carcinoma in post-menopausal women.
Senile vaginitis and vulvitis (topical formulations).

Progestogens alone

Oral contraception.
Dysfunctional uterine bleeding.
Endometriosis.
Menstrual disturbances (for example premenstrual syndrome, dysmenorrhoea).

Oestrogen + progestogen

Oral contraception.
Replacement therapy in ovarian insufficiency.
Menstrual disturbances (for example menorrhagia, metropathia haemorrhagica, dysmenorrhoea).

Hormone replacement therapy (so-called HRT) for menopausal women with severe vaginal atrophy or vasomotor instability and in women with an early natural or surgical menopause (before the age of 45 years) in order to prevent osteoporosis.

Formulations and dosages

Oestrogens alone

There are several proprietary formulations for oral use containing oestrogens only. Ethinyloestradiol is the oestrogen of choice.

Menopausal symptoms: 10–50 micrograms orally t.d.s., reducing to 10–20 micrograms o.d. or b.d. according to symptoms.

Primary amenorrhoea: 150 micrograms orally o.d.

Breast carcinoma: 1–3 mg orally o.d.

Progestogens alone

There are several proprietary formulations for oral use containing progestogens only. We give here the recommended dosages for norethisterone.

Oral contraception (progestogen alone): 350 micrograms (one tablet) orally o.d. at the same time of day each day (preferably in the evening), starting on the first day of the cycle.

Dysfunctional uterine bleeding: to stop bleeding 5 mg orally t.d.s. for 10 d; to prevent bleeding 5 mg orally b.d. from days 19 to 26 of the cycle.

Endometriosis: 10 mg orally o.d., starting on day 5 of the cycle, increasing if required to 25 mg daily in divided doses to prevent breakthrough bleeding; continue for at least 6 months.

Premenstrual syndrome: 10–15 mg orally o.d. from day 5 to day 25 of the cycle.

Dysmenorrhoea: 5 mg orally t.d.s. from day 5 to day 25 for 3–4 cycles.

Combined oestrogen/progestogen formulations

Many combination formulations are available, mostly intended for use as oral contraceptives. These are discussed in Chapter 12 (p. 147).

In replacement therapy for ovarian insufficiency sequential therapy is given, starting with an oestrogen (for example ethinyloestradiol 10 micrograms orally o.d.) for 21 d, and giving a progestogen (for example norethisterone 5 mg orally o.d.) on days 17–21.

In HRT an oestrogen (for example ethinyloestradiol 10 micrograms orally o.d.) is given for 21 d; alternatively oestradiol can be given in a transdermal formulation, one patch (25–100 micrograms) every 3–4 d. In women with a uterus a progestogen (for example norethisterone 5 mg orally o.d.) is given for 10 d in the second half of the cycle, to reduce the risk of endometrial carcinoma. For the symptomatic relief of menopausal symptoms treatment can continue for a year or more; in women whose menopause is early it should be given until they are 50 years old or perhaps even longer.

Other formulations

Oestrogens are available for parenteral and topical administration.

Parenteral oestrogen preparations

These are used in women requiring prolonged oestrogen treatment (for example in primary amenorrhoea or breast carcinoma) and are available as oily injections (given i.m. every 1–14 d) or an implant (given once every several weeks, the exact time interval depending on the dose; for example, a 25 mg implant of oestradiol has a duration of effect of 36 weeks).

Topical oestrogen preparations

These are used for treating atrophic vaginitis and vulvitis, for example dienoestrol cream 0.01–0.025 per cent applied by special applicator o.d.

Parenteral progestogen preparations

Some progestogens are also available as depot injections and have been used both for long-term contraception (medroxyprogesterone, a controversial use of depot progestogens) and to try to prevent abortions in pregnant women with a history of habitual abortion (hydroxyprogesterone, efficacy not proven).

Kinetic data

The commonly used oestrogens and progestogens are well absorbed after oral administration. However, ethinyloestradiol is subject to extensive first-pass metabolism, mostly in the gut wall, and has a systemic availability of about 40 per cent.

The interactions of oestrogens and progestogens with their binding proteins are very complex and their clinical significance is not fully understood. They are highly protein-bound (> 90 per cent). Progestogens are bound both to a sex-hormone-binding globulin and to plasma albumin. The capacity of the globulin is low, but is increased by ethinyloestradiol (> 50 μg/d) and by drugs which induce hepatic microsomal drug-metabolizing enzymes (for example phenytoin, phenobarbitone). Ethinyloestradiol is mostly bound to plasma albumin but not to globulin.

Ethinyloestradiol is extensively metabolized, $t_{1/2} = 12$ h, and there is enterohepatic recirculation following deconjugation of conjugated ethinyloestradiol in the gut. There is a great deal of variation in the extent of metabolism from individual to individual and for some women the lower doses of ethinyloestradiol (20 or 30 micrograms) may be just sufficient for therapeutic efficacy; this is especially important in regard to the interaction with enzyme-inducing drugs (see interactions below).

Mestranol is predominantly metabolized to ethinyloestradiol by demethylation.

Norethisterone and levonorgestrel are extensively metabolized. $t_{1/2}$ for norethisterone is 8 h, for levonorgestrel 20 h.

Ethynodiol and lynoestrenol are partly converted to norethisterone.

Important adverse effects

Adverse effects due to oestrogens and progestogens are common and dose-related.

Oestrogens

Oestrogens, when given alone, commonly cause fluid retention and hypertension. They cause painful breasts and endometrial bleeding in women and gynaecomastia in men. There may be impairment of glucose tolerance in diabetics. Oestrogens may precipitate an acute attack of porphyria in susceptible patients (see Chapter 8). Oestrogens can also cause thromboembolic disease and are associated with an increased risk of benign liver tumours and endometrial carcinoma. These are discussed below under oral contraceptives.

Progestogens

Progestogens, when given alone as contraceptives, commonly cause headache, nausea and vomiting, and abdominal or low back pain. They may occasionally cause breast tenderness. When given for breast cancer they may cause amenorrhoea and hypercalcaemia. If used during early pregnancy they may cause virilization of a female fetus. Long-term (2 year) treatment with depot formulations of progesterone results in a high incidence of amenorrhoea.

Combined oestrogens and progestogens

Combined oral contraceptives, in addition to the effects described above due to their separate components, commonly cause headache, vaginal discharge, mental depression and loss of libido, and urinary tract infections. Migraine may be precipitated or made worse, although occasionally it may improve.

Hypertension

A small increase in blood pressure is not uncommon, but in about 4 per cent a moderate or severe increase may occur. This hypertension is reversible on withdrawal.

Thromboembolism

There is an increased risk of thromboembolic disease in women taking combined oral contraceptives. These women are more likely to develop deep venous thrombosis, pulmonary embolism, myocardial infarction, and cerebral infarction. This effect is thought to be related to the oestrogen content. The risk increases with age and is on average about sixfold compared with women not using oral contraceptives. The risk is lower in women taking a 30 microgram oestrogen preparation. Smoking increases the risk of myocardial infarction.

Tumours

There is an increased risk of benign liver tumours in women taking combined oral contraceptives or oestrogens alone. The risk of hepatocellular adenoma increases with age, dose, and duration of use. The risk is low in women taking a 30 microgram oestrogen preparation. If an adverse effect on the liver occurs (for example jaundice or acute hepatitis) an alternative form of contraception is advised.

Oestrogen use during pregnancy is associated with an increased risk of the occurrence in their teens of vaginal adenosis and vaginal adenocarcinoma in the female offspring. There is also an increased risk of fetal malformations.

Oestrogen use during and after the menopause is associated with an increased risk of endometrial carcinoma. The increase is about sixfold and increases with dose and duration of use. It is not clear, however, what the risks are in women taking low-dose (i.e. 30 micrograms oestrogen) oral contraceptives. There is some protection from progestogens if they are taken during the second half of the cycle (see above).

There is a *decreased* risk of benign breast tumours in women taking combined oral contraceptives. The effect is related to duration of use. There is some evidence of an increased risk of breast cancer. The risk of ovarian carcinoma may be reduced and the risk of carcinoma of the cervix increased.

Gallstones

There is an increased risk of gallstones.

Amenorrhoea

Amenorrhoea occurs in about 5 per cent of women after withdrawal of oral contraceptives but usually lasts no longer than a few months. Prolonged amenorrhoea and permanent sterility are rare.

Contra-indications

Oral contraceptives are contra-indicated in women with oestrogen-dependent tumours (such as breast cancer), pregnancy, a past history of thromboembolic disease, liver disease, or porphyria. Relative contra-indications include hypertension, diabetes mellitus, age over 35 y, heavy smoking habit, recent menarche, migraine, recurrent urinary tract infections, gallstones, mental depression, and epilepsy.

Interactions

Drugs which induce the activity of hepatic microsomal drug-metabolizing enzymes (for example rifampicin, phenytoin, phenobarbitone, see Chapter 10) enhance the metabolism of oestrogens and/or progestogens and can cause failure of therapy in those women in whom the lower doses of oestrogen are only just sufficient, say to maintain contraception.

Rifampicin

Rifampicin has a large effect in enhancing oestrogen and progestogen metabolism and while a course of rifampicin is being given alternative forms of contraception should be used.

Phenytoin and phenobarbitone

Phenytoin and phenobarbitone can cause contraceptive failure, perhaps due to enzyme induction, but perhaps also partly due to an increase in protein binding of progestogen (see kinetic data above). The first sign of contraceptive failure will generally be mid-cycle spotting and in such cases the daily dose of ethinyloestradiol should be increased to 50, 80, or even 100 micrograms if necessary.

There are anecdotal reports of pregnancies in women taking combined oral formulations with some antibiotics, notably ampicillin and tetracyclines. Oestrogens are conjugated in the liver and excreted via the bile into the gut, where they are deconjugated by intestinal bacteria and then reabsorbed. Antibiotics which destroy the deconjugating bacteria might therefore reduce this reabsorption. Although this theoretical explanation of the anecdotal observations has not been confirmed in small formal studies, it is wise to advise a woman who is having a course of antibiotics to use another method of contraception for the duration of the course.

3. Male sex hormones and anabolic steroids

Structures

The principal male sex hormone is testosterone, which is mainly secreted by the interstitial cells of the testis under the influence of LH (ICSH). It is also secreted by the adrenals.

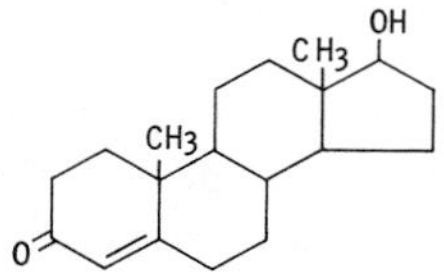

There are several semi-synthetic androgens with different spectra of effects, some (such as methyl-testosterone and mesterolone) with both androgenic and anabolic effects, others (such as nandrolone, stanozolol, and danazol) with principally anabolic effects and less androgenic effect than testosterone. Nandrolone is shown here as an example:

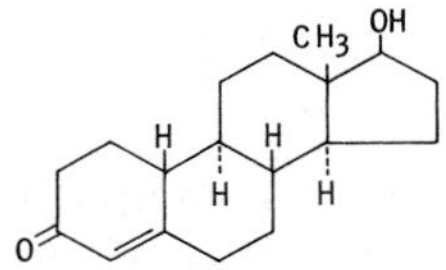

Mode of action

Testosterone has both androgenic and anabolic properties.

The androgenic properties are responsible for producing male attributes. They cause the changes which occur at puberty: growth of the penis, scrotum, and testicles; frequent penile erections; the pubertal growth spurt and eventual fusion of the bony epiphyses; increased thickness and oiliness of the skin with acne; and other secondary sexual characteristics, such as growth of axillary, pubic, and facial hair and deepening of the voice.

The anabolic effects result in increased muscle mass.

Uses

Replacement therapy in testicular or pituitary insufficiency (testosterone, mesterolone).

To increase muscle bulk (for example after debilitating disease: nandrolone, stanozolol).

Osteoporosis in postmenopausal women (nandrolone).

In hereditary angio-oedema (stanozolol).

Dosages
Replacement therapy

Testosterone i.m. is the treatment of choice. Numerous different formulations of different salts are available (for example testosterone propionate, testosterone enanthate, testosterone decanoate) either alone or in combination. The following are examples of suitable regimens:

Testosterone salts (propionate 20 mg/mL + phenylpropionate 40 mg/mL + isohexanoate 40 mg/mL; Sustanon 100®), 1 mL i.m. every 2 weeks.

Testosterone salts (propionate 30 mg/mL + phenylpropionate 60 mg/mL + isohexanoate 60 mg/mL + decanoate 100 mg/mL; Sustanon 250®), 1 mL i.m. every 3 weeks.

Testosterone enanthate 250 mg/mL (Primoteston Depot®), 1 mL i.m. every 3 weeks.

In patients who are unsuitable for i.m. therapy oral treatment may be used, as in the following examples:

Testosterone undecanoate 40–120 mg daily p.o.

Mesterolone 25 mg t.d.s. p.o.

To increase muscle bulk

Nandrolone 25–50 mg i.m. every 3 weeks.

Stanozolol 5 mg orally daily, or 50 mg i.m. every 2–3 weeks.

Osteoporosis in postmenopausal women

Nandrolone decanoate 50 mg i.m. every 3 weeks.

Hereditary angio-oedema

Stanozolol, 2.5–10 mg o.d. to control attacks, reducing for maintenance therapy.

Kinetic data

Testosterone is extensively metabolized in the liver after oral administration and is therefore usually given i.m. The oily solution of testosterone undecanoate is absorbed via the intestinal lymphatics, avoiding first-pass metabolism. Testosterone is extensively bound in the plasma to the sex-hormone-binding globulin.

Nandrolone is given only by i.m. depot injection. It is rapidly hydrolysed in the blood with a half-time of about 4 h, but its kinetics are rate-limited by the depot formulation which is used and it consequently has a half-time of about 8 d.

Stanozolol has not been well studied, but it is thought to be extensively metabolized.

Important adverse effects

The main adverse effects of the male sex hormones are inherent in their actions as virilizing hormones. The virilizing effects are, however, less marked with the specifically anabolic hormones (such as nandrolone) than with testosterone itself.

In children growth may be inhibited by early closure of the bony epiphyses.

In women the virilizing effects cause hirsutism, breast atrophy, acne, clitoral hypertrophy, increased libido, and deepening of the voice.

In men there is increased libido, aggressive behaviour, frequent erections, and occasionally priapism.

Other common effects include sodium and water retention and increased muscle mass (anabolic effect).

Stanozolol can cause liver damage and should be used with care in patients with pre-existing liver disease. Methyltestosterone commonly causes cholestatic jaundice and should no longer be used.

Androgens should not be used in men with prostatic or breast carcinoma. They should not be used in pregnancy, since they may cause virilization of a female fetus, or in breast-feeding mothers.

Interactions

Anabolic steroids may increase the effects of warfarin, perhaps by increasing the affinity of warfarin for its receptor site.

Sodium nitroprusside

Structure

$$Na_2Fe(CN)_5NO$$

Mode of action

Sodium nitroprusside has a direct relaxant effect on the smooth muscle of veins and arteries. Peripheral arteriolar dilatation produces its hypotensive effect. It also reduces ergot-induced arterial vasoconstriction. The haemodynamic effects in acute left ventricular failure are due to the combination of actions on both preload and afterload.

Uses

Accelerated hypertension.
Acute left ventricular failure.
The elective induction of hypotension during surgery.
Ergot-induced arterial vasoconstriction and gangrene.

Dosages

0.5–1.5 micrograms/kg/min by continuous i.v. infusion, increasing as required to 8 micrograms/kg/min. Meticulous and frequent monitoring of blood pressure is required and treatment should therefore be undertaken only in hospital. Sodium nitroprusside must be protected from light during infusion.

Kinetic data

The $t_{1/2}$ of sodium nitroprusside is only a few minutes, and its effects may therefore be rapidly switched on and off by adjustments in the infusion rate. It is metabolized to thiocyanate, which is eliminated in the urine. Thiocyanate toxicity begins at plasma concentrations over 50 μg/mL.

Important adverse effects

Nausea, vomiting, restlessness, headache, palpitation, sweating, retrosternal discomfort, and abdominal pain all occur with over-rapid infusion, as obviously also does hypotension. In patients with renal impairment thiocyanate toxicity may occur. Sodium nitroprusside should not be used in patients with liver disease, aortic coarctation, or arteriovenous shunts.

Spironolactone

Structure

(Compare aldosterone and cardiac glycosides.)

Mode of action

Spironolactone acts through its active metabolite, canrenone, which is an antagonist of the action of aldosterone on the distal convoluted tubule of the nephron. This causes increased sodium and water excretion and potassium retention.

Uses

Fluid retention due to cardiac failure, the nephrotic syndrome, hepatic disease, and malignant ascites. In heart failure and the nephrotic syndrome it is usually used in combination with a thiazide or loop diuretic or both.

In the diagnosis and treatment of primary hyperaldosteronism.

Dosage

100–200 mg o.d. orally.

Kinetic data

Spironolactone is well absorbed. It has a short $t_{1/2}$ (about 10 min) but is metabolized to the active compound canrenone ($t_{1/2} = 16$ h), which is excreted by the kidney. Partly because of the long $t_{1/2}$ of its metabolite spironolactone has a long duration of action and its maximum effects take several days to occur.

Canrenone has been used i.v. as an alternative to spironolactone.

Important adverse effects

Nausea and vomiting are common, especially with high doses. If this proves troublesome it may help to give the total daily dose in two divided doses.

Hyperkalaemia occurs in about 8 per cent of patients, even when a potassium-depleting diuretic is also used.

Gynaecomastia is common and often painful. Other less frequent effects include menstrual disturbances, impotence, testicular atrophy, and peptic ulceration.

Stilboestrol

Structure

(Compare tamoxifen.)

Mode of action

Stilboestrol is a synthetic oestrogen which is twice as potent as oestradiol.

Uses

In the management of postmenopausal oestrogen-sensitive breast carcinoma which fails to respond to tamoxifen.

Although it has been used in the treatment of the symptoms of disseminated prostatic cancer, stilboestrol is being replaced by goserelin and buserelin.

Dosages

Breast carcinoma: 10–20 mg o.d. orally.

Kinetic data

Stilboestrol is well absorbed, but is subject to a high degree of first-pass metabolism. It is highly bound to sex-hormone-binding globulin and to a lesser extent to albumin.

Important adverse effects

Nausea and vomiting occur in about 50 per cent of cases. Tenderness and engorgement of the breasts may occur.

Diethylstilboestrol should not be used in pregnancy because of the association of vaginal adenocarcinoma in female offspring and testicular carcinoma in male offspring.

Diethylstilboestrol may precipitate an acute attack of hepatic porphyria in susceptible patients.

Stilboestrol may cause transient rises in liver transaminases, and it should not be used in combination with other drugs which may damage the liver.

Drugs which induce hepatic microsomal drug-metabolizing enzymes increase the rate of clearance of stilboestrol.

Sulphasalazine and related salicylates

Structures

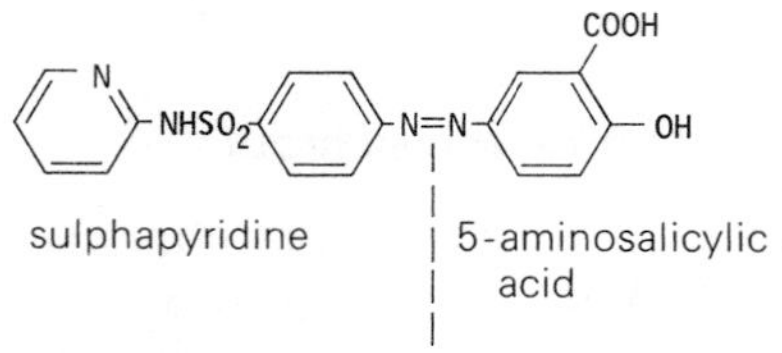

sulphapyridine | 5-aminosalicylic acid

Sulphasalazine is shown here. Mesalazine is the new generic name for 5-aminosalicylic acid. Olsalazine is a compound in which a second molecule of 5-aminosalicylic acid replaces the sulphapyridine in sulphasalazine.

Mode of action

The action of all of these compounds in ulcerative colitis and Crohn's disease is probably through the action of 5-aminosalicylic acid in suppressing the inflammatory reaction in the bowel, perhaps by inhibition of prostaglandin synthesis (see salicylates).

In contrast, in rheumatoid arthritis the sulphapyridine moiety is thought to be the active component, but its mode of action is unknown.

Uses

Ulcerative colitis, both in the treatment of an acute exacerbation and in the maintenance of remission.

Crohn's disease.

Rheumatoid arthritis.

Dosages

Ulcerative colitis

Sulphasalazine, 500–1000 mg q.d.s. orally.

Mesalazine, orally 1.5–3 g a day in divided doses during the acute phase, reducing to a maintenance dose of 0.75–1.5 g a day in divided doses; suppositories, 0.75–1.5 g a day in divided doses; enemas, one at bedtime.

Olsalazine, 1–3 g daily in divided doses.

In arthritis it is usual to introduce sulphasalazine gradually in order to avoid gastrointestinal adverse effects: 500 mg/d in the first week rising to 1 g b.d. in the fourth and subsequent weeks.

Kinetic data

Sulphasalazine is hardly at all absorbed. When it reaches the large bowel it is hydrolysed by colonic bacteria to 5-aminosalicylic acid and sulphapyridine (see structure). 5-aminosalicylic acid is absorbed only about 25 per cent and is mainly excreted in the faeces. Sulphapyridine, on the other hand, is well absorbed from the colon and metabolized as are other sulphonamides (qq.v.).

Olsalazine is also poorly absorbed and is hydrolysed in the large bowel to two molecules of mesalazine.

Mesalazine is well absorbed throughout the bowel and therefore has to be given as special formulations, which do not release their contents until they reach the large bowel. Alternatively, it can be given as suppositories or enemas. After absorption mesalazine is excreted by the kidneys, $t_{1/2} = 1$ h.

Important adverse effects

The adverse effects of sulphasalazine are attributed for the most part to sulphapyridine and commonly include nausea, vomiting, and abdominal discomfort. It may also cause reversible sterility, due to impaired spermatogenesis. Occasional blood dyscrasias require careful monitoring in arthritis. For other adverse effects see under sulphonamides.

Mesalazine may cause adverse effects similar to other salicylates, including an interstitial nephritis; it should not be used in patients with renal impairment. It and its derivatives should not be used in patients who are allergic to salicylates.

Interaction

Lactulose alters the pH of the bowel and so prevents the release of mesalazine from pH-sensitive capsules.

Sulphinpyrazone

Structure

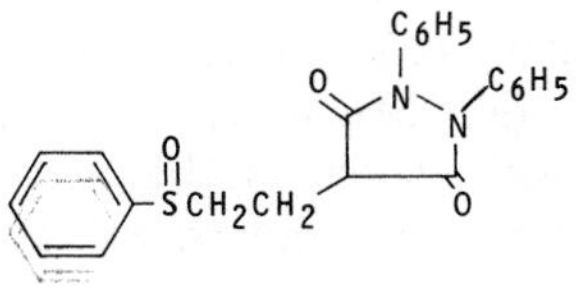

(Compare phenylbutazone.)

Mode of action

Uricosuric effect: by inhibition of the active renal tubular reabsorption of uric acid (Fig. 29.4; see also probenecid and salicylates). Inhibition of platelet aggregation in response to various agents: this might be the basis of its suggested effect in reducing the incidence of reinfarction after myocardial infarct.

Uses

Gout and hyperuricaemia.

Dosage

100–400 mg b.d. orally.

Kinetic data

Sulphinpyrazone is well absorbed. Its $t_{1/2}$ is about 6 h, but its uricosuric effects persist for up to 10 h during maintenance therapy. It is metabolized 50 per cent to a *para*-hydroxyphenyl derivative, which is also uricosuric but has a short $t_{1/2}$ (1 h). Sulphinpyrazone is also excreted unchanged in the urine.

Important adverse effects

Gastrointestinal symptoms occur in up to 15 per cent of patients but are rarely severe. Other adverse effects are rare.

Interactions

The uricosuric effects of sulphinpyrazone and probenecid are antagonized by aspirin at all doses of aspirin. High doses of aspirin are uricosuric and this effect is antagonized by sulphinpyrazone and probenecid. Sulphinpyrazone enhances the action of warfarin and phenytoin, probably by inhibiting their metabolism.

Sulphonamides

Structures

The general structure of the antibacterial sulphonamides is shown here:

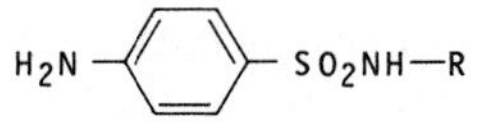

Substitution at R leads to changes in antibacterial activity.

The main sulphonamides in use are sulphadimidine (urinary tract infections) and sulphamethoxazole (see co-trimoxazole).

Sulphonamides which are used for non-infective indications include sulphasalazine (in ulcerative colitis, see separate entry) and sulphapyridine (in dermatitis herpetiformis).

Mode of action

Sulphonamides are bacteriostatic and act by competitive inhibition of the incorporation of *para*-aminobenzoic acid into pteroylglutamic acid (folic acid), which is necessary for bacterial replication. For the effects of a combination of sulphamethoxazole with trimethoprim see under co-trimoxazole.

Uses

The organisms against which the sulphonamides may be active include:

Gram-positive cocci (streptococci, pneumococci, staphylococci);

Gram-negative cocci (meningococci, gonococci);

Gram-negative bacilli (*E. coli, P. mirabilis, H. influenzae*);

Gram-positive bacilli (*B. anthracis, C. diphtheriae*).

Other possibly sensitive organisms are *Nocardia, Actinomyces, Chlamydia,* and *Toxoplasma.*

However, sulphonamides are not so frequently used as previously, because of their adverse effects, the emergence of resistant organisms, their limited antibacterial spectrum, and the introduction of more potent and effective antibiotics. The indications for those sulphonamides still in use are very restricted, for example:

Sulphadimidine (meningococcal meningitis and urinary tract infection with Gram-negative organisms);

Sulphadiazine (meningococcal meningitis, skin infections, nocardiasis, and, in combination with pyrimethamine, toxoplasmosis);

Sulphometapyrazine (chronic bronchitis and urinary tract infection with Gram-negative organisms);

Sulphacetamide (eye infections);

Sulphadimethoxine (trachoma).

Dosages

Examples of oral regimens

Sulphadiazine, 2–4 g initially, then 0.5–1 g q.d.s.

Sulphadimidine, as for sulphadiazine.

Kinetic data

The oral sulphonamides mentioned here are generally well absorbed. They have half-times of 5–10 h and their metabolism is very variable, the major route of metabolism being acetylation, the rate of which is bimodally distributed in the population (see Chapter 8). Sulphadimidine is often used as a reference compound for assessing acetylator status, by measuring the proportion of acetylated metabolite present in an aliquot of urine taken 6 h after an oral dose of 1 g.

Important adverse effects

Allergic reactions are common. These include maculopapular skin rashes, drug fever, and photodermatitis. Much less commonly more severe reactions, such as the Stevens–Johnson syndrome and toxic epidermolysis (Lyell's syndrome), are seen.

Sulphonamide crystalluria, the crystallization of the less soluble sulphonamides in the urine may result in renal damage, but may be prevented by making the urine alkaline with sodium bicarbonate and by maintaining a high urine flow rate. It is not a complication of the more modern, more soluble sulphonamides such as sulphamethoxazole. It is not wise to use sulphonamides at all in patients with renal failure.

Sulphonamides displace bilirubin from plasma proteins and the increase in unbound bilirubin in the circulation may lead to deposition of bilirubin in the brains of neonates (kernicterus). For this reason sulphonamides should not be used for chemotherapy in neonates or pregnant women in the third trimester. However, the affinity of different sulphonamides for the bilirubin-binding protein varies, and sulphasalazine seems to be safe.

Occasionally blood dyscrasias may occur, including agranulocytosis, thrombocytopenia, and aplastic anaemia. Sulphonamides may cause haemolysis in patients with G6PD deficiency (see Chapter 8).

Interactions

Sulphonamides bind to plasma albumin and may displace other drugs such as warfarin, phenytoin, and tolbutamide. The clinical relevance of drug interactions of this kind is discussed in Chapter 10.

Sulphonylureas

Structures

General

$$X \text{—} \langle \text{benzene ring} \rangle \text{—} SO_2NHCONHR$$

(Compare sulphonamides, thiazide diuretics, diazoxide.)

Substitutions at R and X produce compounds with differing pharmacological activities.

Mode of action

Sulphonylureas enhance the release of insulin from pancreatic islet beta cells by closing the ATP-sensitive potassium channels involved in insulin release. This action accounts for their short-term and long-term effects. Some of their long-term effects may also be mediated by an increase in the numbers of peripheral insulin receptors.

Use

Diabetes mellitus of mature onset.

Dosages

All the sulphonylureas are given orally, For the commonly used ranges of dosages see the Table below.

Kinetic data

All the sulphonylureas are well absorbed and extensively metabolized. For half-times see the Table below.

It is a curious phenomenon that although chlorpropamide is more than 50 per cent metabolized its $t_{1/2}$ is prolonged in renal failure and its effects are increased.

	Initial dose*	Usual daily doses	$t_{1/2}$ (h)
Chlorpropamide	250 mg o.d.	100–500 mg o.d.	36
Glibenclamide	5 mg o.d.	2.5–20 mg in divided doses	6
Gliclazide	40–80 mg o.d.	40–320 mg o.d. or divided	10
Glipizide	2.5–5.0 mg o.d.	2.5–40 mg o.d. or divided	3
Gliquidone	15 mg o.d.	45–180 mg in divided doses	6
Tolbutamide	0.5 g b.d.	1–2 g in divided doses	6

*Start with smaller doses in old people

Important adverse effects

Hypoglycaemia is common, particularly with glibenclamide and chlorpropamide.

About a third of patients who take alcohol with chlorpropamide may have a reaction consisting of flushing, vomiting, hypotension, and palpitation. The reaction has also been reported rarely with tolbutamide. Chlorpropamide also causes hyponatraemia by stimulating vasopressin production by the pituitary.

Nausea, vomiting, and a metallic taste in the mouth occur in about 2 per cent of cases, but tend to resolve after a time.

Interactions

β-adrenoceptor antagonists may enhance the hypoglycaemic effects of sulphonylureas and also block most of the symptoms of hypoglycaemia (sweating is an exception).

The hypoglycaemic effect of sulphonylureas is reduced by corticosteroids, thiazide diuretics, and diazoxide.

Cimetidine inhibits the metabolism of tolbutamide.

The chlorpropamide–alcohol interaction has been noted above.

Tamoxifen

Structure

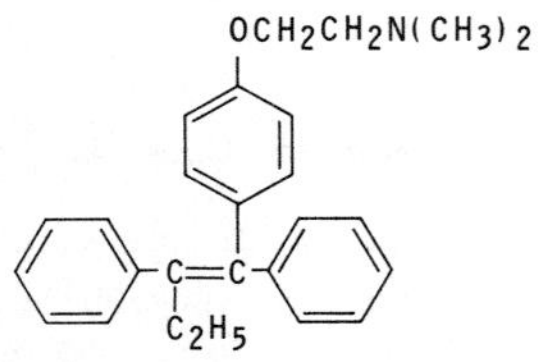

OCH₂CH₂N(CH₃)₂

(Compare stilboestrol.)

Mode of action

Tamoxifen is an antagonist of the effects of oestrogens at tissue receptors. It inhibits the growth of oestrogen-dependent breast cancer cells. In normal pre-menopausal women it decreases plasma prolactin concentrations, perhaps by inhibiting oestradiol-induced prolactin release from the pituitary. In anovulatory women it also increases plasma LH concentrations.

Uses

Breast carcinoma in postmenopausal women.
Stimulation of ovulation in infertility.

Dosages

Breast carcinoma (not to be used in women with functioning ovaries): 10 mg orally b.d. Increase to 20 mg b.d. after 1 month if there is no response.

Treatment of infertility: first exclude pregnancy. If there is regular menstruation give 10 mg b.d. on days 2, 3, 4, and 5 of the cycle, increasing during subsequent cycles to 40 mg b.d. if required. Start treatment at any time if menstruation is not occurring.

Kinetic data

Tamoxifen is well absorbed. It is extensively metabolized by hydroxylation and N-demethylation, but the metabolites are excreted into the gut via the bile and are then hydrolysed to tamoxifen, which is reabsorbed. It consequently has a long half-time during chronic therapy (average 7 d) and it may take weeks or even months to reach steady state during maintenance dose therapy.

Important adverse effects

The major and most common (10–20 per cent) adverse effects of tamoxifen are related to its antioestrogen actions, namely hot flushes, pruritus vulvae, and occasionally vaginal bleeding. Nausea and vomiting are also very common (10 per cent). It may occasionally cause fluid retention and an increase in tumour pain. In women with bony metastases it may occasionally cause hypercalcaemia.

Interaction

Tamoxifen may potentiate the action of warfarin.

Tetracyclines

Structures

Tetracycline

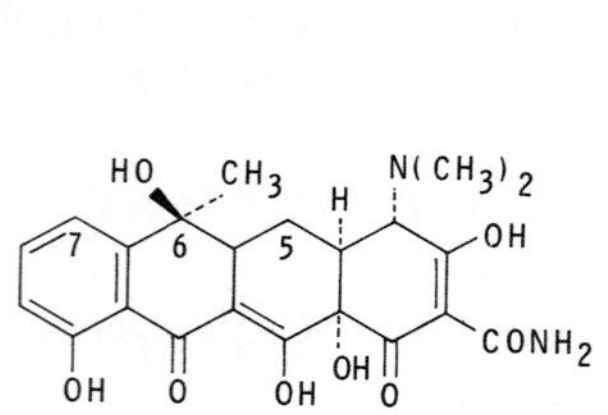

The other commonly used tetracyclines are: oxytetracycline, doxycycline, minocycline, chlortetracycline, and demeclocycline (demethylchlortetracycline).

These compounds are formed by making various substitutions at positions 5, 6, and 7 in the structure shown above (for example oxytetracycline has a hydroxyl group at position 5).

Mode of action

By inhibition of protein synthesis in bacterial ribosomes and disruption of the translation process from RNA to DNA. Tetracyclines are bacteriostatic.

Uses

In Table P8 are listed some of the infectious diseases for which the tetracyclines may be indicated and the organisms with which those diseases are associated.

Tetracyclines are also used as an alternative to rifampicin in the prevention of meningococcal infection in the contacts of those with meningococcal meningitis.

Other uses include the treatment of acne vulgaris and the use of demeclocycline in the syndrome of inappropriate ADH secretion, because of its ability to render the renal tubules relatively insensitive to the effects of ADH.

Dosages

The following are examples of common dosage regimens:

Oral

Tetracycline, 250–500 mg 6-hourly.
Oxytetracycline, 250–500 mg 6-hourly.
Doxycycline, 200 mg initially then 100 mg once daily.
Minocycline, 200 mg initially, then 100 mg 12-hourly.
Chlortetracycline, 250–500 mg 6-hourly.
Demeclocycline, 150 mg 6-hourly or 300 mg 12-hourly.

Intramuscular and intravenous

	i.m.	i.v. infusion
Tetracycline	100–200 mg 6–8 hourly	500 mg over 12 h
Oxytetracycline	100 mg 8–12 hourly	250–500 mg over 12 h

Local application

Tetracyclines are available for local application in creams and ointments, usually containing the antibiotic in a strength of 3 per cent.

∎ **Table P8** The main indications for the use of tetracyclines

Disease	Organism
1. *Tetracycline treatment of choice*	
Acute exacerbation of chronic bronchitis	*Strep. pneumoniae* and *H. influenzae*
'Atypical' pneumonias	
Mycoplasma pneumonia	*Mycoplasma pneumoniae*
Q fever	*Coxiella burnetti*
Psittacosis	*Chlamydia psittaci*
Brucellosis (with streptomycin)	*Brucella abortus*
Leptospirosis (alternative penicillin G)	*Leptospira icterohaemorrhagiae*
Typhus diseases	*Rickettsia* spp.
Lymphogranuloma venereum (LGV)	LGV *Chlamydiae*
Trachoma and inclusion conjunctivitis	*Chlamydia* and *Ureaplasma* spp.
Other rickettsioses (trench fever, rickettsial pox, tick-borne rickettsioses)	
Infections of the skin (local treatment)	
2. *Tetracyclines second-line treatment*	
Syphilis and yaws	*Treponema pallidum* and *T. pertenue*
Actinomycosis	*Actinomyces israelii*
Anthrax	*Bacillus anthracis*
Eye infections (local treatment)	

Kinetic data

The tetracyclines are moderately well absorbed (about 70 per cent) except for minocycline and doxycycline, which are well absorbed (90 per cent). The absorption of tetracyclines is reduced by calcium, aluminium, magnesium, and iron, with which they form insoluble chelates (see interactions).

The values of $t_{1/2}$ differ from tetracycline to tetracycline, partly accounting for the differences in dosage frequency: e.g. tetracycline, chlortetracycline, and oxytetracycline, $t_{1/2} = 8$ h; demeclocycline, $t_{1/2} = 18$ h.

The tetracyclines are widely distributed to body tissues, but of particular importance is their distribution to growing bones and teeth where they may cause discolouration, enamel hypoplasia, and decreased growth of long bones (see adverse effects).

Most of the tetracyclines are excreted in the urine 40–60 per cent unchanged, and renal failure causes decreased clearance and accumulation. Minocycline and doxycycline are excreted in the urine to a much lesser extent and are mostly metabolized in the liver. If a tetracycline has to be used in a patient with compromised renal function doxycycline is the tetracycline of choice.

All the tetracyclines are to some extent excreted in the bile and undergo enterohepatic recirculation.

Important adverse effects

Renal

In patients with compromised renal function, for example patients with renal failure or old people, there may be accumulation of tetracyclines to concentrations in the blood which result in toxic effects, such as anorexia, nausea, vomiting, and diarrhoea. These effects lead to dehydration, which further compromises renal function and leads to the clinical syndrome of acute renal failure.

In addition to this, the *apparent* biochemical degree of renal failure, as judged by the blood urea, may be increased by the antianabolic effects of tetracyclines, resulting in a rise in blood urea without a concomitant rise in serum creatinine.

The indirect adverse effects of tetracyclines on renal function should not be confused with the very special effect of direct renal toxicity caused by tetracycline products formed during excessively long storage with chemical breakdown of the drug. This toxicity results in tubular damage with effects similar to those of the Fanconi syndrome. It is important, therefore, that out-of-date tetracyclines should not be used.

The effect of demeclocycline in producing nephrogenic diabetes insipidus and its consequent value in treating inappropriate ADH secretion has been noted above.

Gastrointestinal

Tetracyclines commonly produce gastrointestinal adverse effects, for example nausea, vomiting, epigastric discomfort, and diarrhoea. Rarely diarrhoea may be caused by superinfection with *Clostridium difficile*, resulting in pseudomembranous colitis (see lincomycin). Oral superinfection with *Candida albicans* may result in thrush (moniliasis), especially in old or debilitated people.

Bones and teeth

Because of the formation of a tetracycline–calcium or tetracycline–thiophosphate complex, tetracyclines are deposited in growing bones and teeth. In the teeth this causes brown discolouration and hypoplasia of the enamel. The deposit in bone may affect bone growth, but this is reversible.

For these reasons tetracyclines should not be given, unless absolutely necessary, to pregnant women (because of effects on the fetus) or to children up to the age of 12 years.

Other adverse effects

Tetracyclines, particularly demeclocycline, may cause the skin to become very sensitive to light in the u.v. range. This effect does not occur with local application.

Intravenous administration may be complicated by thrombophlebitis and large doses i.v. may be hepatotoxic.

Rarely thrombocytopenia, haemolytic anaemia, and eosinophilia may occur.

In infants tetracycline may cause increased intracranial pressure (pseudotumor cerebri) with bulging of the fontanelles. This condition resolves on discontinuation of the drug.

Minocycline may cause vestibular toxicity.

Interactions

Tetracycline absorption is reduced by calcium, aluminium, magnesium, and iron, because of the formation of insoluble chelates. The absorption of the ions is thus also decreased.

Tetracyclines increase the effects of warfarin, probably by an effect on clotting factor activity. In patients deficient in *dietary* vitamin K the removal of *bacterial* vitamin K produced in the gut may be an additional factor.

Thiazide diuretics (benzothiadiazines)

Structures

General

(Compare diazoxide, sulphonamides, sulphonylureas.)

Examples

	R	X
Hydrochlorothiazide	H	Cl
Bendrofluazide	$CH_2C_6H_5$	CF_3
Cyclopenthiazide	$CH_2C_5H_9$	Cl

Mode of action

Diuretic effect: inhibition of sodium and chloride reabsorption in the distal convoluted tubule of the nephron, resulting in increased sodium and free water clearance. The molecular mechanism of this effect may be through the inhibition of a Na/Cl transport system. A secondary effect is the loss of potassium by increased secretion in the distal tubule in response to the increased intraluminal sodium concentration.

Antihypertensive effect: the precise details are not known, but a number of factors appear to be involved. There is initially sodium and water loss, leading to relative hypovolaemia, which may result in lowered cardiac output. However, the hypovolaemia is corrected homoeostatically within a few weeks, while the antihypertensive effect continues. One hypothesis maintains that a lowered sodium concentration in vascular smooth muscle cells leads to a decreased free intracellular calcium concentration, which reduces the reactivity of the vascular smooth muscle to noradrenaline released from sympathetic nerve-endings. Overall, therefore, there is a decrease in peripheral resistance and a fall in blood pressure.

The effect of the thiazides in nephrogenic diabetes insipidus is paradoxical, but may be due to a reduction in extracellular fluid volume and a reduced glomerular filtration rate.

Uses

Oedema due to cardiac failure, liver disease, nephrotic syndrome, and drugs.

Hypertension.

Nephrogenic diabetes insipidus.

Dosages

Hydrochlorothiazide: 50–100 mg o.d. orally.

Bendrofluazide: 5–10 mg o.d. orally.

Cyclopenthiazide: 0.5–1 mg o.d. orally.

The thiazide diuretics are also available in combination formulations with potassium-sparing diuretics (spironolactone, triamterene, and amiloride), with potassium chloride (q.v.) or with β-adrenoceptor antagonists. In such cases the dose is usually the same as that which would be given if the thiazide were being used alone.

Kinetic data

All are well absorbed, and are excreted unchanged by the kidney. The half-times are about 8–12 h. Thus, these drugs should be given in the morning to avoid nocturia.

Important adverse effects

Hypokalaemia, hyponatraemia, and dehydration are the most important adverse effects. Hypokalaemia may be avoided by using potassium supplements or potassium-sparing diuretics (see under 'potassium chloride' for a discussion of the need for potassium supplements in patients taking potassium-wasting diuretics). Hypomagnesaemia may also occur.

Hyperglycaemia occurs but is usually not of clinical importance, although occasionally diabetes mellitus may be precipitated in a susceptible patient. In diabetics increased doses or oral hypoglycaemics may be required. Erectile impotence may occur in men. Hyperuricaemia occurs and occasionally results in acute gout. Hypercalcaemia may occur in susceptible patients, due to reduced urinary calcium excretion.

Rarely bone-marrow suppression may occur, resulting in thrombocytopenia. Pancreatitis has also been reported.

In hepatic insufficiency encephalopathy may be precipitated.

Interactions

Thiazide diuretics reduce the clearance of lithium by the kidney, and lithium dosages should be halved initially and adjusted with careful plasma concentration monitoring (see Chapter 7).

Hypokalaemia potentiates the effects of cardiac glycosides, and alters the effects of antiarrhythmic drugs. Hypokalaemia should be avoided in patients taking antiarrhythmic drugs.

Thyroid hormones

Structures

General

L-thyroxine (T_4): $X = I$.
L-triiodothyronine (T_3): $X = H$.

Mode of action and uses

Thyroxine and triiodothyronine are the naturally-occurring thyroid hormones, and are therefore used as replacement therapy in hypothyroidism of any cause and in hypothyroid coma. Because an increase in circulating thyroid hormone causes feedback inhibition of TSH output from the normal pituitary they are also used in the treatment of diffuse non-toxic goitre, subacute thyroiditis, Hashimoto's thyroiditis, and thyroid carcinoma.

Dosages

20 micrograms of T_3 is equivalent to 100 micrograms of T_4.

Intravenous: use triiodothyronine in severe hypothyroidism. There is controversy about the correct dosage of triiodothyronine in the condition. We recommend 5–20 micrograms 4–12 hourly. A glucocorticoid should also be given (for example hydrocortisone 100 mg i.v. once daily). (See the treatment of thyroid disease, p. 371.)

Oral: triiodothyronine is used when first treating severe hypothyroidism. After initial treatment one would generally switch to thyroxine. Triiodothyronine: 5 micrograms once daily initially increasing at weekly intervals; when a dose of 60 micrograms is reached change to thyroxine. Thyroxine: 25–50 micrograms once daily initially, increasing as required in 50 microgram increments every four weeks up to 300 micrograms daily if required.

Kinetic data

Both are well absorbed and very highly bound to plasma proteins (> 99 per cent). Triiodothyronine $t_{1/2} = 36$ h; thyroxine $t_{1/2} = 7$ d. The $t_{1/2}$ of thyroxine is shortened in hyperthyroidism and prolonged in hypothyroidism.

Important adverse effects

In the early stages of treatment of hypothyroidism patients may suffer angina pectoris, myocardial infarction, or cardiac arrhythmias, especially if they have pre-existing cardiac disease. Later on the signs and symptoms of hyperthyroidism occur if the dose is excessive. Treatment of hypothyroidism with thyroid hormones can be monitored by measuring serum concentrations of triiodothyronine (reference range 1.5–3.0 nmol/L) or thyroxine (50–150 nmol/L) and TSH (0–6 mu/L).

Triamterene

Structure

Mode of action

Triamterene acts in a manner similar to amiloride. It inhibits the movement of sodium through channels in the late distal tubule and collecting tubule which permit the passage of sodium from the urinary space into the tubular cells. This inhibition causes hyperpolarization of the apical plasma membrane, which discourages the secretion of potassium.

Uses

In combination with potassium-depleting diuretics in the treatment of oedema due to cardiac failure, liver disease, nephrotic syndrome.

Dosages

150–250 mg daily in divided doses orally.

Kinetic data

Incompletely but fairly rapidly absorbed from the gastrointestinal tract. Extensively metabolized before urinary excretion, $t_{1/2} = 2$ h. Variable biliary excretion.

Important adverse effects

Hyperkalaemia, dehydration, and hyponatraemia are common. The incidence of hyperkalaemia (about 5 per cent) is unaffected by concurrent administration of potassium-depleting diuretics. Nausea and vomiting occur occasionally.

Triamterene may rarely cause an interstitial nephritis, particularly when used in combination with thiazide diuretics.

Interactions

The potassium-retaining effects of the ACE inhibitors are potentiated by triamterene and this combination should be avoided. Triamterene should not be used in combination with potassium chloride supplements or other potassium-sparing diuretics.

Triamterene may inhibit the urinary excretion of amantadine.

Renal prostaglandins may protect the kidney against triamterene-induced damage and this protection may be lost if patients also take non-steroidal anti-inflammatory drugs, such as indomethacin.

Tricyclic antidepressants

Structures

General

Examples

	X_1-R	X_2*
Amitriptyline	C = CHCH$_2$CH$_2$N(CH$_3$)$_2$	C
Imipramine	N-CH$_2$CH$_2$CH$_2$N(CH$_3$)$_2$	C
Nortriptyline	C = CHCH$_2$CH$_2$NHCH$_3$	C

*In other compounds X_2 may be O (for example doxepin) or S (for example dothiepin).

Mode of action

Tricyclic antidepressants inhibit the reuptake of noradrenaline and 5-hydroxytryptamine (5-HT) at central monoaminergic synapses. The relative potency of inhibition of noradrenaline and 5-HT reuptake varies from drug to drug. Exactly how this action is then translated into an antidepressant effect is not clearly understood. However, it is generally agreed that tricyclic antidepressants take a week or more to show their antidepressant effects, and so attention has recently been directed towards those pharmacological changes in the brain which might occur subsequent to the rises in concentrations of monoamines in the synaptic cleft, i.e. adaptive responses. In experimental animals many such adaptive changes have been found and include down-regulation (i.e. a reduction in the numbers) of cortical β-adrenoceptors, α-adrenoceptors, and 5-HT receptors. What these changes mean in functional terms is still unknown, but is is now apparent that several adaptive responses occur in the brain as a result of the effects of tricyclic antidepressants, and that perhaps their therapeutic activity is dependent upon this spectrum of adaptive responses.

Although not perhaps relevant to their antidepressant effects, these drugs also have central and peripheral anticholinergic effects of importance in poisoning (for example causing cardiac arrhythmias) and in causing some of the common adverse effects (dry mouth, urinary retention). They also have histamine (H_1) receptor blocking actions, which may be responsible for drowsiness during the early stages of therapy.

Uses

Depression (most effective in the endogenous type).

Panic attacks (may cause initial exacerbation).

Nocturnal enuresis (mechanism of action unknown).

Postherpetic neuralgia (in combination with an anticonvulsant such as carbamazepine or valproate).

Dosages

These drugs are probably best given in one daily oral dose at night. Their effects last sufficiently long to allow once-a-day dosage and the impact of the anticholinergic and antihistamine effects may be minimized by taking the tablets last thing at night. Treatment is usually started at a low dosage and increased gradually as required to a maximum. Individual dosages are:

Daily dosage	Amitriptyline	Imipramine	Nortriptyline
Initially	25–75 mg	75 mg*	30 mg
Maximum	225 mg	225 mg	100 mg

*25 mg initially for panic attacks, increasing in steps of 10 mg.

Dosages should not be increased at more than two-weekly intervals, because of the long time taken to achieve a therapeutic effect.

Kinetic data

Tricyclic antidepressants are well absorbed but have variable first-pass metabolism. Amitriptyline and imipramine are metabolized in the liver by demethylation to nortriptyline and desipramine respectively, both metabolites being pharmacologically active. Further metabolism by the liver to inactive compounds follows. Metabolism of these compounds is undoubtedly their most important route of elimination and rates of clearance vary widely from individual to individual, possibly for pharmacogenetic reasons. In addition, their apparent volumes of distribution are very high (for example 15 L/kg for imipramine) because of extensive tissue distribution, which is also very variable. This wide variability in both clearance and apparent volume of distribution results in very wide variations in $t_{1/2}$. For amitriptyline a very wide range of values of $t_{1/2}$ has been reported (between 5 and 161 h) and the average is about 40 h. Values for the other drugs are: nortriptyline, 15–95 h; imipramine, 6–20 h; desipramine, 8–28 h.

All this variability leads to a wide variation in the optimum therapeutic dose in an individual (see above).

Important adverse effects

Anticholinergic effects are very common and include dry mouth, blurred vision, constipation, and difficulty with micturition. However, tolerance may develop and patients should be encouraged to persist with treatment. Taking the dose last thing at night may help to minimize these effects. Care should be taken in patients with prostatic enlargement or closed-angle glaucoma.

Cardiovascular effects include tachycardia, ventricular arrhythmias, heart block and hypotension. Some cases of sudden death in patients on tricyclic antidepressants have been attributed to cardiac arrhythmias.

Care should therefore be taken when considering prescribing antidepressants for patients who have had a myocardial infarction. It may then be advisable to prescribe an antidepressant drug with fewer effects on the heart (see Chapter 31).

Care should also be taken in prescribing tricyclic antidepressants for patients with epilepsy, since they lower the seizure threshold.

Confusional states may result from tricyclic antidepressant therapy, especially in old people.

There is some evidence that high doses of nortriptyline may cause a worsening of depression (see Chapter 7).

Tricyclic antidepressants may initially exacerbate symptoms in patients with panic attacks. Very low starting doses should be used when treating panic attacks with antidepressants (usually imipramine 25 mg).

Interactions

The tricyclic antidepressants diminish the antihypertensive effects of clonidine and the adrenergic neurone-blocking drugs, debrisoquine, bethanidine, and guanethidine.

They potentiate the central depressant effects of alcohol.

They potentiate the effects of other anticholinergic drugs.

They potentiate the effects of adrenaline and noradrenaline (to be noted particularly when administering lignocaine local anaesthetic preparations containing adrenaline: this interaction can be fatal). Occasionally a similar interaction can occur with phenylpropanolamine in 'cold cures' and with amphetamine.

The dose of replacement thyroid therapy may need to be reduced.

Valproate sodium

Structure

$$(CH_3CH_2CH_2)_2CHCOO^- Na^+$$

Mode of action

It is not clear what aspects of the actions of valproate are related to its therapeutic effect, but several actions are known. It inhibits γ-aminobutyric acid (GABA) transaminase and prevents GABA reuptake.

This results in an increase in brain GABA concentrations; it increases the sensitivity of GABA receptors to GABA; it reduces the concentrations of the excitatory neurotransmitter aspartate; and it may open potassium channels, thus stabilizing neuronal cell membranes.

Uses

As an anticonvulsant in:

Generalized seizures

Absences (petit mal).
Tonic–clonic seizures (grand mal).
Myoclonic seizures.

Partial seizures

Psychomotor epilepsy (temporal lobe epilepsy).

Postherpetic neuralgia

In combination with a tricyclic antidepressant.

Dosages

Initially 200 mg t.d.s orally, increasing by 200 mg a day at 3-d intervals to a maximum of 2600 mg/d according to the response. Usual maintenance dosage, 1000–1600 mg/d.

Kinetic data

Valproate is well absorbed. It is very highly protein bound in the plasma and is mostly metabolized in the liver, $t_{1/2} = 12$ h. Plasma concentrations should be up to 700 µmol/L (100 µg/mL), but there is not a very good relationship between the plasma concentrations of valproate and its therapeutic effect.

Important adverse effects

Early on gastrointestinal symptoms, such as nausea and vomiting, are common, but they resolve on lowering the dose and may be lessened by the use of enteric-coated formulations and by taking the tablets with food. Later on tolerance develops and the dose may be increased without adverse effect.

Ataxia, incoordination, tremor, and drowsiness may occur as toxic effects.

Transient hair loss, oedema, and thrombocytopenia occur infrequently.

Valproate has been reported to impair liver function and in a few patients has led to fatal hepatic failure. It should therefore be used with caution in patients with pre-existing liver disease and liver function tests should be carried out before treatment is started, and every 2 months thereafter for up to 6 months. If abnormalities in liver function occur the drug should be withdrawn.

Interactions

Valproate displaces phenytoin from plasma protein binding sites, which causes an increase in phenytoin clearance (see Chapter 10). However, it also inhibits its metabolism, and thus the interaction is complex and unpredictable.

Valproate increases plasma concentrations of phenobarbitone and primidone, perhaps by inhibiting their metabolism.

Vancomycin

Structure

Vancomycin is a complex glycopeptide containing an aminodisaccharide (vancosamine) and several amino acid moieties. Its structure is summarized below.

Mode of action

Vancomycin is bacteriocidal and acts by inhibiting bacterial cell wall synthesis.

Uses

Pseudomembranous colitis (infection with *Clostridium difficile*, see lincomycin, p. 628).

Severe staphylococcal infections.

As an alternative to penicillins in the prophylaxis of infective endocarditis, before dental procedures and cardiac surgery.

As an alternative to penicillins in the treatment of infective endocarditis due to streptococci, enterococci, staphylococci, *Haemophilus* spp, and *Proteus* spp.

Dosages

Oral (pseudomembranous colitis): 500 mg 6-hourly.

Intravenous (infective endocarditis prophylaxis): 1 g 30 min before surgical procedures (see Table 22.13), and after cardiac surgery 1 g i.v. 12-hourly for four doses.

Intravenous (infective endocarditis treatment): 500 mg i.v. 6-hourly.

Vancomycin is very irritant to veins and should be diluted in 200 mL of 5 per cent dextrose or 0.9 per cent saline before i.v. administration.

Infusion should be carried out over 20–30 min.

Kinetic data

Vancomycin is very poorly absorbed from the gastrointestinal tract. It is almost completely eliminated unchanged in the urine, $t_{1/2} = 8$ h, and because of its toxicity it should not be used i.v. in patients with renal impairment (creatinine clearance below 50 mL/min). Renal failure is not a contra-indication to its oral use.

Important adverse effects

Vancomycin is both ototoxic and nephrotoxic. Both of these effects are dose-related, and i.v. vancomycin should not be used in patients with renal impairment (see above) or in patients with pre-existing hearing impairment. If tinnitus occurs the drug should be withdrawn. If the facilities are available plasma concentration measurement should be used to monitor therapy. Plasma concentrations should be below 30 µg/mL.

Extravasation with i.v. infusion causes tissue necrosis and care should be taken to infuse vancomycin into large veins.

The effects of vancomycin on the fetus are unknown and it should not be used i.v. in pregnancy.

Other common adverse effects are hypersensitivity reactions (fever, rash, eosinophilia, anaphylaxis), and nausea.

Interactions

Care should be taken when administering vancomycin i.v. with other nephrotoxic antibiotics (for example aminoglycosides, polymixin B, colistin).

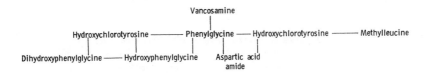

Vasopressin and its analogues

Structures

Vasopressin is a nonapeptide whose alternative name is antidiuretic hormone (ADH). The naturally-occurring human vasopressin is arginine vasopressin:

$$\underset{1}{Cys} - \underset{2}{Tyr} - \underset{3}{Phe} - \underset{4}{Gln} - \underset{5}{Asn} - \underset{6}{Cys} - \underset{7}{Pro} - \underset{8}{Arg} - \underset{9}{GlyNH_2}$$

There are also semi-synthetic vasopressins, including desmopressin (DDAVP or 1-deamino-8-D-arginine vasopressin) and felypressin (2-phenylalanine-8-lysine vasopressin). Lypressin (8-lysine vasopressin) is the naturally-occurring porcine vasopressin.

Mode of action

Vasopressin is synthesized in the hypothalamus and transported to the posterior pituitary. It is then released in response to increases in plasma osmolality and decreases in extracellular fluid volume. It acts on the cortical and medullary segments of the distal part of the nephron in the kidney, where it increases permeability to water and thus enhances water reabsorption without altering solute transport.

Vasopressin also has effects on the cardiovascular system but at considerably higher concentrations than are required to inhibit diuresis. It causes vasoconstriction of arteries and arterioles, including the coronary, pulmonary, and splanchnic arteries.

Vasopressin acts on V_1 and V_2 receptors, causing pressor and antidiuretic effects respectively. The relative potencies of vasopressin and its analogues as antidiuretic agents and as vaso-constrictors are shown in Table P9. Vasopressins which have vasopressor actions also cause smooth muscle contraction elsewhere, notably in the gastrointestinal tract and uterus, and those effects form the basis of some of the adverse effects of high-dose vasopressin.

Uses

Cranial diabetes insipidus (long-term, desmopressin; short-term, vasopressin, desmopressin, lypressin).

To arrest bleeding from oesophageal varices (vasopressin).

With local anaesthetics, to delay their absorption and thus potentiate their effects (felypressin).

Dosages

Cranial diabetes insipidus

Desmopressin, 10–20 micrograms b.d. intranasally (100 microgram/mL solution); in short-term treatment desmopressin can be given i.m. (1–2 micrograms o.d.).

Lypressin, 2.5–10 i.u. three to seven times a day intranasally (rarely used).

Vasopressin, 5–20 i.u. s.c. or i.m. at least twice daily. Rarely used.

Oesophageal varices

Vasopressin is given either in single doses (20 i.u. in 100 mL of 5 per cent dextrose infused over 20 min) or by continuous i.v. infusion (0.4 i.u./min for 24 h).

Terlipressin, 2 mg initially i.v. followed by 1–2 mg 4–6 hourly for up to 72 h.

■ **Table P9** The relative potencies of vasopressin and its analogues as antidiuretic agents and as vasopressors.

Drugs	Relative activity (arginine vasopressin = 1)	
	Antidiuretic	Vasopressor
Arginine vasopressin	1	1
Lypressin	0.8	0.6
Desmopressin	12	0.004

Local anaesthesia

Prilocaine 3 per cent is formulated with felypressin 0.03 i.u./mL. The maximum dose is 20 mL.

Kinetic data

Vasopressin and lypressin are rapidly cleared from the body after i.v. administration ($t_{1/2}$ 10 min), but desmopressin has a much longer halftime (75 min) and can be given less frequently than the other vasopressins.

Elimination of vasopressin is by metabolism by the tissue peptidases (for example in liver and kidney).

Important adverse effects

Adverse effects are few in low dosages and are limited to nausea and occasionally abdominal cramps. The nasal formulations may cause nasal congestion and ulceration.

In the i.v. doses of vasopressin used to stop bleeding from oesophageal varices adverse effects are common and consist of abdominal and uterine cramps and the urgent need to defaecate. Because it can cause coronary artery spasm vasopressin should not be used in patients with a history of coronary artery disease. Care should be taken in patients with a history of hypertension. Drugs have been largely replaced by endoscopic techniques in the management of varices.

Hypersensitivity reactions can occur occasionally.

Interactions

Various drugs can stimulate the secretion of vasopressin by the pituitary and cause the syndrome of 'inappropriate ADH secretion'. These drugs include chlorpropamide, clofibrate, cyclophosphamide, tricyclic antidepressants, and vincristine. Ethanol and phenytoin are inhibitors of vasopressin secretion.

Some drugs are antagonists of the effects of vasopressin on the renal tubule, notably lithium and demethylchlortetracycline, which can thus cause nephrogenic diabetes insipidus. Demethylchlortetracycline has been used to treat the syndrome resulting from increased secretion of ADH.

Chlorpropamide and carbamazepine increase the effects of vasopressin on the renal tubule and may therefore be used in mild cases of nephrogenic diabetes insipidus.

Vigabatrin

Structure

$$H_2C = CH \quad CH_2 \quad COOH$$
$$CH \quad CH_2$$
$$NH_2$$

Mode of action

Vigabatrin (γ-vinyl GABA) is an irreversible inhibitor of GABA-aminotransferase, the enzyme which degrades GABA. The concentration of GABA in the brain is increased, causing an increase in inhibitory synaptic activity.

Uses

As a supplement to existing therapy in patients with refractory partial and generalized seizures.

Dosages

Adults: 2 g initially once or twice daily. The dose may be increased by increments of 0.5–1 g but should not exceed 4 g/d.

Children: 1 g/d if aged 3–9 years; 2 g/d if older.

Dosages should be reduced in old people or in those with impaired renal function.

Kinetic data

Vigabatrin is well absorbed and is eliminated unchanged in the urine, $t_{1/2} = 8$ h. Its effect continues until GABA-aminotransferase is resynthesized.

Important adverse effects

Psychosis, drowsiness, headache, and ataxia all occur occasionally. Nausea and weight gain have also been reported. Vigabatrin should be used with caution in patients with a background of psychosis or behavioural disturbance. Psychosis and increased seizures may occur on stopping vigabatrin. Myelin oedema and vasculation found in animals have not been reported in humans. Dosages should be reduced in patients with renal impairment.

Interactions

Vigabatrin causes a 20 per cent reduction in the plasma phenytoin concentration; the mechanism is unknown and does not seem to be related to altered metabolism of phenytoin.

Vinca alkaloids

Structures
General

Examples
Vinblastine: $R = CH_3$; vincristine: $R = CHO$

Mode of action

The effects of these drugs may be related to their ability to bind specifically to tubulin, the protein found in cellular microtubules. This results in inhibition of cell division in the metaphase of the mitotic phase, for which they are specific.

Uses

Acute leukaemias (vincristine).
Malignant lymphomas, especially Hodgkin's disease (vincristine and vinblastine).

Dosages

Extreme care must be taken in calculating and administering doses of vincristine and vinblastine. Dosage regimens vary according to age, the disease being treated, and other concurrent therapy. Administration is by the i.v. route and single doses are usually given once weekly for a set number of times.

It is essential that specialist advice be sought on precise dosage regimens, because incorrect dosage can result in serious toxic effects.

Kinetic data

Both are poorly absorbed, and are therefore given i.v. They are cleared rapidly from the blood, metabolized in the liver, and excreted in the bile, $t_{1/2} = 3$ h.

Important adverse effects

The most frequent adverse effect is superficial thrombophlebitis at the site of intravenous injection or a local cellulitis if the drug leaks outside of the vein. To avoid this the drug should, if possible, be injected via the tubing of a fast-running i.v. infusion of saline, after reconstitution of the powdered drug in the diluting solution provided by the manufacturer.

Bone-marrow suppression is dose-related. It is more frequent with vinblastine than with vincristine in the dosages commonly used, and generally affects the neutrophils.

Alopecia is very common.

Peripheral neuropathy is common, more so with vincristine, and generally involves peripheral sensory and motor fibres. Occasionally autonomic innervation of the bowel may be affected, leading to constipation and intestinal obstruction. A routine prophylactic laxative is indicated and abdominal pain should be carefully investigated in such patients.

Rarely inappropriate ADH secretion occurs.

Interaction

For the possible interaction with live vaccines see p. 251.

Vitamin B$_{12}$

Structures

There are several different forms of vitamin B$_{12}$, but their structures are too complex to illustrate here. Hydroxocobalamin (vitamin B$_{12a}$) is the most commonly used form in therapy. Cyanocobalamin is not now recommended for general use in the treatment of pernicious anaemia for two reasons: firstly, because of the remote risk of worsening tobacco amblyopia and Leber's optic atrophy; secondly, because hydroxocobalamin has a slower rate of clearance.

Mode of action

Vitamin B$_{12}$ is required during the synthesis of purine and pyrimidine bases and their incorporation into DNA. In vitamin B$_{12}$ deficiency maturation of the erythroid series in the marrow is slowed and a megaloblastic, macrocytic anaemia results.

Uses

Vitamin B$_{12}$ deficiency from any cause.

Dosages

Pernicious anaemia: 1 mg initially i.m., repeated every 2–3 d to a total of 6 mg. Maintenance dose, 1 mg i.m. at 3-monthly intervals.

Treatment of other causes of vitamin B$_{12}$ deficiency is generally the same as for pernicious anaemia, but other therapy may be required (for example folic acid, iron, and treatment of the underlying cause).

Kinetic data

Vitamin B$_{12}$ is not absorbed from the gastrointestinal tract unless it is bound to a cobalamin-binding glycoprotein called intrinsic factor, which is secreted by the gastric parietal cells. Intrinsic factor is absent in pernicious anaemia and after total gastrectomy; its secretion is reduced in chronic gastritis. Absorption of the vitamin B$_{12}$–intrinsic factor complex takes place mainly in the ileum.

Total body stores of vitamin B$_{12}$ are 3–5 mg. Daily losses are 0.1 per cent of total body stores (i.e. $t_{1/2} = 2$ years). Thus, when total body stores are normal daily requirements are 3–5 micrograms. There is an enterohepatic recirculation of 0.5–9 micrograms a day, the reabsorption of which depends on intrinsic factor, so that daily losses may be slightly greater in pernicious anaemia when total body stores have been replenished.

About 1 microgram of the body's vitamin B$_{12}$ is in the plasma, mostly bound to binding proteins (transcobalamins). Tissue binding and protein binding become saturated when i.m. doses of over 100 micrograms are given and then unbound hydroxocobalamin and cyanocobalamin are excreted unchanged in the urine. Since hydroxocobalamin is bound more tightly by the binding proteins than cyanocobalamin its renal clearance is less rapid and it accumulates to a greater extent.

Important adverse effects

Rarely an allergic reaction may occur to hydroxocobalamin.

Vitamin D analogues

Structures

The group of D vitamins includes the following compounds:
  ergocalciferol (calciferol or vitamin D$_2$);
  cholecalciferol (vitamin D$_3$);
  dihydrotachysterol;
  25-hydroxycholecalciferol (calcifediol);
  1α-hydroxycholecalciferol (alfacalcidol);
  1α,25-dihydroxycholecalciferol (calcitriol);
  24,25-dihydroxycholecalciferol.

We illustrate here the active form of vitamin D, 1,25-dihydroxycholecalciferol (calcitriol):

Mode of action

Vitamin D plays a central role in regulating calcium homoeostasis. It is found in the diet and is also synthesized by the skin under the influence of ultraviolet light. Vitamin D_2 (ergocalciferol, found in plants) and vitamin D_3 (cholecalciferol, found in animal tissues) are pharmacologically inactive and have to be converted to active compounds (Fig. P9).

Cholecalciferol (vitamin D_3) is hydroxylated in the liver to 25-hydroxycholecalciferol, which is weakly active. This is then further hydroxylated in the kidney, either to 24,25-dihydroxycholecal- ciferol, which is also weakly active, or to 1α,25- dihydroxycholecalciferol, the most active form of vitamin D. Under the influence of parathyroid hormone, and in vitamin D or calcium deficiency, the formation of 1α,25-dihydroxycholecalciferol is preferred. Orally administered 1α-hydroxy- cholecalciferol is rapidly converted in the liver to 1,25-dihydroxycholecalciferol.

The main effects of vitamin D are to promote the absorption of calcium and phosphate from the gut and to enhance their reabsorption by the proximal renal tubules. These effects increase plasma concentrations of calcium and phosphate and make them available for mineralization of bone.

Uses

Vitamin D deficiency secondary to inadequate diet, malabsorption, and repeated pregnancy.

Hypoparathyroidism (alfacalcidol).

Renal osteodystrophy (alfacalcidol and cal- citriol).

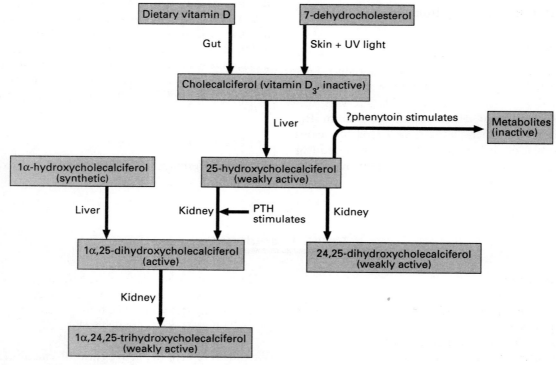

■ **Fig. P9**   The metabolic pathways of vitamin D.

Anticonvulsant-induced osteomalacia.
Congenital rickets.

Dosages

Daily dietary vitamin D requirements are satisfied by 400 i.u. (= 10 micrograms).

In adults over 30 years of age 200 i.u. day are sufficient.

Prevention of rickets in children and of osteomalacia in adults

Cholecalciferol or ergocalciferol, 400 i.u./d; dihydrotachysterol 0.5 mg daily.

The usual formulation for this purpose is ergocalciferol tablets, which also contain calcium lactate 300 mg and calcium phosphate 150 mg.

Dietary insufficiency with rickets or osteomalacia

Cholecalciferol or ergocalciferol 3000–5000 i.u. orally o.d. until healing has occurred, then tapering to daily requirements.

Dihydrotachysterol, 1–3 mg daily for 3 d, reducing to a maintenance dosage of 0.25–2 mg daily.

Malabsorption

Dosage requirements vary enormously and may be as high as 500 000 i.u. of vitamin D_3 per day. Alternatively, alfacalcidol may be used in ordinary dosages (see below). Oral calcium salts are also usually given in malabsorption, but care must be taken to avoid hypercalcaemia.

Hypoparathyroidism

Alfacalcidol, 1 microgram orally daily initially. The dosage may be increased to 2 or 3 micrograms daily, and when the full clinical effect has occurred a maintenance dosage of 0.5–1 microgram daily should be sufficient.

Renal osteodystrophy

Alfacalcidol, as above.

Calcitriol, 1–2 micrograms orally daily initially, increasing in increments of 0.25–0.5 micrograms at weekly intervals to a total of 2–3 micrograms daily depending on response.

Kinetic data

The absorption of vitamin D from the gastrointestinal tract is good. However, vitamin D is fat-soluble and its absorption is reduced in steatorrhoea. Bile is also necessary for its absorption which is therefore reduced in obstructive jaundice.

The metabolic pathways whereby vitamin D_3 is activated to $1\alpha,25$-hydroxycholecalciferol are discussed above.

The main route of excretion of vitamin D is via the bile, with enterohepatic recirculation, and vitamin D is stored in the body for about 6 months. In malabsorption this enterohepatic recirculation is reduced. The half-time of alfacalcidol in the body is 14 d and of calcifediol 19 d.

Important adverse effects

The most important adverse effect of the vitamin D analogues is hypercalcaemia, which is dose-related. Careful monitoring of the plasma calcium concentration is necessary at least once a week during initial therapy and regularly during maintenance therapy.

Because alfacalcidol has a shorter half-time in the body hypercalcaemia is corrected more quickly after withdrawing it than with other vitamin D analogues. When the calcium returns to normal treatment should be started again, if required, at half the previous dosage.

Interactions

Phenytoin and phenobarbitone can cause osteomalacia, perhaps because of enhanced metabolism of cholecalciferol and calcifediol (see Fig. P9). The metabolism of alfacalcidol is also enhanced by these drugs and increased dosages (up to 5 micrograms daily) may be required.

Vitamin K

Structure

Vitamin K_1 (phytomenadione, cf. warfarin):

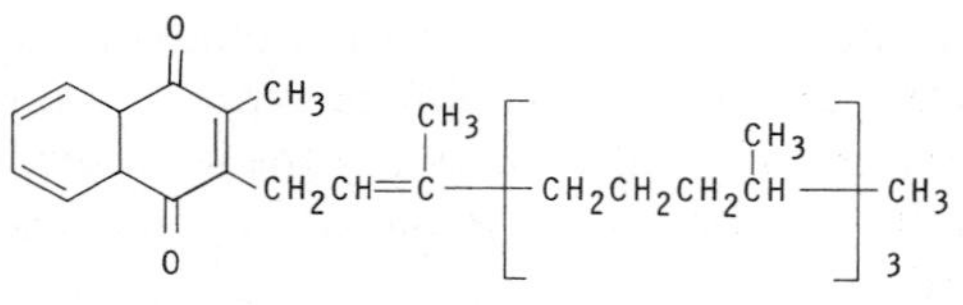

Mode of action

Vitamin K is a cofactor in the synthesis of clotting factors II, VII, IX, and X. It reverses the effects of the coumarin anticoagulants (see warfarin) by acting as a competitive inhibitor of their effects.

Uses

Impaired clotting factor synthesis because of hepatocellular disease, biliary obstruction, or coumarin anticoagulant toxicity.

Vitamin K deficiency from any cause.

Dosages

Vitamin K is available as phytomenadione (vitamin K_1; tablets and injection for i.m. and i.v. administration), and as the synthetic analogue menadiol sodium diphosphate, which is water-soluble (tablets and injection for i.m. and i.v. administration).

Biliary obstruction (for example before gall bladder surgery), for hepatocellular disease (for example before liver biopsy), and coumarin anti-coagulant overdose: 10 mg of phytomenadione i.v. slowly.

Vitamin K deficiency with malabsorption syndromes and hepatic cirrhosis: 10 mg of the water-soluble menadiol once daily.

Vitamin K deficiency in neonates: 1 mg of phytomenadione i.v. (NB Synthetic analogues such as menadiol should not be used in neonates, because they may cause haemolysis, resulting in hyperbilirubinaemia and kernicterus).

Kinetic data

Vitamin K is moderately well absorbed and its absorption may be saturable and dependent on bile salts. It is highly bound to β-lipoproteins. It is metabolized to vitamin K epoxide, which is then reconverted to vitamin K by vitamin K epoxide reductase (see warfarin). Other metabolites are excreted via the bile, $t_{1/2} = 2$ h.

Important adverse effects

If vitamin K is given by fast i.v. injection it can cause an anaphylactoid reaction resulting in flushing, bronchospasm, tachycardia, and peripheral vascular collapse; this may be due to its vehicle, a polyethoxylated castor oil. Intravenous administration should therefore be slow. Use of the i.m. route may lead to haematoma formation at the injection site if clotting is impaired.

Interaction

Vitamin K reverses the effects of the coumarin anticoagulants (for example warfarin).

Warfarin

Structure

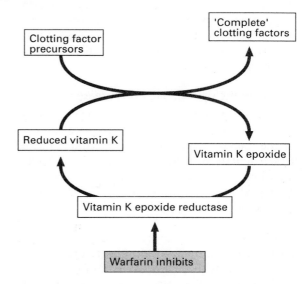

(Compare vitamin K_1.)

Mode of action

Consider first the synthesis of the clotting factors II (prothrombin), VII, IX, and X. These are synthesized in the liver and their synthesis requires vitamin K. Although the precise role of vitamin K in the synthesis of these clotting factors is not known, it is clear that its action is required in the γ-carboxylation of clotting factor precursors before their release from the liver into the circulation, and their eventual activation via the clotting cascade.

During the γ-carboxylation of clotting factor precursors the reduced form of vitamin K is required. It donates protons and is itself converted to the vitamin K epoxide. The oral anticoagulants, of which the coumarin warfarin is now the most commonly used, act by preventing the resynthesis of the reduced form of vitamin K from the vitamin K epoxide, by acting as inhibitors of the vitamin K epoxide reductase (see Fig. P10).

There are two aspects of the effect of warfarin on the prothrombin time during therapy.

The direct effect of warfarin

The actual *degree* of inhibition of the vitamin K epoxide reductase depends on the concentration of warfarin in the liver, which itself depends on the dose and the pharmacokinetic characteristics of the drug in the individual.

The *rate* at which warfarin produces this degree of inhibition depends on the rate of accumulation of the drug and that depends on its $t_{1/2}$ (see below).

Clotting factor clearance

Obviously once warfarin has stopped clotting factor synthesis the rate at which an anticoagulant effect appears (as judged by the prothrombin time, which is used to assay the various clotting

▮ **Fig. P10** The effect of vitamin K on clotting factor synthesis and the mechanism of action of warfarin in inhibiting the synthesis of factors II, VII, IX, and X.

factors) will depend upon the rate at which the amount of each of the clotting factors already present in the body falls. The half-times of the clotting factors in the blood are: factor VII, 6 h; factor IX, 24 h; factor X, 40 h; factor II, 60 h. Because of these differences and the long half-times of some of the factors there is a delay before the full effect of a given dose of warfarin on the prothrombin time is seen.

Uses

Deep venous thrombosis and pulmonary embolism, prophylaxis and treatment.

Prevention of emboli in:

(1) patients with atrial fibrillation, particularly when accompanied by mitral stenosis;

(2) patients with prosthetic heart valves;

(3) patients undergoing elective cardioversion for atrial fibrillation;

(4) patients undergoing hip surgery.

The use of anticoagulants in the secondary prevention of myocardial infarction is controversial.

Monitoring therapy

Therapy with warfarin is monitored by measuring the prothrombin time as a measure of the effect of warfarin on clotting. There are various ways of measuring the prothrombin time and of expressing the results.

Thrombotest with II, VII, and X reagents

This test measures the extrinsic thromboplastin clotting system and depends on the measurement of the time to clotting of a blood sample related to the activity of factors II, VII, and X after the addition of thromboplastin. The result is expressed as a percentage, being the dilution of control blood which yields the same clotting time as the patient's blood. For example, if the prothrombin time is reported at '20 per cent' that means that the time to clotting is the same as would occur with a 20 per cent solution (i.e. a 1 in 5 dilution) of control blood. The optimum range during therapy is 10–20 per cent.

Prothrombin and proconvertin time (Owren)

This test is similar to the thrombotest with II, VII, and X reagents, but before carrying out the clotting time measurement the blood samples are diluted. This has the effect of diluting out the effect of any heparin in the sample but does not alter one's ability to detect the clotting factors. In fact the sensitivity for some of the factors is *increased*. This test is therefore used in patients taking both heparin and oral anticoagulants. The haematologist carrying out the test must be told if the patient is taking heparin, since a falsely low result will be obtained if this dilution is not carried out. The result of the Owren test is expressed in the same way as for the II, VII, X test and the optimum range during therapy is 10–20 per cent.

One-stage prothrombin time (Quick's)

In this test factor V and fibrinogen are detected besides factors II, VII, and X, and this test is usually reserved for patients with other causes of clotting factor defects besides oral anticoagulants. The test has the additional disadvantages that it has to be performed within an hour or two of taking the blood sample and is sensitive to heparin. It is reported as the ratio of the clotting time of the patient's sample to that of the control. The optimum range during therapy is 2–3 times control.

International normalized ratio (INR)

Because the thromboplastin used in the prothrombin tests varies from laboratory to laboratory, an attempt has been made to standardize prothrombin time measurement internationally by the issue of a standard thromboplastin to all laboratories. Each laboratory then calibrates its own thromboplastin against the standard and translates a test result found with its own thromboplastin (for example in the II, VII, X test) into the equivalent INR value using the calibration curve. The result is expressed as the ratio of the clotting time of the patient's blood to the clotting time of the control sample. The optimum range during therapy depends on the condition being treated (see Table P10).

■ **Table P10** Suggested ranges of the INR in the treatment of some conditions with oral anticoagulants

INR	Condition
2.0–2.5	Prophylaxis of deep vein thrombosis, including surgery on high-risk patients (2.0–3.0 for surgery to hip and fractured femur)
2.0–3.0	Treatment of: Deep venous thrombosis Pulmonary embolism Systemic embolism Prevention of: Venous thromboembolism in myocardial infarction Embolism in mitral stenosis Transient ischaemic attacks with embolism in atrial fibrillation
3.0–4.5	Recurrent deep venous thrombosis and pulmonary embolism Arterial disease (including myocardial infarction) Prosthetic heart valves

Dosages

The following is a suggested regimen of treatment with warfarin:

1. Measure the prothrombin time to check its pretreatment value. Primary liver disease and congestive cardiac failure with hepatic congestion can alter the prothrombin time and reduce warfarin requirements (see below under adverse effects).

2. Initial doses. 10 mg once daily orally with daily measurements of the prothrombin time. Change to a maintenance dose when the prothrombin time has changed to the following values:

   prothrombin time (II, VII, X), 20–30 per cent;

   prothrombin time (Owren), 20–30 per cent;

   prothrombin time (Quick's), 2–4.5 times control value;

   INR, 2–4.5 times control value.

   (These different measurements are discussed above under 'Monitoring therapy'.)

   The total initial dose required to produce these changes is usually 20–30 mg, but some patients may require more.

3. Maintenance dosage. This is usually one quarter to one fifth of the total initial dose. For example, if after 3 d of treatment with warfarin 10 mg daily (i.e. a total initial dose of 30 mg) the INR has risen to 2.5, a daily maintenance dose of 7 mg could be given. One would then expect the INR to rise to between 3 and 4 within the next 2–3 d without further change in dosage. However, further small dosage adjustments may be necessary because of interpatient variability. Maintenance doses usually vary between 3 and 8 mg daily.

All this sounds complicated and dangerous, but in practice it turns out to be reasonably efficacious and safe if these guidelines are followed.

If after initial stabilization a change in dosage is made then it takes about 5 d for the prothrombin time to stabilize again, and dosages should generally not be altered again during that time.

Drug interactions and the effect of various diseases may alter warfarin dosage requirements (see below).

Kinetic data

Warfarin is administered as a racemic mixture of its two enantiomers, the R(+) and S(−) warfar-

ins. Both are well absorbed but differ in other respects:

Both are extensively metabolized, but at different rates. The S form is metabolized to 7-hydroxywarfarin and has a shorter $t_{1/2}$ (32 h) than the R form (54 h). The R form is metabolized to warfarin alcohols, which may have some anticoagulant effects.

The S form is about four times more potent as an anticoagulant than the R form.

These differences are important in some drug interactions with warfarin.

Important adverse effects

The commonest adverse effect is bleeding from any organ of the body. This effect is dose-related and usually resolves after withdrawal of the drug.

Various fetal abnormalities occur in association with the use of warfarin in pregnancy. Its use during the first trimester is associated with a small risk of the syndrome known as chondrodysplasia punctata, in which the formation of cartilage and bone is abnormal, resulting in epiphyseal stippling and nasal hypoplasia. It use during the third trimester, particularly after 36 weeks of gestation, is associated with retroplacental bleeding and fetal intracerebral bleeding, since fetal concentrations of clotting factors are low in comparison with maternal concentrations. It is therefore recommended that warfarin be used only during the 13th to 36th weeks of pregnancy, and that heparin, which does not cross the placenta, be used instead during the first trimester and after 36 weeks.

Influence of diseases on warfarin dosage requirements

Some diseases cause reduced warfarin requirements and measurement of the prothrombin time before starting treatment is important.

Impaired liver function

Impairment of hepatocellular function both acutely (for example viral hepatitis) and chronically (for example cirrhosis) reduces warfarin requirements, because of interference with clotting factor synthesis.

In obstructive jaundice there is also reduced vitamin K absorption because of a lack of bile salts, necessary for vitamin K absorption, in the intestinal lumen.

Congestive cardiac failure

Hepatic congestion associated with heart failure results in reduced warfarin requirements and choosing the correct dosage may be very difficult if the heart failure is successfully treated at the same time as anticoagulation is being carried out.

Thyroid function

In hyperthyroidism warfarin requirements are reduced and in hypothyroidism they are increased. The mechanism is not clear, but may involve alterations in the rates of clearance of clotting factors from the blood. Treatment of the thyroid disease results in a return to normal of dosage requirements.

Interactions

Drug interactions occur commonly with warfarin and can be classified by mechanism (see also Chapter 10).

Absorption

The absorption of warfarin and its reabsorption after biliary excretion may be reduced by cholestyramine and colestipol, which bind it in the gut.

Protein-binding displacement

Warfarin is very highly protein bound (99 per cent) and it is displaced from its protein binding sites by salicylates, chloral hydrate derivatives, sulphonamides, and phenylbutazone. The clinical relevance of such interactions is discussed in Chapter 10.

Inhibition of metabolism

Phenylbutazone inhibits the metabolism of s-warfarin but induces the metabolism of R-warfarin. The overall clearance of the racemic mixture is therefore unaffected. However, because s-warfarin is more potent than R-warfarin, there is potentiation of the pharmacological effect of warfarin, and serious bleeding may occur. (Phenylbutazone interacts with warfarin in other ways: it inhibits platelet aggregation, increases the likelihood of peptic ulceration, and may cause thrombocytopenia.)

Other drugs which inhibit warfarin metabolism, and therefore increase its effects, include metronidazole and azapropazone (inhibition of s-warfarin metabolism), amiodarone, chloramphenicol, cimetidine, disulfiram, isoniazid, and alcohol (acutely).

Induction of metabolism

The metabolism of warfarin is increased, and its effects reduced, by drugs which induce hepatic microsomal drug-metabolizing enzymes. These include phenytoin, phenobarbitone and primidone, carbamazepine, rifampicin, and griseofulvin. If a patient is taking warfarin and an enzyme-inducing drug is introduced, warfarin requirements will increase over the following few weeks. On stopping the inducing drug bleeding may occur if the dosage of warfarin is not again reduced.

Potentiation of the pharmacological effect

Several drugs may increase the pharmacological effect of warfarin by effects at the site of action in the liver. Such drugs include clofibrate, tetracyclines, anabolic steroids, and D-thyroxine. The mechanisms whereby these drugs potentiate the effects of warfarin are not at all clear, but the following hypotheses have been suggested:

increased affinity of warfarin for its receptor site (clofibrate, D-thyroxine, anabolic steroids);

decreased synthesis or increased catabolism of clotting factors (anabolic steroids);

modification of the activity of clotting factors (tetracyclines);

decreased availability of vitamin K secondary to decreased plasma lipids (D-thyroxine, anabolic steroids).

It has also been suggested that antibiotics may reduce the availability of vitamin K by inhibiting its production by bacteria in the gut. This is unlikely to occur for two reasons: firstly, bacterial vitamin K production occurs principally in the large bowel, so that only poorly absorbed antibiotics would be likely to have this effect; secondly, bacterial vitamin K accounts for only about one-third of total intake, the rest coming from food. However, there have been reports of potentiation of warfarin by antibiotics in patients in whom there was some other reason for vitamin K deficiency (for example poor diet). None the less if an antibiotic does not potentiate the effect of warfarin by some other mechanism (for example chloramphenicol, tetracyclines, sulphonamides, see above) it is unlikely to participate in an adverse interaction. Thus, antibiotics of the aminoglycoside, penicillin, and cephalosporin groups should generally be safe to use.

Indirect interactions

In patients taking warfarin the tendency to bleed may be enhanced and haemostasis reduced by drugs which impair platelet aggregation (for example dipyridamole, sulphinpyrazone, and most non-steroidal anti-inflammatory drugs, such as aspirin).

Drugs which cause peptic ulceration provide a site for potential bleeding in patients on warfarin. These include most non-steroidal anti-inflammatory drugs.

Unknown mechanisms

The mechanism whereby quinine and quinidine potentiate the action of warfarin is unknown.

Safe drugs

So numerous are drug interactions with warfarin that it is worth mentioning some drugs which appear to be safe to use in patients taking warfarin.

Analgesics

For mild or moderate pain use paracetamol. For more severe pain opiate analgesics such as morphine, diamorphine, and buprenorphine are safe.

Anti-inflammatory drugs

All are hazardous because they may cause gastrointestinal ulceration, and some inhibit platelet aggregation or displace warfarin from protein binding sites. Naproxen, ibuprofen, and indomethacin seem to be relatively safe, but whatever anti-inflammatory drug is prescribed the prothrombin time should be monitored carefully for the first few days and careful watch should

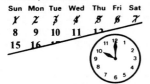

TAKING YOUR TABLETS

Remember the name and strength of the anticoagulant you are taking and always take the correct dose. Take your tablet(s) at the same time(s) each day. If necessary, use a calendar and mark off each dose by a line through the date. In this way you will be unlikely to miss a dose.

Sun	Mon	Tue	Wed	Thu	Fri	Sat
1	2	3	4	5	6	7
8	9	10	11	1̶2̶		
15	16					

Always make sure that you have at least a week's supply of tablets in hand so that you will not run short.
NEVER miss a dose; if you do, don't take a

double dose to make up for it, but tell the clinic doctor when you next go for a blood test. If more than one dose is missed, contact your general practitioner as soon as you can for advice.

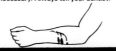

ILLNESS OR BLEEDING

In the event of illness, bleeding or apparent severe bruising, consult your general practitioner immediately. If you consult another doctor who might not know that you are having anticoagulant treatment, you must tell him, especially if an operation is necessary. Always tell your dentist.

OTHER MEDICINES

Aspirin and some other pain relieving medicines affect the clotting power of blood.

You should not take them unless they have been prescribed for you by the doctor who adjusts your anticoagulant dose. Aspirin may be an ingredient of other medicines, so when purchasing medicines always tell the pharmacist that you are taking an anticoagulant. Some other medicines may also interfere with the action of your anticoagulant so when you see the doctor who adjusts your anticoagulant dose always tell him about any new treatments or medicines and mention any changes, even a change of dose. If you have any doubts about your medicines ask the pharmacist or doctor.

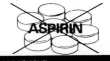

TREATMENT

The success of your treatment depends on your taking the correct dose of anticoagu-

lant, which varies from person to person. The dose is decided by the clinic doctor after testing your blood.

BLOOD

Blood does not usually clot (coagulate) within the blood vessels. When this happens (and it may do so following illness or operation), anticoagulants are used to treat or prevent the condition by reducing the clotting power of the blood to safe levels.

FOOD AND ALCOHOL

Keep to your normal diet and do not make big changes. You may drink moderate amounts of alcohol; do not make big changes in your food and alcohol consumption.

PREGNANCY

Oral anticoagulants taken in the early weeks of pregnancy carry a small but proven risk of damaging the unborn child. If you are a

woman of childbearing years receiving oral anticoagulants, you should not embark upon a pregnancy without consulting your doctor who will be able to decide whether or not you should discontinue the anticoagulant treatment. If you find that your period is two weeks overdue and you consider that you may be pregnant while taking anticoagulants, you should make an early appointment to see your doctor.

Published by The Pharmaceutical Society of Great Britain, 1 Lambeth High Street, London SE1 7JN.

KEEP YOUR TABLETS IN A SAFE PLACE WELL OUT OF THE REACH OF CHILDREN

ADVICE FOR PATIENTS ON ANTICOAGULANT TREATMENT

Always carry this card with you and show it to your doctor or dentist when obtaining treatment. Show it to your pharmacist when you are having a prescription dispensed and when purchasing medicines. As the pharmacist can advise you, it is in your own interest that you purchase all medicines from a pharmacy. Also show it to anyone giving treatment which may result in bleeding.

NAME OF YOUR ANTICOAGULANT

■ **Fig. P11** An example of the kind of warning card which should be issued and carried by a patient taking anticoagulants. (Reproduced with the permission of The Pharmaceutical Society of Great Britain.)

be kept for signs of gastrointestinal ulceration or bleeding.

Psychoactive drugs

Benzodiazepines are safe. The effects of tricyclic antidepressants are small and do not constitute a contra-indication to the use of warfarin; however, warfarin dosage requirements may be slightly reduced and prothrombin time monitoring during the first week or two will allow adjustment of dosages. There is little information about other antidepressants, but maprotiline seems to be safe.

Antibiotics

These are discussed above. Penicillins, cephalosporins, aminoglycosides, nitrofurantoin, nalidixic acid, and lincomycin and clindamycin are all safe. However, lincomycin and clindamycin may cause pseudomembranous colitis with consequent bleeding and care should be taken.

Antihypertensive drugs

Most drugs in this category are safe, including most diuretics, β-adrenoceptor antagonists, methyldopa, and vasodilators (for example hydralazine, prazosin).

Antiarrhythmic drugs

Most drugs in this group are safe, the important exceptions being quinidine and amiodarone.

Digitalis

The cardiac glycosides are safe.

Bronchodilators

Drugs of this type are safe, but proprietary combinations containing a barbiturate should be avoided.

Hypoglycaemic drugs

Insulin is safe. Most sulphonylureas are safe, but careful monitoring of prothrombin time and blood glucose is necessary, especially early on. Metformin is fibrinolytic and may indirectly enhance the effects of warfarin without a change in prothrombin time. It is probably best avoided (as are other biguanides).

Xanthine derivatives (theophylline and related drugs)

Structure

Theophylline

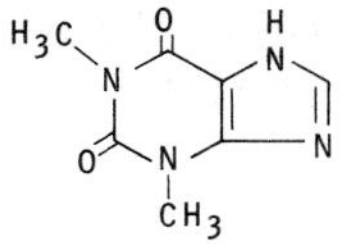

Mode of action

Xanthine derivatives are inhibitors of the enzyme phosphodiesterase and thus inhibit the metabolism of cyclic AMP. It is not certain, however, that this effect totally underlies their mechanism of action, since the concentrations achieved at the site of action may not be sufficiently high. Attention has also been paid to the effect of theophylline as a competitive inhibitor of the actions of adenosine on A_1 and A_2 receptors, but the link between this action and the therapeutic effect of xanthines is not clear, since not all bronchodilatory xanthines are adenosine antagonists.

Uses

Reversible airways obstruction (for example in bronchial asthma).

Left ventricular failure:

acute left ventricular failure accompanied by pulmonary oedema;
in preventing attacks of acute left ventricular failure.

Dosages

Because theophylline itself is poorly soluble and therefore poorly absorbed, it is often linked to one of a wide variety of compounds which enhance its solubility. The following compounds are in clinical use, in addition to theophylline itself, and they illustrate this principle: aminophylline (theophylline ethylene-diamine); choline theophyllinate (choline salt); diprophylline (dihydroxypropyl derivative); proxyphylline (hydroxypropyl derivative).

The amounts of theophylline equivalents in these formulations vary, and this accounts in part for differences in dosages.

The main advantages of these formulations

for oral use are improved absorption and fewer gastrointestinal adverse effects. The latter can also be reduced by using slow-release formulations, and these formulations have also been shown to produce a plasma concentration/time profile with adequate therapeutic concentrations for up to 12 h after a dose, despite the short $t_{1/2}$ of theophylline.

Aminophylline and diprophylline are also formulated for i.v. administration.

Oral

Aminophylline, 100–300 mg repeated as necessary.

Aminophylline slow-release formulations: Pecram® and Phyllocontin.

Continus®, 225–450 mg b.d.

Diprophylline, 200–400 mg, 3–4 times daily.

Choline theophyllinate, 200 mg 2–3 times daily.

Proxyphylline, 300 mg t.d.s. and 600 mg at night.

Theophylline slow-release formulations: Biophylline® 500 mg b.d.; Lasma® 300 mg b.d.; Nuelin SA®, 175–500 mg b.d.; Pro-Vent®, 300 mg b.d.; Slo-Phyllin®, 250–500 mg b.d.; Theo-Dur®, 200 mg b.d.; Uniphyllin Continus®, 200–300 mg b.d.

Intravenous

Aminophylline, as an immediate injection given over 10 min, 250–500 mg (i.e. 5–6 mg/kg); usual maintenance dose 0.9 mg/kg/h by continuous infusion, but dosages vary in disease (see Table P11). Take care when giving i.v. aminophylline to patients who have been taking theophylline previously (see p. 311).

Kinetic data

All the derivatives mentioned above are first converted to theophylline, which is itself metabolized to inactive xanthine derivatives. Its average $t_{1/2}$ is 6 h but is very variable and is affected by many factors, including diet, smoking, coffee-drinking and tea-drinking, and liver disease (see Table P11).

Plasma concentrations of theophylline most likely to be associated with a therapeutic effect in the acute treatment of bronchial asthma are 55–111 μmol/L (10–20 μg/mL).

Important adverse effects

Adverse effects are dose-related. Nausea, vomiting, fine tremor, anxiety, and nervousness may be the first symptoms; at higher doses tachycardia and other cardiac arrhythmias, convulsions, and coma may occur.

Interactions

Theophylline potentiates the effects of β-adrenoceptor agonists in the heart and it is thought that cardiac arrhythmias are more likely when this combination is used.

Some drugs inhibit the metabolism of theophylline (see Table P11).

■ **Table P11**   Factors which affect the clearance rate and dosages of theophylline

1. *Factors which increase the clearance rate of theophylline*
   Age: 1–16 years
   Diet: Low carbohydrate, high protein intake
               Charcoal broiled meats
   Cigarette smoking

2. *Factors which reduce the clearance rate of theophylline*
   Age: <1 year
   Diet: High carbohydrate intake
               High methylxanthine intake (for example coffee and tea)
   Obesity   (base dosages on estimated lean body weight)
   Diseases: Hepatic cirrhosis
               Congestive cardiac failure
               Chronic obstructive airways disease
               Acute pulmonary oedema
               Pneumonia
               Acute febrile illnesses
   Drugs: Cimetidine
               Oral contraceptives
               Erythromycin
               Troleandomycin
               Ciprofloxacin

3. *Maintenance dosages of i.v. aminophylline (for example in asthma) as modified by different circumstances*

Modifying Circumstance	Rate of infusion (mg/kg lean body wt/h)
Age	
Neonates	0.15
<6 months	0.47
6–11 months	0.8
1–9 y	0.9
Adults <50 years	0.9
Adults >50 years	0.7
Coexisting chronic obstructive airways disease	0.6
Coexisting congestive cardiac failure	0.5
Impaired liver function (depends on severity)	0.1–0.5
Drugs (see above)	0.3

Zidovudine

Structure

Mode of action

Zidovudine (azidothymidine, AZT) is a nucleoside, a pyrimidine analogue, which is phosphorylated by cellular kinases. Zidovudine triphosphate inhibits viral reverse transcriptase, for which it has an affinity 100 times greater than for cellular α-DNA polymerase. Zidovudine triphosphate is also incorporated into viral DNA and thus acts as a DNA chain terminator.

Uses

Zidovudine is used in the treatment of HIV infection and produces clear benefit in those with symptomatic disease, prolonging survival. Early evidence also suggests that it will delay progression to AIDS in asymptomatic patients with low CD4 lymphocyte counts. It is also effective in the treatment of HIV-induced thrombocytopenia.

Dosages

The standard dosage in the UK is 250 mg 6-hourly orally. A dosage of 250 mg 12-hourly may have fewer adverse effects, but its efficacy is uncertain.

Kinetic data

Zidovudine is moderately well absorbed (60–70 per cent) after oral administration. It is metab-olized in the liver to a 5-glucuronide metabolite, 50–80 per cent of which is renally excreted. Another 10–20 per cent of the parent drug is excreted in the urine; $t_{1/2} = 1$ h. The fate of the intracellular phosphorylated derivatives (nucleotides) is unknown.

Important adverse effects

Minor problems, such as headache, myalgia, insomnia, and nausea, are not uncommon but often wear off with continued treatment. However, some patients may be unable to tolerate zidovudine because of these effects.

Haematological toxicity is the most serious adverse effect, usually leading to a macrocytic anaemia but occasionally causing a pancytopenia. The anaemia first appears about 6 weeks after starting therapy and is more likely to occur in patients with AIDS than in less immunocompromised patients. It is also more likely in those with pre-existing anaemia.

Some patients may develop a painful myopathy on long-term zidovudine; this usually reverses when the drug is withdrawn.

Interactions

The marrow suppressive effects of zidovudine may be compounded by the concomitant administration of ganciclovir, with an increased risk of neutropenia. Occasionally, similar problems may arise with folate antagonists, such as sulphamethoxazole or pyrimethamine.

The glucuronidation of zidovudine in the liver may be inhibited by other drugs which are glucuronidated (for example morphine), but the clinical significance of this is uncertain.

Probenecid delays the excretion of zidovudine by the kidney, but the clinical value of giving probenecid in routine therapy has not been proven (cf. penicillins).

Index